Veteran and Military Mental Health

Christopher H. Warner • Carl A. Castro
Editors

Veteran and Military Mental Health

A Clinical Manual

Springer

Editors
Christopher H. Warner
Clin. Associate Professor of Psychiatry
Uniformed Services University of the Hea
Bethseda, MD, USA

Carl A. Castro
Professor of Social Work
University of Southern California
Los Angeles, CA, USA

ISBN 978-3-031-18008-8 ISBN 978-3-031-18009-5 (eBook)
https://doi.org/10.1007/978-3-031-18009-5

This Springer imprint is published by the registered company Springer Nature Switzerland AG
The registered company address is: Gewerbestrasse 11, 6330 Cham, Switzerland

In honor of the remarkable men and women who past, present, and future donned the uniform in defense of our nation, their families who have sacrificed so much, and the dedicated professionals, communities, and organizations who are committed to enhancing their well-being.

– Christopher H. Warner; Carl A. Castro

Foreword

As we were completing the final chapters for this volume and beginning the publication process, we watched, along with the rest of the world, several key military actions unfold that will have significant impacts on not only current military service members and veterans but also future ones. The first was the rapid and complete collapse of the United States (US) installed Afghanistan government and the US trained and equipped Afghanistan military as the US military completed its withdrawal from Afghanistan. The Taliban whom the US and its NATO allies had been fighting for 20 years retook control of the entire country in less than a fortnight. The images of American diplomats and Afghan supporters fleeing Kabul, countless Afghani citizens who were supportive of the US and NATO effort desperately trying to escape the country, and the Taliban entering the capital sparked comparisons to the fall of Saigon. During that time, 13 US service members were killed in renewed terrorist attacks in Afghanistan, and countless efforts were initiated by veteran led organizations and groups to help evacuate American citizens who remained in the country and numerous Afghani citizens who were sympathetic to the US and NATO effort.

The second event occurred in early 2022 when the world was shocked to again see war among nation states in Europe as Russia launched a major invasion into Ukraine. Russia's intent was to swiftly overrun Ukraine, depose its government, and to end any intent of Ukraine joining the NATO alliance. The result has been quite different. While NATO and European allies have not committed military forces, they have provided significant assistance in the form of equipment, intelligence, and support while also using their diplomatic, economic, and information instruments of power to support Ukraine. As a result, we have seen prolonged fighting in cities, significant loss of life on both sides, and an increasingly worsening displaced population issue within Eastern Europe. As this conflict progresses, we see continued destabilization of a long-held peace and many experts prognosticating that a large-scale World War is becoming increasingly likely.

Both of these situations highlight the psychological challenges that modern warfare presents. Civilians are again being targeted, citizens are being drafted to fight with little or no training, and the horrors of war are impacting both those who are serving and their families. The images and news reports from Afghanistan and Ukraine have sparked numerous debates and emotions. What is our purpose when we choose to go to war, what obligations and commitment do we have to our allies and partners, and what is the value that we place on our military service members.

For our military service members and veterans, the reactions to these events ranged from anger and astonishment to feelings of grief and betrayal, and for some relief. It is never easy for a nation to choose to go to war or to feel that they lost a war.

It is more difficult for those who participated to perceive that they lost a war. Over 2000 American service members died fighting in Afghanistan, with tens of thousands more permanently wounded, and currently receiving disability benefits for their injuries. The lives of thousands of families were permanently impacted by the demands of this war. Many veterans have experienced seeing their closest friends killed or severely wounded while fighting to bring peace to the people of Afghanistan and safety to the world from terrorism.

Inevitably, many will ask whether it was worth it. The fall of Kabul will lead some to feel that all the sacrifices were pointless and achieved nothing. For certain, many veterans of the Afghanistan War will feel betrayed. That the Nation, its leaders, and in the eyes of some, its people, simply did not care enough about the sacrifices the few were making to bring about victory. At the same time, there are many who are upset that we are not doing more to protect our Allies who are currently under attack in Ukraine.

There are lessons to be derived from the work of Jonathan Shay with veterans from the Vietnam War where he so touchingly described in his landmark book on moral injury entitled, *Achilles in Vietnam*. The lessons he distilled from the experience of veterans in Vietnam must not be forgotten. Many of these are lessons we have known for millennia. War is always traumatic. In every war people are killed, injured, and their lives permanently and irrevocably altered. War leads to feelings of unnecessary suffering and betrayal, and these feelings are magnified when the war is lost and when the sacrifices go unacknowledged. This book is part of the effort to ensure those lessons are not forgotten.

As we look to the future and the mental health demands for this population, the impact of losing the war in Afghanistan on the moral and mental health of those who served in Afghanistan is unknown. Further, the threat of future wars grows more imminent as we see the events of Ukraine and the reverberations already occurring with other nations requesting entry into NATO and further posturing about expanding the war to other nations. The impacts these events may have on the willingness to seek assistance, the military culture, and the trust of these personnel in the government provided medical resources are unclear. As clinicians and those who have chosen to care for these veterans, like the care and support we provide to everyone, we must remain sensitive to each veterans' personal experience. Veterans will process losing the Afghanistan War differently, as will military service members about their prior experiences and their concerns about those to come. As providers we must assess the unique needs of each veteran and meet them where they are. Where veterans are on the road to recovery and the path they will take will be influenced by many factors. The lost war in Afghanistan is just one of many, and the recent events in Ukraine show us that there are more wars to come. Being aware of these factors and responding appropriately will be essential in aiding them in healing.

Bethesda, MD, USA Christopher H. Warner
Los Angeles, CA, USA Carl A. Castro

Preface

The horrors and psychological impacts of warfare and military service have been documented throughout our history. From Odysseus and his trauma of the Trojan War to Hemingway's psychological scars from World War I, these impacts have been documented through books, stories, and more recently films and documentaries. Over the past two centuries, our understanding of that psychological impact and specific mental health conditions has evolved significantly. In the Civil War, early signs and symptoms of anxiety and trauma disorders were documented as Da Costa's syndrome, later becoming "shell shock" during World War I, and eventually establishing our understanding of present-day Posttraumatic Stress Disorder.

In the United States, another significant shift has occurred that informs and impacts these psychological effects, and that was the shift from a draft-based military to an all-volunteer force. Initiated in the 1970s in the aftermath of the politically and publicly unpopular Vietnam War, the United States military restructured in part to account for this new system but also to combat internal problems with indiscipline and reliability due to drug and alcohol problems and growing concerns about the ethical conduct of service members on the battlefield. The result was the establishment of a military career field in our society and resulting requirement for our military services to be concerned not only about our service members but their families as well.

Through the remainder of the Cold War, these military forces trained and operated in largely static locations, some within the United States and some operating in partner nations such as Germany and Korea, but few were deployed for extended of periods of time. However, after the fall of the Soviet Union, the United States continued to maintain a large military force which became more frequently deployed. This change in posture initially occurred with the Persian Gulf War in 1990–1991 when a large military force was sent to the Arabian Peninsula to liberate the nation of Kuwait. Subsequently, throughout the 90s, military forces were frequently asked to participate in stability and peacekeeping operations in locations including Somalia, Haiti, Bosnia, and Kosovo. Additionally, during this time, our military forces and other governmental agencies found themselves targets abroad to growing terrorist threats.

In the aftermath of this terrorist threat striking our nation on September 11, 2001, our nation embarked on a global war on terror that included a war in Afghanistan that has been enduring since 2001 and only now coming to a conclusion, a war in

Iraq that lasted from 2003 to 2011, and more recently ongoing operations in Iraq/Syria/Horn of Africa. With the United States choosing to continue to execute these wars with an all-volunteer force, there was a heavy dependence on National Guard and Reserve forces to mobilize and deploy in support of these wars and for service members to complete recurrent and multiple tours of duty through the war zones to meet the mission. As of the beginning of 2020, more than 2.7 million service members had completed over 5.4 million deployments to Afghanistan or Iraq with more than half completing multiple deployments. Additionally, the force structure saw some dramatic shifts during this time with women accounting for over 10% of the deployed force, the opening of combat missions and military occupational specialties to women, and the ability for LGBTQ service members to be able to openly serve, all occurring during these wars.

Throughout this time, mental health teams have actively deployed to combat zones with these service members providing the first near real time mental health impact data from the combat environment. Coupled with dedicated efforts from Department of Defense, Veteran's Administration, academia, and Military/Veteran advocacy groups, countless studies and information were gathered throughout to better understand the mental health effects of war. This has led to a broader understanding of not only the short-term impacts, but has led to improved screening and identification processes, enhanced treatment, and a better understanding of the impacts not only on service members but also their families. The result is a significant increase in demand for mental health services as post-deployment screening has shown that up to 20% of all redeploying service members are dealing with some mental health issue from their experience. While the Department of Defense and Veterans Affairs mental healthcare systems have adapted and adjusted to meet these demands, these veterans are completing their military service and transitioning to post-military lives throughout our nation.

Further, the increased awareness associated with the veterans of the Global War on Terror has brought to light the continued need for resources for our veterans of prior wars. Presently, the Department of Veterans Affairs reports that there are 20.8 million veterans in our population, and while estimates do expect a 1.8% decline in the Veteran population between now and 2045, Veterans are expected to have a much younger average age and the percent of female veterans is expected to increase significantly. Further, the population of families impacted by deployments will continue to grow significantly. While the Department of Defense and Veteran's Administration will continue to provide an avenue for mental health care for these individuals, it is quite likely that most all psychiatrists during the course of their career will encounter and care for a military veteran.

The intent of this book is to provide a manual for mental health professionals to understand the culture and background which may impact their therapeutic alliance, become knowledgeable about unique resources which are available to veterans, and provide an overview of particular clinical issues which have military-specific aspects to them. This is not meant to be a comprehensive textbook but rather a guide for providers to enhance their treatment and care for our nation's military and veteran personnel.

The book opens with an excellent overview of the military culture and community by New York Times' bestselling author, Eliot Cohen, whose father was an Army Psychiatrist and daughter has served as an Army psychologist. The next block of chapters will provide situational understanding to the experience that your patient may have had including deploying to a combat zone, the challenges of seeking mental health care, and the key influence of transitions in the military-veteran paradigm. The second section will create awareness of the government-provided mental health systems for military and veteran patients. These include an overview of the system of care in a deployed environment to community resources available for veterans while also highlighting key systems such as the disability process which provides compensation and medical service availability to potentially eligible veterans and understanding of the limits of confidentiality for those patients who are currently in military service. The next section will highlight unique aspects of mental health conditions such as military posttraumatic stress disorder, traumatic, or moral injury, while also bringing attention to challenges for particular populations such as homelessness in veterans, mental health concerns for LGTBQ service members/veterans, etc.

As many of you may not only care for a service member or a veteran, but also the family member of a service member or veteran, the final section will outline the impact on these populations from deployments, as well as those who are living with combat injured. Each of these chapters are written by outstanding authors who are nationally renowned in these areas and have firsthand experience in caring for these populations. Additionally, many of them are also service members or veterans. Each chapter will be driven by fictional case examples to illustrate key points and a summary of the key takeaways.

As you embark on reading this manual, we hope it will serve as not only an initial read but a reference that you can draw back to in your practice as you encounter these amazing men and women who have sacrificed for our country. We, the authors of this book, thank you for your service in caring for them and hope this will enhance the care that you deliver.

Bethesda, MD, USA — Christopher H. Warner
Los Angeles, CA, USA — Carl A. Castro

Contents

Part I

Understanding the Veteran and Military Mental Health Culture

Transitioning from Military Service Member to Veteran

1

Wilmer A. Rivas, Sara Kintzle, and Carl A. Castro

Vignette

Joe is 32-year-old white male who served in the U.S. Marine Corps for 6 years as an infantryman. He served two tours of duty in Afghanistan, and one in Iraq. While deployed during his first deployment to Afghanistan he saw significant combat. Several members of his unit were killed, with numerous other suffering from significant combat injuries, including others who injuries required amputations. Joe personally performed immediate first aide on several of his injured friends and was credited with saving several lives. For his bravery in combat, and for saving the lives of several of his fellow Marines, Joe was awarded the Navy Commendation medal for bravery, although many Marines in his unit thought the award should have been higher. Joe often thinks about the lives of his friends that he failed to save, and wonders whether all the sacrifices are really worth it. During his last deployment to Iraq, Joe was injured in an IED attack, and was awarded both the Purple Hearth and the Bronze Star, neither of which he felt he deserved, as his injuries were minor compared to those of his fellow Marines, although Joe was hospitalized for 3 weeks due to his combat injuries. In between his second and third deployment, Joe got married. After his third deployment, Joe's wife, who recently had their first baby, told Joe that if he didn't leave the Marines, she was going to leave them, so Joe refused to re-enlist, although he was clearly considered by his superiors to be an outstanding

W. A. Rivas (✉)
Veterans Affairs San Diego Healthcare System, San Diego, CA, USA

S. Kintzle
Suzanne Dworak-Peck School of Social Work, University of Southern California, Los Angeles, CA, USA
e-mail: kintzle@usc.edu

C. A. Castro
Social Work, University of Southern California, Los Angeles, CA, USA
e-mail: carl.castro@usc.edu

C. H. Warner, C. A. Castro (eds.), *Veteran and Military Mental Health*,
https://doi.org/10.1007/978-3-031-18009-5_1

Marine. Joe left the Marine Corps without any idea of what he was going to do to support his family and without any job prospects. Joe and his family moved in with his wife's parents. Joe had great difficulty finding a job. He blamed his failure to find employment on employers not appreciating the skills he obtained in the military. Three months after leaving the military, Joe's wife informed him that she wanted a divorce as she started seeing a former high school boyfriend. Joe subsequently moved in with his sister and her family. Joe began drinking heavily. After 6 months, Joe's sister told him that he needed to get a job or move out. Joe tried to re-enlist in the Marine Corps only to discover that the Marines would not accept him, so Joe spoke to an Army recruiter to join the Army. While he was waiting to enlist in the Army, Joe met his current girlfriend and moved in with her and gave up the idea of joining the Army. He subsequently found a job that paid minimum wage, which angered Joe as he felt that he deserved more, due to the sacrifices he made. Joe's drinking increased as did his anger, which often erupted at unexpected times. Joe has also had difficulty sleeping for which he reports that drinking helps. Joe's girlfriend wants him to get help. She has encouraged Joe to go to the VA to get help. Joe is reluctant to seek help in the VA yet is willing to see a non-VA doctor.

Transitions are a part of life. Everyone experiences transitions, whether you are in the military or not. While service members are still in the military, they also experience a number of transitions. They deploy, they return from deployments. They change jobs, often by physically moving from one state to another, or from one county to another if they are stationed overseas. Life involves transitions. However, during all of these transitions, the service member is supported by the military. When a service member changes jobs, it is usually due to a promotion, or it is career enhancing. Further, service members typically receive a sponsor to help them adjust to the new military community they are joining.

Transitioning from the military back to civilian life is an entirely different type of transition that very few military members or civilians have ever experienced. It is like moving to a foreign country where the separating service member must figure everything out for themselves, with relatively little or no help from the military or the community they are joining. They need to find a job, a place to live, and figure out where they are going to bank and shop. The need to determine where to go for health and dental care. And if they are married and have children, they must figure out how their family will receive health care. Where their children will go to school. And much more. While the service member is on active duty, all these things are figured out or provided for them. While on active duty, service members are fully employed, are provided housing or housing support, universal health care for them and their family, and military installations have schools, shops, gasoline stations and grocery stores for the service members and their families to use. When a service member leaves the military, they typically lose all this support.

Servicemembers often leave the military with unmet physical and mental health needs that may impact their transition back into civilian life [1]. While some veterans may be eligible for care through the Veteran's Administration (VA), many veterans often seek services from community providers for several reasons. For example, some veterans may be ineligible for VA services due to their discharge status from the military, some may be unaware of their eligibility to use VA care, and some may choose not to use it despite being eligible. In the case of Joe, there is no reason to believe that he is not eligible to receive VA care. However, it would be appropriate to ask about his discharge status. Veterans who received a bad conduct or dishonorable discharge would not be eligible for VA care.

Other Veterans—for example rural veterans—may utilize dual care (care from the VHA and the community) more often than other groups of veterans [2]. Additionally, the VA's Veteran's Choice program has expanded access to community care providers at VA expense for millions of eligible veterans since its implementation in 2014. Under the Choice program, eligible veterans can seek services from community providers when they face long wait times for appointments (longer than 30 days), excessive travel distances (when veterans live more than 40 miles from a VA provider), or if they face additional challenges to accessing VA care [3, 4]. Between fiscal years 2014 and 2018, the number of veterans authorized to use community care increased by 41%, and the use of community care from veterans is expected to increase [3]. As a result, millions more veterans may elect to seek care outside of VA settings from providers who may be less familiar with this unique population. Non-VA health care providers who are treating veterans should enquire about reimbursement through the Veteran's Choice program.

Various helping professions have highlighted the importance of cultural competence when working with clients. Although research on cultural competence has primarily focused on ethnic and racial minority groups, it is important to understand that the military is itself a unique culture within society with its own set of values, language, rituals, ideas, norms, and symbols, as well as unique interpretations to legitimize the existing culture within the military [5, 6]. However, previous studies have found that many medical schools and residency training programs lack educational opportunities that focus on military culture and related issues (as cited by [7]). In this chapter we will use a biopsychosocial-financial framework to highlight some of those unique challenges of the U.S. military that are important for health care providers who lack direct military knowledge needed to facilitate the transition of the service member back to civilian life.

It is important to note, however, that culture is not a fixed construct but rather dynamic and can be influenced by individuals' lived experiences in that culture. Furthermore, many subcultures exist within the military, which may result in differing beliefs, attitudes, and customs. For example, there can be differences between the different branches (e.g., Army vs. Marines), the different components (e.g., Active-Duty vs. Reservists), and by occupational specialty (e.g., Infantry vs. Armor). Additionally, servicemembers come from diverse backgrounds with several intersecting identities (e.g., gender identity, race, ethnicity, sexual orientation, religiosity, and more), all of which may impact their experience in the military. The reader is referred Chap. 20 for a more detailed discussion of LGBTQ+ service members and special considerations that health care providers should consider.

Providers must be wary of making stereotypical assumptions when providing services to veterans and be opened to learning about military culture in general, as well as each servicemember's individual experiences. In Joe's case, he is both a Marine and an infantryman. And as an infantryman Marine, Joe experienced a great deal of combat, including watching many of his fellow service members die or suffer from long-term physical injuries. Further, Marines are often viewed as the less "intelligent" of the services, lacking in the necessary skills and experiences to successfully transition from the Marine Corps back to their civilian communities. This is a myth that needs to be actively overcome. The overall aptitude of Marines is no different than that of soldiers or sailors.

Another important aspect of Joe's case deserves mentioning. It was his girlfriend that suggested that he get help. This is not unusual. It is often the wife, husband or a significant other that recommends that a veteran get help. It is rare that a veteran will seek care on their own. There are many reasons for this reluctance to seek care. Chapter 4 discusses the role that stigma may play in impeding veterans from seeking care and ways that this might be addressed.

Biological Concerns

Military transition is a period filled with many lifestyle changes and stressors for veterans as they make the adjustment back into civilian life. These changes can have a significant impact on veterans' health. For example, obesity, which has become a public health epidemic in the general population is especially problematic among veterans, particularly those who have been recently discharged [8–12]. Several factors may contribute to the significant weight gain seen in recently discharged veterans. Changes in a veteran's daily routine such as engaging in less moderate to vigorous regular exercise post-service, stress and disability due to military service, and lack of a requirement to adhere to military fitness standards are just a few examples [8].

Obesity rates are higher among veterans with related diagnoses such as hypertension, diabetes, and sleep apnea, those with mental health conditions such as depression and PTSD, and veterans with lower extremity joint disorders [9, 11]. This is particularly concerning because many veterans may often experience several of these conditions due to their military service and may contribute to poorer health outcomes. In Joe's case, there is no information provided on Joe's weight or overall health. Yet, based on the initial assessment, Joe likely suffers from PTSD, and has a significant alcohol problem, which could contribute to significant weight gain and other health-related issues, such as diabetes and smoking. Assessments should be conducted to ascertain if these issues exist.

As previously mentioned, veterans may often leave the military with unmet physical health needs. This may be due in part to the "mission-first" value held by many servicemembers, in which the needs of the military supersede the needs of the individual which leads to the "embrace the suck" attitude seen in many servicemembers/veterans [7]. Due to this attitude, many individuals may forego seeking treatment for any number of physical health concerns. This can be problematic because one of the most common conditions diagnosed in veterans is musculoskeletal (MSK) injuries such as back and knee pain, among others [13, 14]. The nature of military service puts veterans at increased risk of MSK injuries due to exposure to a number of contributing factors such as intense physical training, patrolling in uneven terrain and mountainous settings, bearing heavy loads, and combat trauma [13, 14]. Furthermore, MSK injuries contribute significantly to the experience of chronic pain [13, 15]. Thus, providers should be wary of issues that may arise from treating veterans with MSK injuries or chronic pain, particularly those who utilize dual care from the community and the VA because poor coordination between community and VA providers can result in unsafe prescribing of medications, and increased risk of death from opioid overdose [2].

In addition to MSKs providers should be aware about the probability of prior Traumatic Brain Injuries (TBIs) among the veteran population. Previous studies have found that TBIs are common among military personnel, with over 400,000 servicemembers being diagnosed with one between 2000 and 2019 [16]. Due to the widespread use of explosives during the wars in Iraq and Afghanistan, along with advancements in body armor and helmets increasing survivability from these types of attacks, TBIs are seen as a "signature wound" of the present-day conflicts [16, 17]. Furthermore, servicemembers are at increased risk of multiple TBIs due to routine exposure to injury, particularly on deployment, and deployed servicemembers are more likely than non-deployed servicemembers to report multiple injuries [16]. This is particularly concerning because individuals who experience multiple TBIs are at an increased risk of developing mental health problems such as depression, anxiety, PTSD, and suicide attempts, may experience difficulty controlling violent behavior, and may experience issues with memory, concentration, and substance use [18, 19]. Chapter 13 provides a detail discussion of TBI and its impact on veterans.

While physical demands and injuries present a significant health risk to veterans, environmental hazards also pose another risk to their health. Veterans of all ages have had to face environmental hazards during service. For example, in World War I veterans dealt with "trench foot" due to fighting in wet trenches, in Korea many veterans suffered from cold-weather injuries such as frostbite and hypothermia due to the extreme cold, and in Vietnam many veterans have suffered as a result of the use of Agent Orange. In the first Gulf War many veterans struggled with Gulf War Syndrome, although it took years for these veterans to receive the help they needed and deserved. Among Post 9/11 veterans, respiratory exposures are a common concern with as many as 95% of deployed servicemembers reporting at least one type of exposure [20, 21]. Common types of exposures included burning trash and feces, excessive dust and sand, diesel, kerosene, and other fumes, smoke from oil fires, and other pollutants. This may be particularly problematic to those who have deployed to countries with lax pollution standards. There is some evidence that respiratory exposures are associated with increased risk of respiratory problems such as sinusitis, bronchitis, and asthma, especially among veterans with a deployment history [20–22].

Joe was physically wounded in combat, requiring him to spend significant time in the hospital. A detailed history of Joe's injuries should be conducted, paying particular care to any long-term lingering effects of his injury. Joe is likely to minimize the extent of his injuries, believing that other veterans who are more seriously injured deserve care first. It should also be determined if Joe has sought a physical evaluation from the VA for his injuries, which given Joe's reluctance to go to the VA is unlikely. Chapter 10 provides a detailed discussion of the VA disability rating process. If Joe is reluctant to undergo the VA disability rating process, the assistance of another veteran might be useful to assist Joe in navigating the VA disability process as well as helping Joe understand the importance of receiving a disability rating. Since Joe is the recipient of the Purple Heart, a medal awarded for a combat injury, connecting Joe to other veterans awarded the Purple Heart would likely facilitate this process, which could lead to significant monetary compensation and accommodation for Joe.

Psychological Concerns

The US has been engaged in the longest period of armed conflict in its history (almost 20 years at the time this chapter was written). During that time, over 2.7 million servicemembers have deployed in support of OEF/OIF, with some servicemembers deploying multiple times [23]. Due to the stressors related to military service in general, and combat, there is an increased risk of veterans suffering psychologically and behaviorally.

Posttraumatic stress disorder (PTSD), which develops as a result of exposure to traumatic events, has been called one of the "signature wounds" of the military's wars in Iraq and Afghanistan. While anyone who is exposed to a traumatic event may develop PTSD, due to the role of the military (that is combat), servicemembers are at increased risk of being exposed to traumatic events [24]. Common types of traumas reported during combat by servicemembers who deployed to Iraq and Afghanistan include having a friend wounded or killed (50%), seeing noncombatants who were dead or seriously injured (45%), witnessing an accident that resulted in death or serious injury (45%), being moved or knocked over by explosions (23%), receiving a blow to the head (18%), and more [25]. A study by Hoge et al. [26] found that 12% of soldiers and Marines who served in Afghanistan and 18% of those who served in Iraq met criteria for probable PTSD. The National Health Study for a New Generation of U.S. Veterans (NewGen), which consisted of a sample of 60,000 veterans of the OEF/OIF era (including 30,000 who deployed and 30,000 who did not deploy) found similar results, with 15.8% of deployed veterans and 10.9% of nondeployed veterans meeting criteria for PTSD [22]. These findings are consistent with previous studies of veterans from different eras reporting higher rates of PTSD than the general civilian population [24, 27, 28]. Chapter 12 provides a more thorough discussion of the issues involving PTSD.

It is very likely based on the case description of Joe that he suffers from PTSD. Joe's difficulty sleeping, anger, and drinking are all likely related to the trauma that Joe experienced during his numerous combat deployments. It is likely that Joe experienced multiple traumas, involving both his own personal experience of being wounded and caring and seeing fellow Marines wounded. Indeed, Joe may have been suffering from PTSD for some time, yet the structure of the Marine Corps allowed him to still function at a very high level. Once he left the military, the lack of structure provided by the Marine Corps unmasked the PTSD symptoms, which may have contributed to the deterioration of his marriage as well as the request of his new girlfriend to seek help. The multiple traumas experienced by combat veterans and its often delayed manifestations are a unique experience of combat veterans that is often overlooked.

Military Sexual Trauma (MST), which refers to sexual assault and harassment that occurs while in the military, is an additional source of trauma for many servicemembers [20, 21, 24]. This behavior, which can range from unsolicited verbal contact of a sexual nature to physical sexual assault (that is, rape) can have a significant psychological and health outcome on those who experience it [20, 21]. While previous studies have found that up to 20.5% of women and 0.8% of men from the OEF/OIF era report experiencing MST, the NewGen study (which includes Veterans that do not access the VA) found significantly higher rates of MST (41% of women and 4% of men) [20, 21]. Barth et al. [20, 21] found some differences between the service branches, with 52% of women in the Marine Corps reporting MST. These traumatizing experiences are made worse by military leadership which has historically failed to appropriately protect those who report experiencing MST (e.g., [29, 30]). Given this high prevalence among OEF/OIF-era veterans, community providers should screen for possible history of MST and provide a referral to appropriate supportive services. Chapter 15 provides a detailed discussion of MST. The most important thing to note here is that even though Joe is a male combat veteran, an assessment of whether he was a victim of sexual assault should be made. One should not assume the absence of sexual assault unless assessed.

Another concerning mental health issue with this population is the rate of suicides, which have significantly increased among OEF/OIF-era servicemembers and veterans [31, 32]. While there is debate about whether combat or deployments directly influences suicide rates in servicemembers, there is some support that deaths by suicide have increased with the increase in poor mental health conditions among servicemembers [31, 32]. For example, Arenson et al. [33] found that veterans with PTSD are at increased risk of suicide, particularly when experiencing comorbid depression. This is particularly concerning because PTSD often co-occurs with other disorders such as depression, anxiety, TBI, and substance use [25, 34]. Furthermore, veterans may become susceptible to negative outcomes such as suicide during the transition from military service to civilian life. Unaddressed physical and mental health needs may present barriers towards successful transition (e.g., difficulty finding employment and forming meaningful relationships) combined with a loss of a shared military identity can contribute to feelings of burdensomeness and not belonging, that may contribute to risk of suicide [31].

While it is important for providers to be aware of the mental health needs of veterans, it is also worth noting that not everyone who serves will experience a mental health disorder, regardless of combat exposure. In fact, the majority of people (civilian and military) that experience a traumatic event do not develop PTSD, though they may experience some symptoms for a period of time after the event [24]. Although not all veterans who are exposed to combat experience mental health issues, they may be changed by the experience [35]. Additionally, even though they may not experience mental health issues, they may benefit from counseling. This counseling does not have to be a formal therapeutic intervention where the goal is to treat a diagnosable psychiatric illness, but rather the goal is to provide social and emotional support, mentoring, academic counseling, financial counseling, and other forms of counseling that can serve to prevent any changes from escalating into a more serious issue (e.g., mental illness, unemployment, homelessness, etc.) [35]. This can also include providing psychoeducation that teaches veterans how traumatic experiences can change an individual as well as useful coping skills to manage these changes. Thus, it is recommended that community providers be aware of organizations that may provide this type of support before issues escalate to more serious issues so that the appropriate referrals can be made in a timely manner. See Chap. 17 for a more detailed discussion on this important topic.

Joe likely has a drinking problem. By his own accounts, he drinks at night to help him sleep. It is well documented that alcohol rather than aiding in improving sleep quality impairs it. Drinking to facilitate sleep might indicate that Joe is suffering from nightmares due to his combat experiences, although this should not be assumed. He might be drinking for other reasons. A psychological evaluation will be necessary to aid in making this determination. It is not unusual for combat veterans to be angry. Since Joe appears to have anger, and possibly aggression issues, the causes of his anger should also be a focus of assessment.

Socio-Cultural-Spiritual Concerns

Military service plays a large role in a servicemember's daily life, as such, the military has often been described as a 'greedy institution' [6, 36]. This is because the military requires 24/7 commitment from its members. Consequently, they relinquish a large amount of their personal privacy and freedom, they may be subject to frequent relocations, may be deployed overseas on short notice, and often experience extended separations from their families [6, 36]. On the other hand, the military offers many benefits to servicemembers and their families, such as a strong sense of community, housing, healthcare, and a host of other benefits. Thus, transitioning out of the military lifestyle can bring many different changes that affect not only the servicemember, but their families as well.

Servicemembers develop a strong sense of military identity and develop close bonds with their peers through many aspects of their military career, such as in basic training, throughout deployments, and more [7]. Often, they may identify with their military identity more strongly than any other identity, even years after they have left the military [7]. While this strong sense of identity is a great source of pride, it may present an issue during the transition period, partly due to a growing military-civilian cultural gap. The military instills certain values such as interdependence, self-sacrifice, discipline, obedience, and commitment to comrades, which at times conflict with civilian values that emphasize individuality, independence, and freedom of choice [37, 38]. At times, servicemembers may report difficulty connecting with civilians for a variety of reasons, including the perception that civilians do not understand them, or that civilians do not appreciate the sacrifices made by veterans and the military, or feeling like they do not fit into the civilian world [37, 39].

As a result of this cultural gap, servicemembers may be vulnerable to a loss of social support during the transition period, as they leave their military peers behind and try to reintegrate to civilian life. Additionally, some mental health symptoms such as irritability, feelings of detachment, depression, and avoidance of social situations may contribute to interpersonal difficulties and the loss of social support [38]. Additionally, some Veterans experience difficulty reintegrating not just into the civilian world, but reintegrating with their families, particularly after a deployment which can at times lead to divorce [37]. To address this potential loss of support, providers should be knowledgeable of and provide Veterans with referrals to support groups, and organizations through which they can connect with others such as veteran organizations and peer groups. Connecting Joe with local or even national veteran groups, especially ones involving Marines would probably be beneficial. Marines who have successfully transitioned back to their community could serve as useful mentors for Joe.

Joe has a child, and Joe is still married, although he is currently seeing someone else. The status of Joe's family situation needs to be explored in more detail. The most important thing to determine is the current relationships that Joe has with his wife and child. Does Joe see his child on a regular basis? Does Joe and his wife plan on divorcing? Marital counseling might be helpful in either preserving Joe's marriage if that is what the couple desire or helping the couple eventually separate while maintaining an effective relationship so Joe may continue to be part of his child's life. Of course, financial support for Joe's child will also have to be addressed.

Financial Concerns

Another key issue to be aware of when working with veterans, is their financial health or status. While on active duty, servicemembers have a steady income, free housing, access to healthcare (primary, mental/behavior, and dental care), access to dining facilities, and several other benefits that are in place to ensure their needs are met. After transition, Veterans lose access to the majority of these benefits. While veterans may be eligible for some benefits post-service, these are limited and may depend on the type of discharge a veteran receives (e.g., veterans with less than honorable discharge may lose access to education, and/or healthcare benefits). Thus, obtaining steady employment before a veteran is discharged, can ensure a more stable transition into civilian life. It is not unusual for veterans leave the military without securing civilian employment before discharge [40] as was the case with Joe. In fact, nearly three-quarters of service members leave the military with no job.

Lack of employment can lead to several negative outcomes such as, financial difficulties, lack of resources, increased psychological distress, and difficulties in family and social relationships [41]. Furthermore, many of these issues place veterans at higher risk of homelessness (see Chap. 19 on veteran homelessness). Metraux et al. [42] found that unemployment, financial difficulties, and loss of relationships contribute to veterans' homelessness. Mental illness and substance can often increase risk of homelessness in military and civilian populations [43]. Joe and his family left the military with no permanent housing having been arranged.

Luckily for Joe, he and his family were able to move in with his in-laws, and when his marriage began to fail, he moved in with this sister. These types of living arrangements are almost always temporary. Eventually, Joe met someone new, and moved in with her even though he did not have a job at the time. Securing employment may be one of the most important factors associated with well-being and success after discharge [1]. There may be several factors which make it difficult for veterans to secure employment. One of these factors, is the military-civilian cultural gap, such as communication differences, difficulty translating military experiences to civilian terms, and other cultural differences that may be perceived as lack of discipline by veterans (e.g., not showing up on time) [44]. Additionally, some veterans may have an expectation that finding employment with adequate pay and benefits will be easy after transition [40].

Many veterans find themselves having to start over in entry-level jobs or returning to school to earn civilian certifications for skills they gained in the military [44]. Additionally, some unresolved physical and mental health issues may contribute to veteran unemployment [45]. Veterans may sometimes face stigmatizing views related to their military experience. For example, Rudstam et al. [46] found that some human resource professionals may be concerned that veterans with PTSD or TBI are more likely than others to be violent, or that hiring them may involve more costs financially, and in manager time. Similarly, Kleykamp's [47] study suggests employers may be less likely to hire veterans who served in combat arms specialties. All these perceptions may contribute to the perception that civilians neither understand, nor appreciate veterans and their service. On the other hand, Keeling et al. [44] identified the need for social support as a facilitator towards employment, particularly from veteran peers, organizations, and family.

Joe eventually found a job, but it only paid minimum wage. This fact angered Joe as he believed that he was deserving of a better paying job. Many veterans often have unreasonably high job expectations when they leave the military. They believe that it is going to be easy to find a high paying, meaningful job. In fact, finding the right job can take time. Many veterans take up to 2 years or longer to finally find the job that suits them [40]. It should also be noted that Joe is eligible for the GI Bill, which would enable him to go to college or technical school to pursue a profession of his choice. The GI Bill is an incredibly generous education and training program that veterans have earned. If Joe continues to struggle finding a job that he is content with, this option should be discussed with him.

A Roadmap for a Successful Transition

A successful transition from the military back to the civilian community requires several elements. These elements are general principles. Every separating service member will encounter different challenges. Yet, if they keep these five elements in mind, the stress of their transition will be greatly diminished.

The first thing a service member and their family should recognize is that a transition is a process. It is not an event. It is not the date you leave the military or even the date you decide to leave the military. Every service member eventually leaves the military and should always be thinking (and planning) for when that day happens. A successful transition can take months and even years to achieve. Service members and their families should be patient. Service members should not think leaving the military is going to be a disaster nor should they think leaving is going to be easy. Prepare for the worst, hope for the best.

Second, the service member and their family will have to figure things out for themselves and how best to meet their own needs and the needs of the family. There are hundreds of veteran organizations to help veterans and their families, and the veteran must not be afraid or embarrassed to ask for help. The VA is a tremendous asset, and every veteran should be fully prepared to utilize any services the VA can offer. There is strength in unity.

Third, leaving the military will undoubtedly result in a loss of identity and prestige for the veteran, and the family. Friendships with those still serving will change. Simply said, veterans will not be as important as they once were after they leave the military. Veterans will need to make new friends, often with those who have never served. This reality will require the veteran to develop a new identity that merges their active-duty military identity with their new identity as a military veteran who is now also a civilian.

Fourth, many veterans believe that they are entitled to certain things because they served their country. Things like being given a high-paying job, a prestigious job with lots of perks. While veterans should be proud of their service, they must never lose their hustle. Life is competitive. Veterans must learn to leverage their military experience to win these competitions, and there are numerous veteran organizations to help veterans do this. As noted previously, veterans need to be prepared to start a level or two below where they think they should. Veterans need to have faith in themselves that they will be quickly identify as a high performer and be advanced more quickly than their civilian counterparts. Yet, a poor attitude will derail any rapid advancement.

Finally, every veteran who leaves the military should have a job offer in hand. Not a plan to get a job, but an actual job offer, with a start date. Of course, this does not apply to veterans who are being medically retired and are physically unable to work. However, most veterans can work and should plan to work upon leaving the military. Taking 30–45 days off before beginning a new job is reasonable. Taking off 2–3 years is not. The longer a veteran is unemployed, the harder it will be for the veteran to land that coveted high-paying, meaningful job with excellent benefits. Forward planning is essential.

Conclusion

In sum, the transition from military to civilian life can be a stressful experience. Veterans are a unique group who may have several unresolved needs that can impact their transition. While some may receive services and benefits from the VA, many may often be seen in civilian primary care settings. In order to better support this community, providers should be aware of the many factors that may impact veterans and their health, and how these often intertwine with each other compounding their impact. However, it should be noted that the previous chapter is not an exhaustive list of factors veterans may face. Nor should it be assumed that all these experiences affect all veterans. Providers must remember that veterans come from all backgrounds, and their military experiences often differ by branch, military occupational specialty, degree of combat exposure and more. These intersecting identities can influence their experiences as well as the resources they have available to help them cope. Thus, while providers should seek to learn more about military culture, they should always seek to gain a holistic understanding of each individual veteran they serve.

Clinical Pearls

- The biopsychosocial-spiritual-financial health framework can be a useful guide to ensuring that a holistic approach is undertaken to determine the needs of a veteran and their family.
- A loss of military identity can make it difficult for many veterans to fit in with their civilian community. Connecting veterans with veteran organizations can be useful in adding them in their transition.
- A successful transition can take time, upwards of 2 years in many cases. However, there are many resources and programs to assist the veteran, particularly the GI Bill.
- Ensure that veterans receive the services and benefits that they have earned. Many of these benefits and programs are provided by the VA, the state, and non-profit agencies. Encouraging veterans to take advantage of these services should be a top priority.

References

1. Kintzle S, Castro CA. Examining veteran transition to the workplace through military transition theory. In: Harms PD, Perrewe PL, editors. Occupational stress and well-being in military contexts. Bingley: Emerald Publishing Limited; 2018. p. 117–27. https://doi.org/10.1108/S1479-355520180000016009.
2. Schlosser J, Kollisch D, Johnson D, Perkins T, Olson A. VA-Community dual care: veteran and clinician perspectives. J Community Health. 2020;45:795–802. https://doi.org/10.1007/s10900-020-00795-y.
3. United States Government Accountability Office. VA health care: estimating resources needed to provide community care. GAO-19-478. Washington, DC: United States Government Accountability Office; 2019.

4. Yoon J, Leung LB, Rubenstein LV, Rose DR, et al. Use of the Veteran's Choice program and attrition from Veterans Health Administration primary care. Med Care. 2020;58(12):1091–7.
5. Reger M, Etherage J, Reger G, Gahm G. Civilian psychologists in an army culture: the ethical challenge of cultural competence. Mil Psychol. 2008;20(1):21–35. https://doi.org/10.1080/08995600701753144.
6. Soeters JL, Winslow DJ, Weibull A. Military culture. In: Handbook of the sociology of the military. Boston, MA: Springer; 2006. p. 237–54. https://doi.org/10.1007/0-387-34576-0_14.
7. Meyer EG, Writer BW, Brim W. The importance of military cultural competence. Curr Psychiatry Rep. 2016;18(26):1–8. https://doi.org/10.1007/s11920-016-0662-9.
8. Bookwalter DB, Porter B, Jacobson IG, Kong SY, et al. Healthy behaviors and incidence of overweight and obesity in military veterans. Ann Epidemiol. 2019;39:36–2.
9. Breland JY, Phibbs CS, Hoggatt KJ, Washington DL, et al. The obesity epidemic in the Veterans Health Administration: Prevalence among key populations of women and men veterans. J Gen Intern Med. 2017;32(Suppl. 1):11–7.
10. Nelson KM. The burden of obesity among a national probability sample of veterans. J Gen Intern Med. 2006;21(9):915–9.
11. Rush T, LeardMann CA, Crum-Cianflone NF. Obesity and associated adverse health outcomes among US military members and veterans: findings from the Millennium Cohort Study. Obesity. 2016;24(7):1582–9.
12. Teachman J, Tedrow L. Veteran status and body weight: a longitudinal fixed effects approach. Popul Res Policy Rev. 2013;32(2):199–220.
13. Haskell SG, Brandt C, Bastian L, Driscoll M, et al. Incident musculoskeletal conditions among men and women veterans returning from deployment. Med Care. 2020;58:1082–90.
14. Haskell SG, Ning Y, Krebs E, Goulet J, et al. Prevalence of painful musculoskeletal conditions in female and male veterans in 7 years after return from deployment in Operation Enduring Freedom/Operation Iraqi Freedom. Clin J Pain. 2012;28:163–7.
15. Taylor SL, Herman PM, Marshall NJ, Zeng Q, et al. Use of complementary and integrated health: a retrospective analysis of US Veterans with chronic musculoskeletal pain nationally. J Altern Complement Med. 2019;25(1):32–9. https://doi.org/10.1089/acm.2018.0276.
16. Traumatic Brain Injury Center of Excellence. Defense and veterans brain injury center research review on multiple traumatic brain injury/multiple concussion. 2020. https://www.health.mil/About-MHS/OASDHA/Defense-Health-Agency/Research-and-Development/Traumatic-Brain-Injury-Center-of-Excellence/Research. Accessed 28 Jul 2021.
17. Terrio H, Brenner LA, Ivins BJ, et al. Traumatic brain injury screening: preliminary findings in a US Army Brigade Combat Team. J Head Trauma Rehabil. 2009;24(1):14–23.
18. Brenner LA, Homaifar BY, Olson-Madden JH, Nagamoto HT, et al. Prevalence and screening of traumatic brain injury among veterans seeking mental health services. J Head Trauma Rehabil. 2013;28(1):21–30. https://doi.org/10.1097/HTR.0b013e31827df0b5.
19. Walker R, Cole JE, Logan TK, Corrigan JD. Screening substance abuse treatment clinics for traumatic brain injury: prevalence and characteristics. J Head Trauma Rehabil. 2007;22(6):360–7.
20. Barth SK, Dursa EK, Boassarte R, Schneiderman A. Lifetime prevalence of respiratory diseases and exposures among veterans of Operation Enduring Freedom and Operation Iraqi Freedom veterans: results from the National Health Study for a New Generation of U.S. Veterans. J Occup Environ Med. 2016a;58(12):1175–80. https://doi.org/10.1097/JOM.0000000000000885.
21. Barth SK, Kimerling RE, Pavao J, McCutcheon SJ, et al. Military sexual trauma among recent veterans: correlates of sexual assault and sexual harassment. Am J Prev Med. 2016b;50(1):77–86. https://doi.org/10.1016/j.amepre.2015.06.012.
22. Barth SK, Dursa EK, Peterson MR, Schneiderman A. Prevalence of respiratory diseases among veterans of Operation Enduring Freedom and Operation Iraqi Freedom: results from the National Health Study for a New Generation of U.S. Veterans. Mil Med. 2014;179(3):241–5. https://doi.org/10.7205/MILMED-D-13-00338.

23. Wenger JW, O'Connell C, Cottrell L. Examination of recent deployment experience across the services and components. Santa Monica, CA: RAND Corporation; 2018. https://www.rand.org/pubs/research_reports/RR1928.html. Accessed 28 Jul 2021.
24. Norris FH, Slone LB. Epidemiology of trauma and PTSD. In: Friedman MJ, Keane TM, Resick PA, editors. Handbook of PTSD: science and practice. New York, NY: Guilford Press; 2014. p. 100–20.
25. Schell T, Marshall G. Survey of individuals previously deployed for OEF/OIF. In: Tanielian T, Jaycox L, editors. Invisible wounds of war: psychological and cognitive injuries, their consequences, and services to assist recovery. Santa Monica, CA: RAND Corporation; 2008. p. 87–115.
26. Hoge C, Castro CA, Messer S, McGurk D, et al. Combat duty in Iraq and Afghanistan, mental health problems, and barriers to care. N Engl J Med. 2004;351(1):13–22. https://doi.org/10.1056/NJEMoa040603.
27. Kang HK, Natelson BH, Mahan CM, Lee KY, et al. Post-traumatic stress disorder and chronic fatigue syndrome-like illness among Gulf War veterans: a population-based survey of 30,000 veterans. Am J Epidemiol. 2003;157(2):141–8. https://doi.org/10.1093/aje/kwf187.
28. Kulka RA, Schlenger WE, Fairbank JA, Hough RL, et al. Trauma and the Vietnam War generation: report of findings from the National Vietnam Veterans Readjustment Study. New York, NY: Brunner/Mazel; 1990.
29. Cooper H, Steinhauer J. Viral video moves sexual harassment in Marine Corps to forefront. The New York Times. 2021. https://www.nytimes.com/2021/02/19/us/politics/lloyd-austin-military-sexual-assault.html. Accessed 28 Jul 2021.
30. Diaz J, Cramer M, Morales C. What we know about the death of Vanessa Guillen. The New York Times. 2020. https://www.nytimes.com/article/vanessa-guillen-fort-hood.html. Accessed 28 Jul 2021.
31. Castro CA, Kintzle S. Suicides in the military: the post-modern combat veteran and the Hemingway effect. Curr Psychiatry Rep. 2014;16:460. https://doi.org/10.1007/s11920-014-0460-1.
32. Kang HK, Bullman TA, Smolenski DJ, Skopp NA, et al. Suicide risk among 1.3 million veterans who were on active duty during the Iraq and Afghanistan wars. Ann Epidemiol. 2015;25(2):96–100. https://doi.org/10.1016/j.annepidem.2014.11.020.
33. Arenson MB, Whooley MA, Neylan TC, Maguen S, et al. Posttraumatic stress disorder, depression, and suicidal ideation in veterans: results from the mind your heart study. Psychiatry Res. 2018;265:224–30. https://doi.org/10.1016/j.psychres.2018.04.046.
34. Trivedi RB, Post EP, Sun H, Pomerantz A, et al. Prevalence, comorbidity, and prognosis of mental health among US veterans. Am J Public Health. 2015;105(12):2564–9. https://doi.org/10.2105/ajph.2015.302836.
35. Castro CA, Kintzle S, Hassan AM. The combat veteran paradox: paradoxes and dilemmas encountered with reintegrating combat veterans and the agencies that support them. Traumatology. 2015;21(4):299–310. https://doi.org/10.1037/trm0000049.
36. Thomas G. The stress effects of military families' transition to civilian life. Ment Health Pract. 2018;21(9):25–9. https://doi.org/10.7748/mhp.2018.e1311.
37. Demers A. When veterans return: the role of community in reintegration. J Loss Trauma. 2011;16(2):160–79. https://doi.org/10.1080/15325024.2010.519281.
38. Drebing C, Reilly E, Henze K, Kelly M, et al. Using peer support groups to enhance community integration of veterans in transition. Psychol Serv. 2018;15(2):135–45. https://doi.org/10.1037/ser0000178.
39. Brewin CR, Garnett R, Andrews B. Trauma, identity and mental health in UK military veterans. Psychol Med. 2011;41(8):1733–40. https://doi.org/10.1017/S003329171000231X.
40. Castro CA, Kintzle S, Hassan AM. The state of the American veteran: the Los Angeles county veterans study. 2014. https://cir.usc.edu/wp-content/uploads/2013/10/USC010_CIRLAVetReport_FPpgs.pdf. Accessed 28 Jul 2021.

41. Hamilton AB, Williams L, Washington DL. Military and mental health correlates of unemployment in a national sample of women veterans. Med Care. 2015;53:S32–8. https://doi.org/10.1097/mlr.0000000000000297.
42. Metraux S, Cusack M, Byrne TH, Hunt-Johnson N, True G. Pathways into homelessness among post-9/11-era veterans. Psychol Serv. 2017;14(2):229–37. http://dx.doi.org.libproxy1.usc.edu/10.1037/ser0000136.
43. Tsai J, Rosenheck RA. Risk factors for homelessness among US veterans. Epidemiol Rev. 2015;37:177–95. https://doi.org/10.1093/epirev/mxu004.
44. Keeling M, Ozuna S, Kintzle S, Castro C. Veterans' civilian employment experiences: lessons learnt from focus groups. J Career Dev. 2019;46(6):692–705. https://doi.org/10.1177/0894845318776785.
45. Horton JL, Jacobson IG, Wong CA, Wells TS, et al. The impact of prior deployment experience on civilian employment after military service. Occup Environ Med. 2013;70(6):408–17. https://doi.org/10.1136/oemed-2012-101073.
46. Rudstam H, Strobel Gower W, Cook L. Beyond yellow ribbons: are employers prepared to hire, accommodate and retain returning veterans with disabilities? J Vocat Rehabil. 2012;36:87–95. https://doi.org/10.3233/JVR-2012-0584.
47. Keyklamp M. A great place to start? The effect of prior military service on hiring. Armed Forces Soc. 2009;35(2):266–85. https://doi.org/10.1177/0095327X07308631.

An Introduction to Military Culture

2

Eliot A. Cohen

It's Not Just About Being Tough

Military service is relatively rare in the United States today; in 2020, the U.S. military included 1.3 million active duty personnel, less than 0.5% of the U.S. population [1]. For many, including health care providers, the armed forces may be an admired but not an easily understood community. Caricatured in the press either as superheroes or as broken victims of foolish leaders or organizations, veterans often view with a mixture of bemusement and resentment their depiction in the news and social media. This is not a new phenomenon: Rudyard Kipling's 1892 poem *Tommy* has an exasperated British soldier say:

> Then it's Tommy this, an' Tommy that, an' "Tommy, 'ow's yer soul?"
> But it's "Thin red line of 'eroes" when the drums begin to roll,

Kipling's Tommy acidly continues, "We ain't no thin red 'eroes, nor we aren't no blackguards too." American society, and particularly middle and upper middle class society is less dismissive of soldiers in peacetime than perhaps the British public was then, but the sentiment is similar. When our son was commissioned as an infantry officer in 2004 upon graduating Harvard, one prosperous neighbor, a very capable doctor, asked my wife and myself "Why on earth would a smart kid do that?" We debated later which was the predominant note—pity or disdain.

The military world is an exceedingly complex and variegated one. No one, even those who study it professionally, should assume that they know all of its byways and norms. Indeed, those evolve over time, and can change abruptly. In the military in which I briefly served in the 1980s, for example, it was entirely routine for

E. A. Cohen (✉)
Johns Hopkins University School of Advanced International Studies, Washington, DC, USA

Center for Strategic and International Studies, Washington, DC, USA
e-mail: ecohen@jhu.edu

C. H. Warner, C. A. Castro (eds.), *Veteran and Military Mental Health*,
https://doi.org/10.1007/978-3-031-18009-5_2

officers and non-commissioned officers to make disparaging remarks about homosexuals, without fear of rebuke. While open homosexuality can still be uncomfortable in the military, that is no longer so. The change has been enormous.

Norms changed, along with, and sometimes in advance of those of the rest of society. The military was, for example, a particularly segregated and in large part racist collection of organizations until President Truman ordered racial integration in 1948. By the 1960s and 1970s, as the sociologist Charles Moskos frequently observed, the United States Army was one of the few organizations where one could routinely see Black men ordering white ones around [2]. More recently, the integration of female service members into virtually every specialty, including those involving combat, represents an enormous and often unappreciated transformation of military culture.

To be sure, there are things that do not change. The American military, like armed forces everywhere, prize the values of service, discipline, self-sacrifice, and collective endeavor. There is, as everyone knows, a code of tough resourcefulness and achievement, although that takes many different forms. It is a set of institutions that at least formally prize the stoic virtues, with obvious implications for the willingness of service men and women to acknowledge psychological stress or difficulty or to accept psychological treatment. But to think it ends there would be a big mistake.

The Tribes

To understand military culture, one should approach it with the eye of a sensitive anthropologist. The military is a collection of tribes as much as it is a Weberian rational bureaucratic organization—indeed, it is more so. Rituals and totems characterize military life, from rites of passage (boot camp, Ranger School, Hell Week, etc.), to standing at attention and saluting at the sound of Retreat on a military base, to the prized ribbons, flashes and badges on a uniform that show status irrespective of rank, to the formalized hilarity of a dining in or to the joyous falling out parade after a unit returns from a deployment. Indeed, it is time well spent to go to such military life events in order to appreciate what military life is all about.

The services have founding myths and even founding anxieties. The Marines, for example, are well aware that no other country in the world has an organization nominally devoted to amphibious warfare that is nearly so large. It is an optional service and knows it—and so therefore has to prove itself by its competence, its versatility, and its readiness to do anything at short notice.

The Air Force, on the other hand, has had since its foundation at the end of World War II an unstated fear that it could be the product of a technological moment—the era of manned flight. In a world of missiles and drones it might not need to exist. Given that it was carved out of the United States Army at the end of World War II, the Air Force is, ironically, the only service that has recently lost a large chunk of its mission and personnel when the Trump administration announced the creation of a new Space Force.

With these technological changes come psychological challenges as well: Indeed, although grainy video of drone strikes have become a hallmark of the Global War on Terror (GWOT), drone operators are often dismissed as video game players rather than "real" combatants like fighter pilots and Navy SEALs, yet in the last 18 years, it is drone operators who have conducted some of the most frequent and—through the miracle of modern optics—up close and personal killing of these wars. The experience of the war in Ukraine suggests that this role will expand greatly, with considerable resulting stress on the individuals operating these machines.

The differences among the basic tribes—the armed services themselves, viz., the Army, Navy, Air Force, Marine Corps and in some measure the Coast Guard as well—are enormous and significant. Their self-understanding, their views of discipline, authority, comradeship, and the meaning of individuality are all very different. Their lived experiences do not resemble one another a great deal, and although it is not uncommon for members of one tribe to spend time with another (Naval officers deployed to Afghanistan as intelligence analysts, for example), those differences endure.

Service culture reflects the forms of combat around each was built [3]. Naval warfare, for example, originally rested on extremely decentralized command systems at the ship level, with the result that the commanding officer of any vessel had unusual disciplinary and other authorities. The courtesy of coming aboard a ship requires that anyone doing so salute the quarterdeck (the captain's traditional location) and request permission to come on board. That goes for admirals too—by contrast no Army general would dream of having to request permission to visit a battalion area. On board the ship, too, for historical reasons the physical and status boundaries between officer and enlisted were always clearly demarked and remained so longer than in other services. Ships still have "Officers' Country," a separate berthing area, and a wardroom for them.

The very notion of officership is different in the different services. In the Air Force, for example, a pilot must first and foremost master the skills required to fly effectively whatever aircraft he or she is assigned. As officers, pilots are, of course, taught to be leaders, but their real leadership opportunities do not come until years later in their careers. In the early phases of their careers they are operators, doing the actual work of combat or other operations. By contrast, in the Army or Marine Corps an officer is first and foremost a leader. From the very beginning of their intake from the service academies, Reserve Officer Training Corps (ROTC) programs on the campuses, or direct entry through an Officer Candidate School (OCS) class, they are taught that their job is to lead. Their first jobs, most likely, will be as platoon leaders, where they will be coached by sergeants who are nominally their subordinates, but who have far greater experience than they do.

The wrinkles here are fascinating and too numerous to be described in an article. Naval aviators (the proper term) are taught that they are naval officers first, pilots second. That has a noticeable effect on pilot culture, and results from the US Navy's decision in the 1920s not to imitate the Royal Navy's example, whereby pilots flying off aircraft carriers were from the Royal Air Force.

In general, but only in general, service cultures reflect different attitudes to risk and to loss, to safety and security. There is a rich vein of military jokes that capture this:

> Ask the Army to secure a building and they will set up a perimeter around it and make sure nobody gets out. Ask the Marines to secure a building and they will charge in, kill everybody inside, and then set up defenses to make sure nobody gets in. Ask the Navy to secure a building and they will turn off all the lights and lock all the doors at 1700.Ask the Air Force to secure a building and they will sign a 10 year lease with an option to buy [4].

The joke has its roots in serious things. The Air Force cannot function without well-developed and well maintained bases from which it can operate. The Marine Corps developed a particularly violent, head on approach to combat in order to successfully assault defended islands in the Pacific before and during World War II.

The Clans

There are tribal differences that permeate the services, particularly when there are traits that are imprinted on virtually all service members. For example, "Every Marine a rifleman" is a motto that the Marine Corps takes seriously; it applies to their lawyers as much as to their infantry. This has real consequences. Whereas the Air Force, for example, tends to view each of its officer fields as distinct and specialized, the Marine Corps believes that it selects officers for leadership, period, and their specialties are of secondary importance. A really good lawyer can (and has) become the commander of such a critical installation as the basic training installation at Parris Island. That would be far less likely even in the Army.

Still, within each tribe there are clans, which are the various specializations. In general, one may say that any of the combat clans—infantry, armor, or artillery in the Army, for example, or surface warfare in the Navy—dominate the services. This makes sense, because the services exist, after all, to fight. As a result, it is difficult, although not impossible, for a logistician or a signals specialist to achieve the highest rank or command. And here too, tribal cultures may differ from one another.

There is, for example, a cult of toughness in the combat arms that are, it is fair to say, less pronounced in specialties such as finance or maintenance. This does not necessarily reflect true risk: at a base under continual rocket fire everyone is pretty much exposed to the same hazards. But it is the case that the particular qualities involved in the combat arms, and above all, the willingness to come to close quarters with an opponent and administer deadly force, are different. From a mental health point of view this might play out in different ways—the military unsurprisingly spends a great deal more effort on developing the mental toughness and resilience of operators than it does on similar conditioning for support personnel. That does not mean that incidence of mental health problems will necessarily be greater in any subgroup, just that it will be different.

Clan differences have an effect on all kinds of outlooks and predispositions. Thus, another old piece of military humor, often attributed to Admiral Ike Kidd, president of the Naval War College in the 1980s, which begins:

> Logisticians are a sad and embittered race of men who are very much in demand in war, and who sink resentfully into obscurity in peace. They deal only in facts, but must work for men who traffic in theories. They emerge during war because war is very much a fact. They disappear in peace because peace is mostly theory. The people who traffic in theories, and who employ logisticians in war and ignore them in peace, are generals.
>
> Logisticians hate generals.

And so on. Whether certain personality types are attracted to particular clans (one has to think they are), it is noticeable that each of the clans has its own characteristic temperament. In some cases this is very pronounced, particularly where formal psychometric evaluations are employed for selection. Submariners, for example, because of their peculiar environment are usually quiet, self-contained, and highly intelligent (although not always happy). You will not hear them roaring about "the spirit of the bayonet," and no one would want them to.

Similarly, anyone dealing with nuclear weapons is likely not to have been selected for a love of risk or razzle dazzle improvisation. Parenthetically one may note that contrary to what one might think, the more dangerous the endeavor in the military the more it often inculcates exquisite management of risk. There are rather few cowboys in the United States military, and not many who get to the top.

No matter what the clan, the traits needed to function in it, whether they were there before or not, eventually become imprinted. The military is what sociologist Erving Goffman calls a total institution, with unlimited claims on an individual's time, loyalties and attention [5]. It is very hard to live in one of these subcultures and disregard its norms and behavioral patterns.

There are undoubtedly variations by personality type and over time, shaped most profoundly by technology. The reckless fighter pilot of World War II, for example, would have no place flying a modern fighter plane whose cost is in the high eight figures. But the kind of focus and snap decision-making that flying a fighter plane requires still does mandate a certain psychological profile, and in particular one that is capable of a great deal of compartmentation—and a great deal of ego. Those qualities, highly desirable in air-to-air combat even today, may be a lot less productive in, say, a marital relationship.

Understanding the Castes

And there are other profound differences among service personnel, most notably driven by the division of the military world into officers, non-commissioned officers, and enlisted personnel; in the last half century or so these have been supplemented by warrant officers, a kind of highly trained senior specialist. With qualifications and caveats, one can say that the castes can be very different indeed.

Again, the caricature. In the cartoon Beetle Bailey, or earlier, in Bill Mauldin's superb World War II drawings the castes are depicted in forms familiar to most

Americans—the hapless privates victimized by the Army, the sergeants bossing them around, and the officers who are, if junior, bewildered and only marginally competent, and if senior, utterly out of touch and clueless. These were exaggerations in the middle of last century and very far from the truth in today's world. But still, there are important differences, in terms of outlook and career aspirations.

Officers are expected, first and foremost, to lead. Because this has implications for character, all kinds of expectations are piled on by the institution. Infractions that would be lesser offenses for enlisted personnel, from bouncing checks, to driving under the influences, to adultery, can be career killers for them. For the most part, non-commissioned officers, the steady backbone of the American armed services, are the ones who manage and shape the organization. Although like officers they are on career paths pointing towards promotion and growth, their chief responsibilities involve the day to day coordination of the individuals they lead. And the enlisted are the ones who do the real labor, the often mechanical and manual work, of keeping military organizations going.

From a psychological point of view this matters as well. NCO's will probably have seen a lot; they are famously cynical about the larger institutions in which they dwell because they so often have to create the informal fixes and workarounds to get things done. An NCO, addressed as "sir" or "ma'am" by the uninitiated, will usually growl back, "Don't call me ma'am! I work for my pay!", an implication that NCOs, not officers—who are correctly addressed as sir or ma'am—do the real work of the service.

Officers may be more ambitious but are in any case always conscious of being on a stage and being observed. Enlisted, who are often only in the military for limited periods of enlistment are, unless they are already thinking of making it a career, hanging in for a period of adventure, escape, or maturing. These perspectives undoubtedly have some effect on how they cope with psychological stress. In some cases, the norms are profoundly at odds with the emotions one must feel.

On numerous visits to war zones in Iraq and Afghanistan, for example, I observed general officers who were invariably cheerful, upbeat and optimistic. In their breast pockets, however, they carried laminated pictures of every service member who had fallen under command. I often wondered how they managed to balance the professional requirement of high level leadership with the losses that, as humans, they felt. John Keegan, in a famous book, referred to "the mask of command" that military leaders must wear [6]. The higher up officers go, the more frozen in place that mask has to be - and the more difficult the moment when the facade cracks.

Community

One of the great advantages and attractions of military life can be community. Visit a military base, even in one of the less prosperous states and one sees middle class respectability that seems straight out of an imagined version of the 1950s. Modest (and sometimes not so modest) but comfortable homes, neatly mown lawns, bustling recreation and shopping centers, and an air of tranquility are throughout. When the United States shifted to an all-volunteer force in the 1970s it underwent a profound change in its physical aspects as well as culture. "Recruit the soldier, retain the family" is an often-heard motto, and the services are acutely aware that they are ever more likely to have a force that is married and that requires robust family support. This has been particularly true in wartime, when units are deployed overseas for extended periods of time.

At the same time, the advent of an increasingly married force, with spouses working off base or from home, means that some of the old self-sufficiency is gone. Military families are often more integrated into general American society than once they were: the downtown of Fayetteville, North Carolina, home to Fort Bragg and the 82nd Airborne Division now has the same kinds of upper end chain restaurants and stores you would expect in any prosperous suburb, and doing a similarly robust business—just filled with extremely fit young men and women with conservative haircuts. Service personnel are on Facebook and Instagram as much as their peers, although they often have their own sites, which are also portals into military culture. One of the most interesting and revealing is taskandpurpose.com. Also worth mentioning is duffelblog.com, a military version of The Onion—although illuminating, its sometimes profane content is not for the faint of heart.

Still, community is an essential part of military life. This has particular strengths in wartime: when a unit returns to home base the celebration is not just of individual parents, spouses, or children, but an entire community welcoming the troops home. Emotionally, it is more like the return of soldiers to their communities at the end of the Civil War than of demobilized soldiers at the end of World War II who more often came back as individuals. The ties of mutual support on the bases today, including in the event of service members being killed or wounded, are profound.

Military humor is a very good way of understanding military community; so too is attention to the argot of military life. Military running cadences, for example, offer no small insights into the wry, and sometimes morbid sense of humor that service members use to insulate themselves from some scary things ("C-130 rolling down the strip, Airborne Daddy on a one way trip," etc.) Within the tribes certain kinds of slang are pervasive. Someone in the Navy who has done a good job will be told "Bravo Zulu" by peers or superiors—in the Navy's old signal flag system the two letters, B and Z, signified well done. The flags may be gone, but the term remains. Or a desk jockey in the Pentagon may nonetheless be warned by an Air Force colleague to "check six," which means to look out for an ambush (in this case, presumably bureaucratic). The term originates from early and mid-twentieth century fighter combat, in which spatial orientation could be imagined as a clock dial. If 12 o'clock is straight ahead, 6 o'clock is straight behind one, and most fighter pilots were shot down by an unseen enemy from behind.

Conversation thick in slang and argot is another way of sustaining community. Leaving that behind can have a way of reminding service personnel that they have left behind a society in which the rules were clear, and the relationships established, for a world which is anything but.

The loss of the sense of community can be one of the most difficult things that service members can feel once they leave service. There is no longer a cocoon:

one's children or spouse will not have close friends who know exactly what they are going through, or what the service member is going through. As other branches of the government (e.g. the State Department) have learned, when individuals redeploy as individuals from a war zone after an extended deployment it can be very tough indeed.

One positive feature of contemporary military communities is the normalization of psychological care and wellness. When one battalion commander returned from Iraq in 2006, where his paratroopers took 135 killed and wounded out of roughly a thousand deployed, he told the soldiers on parade that he was headed for a psychiatric evaluation the next day, and that they should too (personal account of COL Craig Osborne). The military pays acute attention to the problem of suicide by returning soldiers, and has done a great deal to remove the stigma associated with seeking mental health support. But when service members return to civilian life they are no longer in a setting in which PTSD is normalized; pity is not the same thing.

Of course, it was not always thus. What was once stigmatized as mere weakness, then diagnosed as "shell shock" (World War I) or "combat fatigue" (World War II) is now more generally understood as Post-Traumatic Stress Disorder (PTSD). To be sure, the acceptance of the need for psychological care can still run counter to the cult of toughness endemic among certain of the clans discussed above. But the military has come a long, long way. One of the more popular breathing apps in the Apple Store is Tactical Breather, devised by the Defense Health Agency for service personnel. One purpose is simply to help manage anxiety and maintain calm—but it is also to enable service personnel to engage more effectively in combat (particularly true for snipers). As World War II psychiatrists in the US Army noted uncomfortably, mental health in the military is both a good in itself and a means to keeping the force in the best fighting condition possible.

"Most Remarkable Like You"

That is Tommy's final phrase in Kipling's poem. He wants to remind the reader that he is, after all, a human being, with strengths and weaknesses, merely one who is called upon to do unusual things. For many military personnel their service will be the most important experience in their lives. Even for those of us with minimal experience in uniform there are pieces that stick. As the dean of a major division of Johns Hopkins University I often thought about the leadership basics inculcated in an ROTC class "Your priorities are your mission, your people, yourself, in that order." "The person in charge eats last." "Lead by example." "Your subordinates are watching everything you say and do." For those with much more extensive military experience the effects can go much deeper.

But having said that, it is important to remember that the military attracts an extraordinary range of human beings who enter military service for a range of reasons. As Abraham Lincoln, in one of his displays of unillusioned wisdom, put it, soldiers enlist for a number of reasons. "Among these motives would be patriotism, political bias, ambition, personal courage, love of adventure, want of employment, and convenience, or the opposites of some of these [7]."

Most veterans come out of their military service glad that they did it and go on to be more successful than most in their later careers. They will often speak of the enduring lessons of self-discipline, perseverance, resilience, and selflessness that they have carried away from their time service. As Shakespeare's Henry V promises his troops before the battle of Agincourt, "they will remember, and with advantages" what they did and what it meant to them. A great many others will set nostalgia aside and simply get on with their lives.

Many veterans will take back to civilian life confidence about their ability to surmount difficulty. One of the strengths of the American military, after all, is the robustness of training programs designed to instill confidence. Another is an educational and development system predicated on the notion that one can always do better and take on greater things. In this it is different from many other militaries which have much less of the "up or out" culture and organizational incentives towards continual self-improvement. At any given time 10–15% of the armed forces are in some form of individual training or educational program. The more they have adopted military culture, in other words, the more service personnel will be attuned to the possibility of self-development and further achievement.

But there will also be a large number who leave service having been damaged in body or spirit, having lost the anchors and integrating structures that gave their lives meaning, and that insulated them from many forms of distress. For them, and particularly those who have experienced shocking violence or loss, the difficulties can be exacerbated by a conviction that "civilians just don't get it," or, perhaps more perniciously, that civilians are unworthy of the sacrifices they have made, or that they live by codes of conduct less honorable than theirs.

In short, there are very few generalizations that will help mental health professionals understand all veterans equally. Indeed, the beginning of wisdom in this regard is to acknowledge and appreciate the varieties of military experience. And as for clinical care, the fundamental recommendation from a student of the armed forces must be the most basic of all: to be prepared to learn endlessly, and to listen with the utmost care.

References

1. Council on Foreign Relations. Demographics of the U.S. Military. 2020. https://www.cfr.org/backgrounder/demographics-us-military. Accessed 12 Jul 2021.
2. Moskos CC, Butler JS. All that we can be: black leadership and racial integration the army way. New York, NY: Basic Books; 1996. p. 2, 135.
3. Builder CH. The masks of war: American Military styles in strategy and analysis. Baltimore, MD: Johns Hopkins University Press; 1989.
4. Wabo C. The 14 funniest military jokes ever – updated in 2021. 2021. https://www.marineapproved.com/funniest-military-jokes/. Accessed 12 Jul 2021.
5. Goffman E. Asylums: essays on the social situation of mental patients and other inmates. London: Taylor and Francis; 2017.

6. Keegan J. The mask of command. New York, NY: Viking; 1987.
7. Lincoln A. Opinion on the draft (1863). In: Speeches and writings 1859–1865. New York, NY: Library of America; 1989. p. 504.

Eliot A. Cohen is Robert E. Osgood Professor of Strategic Studies at Johns Hopkins School of Advanced International Studies and its former Dean, and the Arleigh Burke Chair in Strategy at the Center for Strategic and International Studies. He has spent nearly four decades studying the US military and working with it in government and counts among former students scores of serving and retired military officers of all ranks. His father served as a military psychiatrist during World War II, and he is the father of a US Army Iraq veteran and a US Navy officer.

3 Enhancing Resilience in Service Members and Military Veterans

Amy B. Adler and Ian A. Gutierrez

The military depends on its service members to be physically and psychologically resilient. Resilience is essential because military service demands long hours, extended time away from family and friends, frequent relocation, endurance in the face of harsh environmental conditions, performance under stress, and courage in life-threatening situations. Soldiers, sailors, airmen, and Marines who are resilient are able to adeptly respond to these challenges, quickly recover from them, and even grow from their experiences.

Most Service Members Are Resilient

While mental health problems represent one of the top reasons for medical evacuations from a deployed setting [1], the majority of service members do not report mental health problems while serving in the military or as veterans following retirement from service. Rates of PTSD are estimated at 5.5% in the overall U.S. military population and 13.2% in operational infantry units, meaning more than four in five service members (82.8–94.5%) do not meet clinical criteria for PTSD [2]. Besides PTSD, 22.3% of service members report clinical levels of depression symptoms [3], 13% report clinical levels of anxiety symptoms [3], and 15.2% report alcohol-related problems [4]. While these rates are substantial, they also suggest that approximately three in four service members have no clinically significant concerns related to mental health problems or alcohol use.

Resilience, however, is more than the absence of mental health problems. There are numerous definitions of resilience, but these definitions typically describe resilience as comprising the inherent individual attributes that enable successful adaptation, functioning, or positive change following adverse events [5, 6]. One relatively

A. B. Adler (✉) · I. A. Gutierrez
Walter Reed Army Institute of Research, Silver Spring, MD, USA
e-mail: Amy.b.adler.civ@health.mil; Ian.a.gutierrez2.civ@health.mil

C. H. Warner, C. A. Castro (eds.), *Veteran and Military Mental Health*,
https://doi.org/10.1007/978-3-031-18009-5_3

simple and straightforward definition of resilience is "the demonstration of positive adaptation in the face of adversity" ([7], p. 6). The Department of Defense similarly defines resilience as "… the ability to withstand, recover, and/or grow in the face of stressors and changing demands" [8].

The fact that militaries like the U.S. Department of Defense have definitions of resilience demonstrates that resilience is central to the concept of military culture, where service members are expected to put "mission first" and move effectively through cycles of preparation for deployment, deployment, reintegration, and recovery before preparing to deploy again. Across the different phases of this cycle, service members are expected to adapt to rapidly changing and uncertain circumstances, to subordinate themselves within a hierarchy, and to navigate volatile, uncertain, complex, and ambiguous (i.e., VUCA; [9]) environments. Although individuals may falter in the face of adversity or need help to recover, the majority of service members consider themselves to be resilient.

In one anonymous survey, for example, soldiers preparing to deploy were asked to rate their own resilience using the Self-Rated Resilience Scale ([10]; Table 3.1). While junior-ranking soldiers reported less resilience than non-commissioned officers or officers, the majority agreed that they bounced back and recovered from adversity. Table 3.1 also illustrates that service members do not uniformly describe themselves as resilient in all ways, consistent with findings from Warner et al. [11] that service members are frank in their responses on anonymous surveys.

This frank self-appraisal is predictive of mental health. In a longitudinal study, soldier ratings of their own resilience prior to deployment was positively associated with their mental health nearly a year after they had returned from a combat deployment [12]. Moreover, soldiers who perceived themselves as highly resilient had better mental health outcomes not only because of their individual capabilities, but also because they actively reached out to others around them when they returned home. These results demonstrate that self-rated resilience is a useful marker of a

Table 3.1 Self-rated resilience by rank category

	% Agree or strongly agree		
Resilience item	Enlisted	Non-commissioned officers	Officers
"I tend to bounce back quickly after hard times"	62.1	75.8	79.6
"I have a hard time making it through stressful events"*	12.7	11.8	9.4
"It does not take me long to recover from a stressful event"	54.3	65.7	70.7
"It is hard for me to snap back when something bad happens"*	8.9	8.4	5.0
"I usually come through difficult times with little trouble"	49.4	58.1	71.1
"I tend to take a long time to get over setbacks in my life"*	10.1	9.4	6.1

Note: Items are from the Self-rated Resilience Scale [10]. Items with * are normally reverse scored in the overall scale. Data are from a study of 2290 soldiers in an anonymous survey conducted in garrison in 2015 service member's ability to withstand the rigors of deployment. Clinicians can leverage this finding by asking service members to rate their own resilience and their use of social connection.

We note, however, that this high level of resilience among service members is potentially influenced by multiple personal and institutional factors. On the one hand, the military might attract service members who are resilient, who are driven to succeed under demanding circumstances, and whose personal goals and values resonate with military culture [13]. On the other hand, the military selection system might also screen for resilient individuals. Certainly, recruits must meet basic standards of mental health prior to enlistment or commissioning, and some mental health conditions preclude individuals from military service. For those who do make the cut, however, military experience and training might help them become more resilient than they were when they joined the service by further developing their existing skills, capabilities, and confidence. Although research has yet to determine which of these factors contributes most strongly to service member resilience, it is likely that service member resilience reflects some combination of these forces.

Selected Components of Resilience

Even though most service members are resilient, they still sometimes falter and need additional support. Risk associated with behavioral health symptoms range from background characteristics, such as adverse childhood experiences [14, 15], to exposure to extreme military stressors, such as combat and atrocities [16, 17]. In this chapter, we limit our focus to four biopsychosocial factors with significant implications for providing clinical care and consultation to service members: sleep, emotion regulation, social cohesion, and leadership. We selected these four because they are well established in the research literature as predictive of quality of life and mental health in the military occupational context.

Sleep

Sleep is vital for service members' physical and psychological resilience [18], and sleep problems can signal an increased risk for subsequent mental health problems [19, 20]. Sleep disorders among service members are discussed in greater detail by Capaldi (this volume); here, we emphasize sleep as a critical foundation for understanding service member resilience. Insufficient sleep is associated with missed work [21], difficulty with cognitive tasks [22, 23], and impaired military performance [24].

Despite the importance of sleep for health, soldiers routinely report sleeping fewer than 7 h/day, the minimal recommended amount of sleep [25]. In one sample of more than 2300 soldiers, 77.2% reported sleeping 6 h or fewer per 24-h period [26]. The epidemic of insufficient sleep is embedded in a larger organizational context where sleep is regarded as something that can take a back seat to mission requirements. Efforts are underway to prioritize sleep within the military [27]. At present, however, service members may underestimate the importance of sleep for building resilience to stress and sustaining performance.

Interestingly, just being aware of the benefits of sleep can improve service members' sleep hygiene [28]. For example, one study showed that service members do not have to have a diagnosable sleep problem to benefit from greater awareness about the importance of sleep [28]. Indeed, the more soldiers know about sleep and the more they make sleep a priority, the better their sleep health [26]. These studies suggest that clinicians should not only limit their evaluation of sleep health to screening for possible sleep disorders among service members (Capaldi, this volume), but should also provide consultation to service members regarding how they can improve sleep for improved physical and cognitive performance.

Emotion Regulation

Lack of sleep is also associated with difficulties in emotion regulation—the ability to appropriately control, manage, or express an emotional response [29]. Service members who can regulate their emotions effectively are able to function well occupationally, socially, and interpersonally. Emotion regulation does not only refer to the ability to control one's temper—it also refers to the ability to express a range of emotions from guilt, sadness, and anxiety, to joy, love, and gratitude.

Within the military culture, emotions are typically held in check, and a certain amount of stoicism is seen as useful to endure the physical and psychological demands that are part of military service [30] (see Box 3.1 for a soldier's description of managing emotions after coming back from a combat deployment). Accepting emotions, rather than acting on them or engaging in problem-solving, is associated with better adjustment [31], even within the context of basic combat training, where new soldiers learn the fundamentals of Army culture. Soldiers refer to this skill of acceptance by using the phrase "embrace the suck." The correlation of acceptance with better adjustment likely reflects the fact that soldiers are confronted with stressors that are largely out of their own control, and acceptance is therefore a more useful tool—if not the only tool—to facilitate adjustment.

Box 3.1 Emotions After Combat

The [transition] from being in a combat zone to home was good and bad. Some of the good reasons were getting out of the fucking desert and heat. Being able to see my family, wear civilian clothes, be with my girl and have actual off time without being on "Stand By." Being able to let loose a little and have some fun without worrying about being in danger. The bad reasons are always feeling like I'm forgetting something. Watching my cousins over there go insane. Feeling like someone is always behind me and not letting my guard down. Talking about my experience with others and not controlling my emotions about it. I've never gone through a transition like this before and I'm not a fan of it. Feeling like something's wrong when it's not, always in a hurry to do things. People telling me I need to relax more. I don't feel like I did anything in Iraq. Just drive around and wait to get blown up. (Soldier 4 months after returning from Iraq)

Restricting emotional expression can be useful in the occupational context, but it can harm service members' ability to create meaningful connections with others outside of work. The ability to express a range of emotions at the right time and place can be useful for building relationships at work, in social settings, and at home [32]. While military culture often encourages the restriction of emotional expression, there are exceptions. Most notably, military culture normalizes and permits the expression of anger. Research shows that service members may perceive anger as helpful in performing their duties (reported as helpful by 48.3% of soldiers in one study; [33]), but this perception is associated with an increased risk of mental health symptoms. Although anger is often viewed as useful or acceptable, evidence suggests that it is actually associated with poorer adjustment [34].

Clinically, service members may need to be coached to address anger in different ways. First, service members should be encouraged to regard anger as just one of many emotions—and one that may not be in their best interest to harbor, particularly at the exclusion of other emotions. Second, they should be encouraged to cultivate awareness of positive emotions, such as love, joy, and gratitude. Simple approaches like a gratitude diary have been associated with an increase in wellbeing and a decrease in anxiety (e.g., [35]). Finally, encouraging flexibility in coping responses can help encourage emotion regulation. Techniques such as mindfulness can help boost a service member's resilience and sustain their cognitive performance (e.g., [36]), and clinical treatments, including mobile applications, have been developed to target anger in service members and veterans [37–39].

Social Cohesion

Numerous studies have documented the role of social connection in establishing a healthy life. Indeed, a lack of social connection is not only associated with poor mental health [40], but a 26% greater likelihood of early death [41]. Social connection lies at the heart of military culture, and serving alongside, protecting, and supporting one's fellow service member is a revered characteristic of military service. The solidarity among soldiers is paramount to the Army profession, as manifested in the Soldier's Creed, which states, "I am a Warrior and a member of a team" and "I will never leave a fallen comrade" ([42], p. B-3). A soldier's connection to fellow battle buddies, or an airman's connection to fellow wingmen, however, extends far beyond the battlefield: The friendships developed in military service can last a lifetime and serve as an important source of support in times of need ([43, 44] [see Box 3.2]).

Box 3.2 Social Cohesion and Loss

I got a tattoo ... dedicated to seven men lost ... so that I will always have my brothers with me. My wife actually helped me in writing out the poem for the tattoo. That helped a lot, made me feel very good inside. I am ready for another deployment and I think that's why my transition has gone so well because I have someone that cares for me and has my back. (Soldier 4 months after returning from Iraq (reported in [45]))

Social connection is the psychological adhesive that binds service members together, transforming them from individuals into a cohesive military unit that works in seamless harmony to advance a shared mission. Unit cohesion has been found to moderate military stressors, including deployment, and individuals who are excluded from this cohesion are at increased risk for mental health problems and suicidal ideation [46]. Resilient service members, then, are those who are able to sustain relationships within and outside of the military culture.

Leadership

The importance of leaders in military culture cannot be overstated. Leaders serve a critical role in establishing shared expectations, pulling groups together, and ensuring the well-being of unit members.

However, just as military leaders can set the stage for their groups to sustain their resilience under pressure, they can also undermine it. Service members are willing to pursue a mission at great personal cost and, in exchange, they expect that the organization will take reasonable steps to ensure their well-being, care for their families, and provide them with the necessary training, equipment, and leadership [47]. When leaders fail to uphold their end of this psychological contract, the sense of betrayal can be profound. Leaders who humiliate others, have others engage in unnecessary risk, or engage in unethical behavior undermine the resilience of their teams.

Service members are likely to serve under a diverse array of leaders. Some of these leaders will likely fall short of expectations, while others will surpass them. Importantly, positive perceptions of leaders are associated with better mental health outcomes, cohesion, and perceived organizational support [48]. Clinically, that means that even as individuals may feel disappointed or even betrayed by their leaders, they may have also experienced positive leadership as well. Good leaders can serve as a great resource—and for those service members who have left military service, the lack of a leader in their life may feel like quite a void. Several studies have found that specific and clearly identifiable leader behaviors are associated with better individual adjustment. For example, platoons leaders—typically junior officers—who ask about the sleep habits of their unit members and encourage unit members to get plenty of sleep have unit members who report getting more sleep [49]. Similarly, leaders who remind unit members about the importance of the mission and encourage them to take time to physically and psychologically reset have unit members who report less emotional exhaustion, a sign of burnout [50]. Thus, clinicians who can work with leaders to encourage targeted behaviors may be able to enhance the resilience of the unit as a whole. Clinicians are encouraged to consider the role of leaders and their potential influence on service members who are seeking clinical care.

Resilience Training

Resilience building is valued within the military and taught both implicitly and explicitly. New recruits receive training designed to test their resilience and build their sense of confidence when they first enter the military, and they continue to receive informal and formal resilience training through their service. Basic training challenges new recruits to manage a great deal of new information and succeed at basic tests of military skills, including marksmanship, navigation, and combat casualty care. Once assigned to a unit, service members routinely train with their teams in increasingly realistic battlefield scenarios. In passing through various career milestones, service members become more confident and resilient at home station and on deployment.

Formal resilience training aims to ensure that all service members have the necessary mental skills for life in the military. Not all service members arrive at their first duty station with the same foundation for navigating life challenges: Notably, service members have a higher rate of adverse childhood experiences than non-military personnel [14]. As such, providing new personnel with essential resilience skills may enable them to manage the demands of military service more successfully. This proactive approach may also be a useful way for the military to reduce attrition, and thus help offset the shortage of eligible recruits [51].

In the Army, resilience training is part of a mandatory curriculum that instructs soldiers on the use of specific cognitive and behavioral skills. Launched in 2008, the Army's Comprehensive Soldier Fitness program (CSF; [52]) comprised several resilience initiatives, including a mandatory self-assessment using the Global Assessment Tool [53] and unit-based resilience training (i.e., Master Resilience Training [MRT]; [54]). MRT provides soldiers with social, cognitive, and behavioral skills for problem solving and effective communication, and incorporates performance psychology skills such as goal setting, self-talk, and energy management [55]. CSF training was also developed for the deployment cycle, particularly post deployment resilience training, and randomized trials of the foundational material have demonstrated the efficacy of this approach [56, 57].

Skills taught in the Army's resilience training programs have corollaries with approaches used in clinical treatment. For example, MRT teaches soldiers to practice anxiety reduction techniques, such as deliberate breathing, and engage in cognitive restructuring to avoid thinking traps. Other skills adapted from psychological research include practicing gratitude (i.e., "Hunt-the-Good-Stuff"; [54]) and responding positively to good news (i.e., Active Constructive Responding; [58]). As the Army updates its resilience training program, certain themes are emerging. First, the goal is to have fundamental skills integrated into formal training environments and taught by expert trainers. Second, the unit-level component of resilience training is shifting to a coaching model, with the emphasis on preparing NCOs to encourage use of resilience skills at certain times and places, rather than provide classroom-based instruction on the skills themselves. Finally, additional validated training is being examined to provide units with options for including additional resilience skills that are an appropriate fit based on a unit's particular needs.

The common language provided by these resilience skills can be leveraged in a clinical context with service members who have been exposed to formal MRT training or to whom these concepts are otherwise familiar. Table 3.2 provides examples of the kinds of resilience skills taught in the Army's program and the foundation of these skills in the literature.

The Navy and Air Force have equivalent resilience-building initiatives (for an early review, see Rand's 2011 Report by Meredith et al. [6]). Currently, the Navy has the 21st Century Sailor, which incorporates a suite of programs that addresses topics ranging from life-work balance to nutrition. While we are not aware of publications detailing the effectiveness of these efforts, Navy-specific studies have identified factors that influence resilience. For example, Burt and Barr [59] identified the influence of leadership in the resilience of Navy recruits, and the role of performance enhancement strategies such as goal setting, emotional control, and attention control in the resilience of Navy Explosive Ordnance Operators [60]. In a Rand technical report from 2010, the Air Force also examined resilience factors related to performance [61] and launched Airman Resilience Training. A program evaluation published by Rand in 2014 documented variability in training implementation and low perceived utility of the program [62]. Currently, the Air Force has materials available under the banner concept of "Air Force Resilience" (see https://www.resilience.af.mil/Prevention-Tools/ for a list of tools ranging from how to manage anxiety and legal problems to how to encourage Airmen and families to thrive) [63], and has developed Wingman Connect, training designed to improve social connectedness.

Although not the focus of the present chapter, we do note that other nations have resilience training programs as well. For example, the Canadian Forces has the

Table 3.2 Sample resilience skills and their clinical corollaries

Resilience skill[a]	Clinical corollary	Comment
Activating Event-Thoughts-Consequences (ATCs)	Cognitive therapy and Activating Events–Beliefs–Consequences (ABC) model	Teaches that thoughts impact emotions and actions; encourages changing automatic thought
Thinking Traps (e.g., them, them, them; me, me, me)	Cognitive distortions (e.g., all-or-none thinking) and challenging cognitive distortions	Identifies common errors in thinking; encourages looking for patterns in response and asking questions to broaden attention to alternative explanations
Icebergs	Deeply held beliefs and core values	Identifies underlying beliefs that can fuel a strong, even disproportionate reaction; provides insight
Hunt the Good Stuff	Gratitude diary	Encourages reflection on positive experiences, supports optimism
Active Constructive Responding	Capitalizing on positive events	Perpetuates the positive emotions experienced by others following a positive experience, builds connection
Deliberate breathing (also called "tactical breathing")	Deep breathing	Anxiety reduction

[a] Based on Reivich et al. [54]

Road to Mental Readiness program, although this training may have limited effect, as demonstrated in a randomized trial with recruits [64]. Similarly, the Australian Defence Force has BattleSMART [65], an integrated program that also begins with recruits as well as other training packages such as self-reflection [66]. Likewise, in the UK, the military has implemented resilience training in various forms [67, 68]. While resilience training is popular across militaries of different nations, the need for continued training development, efficacy testing, and implementation optimization remain priorities for future efforts [69, 70].

Transition and Reintegration

Transitions offer an opportunity for new opportunities, personal growth, and career development, but can also be associated with increased mental health risk (see Castro, this volume, for discussion of transition and mental health). Within the Army, about a third of soldiers who transition into new units report difficulty with transition [71] and this stress is experienced regardless of rank or marital status. Transitioning into the first unit of assignment has also been associated with increased risk of attempted suicide [72].

Transitioning out of the military may also be a challenge to resilience. As service members depart military service, they have to adapt to significant changes to their identities, social rules and roles, their sense of purpose, and their social network [73]. For instance, veterans of the conflicts in Iraq and Afghanistan report struggling to navigate the lack of structure in civilian life and feeling disconnected, unsupported, and directionless as they search for a new sense of normality in their lives [74]. The loss of team orientation and of their importance to others can undermine their ability to find meaning in civilian life. Moreover, the strengths that helped them succeed in the military can challenge their ability to adjust to civilian life if these strengths are not adapted successfully [32]. For example, a sense of duty is a core Army value and can be beneficial for employment and community participation when that sense of duty translates into being reliable, task-focused, and achievement oriented. This same strength, however, can impede adjustment and lead to psychological rigidity and impatience if not adapted carefully for the civilian context. Thus, focusing on transition itself may be valuable for clinicians to consider.

New initiatives within the Department of Defense emphasize the importance of navigating the military-to-veteran transition. Within the Army, one such initiative is the Soldier for Life program. As the program's title suggests, the military offers a place of belonging for soldiers that transcends their specific years of service. The Marines take a similar approach in recognizing that the connection can transcend the formal transition, using the phrase "Once a Marine, always a Marine." However, veterans differ with respect to their identification with the military following their service. When working with veterans, clinicians should discuss the influence that the military has on their understanding of resilience and the military's impact on personal identity.

Resilience in the Clinical Context

If resilience is integral to the military culture, what role does it have in the consulting room, with clinicians, and in therapy? In this section, we review components of resilience and beliefs about resilience that may help clinicians in connecting with, understanding, and creating a treatment plan for service members and veterans.

First, it is important to remember that a service member or veteran would not have been able to complete military milestones without a foundational level of resilience.

Second, it is important to consider the individual's place in terms of military career and deployment cycle. Where is the individual in terms of basic developmental milestones? Where is the individual in the deployment cycle? Depending on the answer, different resilience challenges are likely to be present. For example, performance anxiety may be an issue for those who are anticipating a stressful challenge like deployment, in which case performance psychology skills might be useful to supplement interventions (e.g., self-talk, goal setting, energy management). If the individual is having difficulty in the aftermath of an intense, potentially traumatic experience, other resilience skills may be useful as a supplement to traditional clinical interventions, such as those skills that build social connections. The clinician might also ask what roles, if any, unit members and leaders play in the service member's adjustment trajectory. If the individual is transitioning out of the military, then the challenges include a wider scope of redefining oneself, one's purpose, one's team and one's military family. To address these issues, clinicians may want to discuss these questions with individuals from both a practical and existential perspective, exploring what personal and organizational community supports are available to assist with transition to civilian life, and helping the service member discuss and identify goals for life after the military.

Clinical Pearls

- Bear in mind that most service members are resilient
- Remember resilience is deeply valued
- Consider timing within the military career cycle
- Address sleep problems
- Focus on social connection
- Build emotion regulation skills
- Leverage preference for self-management

Third, service members may prefer self-management (see the chapter on stigma by Ivany, this volume). Rather than being reluctant to see a clinical provider because of stigma or fear of negative career consequences, service members may be reluctant because of a preference for self-care. Surveys show that soldiers prefer to engage in self-management [75, 76]. This preference does necessarily constitute a rejection of treatment. Instead, the treatment can be recast as a form of coaching—a way to help the service member strengthen their own skills and improve their functioning. Adopting a coaching role may be a better match with the service member's preferences and values. Although this self-management preference could be viewed as defensive, being responsible for one's self can also be considered a strength.

Fourth, tackle sleep head on. Be sure that the service member understands the value of their own sleep and the risks to emotion regulation, cognitive functioning, and physical health if sleep is limited. Sleep provides a critical basis for emotion regulation; addressing sleep first will help to promote greater resilience.

Fifth, in a similar vein, address social connection directly. Prioritize the need to cultivate a social network—one that provides meaningful social contact. And for those transitioning out of the military, a social network that can withstand the transition to civilian life.

Sixth, consider introducing mindfulness as a way to build resilience and enhance performance, given the link between self-reported mindfulness and adjustment in military personnel [77] and veterans [78]. Service members and perhaps veterans as well may be open to skills that enhance their performance and readiness. This kind of skill is also consistent with a preference for self-management. Without practice, however, this skill will not likely be valuable, and thus it is important to integrate mindfulness practice into daily routines.

Finally, it is important to take mindset into account. Individuals with what Dweck [79] calls a fixed mindset view their skills and abilities as fixed. In contrast, individuals with a growth mindset view their skills as something they can improve and change. Unsurprisingly, these two different mindsets can influence the degree to which individuals respond well under stress.

Box 3.3 relates the story of two different non-commissioned officers, with two different responses to a setback, integrating the themes highlighted throughout this chapter. When confronted with the same challenge, Staff Sergeant Ryan spirals down while Staff Sergeant Steele gains confidence. Ryan responds with sleep problems and anger, has difficulty regulating his emotions, and is bitter about what he sees as poor leadership. Instead of reaching out, he starts to isolate himself. Ryan has a fixed mindset, believing he (and likely his squad) have a certain set of skills that cannot change. This kind of mindset can prevent his growth and potentially sabotages his future success.

Box 3.3 Soldiers with Fixed and Growth Mindsets

Staff Sergeant Ryan and Staff Sergeant Steele are both squad leaders. Both recently received negative feedback from their Company's First Sergeant in front of the entire formation about their squad's readiness. Staff Sergeant Ryan starts ruminating about what he perceives as his failure, losing sleep, yelling at his squad out of frustration, and shutting himself off from his peers. He knows he's tried his best to motivate his squad but it hasn't worked and now the entire company knows. He feels embarrassed by the First Sergeant, and let down. He didn't think being a squad leader was going to be this difficult.

Staff Sergeant Steele feels the heat too but he takes some deliberate breaths and thinks about what pieces of the problem he can control and what he can't control, and remembers that this issue isn't all-or-nothing. He's had other successes before, he just has to work harder to get there this time. He reaches out to another squad leader for advice and establishes specific goals for his squad. He tells them this is an opportunity to prove themselves and when they do better, he reinforces their pride by listening to their accomplishments.

In contrast, Steele has a growth mindset. He believes that people can cultivate their talents and skills. This perspective encourages him to change his leadership approach and to believe in the ability of his squad to change as well. He uses specific resilience techniques: deliberate breathing to calm down, and thinking about what he can control. He also builds social connection both by reaching out to others and by using active constructive responding with his squad to help them savor their small successes, reinforcing their trust in him and building their resilience.

In this way, resilience can be understood as not simply a variable that impacts individual service member health and performance. It's a capacity that impacts others, from family members to fellow unit members, creating a blueprint for the next generation.

Conclusion

Clinical approaches to providing care for military service members often focus on pathology and dysfunction. However, this perspective overlooks the fact that service members display a remarkable degree to resilience, hardiness, and fortitude in carrying out their duties, and the vast majority of service members do not meet diagnostic criteria for common psychiatric disorders. As the military continues to emphasize resilience-based training, more service members are exposed to ideas and concepts that have useful clinical corollaries that clinicians can capitalize on in treatment.

It may also be useful for clinicians to be mindful of the impact that military culture has on service members, particularly in regards to their sleep health, social relationships, and emotion management. Additionally, treatment providers working with active-duty populations should explore the positive (and negative) effect that military leadership can have on individuals seeking clinical care. Clinicians can also consider using the military culture's emphasis on resilience as a subject of discussion in assessing an individual's wellbeing. Finally, clinicians can consider adopting a coaching perspective in providing treatment in order to match service members' preference for self-management.

Disclaimer

Material has been reviewed by the Walter Reed Army Institute of Research. There is no objection to its presentation and/or publication. The data presented derive from protocols approved by the Walter Reed Army Institute of Research Institutional

Review Board. The opinions or assertions contained herein are the private views of the presenter and are not to be construed as official or as reflecting the position of the Department of the Army or the Department of Defense. The investigators have adhered to the policies for protection of human subjects as prescribed in AR 70–25

References

1. Cohen SP, Brown C, Kurihara C, et al. Diagnoses and factors associated with medical evacuation and return to duty for service members participating in Operation Iraqi Freedom or Operation Enduring Freedom: a prospective cohort study. Lancet. 2010;375(9711):301–9.
2. Kok BC, Herrell RK, Thomas JL, Hoge CW. Posttraumatic stress disorder associated with combat service in Iraq or Afghanistan: reconciling prevalence differences between studies. J Nerv Ment Dis. 2012;200(5):444–50.
3. Lane ME, Hourani LL, Bray RM, Williams J. Prevalence of perceived stress and mental health indicators among reserve-component and active-duty military personnel. Am J Public Health. 2012;102(6):1213–20.
4. Jacobson IG, Ryan MA, Hooper TI, et al. Alcohol use and alcohol-related problems before and after military combat deployment. JAMA. 2008;300(6):663–75.
5. Britt TW, Shen W, Sinclair RR, et al. How much do we really know about employee resilience? Ind Organ Psychol. 2016;9:378–404.
6. Meredith LS, Sherbourne CD, Gaillot SJ, et al. Promoting psychological resilience in the US military. Santa Monica, CA: RAND Corporation; 2011. https://www.rand.org/pubs/monographs/MG996.html. Accessed 13 Jul 2021.
7. Britt TW, Sinclair RR, McFadden AC. Introduction: the meaning and importance of military resilience. In: Sinclair RR, Britt TW, editors. Building psychological resilience in military personnel: theory and practice. Washington, DC: American Psychological Association; 2013. p. 3–17.
8. Chairman of the Joint Chiefs of Staff Instruction. Chairman's total force fitness framework [CJCSI 3405.01]. 2013. https://www.jcs.mil/Portals/36/Documents/Library/Instructions/3405_01.pdf?ver=2016-02-05-175032-517. Accessed 10 Nov 2019.
9. Nindl BC, Billing DC, Drain JR, et al. Perspectives on resilience for military readiness and preparedness: report of an international military physiology roundtable. J Sci Med Sport. 2018;21:1116–24.
10. Smith BW, Dalen J, Wiggins K, et al. The brief resilience scale: assessing the ability to bounce back. Int J Behav Med. 2008;15:194–200.
11. Warner CH, Appenzeller GN, Grieger T, et al. Importance of anonymity to encourage honest reporting in mental health screening after combat deployment. Arch Gen Psychiatry. 2011;68(10):1065–71.
12. Britt TW, Adler AB, Fynes J. Perceived resilience and social connection as predictors of adjustment following occupational adversity. J Occup Health Psychol. 2021;26(4):339–49. https://doi.org/10.1037/ocp0000286.
13. Eighmey J. Why do youth enlist? Identification of underlying themes. Armed Forces Soc. 2006;32(2):307–28.
14. Blosnich JR, Dichter ME, Cerulli C, et al. Disparities in adverse childhood experiences among individuals with a history of military service. JAMA Psychiatry. 2014;71(9):1041–8.
15. Katon JG, Lehavot K, Simpson TL, et al. Adverse childhood experiences, military service, and adult health. Am J Prev Med. 2015;49(4):573–82.
16. Killgore WDS, Cotting DI, Thomas JL, et al. Post-combat invincibility: violent combat experiences are associated with increased risk-taking propensity following deployment. J Psychiatr Res. 2008;42(13):1112–21.

17. Wilk JE, Bliese PD, Kim PY, et al. Relationship of combat experiences to alcohol misuse among U.S. soldiers returning from the Iraq war. Drug Alcohol Depend. 2010;108:115–21.
18. Hirshkowitz M, Whiton K, Albert SM, et al. National Sleep Foundation's updated sleep duration recommendations. Sleep Health. 2015;1(4):233–43.
19. Adrian AL, Skeiky L, Burke TM, et al. Sleep problems and functioning during initial training for a high-risk occupation. Sleep Health. 2019;5:651.
20. Wright KM, Britt TW, Bliese PD, et al. Insomnia as predictor versus outcome of PTSD and depression among Iraq Combat Veterans. J Clin Psychol. 2011;67:1240–58.
21. Hui SKA, Grandner MA. Trouble sleeping associated with lower work performance and greater healthcare costs: longitudinal data from Kansas state employee wellness program. J Occup Environ Med. 2015;57(10):1031–8.
22. Belenky G, Wesensten NJ, Thorne DR, et al. Patterns of performance degradation and restoration during sleep restriction and subsequent recovery: a sleep dose-response study. J Sleep Res. 2003;12(1):1–12.
23. LoPresti ML, Anderson JA, Saboe KN, et al. The impact of insufficient sleep on combat mission performance. Mil Behav Health. 2016;4:356–63.
24. Smith CD, Cooper AD, Merullo DJ, et al. Sleep restriction and cognitive load affect performance on a simulated marksmanship task. J Sleep Res. 2019;28(3):e12637.
25. Watson NF, Badr MS, Belenky G, et al. Recommended amount of sleep for a healthy adult: a joint consensus statement of the American Academy of Sleep Medicine and Sleep Research Society. Sleep. 2015;38(6):843–4.
26. McDonald J, Ganulin M, LoPresti M, Adler AB. Sleep knowledge, goals, and habits in soldiers. Sleep Health. 2019;5:426.
27. Performance Triad (P3). https://p3.amedd.army.mil/. Accessed 13 Jul 2021.
28. Adler AB, Gunia BC, Bliese PD, et al. Using actigraphy feedback to improve sleep in soldiers: an exploratory trial. Sleep Health. 2017;3(2):126–31.
29. Palmer CA, Alfano CA. Sleep and emotion regulation: an organizing, integrative review. Sleep Med Rev. 2017;31:6–16.
30. Hall LK. The importance of understanding military culture. Soc Work Health Care. 2011;50:4–18.
31. Britt TW, Crane M, Hodson SE, Adler AB. Effective and ineffective coping strategies in a low-autonomy work environment. J Occup Health Psychol. 2016;21(2):154.
32. Adler AB, Sowden WJ. Resilience in the military: the double-edged sword of military culture. In: Roberts LW, Warner CH, editors. Military and veteran mental health. New York, NY: Springer; 2018. p. 43–54.
33. Adler AB, Brossart D, Toblin RL. Can anger be helpful? Soldier perceptions of the utility of anger. J Nerv Ment Dis. 2017;205:692–8.
34. Adler AB, LeardMann CA, Villalobos J, Jacobson IG, Forbes D, Millennium Cohort Study Team. Association of problematic anger with long-term adjustment following the military-to-civilian Transition. JAMA Netw Open. 2022;5(7):e2223236. https://doi.org/10.1001/jamanetworkopen.2022.23236.
35. Southwell S, Gould E. A randomised wait list-controlled pre–post–follow-up trial of a gratitude diary with a distressed sample. J Posit Psychol. 2017;12(6):579–93.
36. Jha AP, Morrison AB, Parker SC, Stanley EA. Practice is protective: mindfulness training promotes cognitive resilience in high-stress cohorts. Mindfulness. 2017;8(1):46–58.
37. Cash R, Varker T, McHugh T, et al. Effectiveness of an anger intervention for military members with PTSD: a clinical case series. Mil Med. 2018;183(9–10):e286–90.
38. Morland LA, Love AR, Mackintosh M, et al. Treating anger and aggression in military populations: research updates and clinical implications. Clin Psychol Sci Pract. 2012;19:305–22.
39. Morland LA, Niehaus J, Taft C, et al. Using a mobile application in the management of anger problems among veterans: a pilot study. Mil Med. 2016;9:990–5.
40. Cacioppo JT, Amaral DG, Blanchard JJ, et al. Social neuroscience: progress and implications for mental health. Perspect Psychol Sci. 2007;2(2):99–123.

41. Holt-Lunstad J, Smith TB, Baker M, et al. Loneliness and social isolation as risk factors for mortality: a meta-analytic review. Perspect Psychol Sci. 2015;10:227–37.
42. U.S. Army. The army profession [ADRP-1]. Washington, DC: Headquarters, Department of the Army; 2013. https://usacac.army.mil/sites/default/files/misc/doctrine/CDG/cdg_resources/manuals/adrp/adrp1.pdf. Accessed 2 Dec 2019.
43. Caddick N, Phoenix C, Smith B. Collective stories and well-being: using a dialogical narrative approach to understand peer relationships among combat veterans experiencing post-traumatic stress disorder. J Health Psychol. 2015;20:286–99.
44. Hunt N, Robbins I. World War II veterans, social support, and veterans' associations. Aging Ment Health. 2001;5:175–82.
45. Adler AB, Bliese PD, McGurk D, Salvi A, et al. Mitigating the impact of combat through expressive writing: a randomized controlled trial. In: Adler AB, Bliese PD, editors. Expressive writing after returning from combat: two new studies. 2009 Symposium conducted at the 117th American Psychological Association meeting, Toronto, Canada; 2009.
46. Cacioppo JT, Cacioppo S, Adler AB, et al. The cultural context of loneliness: risk factors in active duty soldiers. J Soc Clin Psychol. 2016;35:865–82.
47. Adler AB, Castro CA. An occupational mental health model for the military. Mil Behav Health. 2013;1(1):41–5. https://doi.org/10.1080/21635781.2012.721063.
48. Lopez AA, Adler AB, Cabrera OA, Thomas JL. Validation of the WRAIR Leadership Scale. Mil Behav Health. 2018;7:1–10.
49. Gunia BC, Sipos ML, LoPresti ML, Adler AB. Sleep leadership in high-risk occupations: an investigation of soldiers on peacekeeping and combat. Mil Psychol. 2015;27(4):197–211.
50. Adler AB, Adrian AL, Hemphill M, et al. Professional stress and burnout in U.S. military medical personnel deployed to Afghanistan. Mil Med. 2017;182:1669–76. https://doi.org/10.7205/milmed-d-16-00154.
51. Laich D. Manning the military: America's problem. Military Times. 2019. https://www.militarytimes.com/opinion/commentary/2019/07/23/manning-the-military-americas-problem/. Accessed 13 Jul 2021.
52. Casey GW Jr. Comprehensive soldier fitness: a vision for psychological resilience in the US Army. Am Psychol. 2011;66(1):1–3.
53. Lester PB, Harris PD, Herian MN, Sowden WJ. A force of change: Chris Peterson and the US Army's Global Assessment Tool. J Posit Psychol. 2015;10(1):7–16.
54. Reivich KJ, Seligman ME, McBride S. Master resilience training in the US Army. Am Psychol. 2011;66(1):25.
55. Adler AB, Bliese PD, Pickering MA, et al. Mental skills training with Basic Combat Training soldiers: a group randomized trial. J Appl Psychol. 2015;100:1752–64.
56. Adler AB, Bliese PD, McGurk D, Hoge CW, et al. Battlemind Debriefing and Battlemind Training as early interventions with soldiers returning from Iraq: randomization by platoon. J Consult Clin Psychol. 2009;77:928–40.
57. Castro CA, Adler AB, McGurk D, Bliese PD. Mental health training with soldiers four months after returning from Iraq: randomization by platoon. J Trauma Stress. 2012;25:376–83.
58. Gable SL, Reis HT. Good news! Capitalizing on positive events in an interpersonal context. In: Zanna MP, editor. Advances in experimental social psychology, vol. 42. New York, NY: Academic Press; 2010. p. 195–257.
59. Burt CS, Barr IE. An inquiry into the resilience of US Navy recruits. Naval Postgraduate School Monterey United States. Defense Technical Information Center Report AD1009097. 2015. https://apps.dtic.mil/dtic/tr/fulltext/u2/1009097.pdf. Accessed 21 Jul 2021.
60. Taylor MK, Rolo C, Stump J, et al. Psychological strategies during military training are linked to resilience in US Navy Explosive Ordnance Disposal Operators. J Spec Oper Med. 2019;19(1):61–5.
61. Meadows SO, Miller LL, Robson S. Airman and family resilience: lessons from the scientific literature. Santa Monica, CA: RAND Corporation; 2015. https://www.rand.org/pubs/research_reports/RR106.html. Accessed 13 Jul 2021.

62. Gonzalez GC, Singh R, Schell TL, Weinick RM. An evaluation of the implementation and perceived utility of the airman resilience training program. Santa Monica, CA: RAND Corporation; 2014. https://www.rand.org/pubs/research_reports/RR655.html. Accessed 13 Jul 2021.
63. Wyman PA, Pisani AR, Brown CH, et al. Effect of the Wingman-Connect upstream suicide prevention program for air force personnel in training: a cluster randomized clinical trial. JAMA Netw Open. 2020;3(10):e2022532. https://doi.org/10.1001/jamanetworkopen.2020.22532.
64. Fikretoglu D, Liu A, Nazarov A, Blackler K. A group randomized control trial to test the efficacy of the Road to Mental Readiness (R2MR) program among Canadian military recruits. BMC Psychiatry. 2019;19(1):326.
65. Forbes D, Metcalf O. Veteran and military mental health: the Australian experience. Int Psychiatry. 2014;11(4):83–5.
66. Crane MF, Boga D, Karin E, et al. Strengthening resilience in military officer cadets: a group-randomized controlled trial of coping and emotion regulatory self-reflection training. J Consult Clin Psychol. 2019;87(2):125–40.
67. Fitzwater JPJ, Arthur CA, Hardy L. "The tough get tougher": mental skills training with elite military recruits. Sport Exerc Perform Psychol. 2018;7(1):93–107.
68. Precious D, Lindsay A. Mental resilience training. J R Army Med Corps. 2019;165(2):106–8.
69. Forbes S, Fikretoglu D. Building resilience: the conceptual basis and research evidence for resilience training programs. Rev Gen Psychol. 2018;22(4):452–68.
70. Vanhove AJ, Herian MN, Perez AL, et al. Can resilience be developed at work? A meta-analytic review of resilience-building programme effectiveness. J Occup Organ Psychol. 2016;89(2):278–307.
71. Adrian AL, Adler AB, Thomas JL, Britt TW. Integrating new soldiers: the role of leaders and unit members. Mil Psychol. 2018;30(2):131–41.
72. Ursano RJ, Heeringa SG, Stein MB, et al. Prevalence and correlates of suicidal behavior among new soldiers in the US Army: results from the Army Study to Assess Risk and Resilience in Servicemembers (Army STARRS). Depress Anxiety. 2015;32(1):3–12.
73. Adler AB, Castro CA. Transitions: a theoretical model for occupational health and wellbeing. Occup Health Sci. 2019;3:105–23. https://doi.org/10.1007/s41542-019-00043-3.
74. Ahern J, Worthen M, Masters J, et al. The challenges of Afghanistan and Iraq veterans' transition from military to civilian life and approaches to reconnection. PLoS One. 2015;10:e0128599.
75. Adler AB, Britt TW, Riviere LA, et al. Longitudinal determinants of mental health treatment seeking by US soldiers. Br J Psychiatry. 2015;207(4):346–50.
76. Britt TW, Jennings KS, Cheung JH, et al. Determinants of mental health treatment seeking among soldiers who recognize their problem: implications for high-risk occupations. Work Stress. 2016;30:318–36.
77. Nassif TH, Start AR, Toblin RL, Adler AB. Self-reported mindfulness and soldier health following a combat deployment. Psychol Trauma Theory Res Pract Policy. 2019;11(4):466–74.
78. Barr N, Davis JP, Diguiseppi G, et al. Direct and indirect effects of mindfulness, PTSD, and depression on self-stigma of mental illness in OEF/OIF veterans. Psychol Trauma Theory Res Pract Policy. 2019;14:1026.
79. Dweck C. What having a "growth mindset" actually means. Harv Bus Rev. 2016;13:213–26.

Stigma and Barriers to Care for Mental Health Treatment for Military and Veteran Populations

4

Joseph F. Meyer, Melissa S. Wattenberg, Katherina A. Kosman, Maggi A. Budd, Martha J. Duffy, Amy Agrawal, Janet S. Richmond, Sigmund Hough, Bruce Meltzer, Abigail Z. Schein, Mark F. Poster, and John C. Bradley

Vignette

A 24 year-old Non-Commissioned Officer (NCO) returning from deployment to Afghanistan where he served as an Infantry team leader receives his health screening at his home station. He endorses significant combat exposure with one of his

J. F. Meyer · M. A. Budd · A. Agrawal · A. Z. Schein · M. F. Poster
Harvard Medical School, Boston, MA, USA

VA Boston Health Care System, Boston, MA, USA
e-mail: Margaret.budd@va.gov; amy.agrawal@va.gov; Abigail.schein@va.gov

M. S. Wattenberg · M. J. Duffy
VA Boston Health Care System, Boston, MA, USA

Boston University School of Medicine, Boston, MA, USA
e-mail: melissa.wattenberg@va.gov; martha.duffy@va.gov

K. A. Kosman · B. Meltzer
VA Boston Health Care System, Boston, MA, USA
e-mail: Katherine.kosman@va.gov

J. S. Richmond
VA Boston Health Care System, Boston, MA, USA

Tufts University School of Medicine, Boston, MA, USA

McLean Hospital, Belmont, MA, USA
e-mail: janet.richmond@va.gov

S. Hough · J. C. Bradley (✉)
Harvard Medical School, Boston, MA, USA

VA Boston Health Care System, Boston, MA, USA

Boston University School of Medicine, Boston, MA, USA
e-mail: Sigmund_hough@hms.harvard.edu; John.bradley7@va.gov

C. H. Warner, C. A. Castro (eds.), *Veteran and Military Mental Health*,
https://doi.org/10.1007/978-3-031-18009-5_4

soldiers killed in action. He endorses some symptoms of PTSD but denies significant impairment. He is offered a referral for further mental health evaluation, but declines citing an expectation that he can handle the symptoms on his own and his desire to continue to excel in his career. He is excited to spend time with his wife and infant child. After a brief honeymoon period with occasional binge drinking to "blow off steam" his wife complains that he is irritable, screaming in his sleep and encourages him to seek help. He tries to reassure her that he can resolve his problems on his own and that he doesn't think he needs mental health care. Silently, he worries that, as a young NCO, his soldiers, peers, and superiors will perceive him as weak if he seeks care and will not entrust him with advancement.

Introduction

The earliest use of the word stigma has been traced to ancient Greece, where it was defined as a marking, spot, or tattoo carved into the body using a sharp stick, or stig. These markings were sometimes, although not exclusively, used to identify ostracized "undesirables" [1], which may have included those with mental illness between the fifth century B.C.E. and second century C.E. [2]. Unsettling records of associations of stigma with mental illness occurred during the late fifteenth century within a theological historical context in which psychiatric distress was conflated with sinfulness and immorality, which was clearly reflected in the *Malleus Maleficarum* [3]. Individuals likely exhibiting symptoms of severe mental illness, such as schizophrenia spectrum and bipolar disorders, were viewed as demonically possessed (or under other Satanic or occult influences) and thus subject to brutal torture tactics and religiously sanctioned murder by Catholic Inquisitors to extract confessions of so-called witchcraft [4].

In Christianity, stigmata are bodily wounds or scars that correspond to the wounds on Christ's hands, feet, chest, and head inflicted by his crucifixion. Stigmata have a revered but controversial place in the Catholic religion, signifying a connection to Christ, but also an affliction that burden's the stigmatic. Some believe the stigmatic to be insane, psychogenic, or factitious. In any case, stigmatics are thought to over identify with Christ's suffering and bear their stigmata with piety and ecstasy. Nineteenth Century neurologist Désiré-Magloire Bourneville [5] wrote in *Science & Miracle: Louise Lateau, ou la Stigmatisée Belge* about saints who professed to bear stigmata. He hypothesized that stigmatics may have been suffering from epilepsy, hysteria, or dissociation.

It was not until the seventeenth and eighteenth centuries that state agencies took on the mantle of caring for the mentally ill, although the nature and quality of many state-sponsored services (e.g., confinement, incarceration, and mass institutionalization) were highly questionable by modern standards [6]. Fast forward to the twenty-first century, and stigmatization of psychiatric illness, as well as its discriminatory consequences, continues across the globe [7, 8].

Mental Illness has carried a stigma throughout the history of humanity. Mental illness has been poorly understood, and can be mystifying for family, friends, and the larger social group. Those who live with a psychiatric condition may find themselves engaging in actions that differentiate them from others, which can make them vulnerable to ostracization from the larger group. The pattern of shunning the most vulnerable likely reflects naturalistic social hierarchies that value predictability—either as an indication of one's capacity to contribute to the collective good, or as necessary to actual survival of the collective. Conversely, a culture may value a person with mental illness when their symptoms are believed to serve a greater purpose, such as offering visions or translating the word of the gods.

When a person's illness is seen as having little utility for the good of the collective, or worse, as posing a threat, the bearer of the illness may be alienated from the group. This alienation is a threat to the livelihood and survival of the person with illness, and by association, those in their family or social group.

Nowhere is the stigma of mental illness more impactful than in the military, where group cohesion is essential for mission accomplishment and survival in combat. The cohesion and camaraderie within military units strengthen their effectiveness in combat and ensure the greatest chance of survival. Threats to the effectiveness, reputation, or survival of the group must be eliminated at all costs.

When we understand how important unit cohesion is to service members, we can begin to understand the impulse to stigmatize, alienate, and eliminate threats to the group. We can also understand how a person who is becoming ill will seek to hide their symptoms from discovery so that they can retain membership in the unit.

In this chapter, we will offer some insights about stigma in both the societal as well as military context. We will examine stigma from the perspective of the individual as well as the larger group. We will also explore some of the social determinants of stigma and describe some of the structural determinants that exist within the military—determinants that are perpetuated after service within the Department of Veterans Affairs. And finally, we will offer some interventions that may reduce the effects of stigmatization, if not address stigma itself. We hope this chapter will provide a roadmap for policy changes and clinical practice that will be more encour aging of help seeking and primary prevention.

Stigma, Its Elements, and Its Impact

Goffman's [9] seminal text "Stigma: Notes on the Management of Spoiled Identity" defines social stigma in terms of *spoiled identity* pervading social connection and interpersonal viability across the spectrum of social functioning. Goffman suggests that a socially accepted identity facilitates the establishment of social ties and the capacity to operate within a mutually understood social context. From this perspective, stigma isolates individuals from the larger culture and community, denies them viable social roles, and deprives them of the norms of social interaction. Whereas a secure, non-stigmatized identity provides relatively safe passage through a variety of social contexts, stigma curtails social access and diminishes social safety. The stigmatized person is marginalized, disqualified, and disenfranchised as far as participation in the larger society. Stigmatized individuals' communications are likely to be ignored, disregarded, discredited, or distorted. Attempts to break through these barriers are likely to be met with derision, scorn, and scapegoating. The resulting attitude toward the self may involve feeling irrelevant, invisible, or shamed for they are considered "the other." Social options then become limited to embracing the stereotypic qualities of the spoiled identity; resorting to artifice to cover the stigmatized characteristic; assuming merely transactional relationships; withdrawing; submerging personal identity within a larger controlled group identity; and the creation of a personally chosen and developed community that is, to an extent, independent of the mainstream stigmatizing context [10]. Instances of this last and more empowering option—personally-chosen and developed communities (which overtly or implicitly counter stigma)—include: the National Alliance on Mental Illness (NAMI) as a resource for families and individuals affected by serious and persistent psychiatric conditions; disability support groups; and artistic communities that embrace creative outliers.

As the study of stigma has evolved, its conceptualization has become more nuanced, with acknowledgment of its variability in a pluralistic society, and the potential for overcoming its impact without denying its harmful consequences. Dovidio et al. [11] note that stigma harms both the stigmatized and the stigmatizers, through "dehumanization, threat, aversion, and sometimes the depersonalization of others into stereotypic caricatures" (p. 1); "Stigmatized individuals are regarded as flawed, compromised, and somehow less than fully human" (p. 3). At the same time, the particulars of what is stigmatized, and the expression of stigma, are often situational rather than absolute across a culture. While the impact can be dire for individuals targeted by stigma, there is increasing awareness that people cope with stigma in much the same way they cope with other hardships—often with considerable resilience [10–12]. This awareness of room to move for stigmatized populations has given rise to advocacy groups, support groups, and stigma-countering movements across a variety of fields. In the field of mental health, the psychosocial rehabilitation perspective and recovery approaches work toward the reversal of stigmatizing self-appraisal and the creation of communities and psychosocial resources that embrace individuals with lived experience of a major psychiatric diagnosis [13, 14].

The loss to society resulting from stigma would have to be considered tragic. Barriers in the areas of work, education, avocation, and social involvement translate into missed opportunities at all levels of society. Additionally, the profound alienation resulting from stigma will almost always incur a sense of shame in the individual (and, by association, the family of the stigmatized individual), undermining confidence in the capacity to contribute within the overall culture. Ultimately, the isolation and hopelessness secondary to both public and internalized stigma may increase suicide risk [15], the ultimate loss for society and the families of the stigmatized person. Regarding risk for violence, the sense of being dehumanized by others can, for some individuals, result in decreased perspective-taking on fellow human beings who no longer appear to be members of a shared society, which may increase potential for fear-based, retaliatory, or alienation-based violence [16]. At the same time, victimization *of* individuals with a serious and persistent psychiatric condition is more common than victimization *by* persons with this lived experience [17]. This pattern of victimization may be related directly or indirectly to the increased vulnerability associated with stigmatized status.

It may be useful to consider Maslow's Hierarchy of Needs [18]. Where does stigma land across those needs? Stigma cuts through the hierarchy at all levels, including physiological and safety needs, as well as the higher order needs of belonging and self-actualization, as individuals are forced to scramble for scarce resources, and struggle with the loss of valued places (whether figuratively, through feeling alienated from essential places, or literally banned from desired locales). The loss in access to place is more profound than mere social alienation, given it is at a need level at which safety (shelter) and physiological needs are threatened; this is a fundamental level at which personhood is denied. The deepest and most dangerous form of stigma occurs when there is no right to safety, and the meeting of physiological needs is denied. The most profound examples may be seen in ethnic cleansing and genocide, and the impact of racism in our neighborhoods. The violation of safety and physiological needs is often clear when the impact of trauma is examined. The loss of predictability and control implied by trauma [19, 20], may contribute to internalized stigma and accompanying shame and humiliation. Janoff-Bulman [21] notes the potential threat of trauma to identity in the context of the naïve "just world" hypothesis: trauma violates the idea that good things happen to good people and bad things do not, leaving an opening for a reappraisal that one is not a good person given the occurrence of trauma. Loss of positive identity in the face of trauma is accompanied by loss of the predictability and control needed to feel safe in valued places and in valued relationships, which tends to affirm self-stigmatizing attitudes. It is notable that the DSM-5 [22] incorporates forms of negative self-appraisal within the criteria for PTSD.

Stigmatized people may also tend to find themselves in stigmatizing places. It is well-known that people with psychiatric disorders disproportionately populate jails and prisons [23, 24], as well as homeless shelters [25, 26], and, of course, psychiatric hospitals. These environments are among the few that 'accept' stigmatized persons, and may often be, unwittingly or systemically, responsible for perpetuating stigma. For stigmatized persons, affiliation with these institutions can serve to reaffirm the original stigma. To be fair, each of these places may have programs to counter the stigmatizing nature of the total institutional experience, which seeks to empower individuals residing within them toward community reintegration. However, there is often a 'bottleneck' at the community, which in a great measure is due to external, or 'public,' stigma. Individuals marked by stigma may find themselves recycling through these environments, in part because these settings are self-perpetuating, and in part because they are where social forces that confer stigma assign stigmatized individuals. Stigmatized individuals may resist any kind of help, including psychotherapy, seeing it as another form of stigmatizing experience.

Because both the military and VA are culturally sanctioned places, people with symptoms of psychiatric disorders may take refuge in these institutions and the identity they provide. While the structure of the military can be protective for persons managing significant symptoms of psychosis or depression, the demands of the military may be hard to manage. However, for VA-eligible persons, the status of veteran provides a refuge and a place of acceptance, to some extent independent of the treatment setting within the VA (in contrast to non-VA mental health care that occurs in settings defined by mental health needs). For veterans who are not eligible for the VA due to their discharge status, the sense of stigma is magnified by the discharge status in addition to the psychiatric label. Ineligible veterans often seek redress to restore VA benefits and services, as well as their status among the honorably discharged. While differences in status among veterans may be conferred by veteran groups, the identity of veteran is generally preserved.

Dimensions of Stigma

Several types of stigma have been identified by psychological researchers, namely, public (or interpersonal) stigma, internalized (or self-) stigma, and structural stigma [27, 28]. Corrigan and Watson [29] define public stigma as consisting of pernicious attitudes and beliefs about mental illness endorsed by public laypeople. When members of the public behave in accordance with these perspectives toward people with lived experiences of mental illness, the latter will experience stigma first-hand, which may result in internalized stigma [30].

"Stigma is relationship- and context-specific; it does not reside in the person but in social context." ([31], p. 395). Self-stigma is derived from the phenomenological literature [32]. According to contemporary social cognitive models of self-stigma (see [33–35]), people with mental illness may directly experience stigma by way of being discriminated against and/or labeled in a derogatory manner, which may contribute to a dysfunctional acceptance of negative self-stereotypes and/or perceptions of discrimination as deserved or justified. This resulting self-stigma, which has been discussed at length in the peer-reviewed literature, is associated with a broad array of negative outcomes, including increased social withdrawal, an exacerbation of various psychiatric symptoms, diminished self-esteem, loss of hope, demoralization, shame, ineffective avoidant coping behaviors, impaired symptom management, and delayed recovery [36, 37].

Linguistics of Stigma

Most modern-day stigmatizing labels applied to mental illness appear to take the linguistic form of *generics*, or quintessential categorical generalizations that give rise to stereotypes [38]. These may range from overtly essentialist cognitive heuristics, such as "schizophrenics are dangerous" [38], to more subtle clinical language, like referring to a patient as a treatment "failure" [39].

Stigmatizing generics are not unique to the United States, nor are they unique to military veterans. Detailed qualitative analyses of national and local British newspapers covering homicide-suicide events revealed strikingly pejorative labels such as "nut," "psycho," and "psychopath" applied to people with mental illness [40].

Unfortunately, the application of pejorative labels to people with lived experiences of mental illness does not appear to be exclusive to the public spheres. Academics and clinicians have been called out for arguably similar behaviors in professional journals (see [41], p. 1218, for an example of a published article title including the words "Difficult Patients").

It is highly unlikely that isolated efforts to alter linguistic generics (absent accompanying stigma-reduction strategies) will attenuate the presence and impact of public and internalized stigma long term. Extant evidence appears scant in support of lasting positive changes in public attitudes and behaviors toward people with mental illness following changes in linguistic nomenclature. For example, altering disorder labels alone (e.g., simply replacing "schizophrenia" with "salience syndrome") seems to have a marginal impact on reducing stigmatizing attitudes of people who are largely unfamiliar with mental illness, and beneficial aftereffects appear transient [42]. Moreover, merely replacing pejorative labels with more palatable descriptors (e.g., substituting "person with a substance use disorder" for "addict") has been associated with minimal influence on recovery-related outcomes [43], although the use of such language has value in that it is more respectful.

Complicating matters further is the apparent disagreement among people with mental illness, psychiatrists, and other healthcare providers regarding "best" descriptive language and summary terms [42]. As cogently summarized by Corrigan [44], "words matter," but contemporary research continues to fall short of arriving at a consensus on "best words" to represent and describe mental illness.

Optimal approaches to eroding stigmatizing language barriers in mental health remain elusive and undoubtedly will continue to raise challenging research inquiries well into the future. Additionally, substantial uncertainty continues to surround the identification of effective communication strategies holding promise for mobilizing public support for potentially beneficial mental health policies (e.g., medication-assisted treatment for opioid use disorders and harm reductions policies) [45]. Because stigmatizing mental health language appears to be a potent intervening variable that not only weakens public support for such policies [46], but also may elicit legally punitive attitudes toward, for example, people with substance use disorders [47], it may be fruitful to discern communication methods that simultaneously garner positive public support while minimizing stigmatizing perceptions (e.g., sympathetic human narratives of lived experience combined with affirming messages of treatment effectiveness and recovery) [45].

Euphemisms for Psychiatric Illness and Care

"Euphemism" is derived from the Greek word eupheme, meaning to use language to affect a "good omen" [48]. The intention is to reduce the negative expressive potential of a concept because one believes that a more direct expression may be disturbing to the hearer or the speaker [49]. Euphemisms serve both the giver and the receiver—the speaker avoids potential discomfort with delivery, and the receiver is palliated by an otherwise harsher expression. However, research has shown that those who generate the euphemism benefit more than the receiver, and euphemisms are used more when conversations are face to face [50]. There is debate as to whether employing euphemisms in psychiatry is helpful, harmful, or simply ineffective.

On the one hand, data suggest relabeling psychiatric diagnoses can have the powerful effect of shifting psychiatric practice and public opinion. A compelling example hails from Japan where schizophrenia was renamed "integration disorder" in 2002 after it had been called "mind-split disease" for generations [51]. After the change, surveys indicated that patients were more likely to be informed of their diagnosis, consent to treatment, engage in care, experience less stigma, and achieve greater social integration [52].

On the other hand, some feel renaming has a high cost to patient care. Fred Frankel [53] asserted that repeated avoidance of the term "mental illness" causes harm to people with mental illness by perpetuating a denial about their condition and the effect on others. Others suggest euphemisms that were designed to avert offense may cause offense. For example, a study using vignettes to manipulate characters as having no label, a label with a specific disability, or labeled as "special needs" showed participants exhibited negative associations with the term "special needs" more than associations with "disability" or other direct terms. The authors concluded that "special needs" is an ineffective euphemism due to its imprecision and connotation with segregation, resulting in a dysphemism [54].

Stephen Pinker's [55] description of the "euphemism treadmill" deems euphemism's effects short-lived. Over time, the new name given to a softened concept will eventually become colored by the original concept, so renaming something does not change the essence of the thing in question.

Euphemisms likely persist due to societal pressures to be politically correct, and euphemisms alone will not eliminate societal or intrapersonal stigma associated with mental illness. The American Psychiatric Association offers guidance with wording when reporting to the media about mental health conditions, including putting the person first (e.g., person with schizophrenia), naming the specific disorder whenever possible (e.g., saying "bipolar" rather than "mental illness"), and avoiding derogatory terms (e.g., "crazy", "junkie", "victim") (see Words Matter: Reporting on Mental Health Conditions at psychiatry.org [56]).

Who Gets to Decide on Nomenclature?

A significant stigma in mental health care may also include fear of being labeled or receiving a psychiatric diagnosis in one's chart. At the same time, the role of correct diagnostic terminology is also critical case definition, applying effective and appropriate treatment, and facilitating communication among clinicians and researchers, as well as establishing accurate billing codes for reimbursement [57]. The topic of diagnostic nomenclature is complicated by the shifting landscape and controversies in mental health classification, fueled by a centuries-old debate with evolving theories about the phenomenology, etiology, and course defining each condition. As far back as the 1800s, European physicians Kraepelin and Alzheimer sought to differentiate presentations such as dementia, schizophrenia, and other psychiatric illnesses [57].

In the United States, psychiatry was first recognized as a medical specialty in 1844, but initially disjointed as a field across diagnostic systems, psychoanalysis, and the role of biological research [57]. The initial impetus for developing a classification system of mental health diagnosis was to collect statistical census information. In 1917, the American Medico-Psychological Association (with a name change to the American Psychiatric Association [APA] in 1921), began to develop a classification plan, but with the intent for administrative record keeping and statistics, rather than a focus on treatment of mental illness [56]. Related to work among veterans, a subsequent broader classification system was developed by the US Army (and modified by the Veterans Administration) to reflect outpatient presentations of World War II veterans. This work influenced the World Health Organization (WHO) edition of the International Classification of Diseases-6 containing psychiatric categories, which influenced the publication of the first Diagnostic and Statistical Manual of Mental Disorders (DSM) in 1952 [56].

The role and definition of psychiatric labels continue to evolve. Subsequent DSM iterations included controversial changes, including a shift to re-medicalize psychiatry and with a focus on research criteria [56, 58]. Beginning in 2000, work groups were formed to synthesize the current state of psychiatric science and to identify gaps in current research. These efforts culminated in the formation of 13 work groups focused on various disorder areas, the DSM-5 APA Task Force in 2007, and the publication of the DSM-5 in 2013 [56].

Criticisms across the iterative development of the DSM include increasing length of time of Task Force deliberation to produce revisions, as well as a perceived increase in financial ties of its developers to the pharmaceutical industry, with industry ties of the Task Force increasing from 57% in DSM-IV to 72% in DSM-5 [59]. Additional criticism of the DSM includes practical limitations when attempting to administer comprehensive diagnostic interviews within the narrow confines of real-world encounter times [57]. Of importance, the threshold of diagnostic criteria for many disorders in the DSM-5 were lowered, with debate around what constitutes pathology threshold in psychiatry as well as societal and cultural norms [60, 61].

Adding to these debates, the DSM-5 is primarily used in the United States, while the ICD is principally utilized internationally and for insurance coding purposes. Although the DSM is used in research internationally, it is less widely accepted by clinicians outside of the United States. European clinicians favor the use of the ICD system likely in part that their governments require its use for reimbursement [62].

Given the power that the DSM wields in psychiatric diagnostic labeling, these controversies and debates are important to consider when exploring the stigma and fear that individuals may have in seeking mental health care [60].

The "D" in PTSD and Other Efforts to Destigmatize MH Care in the DoD

The Military has attempted to embrace discussions about mental illnesses related to combat experience in an effort to acknowledge that they are occupational hazards. It has actively sought to destigmatize these illnesses, and to encourage help-seeking behaviors among service members. One notable effort was advocacy to eliminate the "D" in PTSD, which was rooted in the presumption that posttraumatic stress was a normal response to exposure to combat and death. Some leaders went so far as to relabel the condition Posttraumatic Injury, citing the causative nature of the traumatic exposure. There was even serious debate surrounding the question of whether Posttraumatic Stress Disorder should be acknowledged as meriting a Purple Heart as had been done for Traumatic Brain Injury and as had been done in Canada. Interestingly, service members did not wholly welcome this destigmatization campaign as it was seen as having the potential to deny them the benefits of service-connected disability.

In the context of the wars in Iraq and Afghanistan, military leaders were seeing an increase in the rates of suicide by active service members. This acknowledgement was met with a call to arms to combat this threat to the troops. An aggressive mental health destigmatization campaign was initiated to raise awareness about suicide and its potential causal factors. One of the strategies employed was self-disclosure by respected leaders in public service announcements. Another was a psychoeducation campaign. Both were intended to normalize the fact that "stress" is ubiquitous and that anyone can develop symptoms when exposure is significant. These campaigns aimed to normalize help-seeking as routine maintenance for the warfighter, analogous to preventive maintenance of vehicles and weapon systems.

These efforts to normalize help-seeking for mental illness were limited by centuries of warrior culture valuing stoicism and toughness. Additionally, the pervasive attitudes around unit esprit de corps and group cohesion dictate that a unit is only as strong as its "weakest link." Stoicism combined with toughness and cohesion create an environment where no member dares to be the first to admit any weakness for fear of losing their standing in the group, thereby perpetuating the stigma associated with admitting psychological symptoms and seeking help.

Barriers to Care

Barriers to care may arise from internal prohibitions or external sources. Internal barriers can be the result of internalized perceptions about mental illness itself, the attitudes about those dealing with illness, or from beliefs about the impact of illness on one's life, relationships, and career. External barriers emplaced by families, cultures, or professions only serve to reinforce internal barriers.

Shame

At the moment at which Cognitive Behavioral Therapy was gaining favor over psychoanalysis, Helen Block Lewis [63] put the emotion of shame on the map. The founder of psychoanalytic psychology, Lewis confronted the emotion that other analysts had avoided. She wryly pointed out the embarrassment that shame presented to both patient and therapist, and how social convention and politeness often limited its analysis. She noted that guilt was often the subject of analysis, while shame was rarely addressed. It might be said that the permission to address shame set the stage for the acknowledgement of trauma. Perhaps not entirely coincidentally, her daughter, Judith Herman, was one of the first writers in the field to acknowledge childhood trauma [64], eventually starting one of the early trauma treatment centers in the Boston area [65]. While Lewis does not discuss stigma specifically, she notes loss of face and esteem as a result of shame. She notes that while guilt is about what a person has done, shame is about who the person is. Since her seminal work, acknowledgement of the role of shame has proliferated in research and clinical practice [66, 67], including in the diagnostic criteria for PTSD [22]. Wurmser described the vicious circle (*circulus vitiosus*) of shame, resentment, and revenge, clinically resulting in massive condemnation of self and others [68].

Symptoms experienced by individuals diagnosed with psychosis often are suffused with shame-based dialogue and convictions that are likely influenced by stigma. Hallucinations tend to be persecutory, with an emphasis on derogatory and degrading utterances about the individual's identity—whether sexual, spiritual, or racial. Suicidality is highly stigmatized by Eurocentric society. Due to the taboos around suicide, people who have suicidal thoughts may fear that they will be shamed because of their thinking. They may be ignored or invalidated by people who do not appreciate that the thoughts are often uncontrollable and are connected to intense emotions. This misunderstanding or mishandling of a person with suicidal thoughts may increase shame and escalate thoughts into suicidal behavior. Therefore, it is important for society to foster the kind of environment where people with suicidal thoughts can discuss their thoughts safely without stigma driving an exacerbation of mental health symptoms.

People with high suicide risk are often admitted for psychiatric assessment and stabilization. This intervention may compound the person's shame and stigma by overriding their personal autonomy with an involuntary psychiatric hold, and cause embarrassment, loss of work, and negatively impact certain rights and privileges. The fear of involuntary hospitalization may cause some people to minimize the seriousness of their suicidal thoughts. This dynamic must be understood by clinicians so that appropriate suicide risk assessment can be performed.

Humiliation

Humiliation is a stigmatizing act perpetrated by another. Lazare [69] makes a distinction between shame and humiliation. Shame is an internal, private sense of inadequacy or failure. Humiliation is interpersonal and public; it is an act of aggression (whether conscious or unconscious) that renders the victim helpless, exposed, and vulnerable. Lazare opines that humiliation is an aggressive act akin to "murdering" the soul of the injured person. Responses to this aggression are strong and may include physical violence directed toward others. Humiliation may compound and eclipse the original trauma to be the primary symptom of illness.

Military and Veteran Culture

Stigma, military membership, and veteran status interact in a variety of ways. For some members, the military offers opportunity for education and career not available in their community, for others refuge from poverty, homelessness, and abuse. Navigating the military environment may result in a new sense of belonging and destigmatization given the clear rules and avenues to promotion. Positive status as a military member can replace shame with an honored position in society (depending on the historical moment and the specific post-military or nonmilitary community to which the individual belongs).

Sources of stigma stemming from within the military service experience range from being outcast from one's peer group, to being subject to bullying and/or military sexual trauma (MST). Another source of stigma and shame is related to combat trauma exposure, especially if PTSD or other symptoms develop. Individuals may feel a loss of self-worth if they perceive themselves as "weak," especially if others directly or indirectly affirm that appraisal. Help-seeking, while it may be encouraged, may also be viewed as a stigmatizing sign of weakness [70, 71]. Additionally, survivors of combat often report a reaction to recognizing that they are *expendable* in the context of the overall mission. Depending to an extent on the perceived value of the mission, there may be a sense of pride at being essential to the mission, or a sense of shame that one's life is not worth more than the mission. This awareness of expendability can be a source of shame in future life and may be hard to shake or transform into a renewed sense of worth, conferring a sense of stigmatization for a subset of veterans.

Gender/Sex Bias

Women are underrepresented in the military and the VA. Specialized women's health programs have been developed to make them feel welcomed and to address their healthcare needs. Women represent 52% of the general United States population, but only 16% of the active military and 10% of the overall veteran population [72]. However, women are the fastest growing segment of VA populations [73]. Clinicians well-versed in gender considerations and women's mental health are needed to promote a willingness to listen to experiences and decrease stigma in seeking care. From a psychosocial perspective, female veterans experience significantly more sexual harassment and sexual assault prior to and during military service compared to males [74]. Most early research on trauma and PTSD focused on men [75], yet gender differences are important to consider. Statistically, women are twice as likely to experience PTSD as men following traumatic exposure [76]. An array of more recent scientific literature has begun to explore gender differences in neuroendocrine stress response and rates of psychiatric presentations. From a psychotherapy perspective, gender bias and gender considerations are also important to consider, as therapists may also fail to effectively address gender and power considerations in therapy interactions [77].

Structural/Systemic Stigmatization

No discussion of stigma is complete without mention of policy and cultural norms which nurture, propagate, and allow stigma to entrench itself within us as individuals and as a society. Until recently, psychological research on stigma focused on individual-level micro interactions: either within oneself, termed individual, or internalized stigma; or, between two people, termed interpersonal stigma [28]. In the past decade, more research has shifted to understanding a higher level of stigma, termed structural stigma, which encompasses broader cultural norms, social constructs, and all levels of policy which allow stigma to entrench. Structural stigma has roots in the related concept of institutional racism, which highlights how racism is perpetuated through institutional policies and cultural ideologies. Structural stigma is an encompassing term, of which institutionalized racism is one type of structural stigma [28]. Other examples of structural stigma can be found in LGBTQ+ populations, immigrant populations, disabled populations, and many other marginalized groups. For a more in-depth discussion of LGBTQ+ issues in the military and veteran population, please see the chapter dedicated to this topic.

Several recent studies have identified the link we may intuit: in societies with high levels of structural stigma (in the form of written policy or cultural norms), stigmatized individuals are more likely to internalize negative attitudes toward themselves and conceal their stigmatized condition [28, 78–80]. Perhaps most importantly, many studies have begun to identify downstream negative health effects of structural stigma on stigmatized groups. This critical research has begun to accrue evidence in support of what we know from personal experience: that policies and cultural norms that stigmatize individuals based on any number of factors—from race, gender, sexual orientation, ability, primary language, body size, or mental health condition—will have significant negative health repercussions. New research has also noted that abolishing policies that create stigma will reverse this effect and improve the health of stigmatized individuals [28].

Military and veteran personnel have been exposed to their own specific set of cultural norms and structural stigma due to their military background. One prominent example of structural stigma can be found in the former US military policy banning homosexuality, and the more permissive Don't Ask, Don't Tell (DADT) policy which, despite its repeal in 2011, has continued to exert a negative cultural influence toward LGBTQ+ individuals. The proportion of LGBTQ+ service members who are out to peers and medical providers has increased since the repeal of DADT, but many veterans report a lasting cultural legacy of "otherness" [81]. In 2016, the Department of Defense announced a policy to formally allow transgender individuals to openly serve in the military. However, this policy toward inclusion was quickly rescinded by the Trump administration in 2017, and after extensive legal challenges, the transgender ban went into effect in 2019. The fraught policy around transgender individuals serving in the military continued until January 2021, when the new Biden administration signed an executive order overturning the ban, once again allowing transgender individuals to serve openly in the US military. Policies like these exert a heavy influence on the culture of the US military and have significant stigmatizing effect.

As we move forward as individuals and clinicians, it is imperative that we challenge structural stigma by identifying and dismantling policies which "constrain the opportunities, resources, and wellbeing of the stigmatized" [82]. As the DOD healthcare system is part of the overall military subculture, it has tended to be relative weak in training clinicians in the cultural competencies for the care of racial, ethnic, sexual and gender minorities. This lack of cultural competency serves to perpetuate stigma against these groups, self-stigma of these people, and entrench barriers to help-seeking for mental illness.

Stigma Within Healthcare Systems

It is important to recognize that stigma toward people with mental illness extends to healthcare professionals. We must acknowledge that mental health professionals also suffer from the widespread cultural message that people with mental illness are undesirable. Mental health clinicians, despite an abundance of training and exposure to those with mental illness, have similar levels of stigmatizing attitudes as laypeople [83–85]. Stigma from healthcare professionals toward those they are charged to serve is highly problematic and creates additional barriers to care. Clinicians must confront their own implicit bias and stigma to effectively serve their patients. Furthermore, efforts to reduce mental health stigma that permeates our society will never succeed if clinicians do not confront their own negative attitudes.

Mental health professionals may find themselves in a position of being disparaged by fellow clinicians when they work with patients whose lived experience includes potentially disabling diagnoses of schizophrenia, bipolar disorder, or depression with psychotic features [67, 84]. Indications of *secondary stigma* (or stigma by association) may be subtle or obvious; they may be embedded in comments from colleagues, and inherent in systemic attitudes and practices. Even within mental health, there can be a stratification of patient populations such that attitudes and behaviors differentially allocate respect and resources to the patients and the clinicians that treat them.

Stigma Within the Department of Defense

Healthcare service utilization is often used as a proxy for self-stigma among returning soldiers; it is easier to quantify than other measures such as quality of life, well-being, and treatment success. The soldiers most in need of services are also those who report the most barriers to care [86]. Multiple studies suggest only about half of returning veterans get treatment for post-traumatic stress disorder, alcohol use disorder, anger problems, physical health problems, and suicidal ideation [87]. About a fifth of people returning from the wars in Afghanistan and Iraq are reporting symptoms of PTSD or major depression, but only about half seek treatment. A major reason many service members do not seek treatment is the self-stigma associated with receiving mental health care [88].

Aspects of self-stigma may lead to overvalued assumptions about social stigma. Contrary to assumption, negative career consequences for seeking mental health services while in the military are uncommon. One study found that 97% of people who self-referred experienced no career impact; only 3% of people who referred themselves for mental health treatment had a negative career impact. However, untreated mental illness, when sufficiently symptomatic to result in behaviors observable by others can have serious occupational consequences. When a commander refers a service member for a mental health evaluation, up to 39% experience negative career impact [89].

Britt et al. [90] evaluated the question of what barriers predominate amongst members of a US Brigade Combat Team of over 2000 soldiers when considering mental health care. These troops most frequently endorsed a preference for handling problems oneself as the primary determinant for a decision to seek care. Additionally, they declined care believing that symptoms will go away on their own. An important factor informing their decision not to seek care was a concern with being seen as 'broken' by their unit. This paralleled their belief system around physical health where the three most frequently endorsed barriers treatment were a preference for handling problems oneself, fear of being seen as broken by one's unit and a concern of treatment harming the soldier's career.

Interestingly, when examining how leadership attitudes and behaviors impact a servicemember's self-stigma and willingness to self-identify and self-refer for mental health care, Britt et al. [91] identified that positive and negative NCO and officer leader behaviors were predictive of overall stigma and barriers to care, but that NCO attitudes and behaviors were most influential. NCOs play an important role as gatekeepers within unit structure and can actively encourage or dissuade allowing time for health care.

Kelley et al. [92] found that perceived organizational support may lessen stigma and serve as a protective factor for soldiers returning from combat. Barnes et al. [93] found that higher levels of perceived organizational support predicted lower levels of PTSD before, during, and after deployment. The opportunity for stigma intervention in theater by deploying mental health providers with military units and enabling them to become credible "known entities" among the command leadership positively affected self-stigma related to help-seeking among returning soldiers [94]. Although this strategy primarily sought to decrease barriers to care, it also may have affected potentially stigmatizing beliefs, attitudes, and behaviors at the military unit level [94].

In our vignette, our NCO described previously was deeply concerned about how he would be perceived by members of his unit. His direct superior was highly respected and appeared to embody all of the attributes of a super soldier. He appeared tough, capable, and demanding of excellence. Our NCO sought to model himself after him. He feared that if he revealed any attribute other than strength and resilience, he would no longer be worthy of mentorship by his NCO. Our NCO also witnessed in a sister unit how a junior NCO became mocked and alienated when he sought mental health care. Here we see how the perceived attitudes of leaders can negatively impact help seeking behavior.

Britt et al. [95] further examined the role of four different stigma perceptions amongst soldiers: perceived stigma to career, perceived stigma of differential treatment, self-stigma from seeking treatment, and stigmatizing perceptions of soldiers who seek treatment. While each perception played a role in help seeking, stigmatizing beliefs about those who seek treatment were most influential regarding decisions to seek care. Concerns about the impact of treatment on one's career and differential treatment from others, were associated with an increased probability of dropping out of mental health treatment, but self-stigma from treatment seeking was the only unique predictor of dropout.

In the initial phase of the land combat study, Hoge et al. [96] observed that of soldiers returning from combat who endorsed symptoms of a mental disorder, only 38–45% indicated an interest in receiving help, but only 23–40% sought mental health care. Those whose responses were positive for a mental disorder were twice as likely as those whose responses were negative to report concern about possible stigmatization and other barriers to seeking mental health care.

In a more recent study [97], Of 4674 cohort soldiers referred to mental health care at a military treatment facility post-deployment, 75% followed up with this referral. The soldiers who received a PTSD diagnosis had a high dropout rate, with 22% attending only one mental health care visit and 41% received minimally adequate care (eight or more encounters in 12 months). Of those soldiers a PCL-17 score above 50, 24% dropped out of care. Reported reasons for dropout included soldiers feeling they could handle problems on their own, work interference, insufficient time with the mental health professional, stigma, treatment ineffectiveness, confidentiality concerns, or discomfort with how the professional interacted.

From the vignette, the NCO's spouse eventually expressed how distressed she had become watching him continue to demonstrate symptoms of irritability, anger control, and drinking and how he had been unsuccessful at managing his reintegration on his own. She implored him to seek help and threatened to leave him if he continued on his current path. He realized that his problems weren't resolving on their own as he hoped, but he was fearful of being seen as "that guy (who can't handle himself)" by his unit. One day, he received a citation from the MPs for drunk driving and was confronted by his NCO. He learned that after his respected leader's first deployment, he demonstrated a similar pattern of poor reintegration. His leader was convinced by his First Sergeant to self-refer for mental health care. This NCO reluctantly went into treatment and achieved support and remission of his symptoms that allowed him to regain his ability to lead effectively. The NCO demonstrated exactly the positive attitudes and behaviors around help-seeking that enabled our junior NCO to receive effective treatment.

If social stigma is an imputation, mark of disgrace, or stain associated with a particular person, quality, or circumstance, perhaps it can also be understood by considering its opposite: esteem, honor, respect, and acceptance. While institutional and social stigma remain difficult to quantify, one marker of the desire for culture change may be seen in DoD's policy development aimed at reducing stigma [98]. Awareness of the VA's list of common challenges and solutions or the MilitaryOneSource database of websites facilitating civilian life transitions may raise awareness of social understanding and acceptance and thereby decrease both social and perceived stigma.

Fitness for Duty

The Military has well-established standards of medical fitness. The standards are in place to ensure that each member is able to function in austere conditions under extreme duress. The military effectiveness of the operational unit depends upon adequate staffing and well-functioning interdependent parts. If members are lost on the battlefield to illness, the military operation may fail. Medical personnel within these formations have a duty to serve the needs of the service as well as the needs of the individual member. This creates the potential for ethical conflict as well as a barrier to care. Military mental health officers are required to continually ensure service members meet current standards of fitness, and soldiers know that accessing medical or mental health care can place them at risk of restrictions to duty or discharge from the service, which often is at odds with service members' desires.

Service members are keenly aware of the risks of seeking care within a system that could cause harm to their career aspirations. There is often deep mistrust for all but emergency and battlefield care. Mental Health care is the most deeply stigmatized form of healthcare as it is often viewed as contrary to the highly valued ideals of stoicism and toughness.

Operational Readiness

One unique aspect of military psychiatry is the fact that mental health professionals of all disciplines deploy to theaters of combat with the soldiers they treat. The rationale for having them in the theater of combat is to provide triage and care as close to the front as possible. The clinician's role is to ensure far forward treatment in order to optimize the potential to return the soldier to duty. This treatment is delivered with the expectation that the soldier will be restored to health and returned to duty [99]. Those soldiers who do not recover quickly are evacuated to a higher level of care and often are returned stateside with little prospect of returning to their unit. This loss of status created by becoming a psychiatric casualty can be highly stigmatizing, both by the soldier's unit and within the medical evacuation system also caring for those who were wounded in action, setting up distinct classes of casualties.

Commanders are keenly aware of the potential for soldiers under duress to be medically evacuated from the combat zone. As unit cohesion depends on the willingness of each member to tolerate danger and distress, a culture develops in which members wish to demonstrate their commitment to the group and will sacrifice their personal needs and desires. This warrior ethos creates an unspoken taboo about focusing on individual needs and help-seeking behavior, and this taboo in turn prohibits seeking medical or mental health care except when the needs are dire. To actively lower the threshold for primary prevention, ease of access, and early intervention, the DoD Combat Operational Stress Control doctrine provides front-line mental health teams to serve as consultants to commands to enhance primary prevention and clinicians for troops for early intervention.

Administrative Separation

When a service member has a substance use disorder, adjustment disorder, personality disorder, and/or pattern of misconduct; and they are unable to refrain from problematic use or behavior, the military command may choose to discharge them from service. This option requires the service member to receive a formal mental health evaluation, a course of treatment, and efforts to restore health. The evaluation serves to establish a diagnosis (if any) and to ensure that a major psychiatric illness does not exist that would account for the behavior and qualify the member for medical retirement. Administrative separation is usually characterized as an honorable or general discharge but does not qualify the veteran for retirement benefits. Administrative separations are highly stigmatized in that they imply that the service member could not perform at the level expected. This process has a complex history being abused to discharge soldiers who should have rightly been afforded treatment and/or medical disability retirement. There is a loss of prestige that would normally accompany a completed enlistment or term of service. Under some circumstances, the administrative separation also includes a bar to reenlistment. This type of discharge carries a stigma when seeking employment as most employers hiring former service members will ask to see the discharge paperwork when making a hiring decision. The stigma can also be experienced by friends and family, who may be disappointed with the lack of completion of a successful term of enlistment, diagnosis notwithstanding.

Medical Retirement

When a service member develops a psychiatric illness that is disabling or otherwise unfitting for unrestricted military service, they are offered up to 1 year of intensive treatment to recover an acceptable level of functioning. If the recovery is not sufficient to meet medical fitness standards, or if the condition includes severe psychotic, cognitive, or behavioral symptoms, then the member is discharged with a medical retirement. This type of discharge affords the member ongoing medical benefits as well as retirement compensation. The Departments of Defense and Veterans Affairs coordinate their efforts to determine what service-connected conditions qualify for a disability rating and potential benefits through the Integrated Disability Evaluation System (IDES).

Medically retired service members are eligible for care in the community using their retirement benefits, and they are also eligible for care within the VA. Medical retirement includes a determination of the lifetime risk of ongoing disability. This disability rating determines the percentage of "service-connection" and retirement pay. The medically retired service member can now seek care and further disability determination by the Veterans Benefits Administration.

There are many forces at play in the medical disability process. The service member may be motivated by their warrior ethos to minimize any illness in an attempt to remain on active duty and continue to serve, thereby avoiding the stigmatization of a medical discharge. Alternatively, the service member might be seeking separation from the military and long-term disability compensation. The physician conducting the medical retirement examination must be aware of the dynamic forces at play and the potential for malingering and other secondary gain issues. The physician attempts to remain objective but can be influenced by personal biases, military cultural influences, and the patient's interests. Implicit biases against psychiatric illness may unwittingly color physicians' views of the service member and either push for expeditious discharge from the ranks or minimize the psychiatric illness as not deserving of retirement benefits. Thus, the patient's interests may conflict with those of the military, and the physician must reconcile any biases to serve both professional obligations to the patient and the government.

Once service members are retired from the military with a disability, they are referred to the Department of Veterans Affairs automatically for enrollment. This ensures that service members/veterans become eligible for all applicable benefits. These benefits include access to health care for the service-connected disability, and a host of financial benefits and disability compensation.

Disability Determination

Veterans are increasingly using the VA to avail of the benefits that they have earned and deserve. One half (9.8 out of 20.0 million) of all veterans used at least one VA benefit or service in 2017, an increase of almost 11 percentage points since 2008. Of the 9.8 million users, 45% used multiple benefits which is up from 33% in 2008.

The percent of female veterans who used VA benefits increased from 36% in 2008 to 50% in 2017. The corresponding rate among male veterans in 2008 and 2017 was 39% and 49%, respectively. VA Health Care and/or Disability Compensation users accounted for 76% of all VA users in 2017, up from 69% in 2008. The median age of male veterans who used at least one VA benefit is 64; median age of male non-users is 58 [73].

Stigma and shame can be a barrier preventing a veteran from accessing their earned benefits. Some veterans feel shame is applying for benefits or seeking care, falsely thinking of these benefits as welfare or a hand-out. Other veterans may be apprehensive about the prospect of being invalidated by the medical disability system, particularly for psychiatric illnesses with few objective diagnostic findings. The stigmatization of invisible disabilities (such as mental illness, including post-traumatic stress disorder, anxiety, or depression) creates challenges for veterans as they transition into civilian life [100, 101]. Despite State and Federal Law protecting those with disabilities, discrimination still exists in terms of hiring, housing and other opportunities related to false beliefs or stereotypes about disabilities.

On balance, being service connected represents the privilege of sharing in a historical reflection on events, tragedy, heroism, and unspoken emotions. Being service connected is the honor of being a survivor from which the true meaning of "Thank you for your service" is derived [102].

A robust literature base specifically identifying and testing social stigma-reduction interventions for returning service men and women is lacking. Efforts to assess the sources of self- and societal stigma upon returning troops, attitudes and beliefs, and the societal structures that enable people to impose attitudes and beliefs onto others, are difficult to measure. Efforts to measure change in these fundamental experiences are methodologically complex. Most studies identified in review articles had small sample sizes, did not follow-up to assess whether observed reductions in self-stigma were maintained postintervention, and used an incomparable methodology [103, 104]. Please also see the chapter on the DoD and VA Medical Disability system for a more in-depth discussion of this topic.

The VA and Stigma

In 1865, President Abraham Lincoln directed the United States in his second inaugural address "to care for him who shall have borne the battle, and for his widow, and his orphan." [105] After the Civil War, individual states took on the mission to care for veterans through the creation of Veterans' Homes. It was not until after World War I when the Federal Government assumed responsibility for the care of veterans through the establishment of three separate agencies to provide for their needs. Congress created the National Home for Disabled Volunteer Soldiers, the Veterans Bureau, and the Bureau of Pensions of the Interior Department. These three agencies were consolidated into the Veterans Bureau in 1921 and assimilated the Public Health Service Veteran's Hospitals. In 1930, President Hoover elevated the Veterans Bureau to become the Veterans Administration (VA) and named

Brigadier General Frank T. Hines to be the first Administrator. It was thought that a military officer would best administer this new agency and create a culture that might attract veterans to its services. After World War II, the Veterans Administration was expanded to 125 hospitals, and new benefits were developed with the goal to help veterans successfully transition and integrate back into civilian life. President Reagan raised the Veterans Administration to a Cabinet-level Department of Veterans Affairs. The United States Department of Veterans Affairs (VA) is now comprised of three divisions: The Veterans Health Administration (VHA), the Veterans Benefits Administration (VBA), and the National Cemetery Administration (NCA) [106].

The Veterans Administration, as the largest public healthcare system in the nation, is complex in its image, and its meaning to veterans and the community. It serves a panoply of healthcare, research, and training functions. It is extraordinary in its scope and impact. The VA boasts hundreds of university affiliations across the country and offers training across many professions. It can be seen as monolithic; yet there is the common quip that "If you've seen one VA … you've seen *ONE VA*" (suggesting strong local character—and sometimes inconsistency—within the monolith). As a pluralistic setting, the VA has had impact on stigma from a variety of directions, through a variety of mechanisms. The VA has also varied over time in its relationship with mental health stigma, often coming to the table late but disseminating counter-stigma policies once adopted.

As the field of mental health grew more central to American culture, its influence was seen in the military and in the VA during and following World War II, in the form of both assessment and psychotherapy. The presence of stigma in the VA has paralleled the culture in general, For example, when deinstitutionalization occurred in the late 1960s and again in the 1970s with the advent of psychotropic medication, the VA and many other mental health organizations provided day treatments aimed at assuring the transition to outpatient care. Many programs initially developed more conservative versions of Fountain House, the first identified peer-run club house for people with lived experience. Programs offered creative therapies, sheltered employment, and a full range of group therapies. The first evidence-based practices for psychosis emerged, and behavioral family therapy was developed [107]. However, a shift in the field toward a medical, brain-science model in the late 1980s led to diminished valuing of psychotherapy, and hyper-valuing of psychopharmacological interventions. This trend occurred at a time when the field was also influenced by an economic value system that emphasized gainful and substantial employment as a signal of health. While idealistic movements such as psychosocial rehabilitation [108] radically put forward the value of work and rehabilitation programs for people with serious psychiatric diagnoses, hospital administrators, including in VA, sometimes responded by cutting programs serving this population. In one large VA medical center, a fully staffed, multifaceted, model day treatment program serving over 350 veterans was replaced by a nonclinical drop-in center and assigned to a single social work associate, with the rationale that the high-need, vulnerable veterans in this program were unlikely to progress in an economically meaningful way, and simply needed to be monitored on a daily basis.

As the pendulum swung toward recovery, supported employment, peer support, and honoring the potential of individuals with psychiatric conditions, programs such as the PRRCs have taken hold in VA's across the nation. The recognition of PTSD as a mental illness has likely contributed to acknowledgement of other mental illnesses. The emergence of the PTSD diagnosis in the Diagnostic and Statistical Manual, third edition [109] established the first diagnosis based on human experience of trauma. As PTSD grew in acceptance in VA and elsewhere throughout the 1980s and 1990s, interest in and respect for lived experience began to partially counter the ongoing stigma of mental illness.

World War II veterans were for many years the most prominent and outspoken utilizers of the system, while veterans of peacetime service and the wars in Southeast Asia (e.g., the Korean War and the War in Vietnam) often felt themselves relegated to a secondary status. The notion of a war that was vast, 'heroic' and 'won' by the U.S. overshadowed the mental health issues of World War II survivors, a portion of whom were hospitalized long-term in VA hospitals with little recognition of their post-combat conditions (and in the absence of a specific diagnosis to describe their conditions) [110]. Paradoxically, the War in Vietnam led to greater recognition of the lived experience of combat survivors, although the Vietnam veterans were themselves stigmatized across contexts from work to media representations to treatment in VA, The cultural attitude toward Vietnam veterans shifted gradually with the appreciation of trauma as a reality, in a jagged dialectic process. Since at least the Persian Gulf War in 1990, the VA has transformed toward embracing and providing state-of-the-art mental health treatments for combat veterans. The early work on establishing the diagnosis and treatment of PTSD had its roots in the VA. The identification of PTSD as a way to describe certain symptoms, behaviors, and challenges in relationships had a destigmatizing impact not only on people diagnosed with combat trauma-related symptoms, but on the field in general. It was the first diagnosis that clearly acknowledged the impact of trauma in human suffering, rather than suggesting character frailty as the source of psychological distress. As combat-related PTSD is now among the most accepted mental illnesses treated in the VA, other psychiatric disorders such as schizophrenia and bipolar disorder may be subject to greater stigma.

Veterans within the VA often experience the VA as validation of their military service and their value in society. Veterans' criticisms are proprietary rather than dismissive. For example, while there is ample anecdotal evidence of the VA responding inadequately to the needs of Vietnam Veterans immediately after the war, there is also ample evidence of a shift to meet these veterans' needs. The literature indicates that Vietnam veterans with PTSD ended up utilizing VA services substantially to cope with PTSD symptoms [111, 112]. For veterans with significant mental illnesses, veteran status offers a source of self-esteem and identity not afforded to nonveterans diagnosed with serious and persistent psychiatric conditions. Given the loss of identity experienced with serious psychiatric conditions [9], the identity as a veteran has a strong advantage to individuals in this system. There can be a downside to this identification, as veterans experiencing internalized stigma (and fearing external stigmatization) may then find it difficult to venture outside the system into even accepting organizations. This limiting factor may actually result in greater self-stigma in the long run, given that veterans may not afford themselves the *dignity of risk* of trying out new and potentially destigmatizing experiences in the community. Veterans have been known to comment, after visiting non-VA social clubs and recovery centers, "I like it better here (at VA program)"—even when the alternate setting is relatively attractive, and welcoming.

In 2006, the VHA responded to a national call to transform mental health care [113] with an array of requests for proposals (RFP's) aimed at empowering individuals with serious and persistent psychiatric conditions, and countering their experience of public and internalized stigma. The RFP's funded projects for: intensive treatment for serious and persistent psychiatric disorders, peer education and support, family therapy for veterans with serious psychiatric conditions; and supported employment. Over the next several years, VA embraced a recovery rather than maintenance model, and took a counter-stigma stance within a strengths-based psychiatric rehabilitation approach. This wave of recovery-based treatment brought with it investment in evidence-based practices for psychiatric conditions, including Social Skills Training [114], and Illness Management and Recovery [115]—allowing veterans with lived experience access to respectful and viable treatments. At this same time, Peer Education and Support was introduced into the VA, both within recovery programs and independently. These initiatives began to bring the VA in line with the recovery community outside the VA, moving the VA from a traditional medical model toward a more equitable and respectful stance. The following decade saw the VA adopting, and training staff in, a whole health approach that embraced a broad range of integrative interventions, and introduced a "patient-centered care" philosophy in which the veteran served is a key member of the treatment team and a central medical decision maker. Similarly, the VA embraced a "housing-first" approach, supporting veterans toward obtaining and keeping apartments in the community. This acceptance-based resource also helped to reduce stigma and validated the right of persons with lived experience to obtain and keep housing. The VA, through embracing these progressive, person-centered initiatives, played a part in legitimizing them and contributing to reduction of stigma.

Interventions to Reduce Stigma

Anti-stigma work is an incredibly heterogeneous area, with programming that varies by context, approach, audience, method, and outcome measurement. Research in on stigma reduction has not yet produced high-quality evidence to identify interventions that successfully achieve long-term reduction in stigmatizing attitudes [116]. Broad categories of anti-stigma interventions include education (e.g., replacing myths with accurate knowledge), contact (i.e., face-to-face interactions with people who have mental illness to challenge preconceived biases), and protest aimed at suppressing negative attitudes about mental illness [117].

Anti-stigma work is increasingly visible. Public campaigns to increase mental health awareness include large organizations like National Alliance on Mental Illness (NAMI), Mental Health America (MHA), and scores of other organizations dedicated to a multitude of mental health diagnoses. Many large mental health advocacy groups in the United States and internationally have dedicated anti-stigma work.

Interventions to reduce stigma must include those targeted toward healthcare professionals and their own biases about mental illness. A culture of nondisclosure among clinicians may perpetuate stigma [118]. Clinicians may be hesitant to admit personal struggles with mental health due to possible licensure repercussions. This culture of denial contributes greatly to clinician silence and further compounds the isolation and "otherness" of those with mental illness.

Healthcare Literacy

The current state of research results on attenuating public stigma and self-stigma with mental health literacy initiatives can be described as cautiously optimistic. A widely cited meta-analysis published by Corrigan et al. [119], which spanned 72 research articles with 38,364 community participants drawn from 14 countries, revealed that adults participating in public anti-stigma initiatives (i.e., those involving face-to-face contact with people with severe mental illness) evidenced the greatest changes in positive attitudes and behaviors. This contact-based approach was found to be superior to traditional educational efforts focused on debunking common myths of mental illness, and this finding was most salient in studies employing randomized controlled trial (RCT) designs, which bolsters confidence in the internal validity of causal inferences.

Another notable result of the Corrigan et al. [119] study was that education alone seemed to reduce stigmatizing attitudes more effectively among adolescents compared to adults, perhaps due in part to more inchoate beliefs at younger ages. Other studies, however, have suggested that adults may likewise be positively swayed by more traditional information dissemination approaches. For example, a recent mental health first aid program provided to family members of Australian Defense Force veterans diagnosed with psychiatric illnesses was associated with significantly increased knowledge of mental illness in addition to significantly decreased social distancing attitudes [120]. A limitation of this finding is that increased social approach behaviors may be confounded with pre-existing closeness between family members, in this case, spouses (as opposed to between strangers).

Specific mechanisms of action by which educational approaches alleviate public stigma remain unclear. One recently proposed mechanism entails a magnification of perceived similarities between psychologically healthier people and people with severe mental illness, thereby blurring previously salient in-group/out-group differences [121], although this inference remains somewhat conjectural and is in need of further replication. As discussed in detail by Corrigan, the concept of celebrating differences with affirming attitudes, as opposed to simply spotlighting similarities, may also facilitate stigma reduction (i.e., viewing people with mental illness as different and respected members of society in a "parity, not pity" cultural paradigm as a healthier and less prejudicial alternative to mainstream media-driven reification and sanctification of disempowered victimhood; for a thoughtful elaboration on this perspective). How the public perceives similarities and differences between themselves and those with mental illness, and the degree to which these perceptions may be beneficially modified with education is an understudied, albeit potentially fruitful, anti-stigma research area.

Research on reducing self-stigma via contact-based methods has yielded similarly encouraging results. For example, a comprehensive literature review on stigma and severe mental illness conducted by Yanos et al. [122] revealed six primary group intervention strategies addressing self-stigma. These included a manualized, 16-week Self-Stigma Reduction Program [123]; a structured, 20-session, manual-based Narrative Enhancement and Cognitive Therapy group [124]; and a manualized, 3-session Coming Out Proud peer-led group [125], among others. The literature review indicated that all of these contact-based intervention programs emphasized psychoeducation (e.g., challenging myths about mental illness), which was viewed by the authors as a valuable tool for enhancing critical thinking skills while facilitating the recognition and rejection of inaccurate and damaging stereotypes [122]. However, as acknowledged by the authors, the extent and stability of outcomes related to self-stigma mitigation remain unclear and warrant further research.

Another potentially productive direction for weakening the impact of stigma may be through the use of cognitive-behavioral and acceptance-commitment strategies adapted for enriching self-concept and personally meaningful values beyond the confines of psychiatric symptoms, which may simultaneously and more naturalistically challenge the veracity of harmful stereotypes and self-stigmatizing beliefs [37]. Although these therapeutic approaches have not been explicitly framed as such in the literature, the authors of this chapter would propose conceptualizing them as indirect, clinically pragmatic forms of mental health literacy by way of reinforcing more accurate self-knowledge vis-à-vis symptoms in the broader context of the life narrative (e.g., educational symptom clarification via functional analysis in tandem with self-empowering, big-picture values clarification).

Although research in this area remains in its early phases as of the writing of this chapter, exploratory studies and smaller-scope literature reviews have furnished promising results. For example, cognitive restructuring has been identified as a possible method for weakening self-stigma and increasing help-seeking behaviors among combat veterans [126]. In addition, a systematic review of 15 studies indicated that ACT-based interventions were consistently associated with post-treatment reductions in stigma, perhaps by way of gradually improving psychological flexibility [127]. Furthermore, the practice of self-compassion, which is often practiced in mindfulness and acceptance-based approaches, appears to bestow a small but clinically important protective function against the psychological internalization of perceived public stigma, thus promoting increased resilience in the face of negative societal attitudes toward mental illness [128].

As compellingly argued by Corrigan, several caveats are in order when considering mental health literacy initiatives, including (but not limited to) wariness of (a) overconfident educational positivism, (b) unanticipated public psychological reactance, (c) the lure of slacktivism, and (d) unfounded faith in public service announcements (PSAs). Educational positivism is a term proposed by Corrigan [44] referring to the democratic dissemination of knowledge by way of pedagogy that may become prone to misguided professional overconfidence in a "more-is-better" bias regarding information dissemination. Overly ambitious educational interventions may inadvertently overwhelm cognitive processing capacity and thus foment confusion via information overload, and they may fail to impart a lasting impression or motivate behavior change due to a lack of emotional significance [129].

In the face of novel educational information that is perceived as a threat to personal freedom of choice, an attitude rebound, or "boomerang" effect termed psychological reactance is also possible. This unfortunate effect has been observed in response to anti-smoking campaigns in South Korea, which were paradoxically associated with increased anger and negative attitudes among smokers toward public smoking cessation initiatives [130]. A similar "don't tell me what to think" reaction may be elicited if the public feels lectured into a corner about mental health stigma, especially when such lectures are associated with authority figures ([44], pp. 117–118).

Posting educational information and/or giving a shoutout to a noble political cause on social media may feel emotionally gratifying, but it may sometimes devolve into what has been termed *slacktivism* as opposed to more behaviorally rich activism [131]. Corrigan [44] defines slacktivism in the context of mental health stigma as "feel-good fecklessness" (p. 113) in the form of electronically posting emotionally meaningful social justice endorsements online with little effort and with very little, if any, discernible or measurable real-world impact. This is contrasted with the hard work and rigorous behavioral engagement inherent in contact-based educational outreach efforts described in preceding paragraphs.

Finally, cautious scrutiny is warranted in the face of commercially lauded, and often expensive, mass public education endeavors. A prime example of this is the PSA. PSAs are often disseminated through various media outlets, including radio, television, and online social media, and have been touted by social marketing experts as an effective form of public education for decreasing stigma ([132]; see also [44], for a detailed review and synthesis of the literature on PSAs targeting mental health stigma). Although PSAs appear to succeed in penetrating populations to varying degrees (i.e., rendering target audiences more aware of stigma), their degree of real-world mitigation of prejudicial attitudes and behaviors toward people with mental illness in society is uncertain [133].

Wellness Interventions

A wellness approach to treating mental illness moves away from conventional psychiatric medicine towards a more holistic perspective. In 1977, George Engel presented a framework to view health and wellness *not* as an absence of disease, but a balance of psychological, physiological, and social factors. The biopsychosocial model [134] espouses that medicine should not solely adhere to a medical or disease model. Instead, psychosocial, and environmental factors must be considered along with medical factors because people suffer as a whole, and not as isolated organs. The World Health Organization incorporates Engel's biopsychosocial model and defines health as "a state of complete, physical, mental, and social well-being and not merely the absence of disease or infirmity." Engel's model has continued to evolve and includes other domains such as spiritual, financial, and recreational health.

Lancet Psychiatry published a robust argument from Sarris et al. [135]. Declaring that diet and nutrition are central determinants of psychiatric health, and we should consider diet and nutrition for psychiatric disorders the same as we do for cardiac and other diseases. In addition, Schuch et al. [136] meta-analysis showed exercise as an effective strategy to treat depression. Sufficient evidence and research support the use of medications to treat mental illness. However, positive and lasting effects have only been modest, and the burden of mental illness will continue without alternative or adjunctive efforts [135]. The biopsychosocial model provides a helpful framework to contemplate wellness activities as interventions, and/or as supplemental to other treatment modalities for optimizing mental health.

Promoting health and wellbeing through wellness interventions can be cost-effective, and the non-trauma focus can be appealing to populations who may not otherwise seek mental health treatment, such as people who live in rural areas [137] or veterans, for example. Veterans particularly have been reluctant to seek mental health services and have been shown to be an important target population for wellness interventions [138].

Veterans may prefer wellness interventions over traditional treatments as a way to avert re-experiencing trauma [139, 140], or associated stigma [141, 142]. In contrast to frequent dropouts in traditional interventions, Mori et al.' [139] wellness program with veterans with PTSD showed no absences and positive endorsements from the participants. The National Strategy for Preventing Veteran Suicide [143] acknowledged the importance of promoting Complementary and Integrative Health (CIH) approaches as a way to expand the repertoire of services that at-risk veterans may be more inclined to utilize. Vitale et al. [140] also had high engagement and success with veteran participants in a CIH group with direct intentions to introduce CIH as a strategy to reduce stigma associated seeking mental health treatments.

Overall, wellness interventions appear to be valuable in getting people involved in activities that promotes self-efficacy and general well-being, despite the challenges with assessing positive outcomes. It is important to appreciate the bidirectional relationship between causal effects between complementary interventions and mental health [144, 145]. For example, we can perceive lack of social connectedness as both a cause and a symptom of depression [144]. Furthermore, depression can induce short sleep durations, and short durations of sleep can be a risk factor for depression onset [145]. Nevertheless, there is sufficient and expanding evidence for the benefits of wellness interventions.

Researchers are moving more toward studying the implementation of multiple wellness domains, rather than singular wellness activities, with good results [136, 140]. Rolin et al. [146] created a multidomain program and published a longitudinal, prospective, open-label clinical trial and outcomes after implementing it with individuals with mild to moderate mental illness. The program, called "WILD 5", stands for "Wellness Interventions for Life Demands." Five domains associated with holistic wellness are the core focus—physical exercise, restorative sleep, mindfulness through meditation, social connectedness, and optimal nutrition. After 30 days of the program, participants reported statistically significant improvement on all domains and even a potential pathway toward remission. There is much empirical evidence in the literature supporting a multifactorial approach to mental health and wellness activities are showing to be a patient-centered approach that carries less stigma and perhaps more success than conventional psychiatric treatment alone.

Many studies focus on one or more wellness modality, with different outcome concentrations. To conserve space, the reader is referred to Table 4.1 that lists empirical literature on specific wellness interventions (e.g., exercise, nutrition, sleep hygiene, mind-body practices, social connectedness, spirit, and soul) and associated improved mental health.

Mindfulness, Whole Health and the Circle of Health

The concept of wellness is defined as the process of developing conscious and deliberate (mindfulness) behaviors that lead toward more satisfying lives (i.e., "well-being") through improved emotional, physical, social, spiritual, environmental, and intellectual health [147]. The emphasis is on a person's strengths and one's own role in maintaining one's mental and physical health. One comprehensive example is Veterans Health Administration (VHA) Office of Patient Centered Care and Cultural Transformation that offers veterans treatment that places the veteran at the center of their care and teaches veterans mindful management of their well-being and health. The overarching vision is for a transformation within VA healthcare from a problem-based disease system to healthcare that is patient-centered and focused on "Whole Health" (https://www.va.gov/wholehealth/). The goal is to provide proactive, personalized, patient-driven health care. The interconnectivity of all-inclusive aspects of an individual person in the context of their community, and use of conventional, preventative, and complementary treatments affects a person's overall physical, emotional, spiritual, mental health and well-being (see Fig. 4.1, The Circle of Health). Improving specific areas in one's life can benefit other areas. In this initiative, Veterans identify areas in their "whole" life that matter most to them, learn to set goals, and are taught to mindfully make meaningful life changes.

Table 4.1 Published wellness interventions and targeted mental health outcomes

Wellness intervention	Supportive literature	Mental trait/ outcome measures
Exercise	Hall, K. S., Morey, M. C., Beckham, J. C., Bosworth, H. B., Sloane, R., Pieper, C. F., & Pebole, M. M. (2020). Warrior wellness: A randomized controlled pilot trial of the effects of exercise on physical function and clinical health risk factors in older military veterans with PTSD. *The Journals of Gerontology. Series A, Biological Sciences and Medical Sciences, 75*(11), 2130–2138. https://doi.org/10.1093/gerona/glz255	Depression
	Schuch, F. B., Vancampfort, D., Rosenbaum, S., Richards, J., Ward, P. B., & Stubbs, B. (2016). Exercise improves physical and psychological quality of life in people with depression: A meta-analysis including the evaluation of control group response. *Psychiatry Research*, 241, 47–54. https://doi.org/10.1016/j.psychres.2016.04.054	PTSD Meta-analysis Depression
Health and wellness group	Drapalski, A. L., Lucksted, A., Brown, C. H., & Fang, L. J. (2021). Outcomes of ending self-stigma, a group intervention to reduce internalized stigma, among individuals with serious mental illness. *Psychiatric Services (Washington, D.C.), 72*(2), 136–142. https://doi.org/10.1176/appi.ps.201900296	Schizophrenia Schizoaffective disorder Bipolar disorder
Nutrition Exercise	Sarris J., Logan A. C., Akbaraly T. N., Amminger G. P., Balanzá-Martínez V., Freeman M. P., … Jacka F. N. on behalf of International Society for Nutritional Psychiatry Research. (2015). Nutritional medicine as mainstream in psychiatry. *Lancet Psychiatry*, 2, 271–274	Psychiatric disorders
Sleep	Sun Y., Shi L., Bao Y., Sun Y., Shi J, Lu L. (2018). The bidirectional relationship between sleep duration and depression in community-dwelling middle-aged and elderly individuals: Evidence from a longitudinal study. *Sleep Medicine*, 52, 221–229.	Depression; mood regulation
	Herring M. P., Kline C. E., O'Connor P. J. (2015). Effects of exercise on sleep among young women with Generalized Anxiety Disorder. *Mental Health and Physical Activity*, 9, 59–66	Generalized anxiety disorder
Meditation	Seppälä, E. M., Nitschke, J. B., Tudorascu, D. L., Hayes, A., Goldstein, M. R., Nguyen, D. T. H., Perlman, D., & Davidson, R. J. (2014). Breathing-based meditation decreases posttraumatic stress disorder symptoms in U.S. military veterans: A randomized controlled longitudinal study. *Journal of Traumatic Stress*, 27(4), 397–405. https://doi.org/10.1002/jts.21936	PTSD

(continued)

Table 4.1 (continued)

Wellness intervention	Supportive literature	Mental trait/ outcome measures
Social connectedness	Saeri A., Cruwys T., Barlow F. K., Stronge S., Sibley C. G. (2017). Social connectedness improves public mental health: Investigating bidirectional relationships in the New Zealand attitudes and values survey. *Australian and New Zealand Journal of Psychiatry*, 52, 365–374.	General mental health; distress
Music and creative arts	Levy, C. E., Spooner, H., Lee, J. B., Sonke, J., Myers, K., & Snow, E. (2018). Telehealth-based creative arts therapy: Transforming mental health and rehabilitation care for rural veterans. *The Arts in Psychotherapy*, 57, 20–26. https://doi.org/10.1016/j.aip.2017.08.010	Depression Anxiety Quality of life
Mind-body (acupuncture; meditation; mindfulness) Expressive arts (writing: music) Exercise (dance; yoga) Sleep hygiene Spirit and soul Nutrition Life skills	Vitale, A., Byma, L., Sun, S., Podolak, E., Wang, Z., Alter, S., Galfalvy, H., Geraci, J., Langhoff, E., Klingbeil, H., Yehuda, R., Haghighi, F., & Feder, A. (2021). Effectiveness of complementary and integrative approaches in promoting engagement and overall wellness toward suicide prevention in veterans. *The Journal of Alternative and Complementary Medicine (New York, N.Y.), 27*(S1), S-14-S-27. https://doi.org/10.1089/acm.2020.0245	Suicidal ideation Depression Anxiety PTSD
Exercise Nutrition Meditation Sleep hygiene	Schuch F. B., Vancampfort D., Richards J., Rosenbaum S., Ward P. B., Stubbs B. (2016). Exercise for the treatment of depression: A meta-analysis adjusting for publication bias. *Journal of Psychiatric Research*, 77, 42–51.	Meta-analysis Depression
Exercise nutrition Sleep Meditation Social connectedness	Rolin, D., Fox, I., Jain, R., Cole, S. P., Tran, C., & Jain, S. (2020). Wellness Interventions in Psychiatrically Ill Patients: Impact of WILD 5 Wellness, a Five-Domain Mental Health Wellness Intervention on Depression, Anxiety, and Wellness. *Journal of the American Psychiatric Nurses Association, 26*(5), 493–502.	Depression; generalized anxiety disorder; sleep outcomes

Recovery-Based Approaches and Stigma

As an intended antidote to stigma and its impact, the strengths-based model of the psychiatric rehabilitation movement [108, 148, 149] seeks to empower stigmatized individuals by way of reestablishing meaningful roles in the community, intentionally confronting and overcoming stigma-based biases and barriers, and establishing safe harbor in which a secure, integrated identity can be developed or restored. Fountain House, established in the 1940s, and Boston University's Center for Psychiatric Rehabilitation, established in 1979, are two renowned examples of centers developed to offer validation, safety, support, and a network of places for

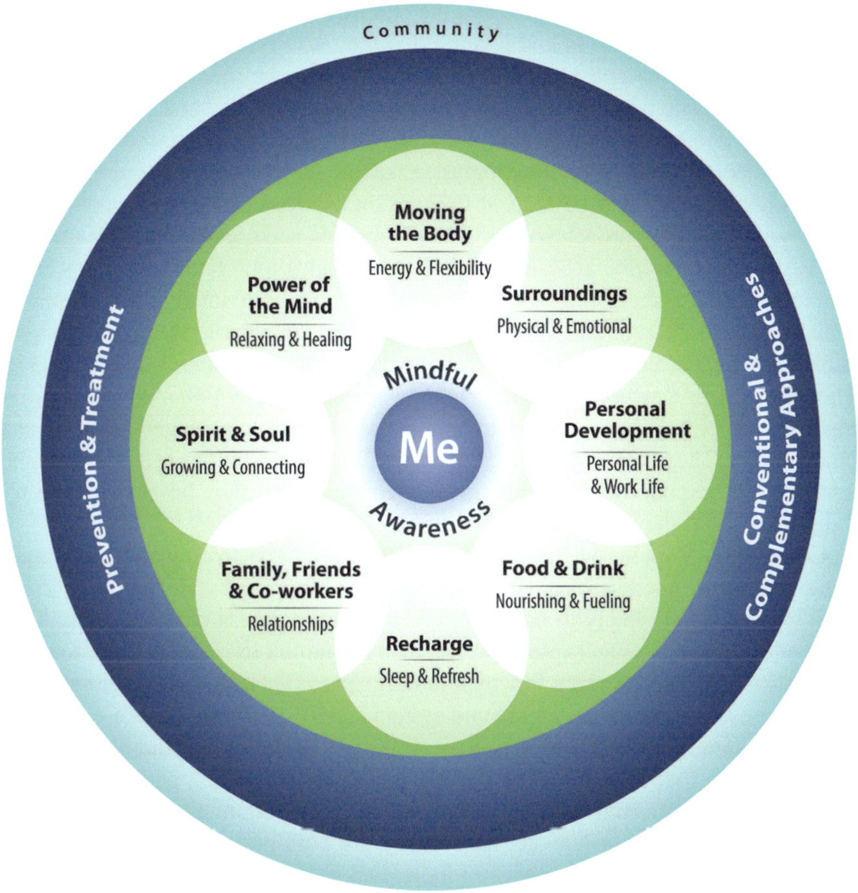

Fig. 4.1 VA whole health care—the circle of health

individuals diagnosed with serious psychiatric conditions. The recovery movement has promoted peer-run Recovery Learning Centers and social clubs.

As safe havens have developed, a dialectic process has occurred alongside them, fueled by the potential pervasiveness of stigma: Do these places improve society by normalizing psychiatric disorders and creating stigma-free outlets? Or do they further segregate individuals with psychiatric diagnoses, perpetuating their stigmatization? Do these organizations facilitate participation in the larger culture, reducing stigma through an integrative process promoting entry in the culture and generating awareness within the culture? Do they obstruct a possible re-entry process through suggesting that the safe havens are the only safe places? Or do they expand what our culture has to offer and provide practice with living stigma-free? This natural apposition recurs as the individual and the culture struggle with the "stickiness" of stigma, offering alternatives and healing that may also present as potentially self-perpetuating patterns and practices. This struggle can be seen in the attempts to change use of stigmatizing language, as each new term becomes suspect and is replaced by another more neutral or positive word (only to be replaced as it begins to be used pejoratively or patronizingly).

This conflict can also be seen in the tension between skills-based models and "community first" approaches. Skills-based models such as Illness Management and Recovery [115], Social Skills Training [114], Behavioral Family Therapy [150] promote 'safe passage' into society through arming individuals with increased social capacities. Community first approaches prioritize entering the community of choice and then selecting work on the skills needed for community longevity [13]. The former takes a protective stance based on a relapse-prevention model emphasizing the cost of negative experiences for people already challenged by self- and other-stigma. The latter touts *the dignity of risk*, that people with serious and persistent psychiatric conditions are like everyone else in that they have a right to try things out, and if they fail, fine-tune it, and try again.

Community mapping [13], as a community-first approach, emulates other community advocacy models (e.g., Participatory Asset Mapping by HealthCity; [151]). Individuals who are likely to have limited community access chart a course of re-entry or entry, much as an explorer would map unfamiliar territory in order to make it a known and familiar place in which to participate. This approach highlights the importance of a sense of belonging and systematically confronts the sense of alienation and shame resulting from a history of being rebuffed in the community.

Shifting the focus of evaluation to the stigmatized individual, participants identify needed and preferred resources, and evaluate their communities to identify not only where they are, but how accessible they are both physically and in terms of comfort level. It is not enough that an individual superficially access a resource in the community, feel uncomfortable, and quickly leave; it is essential that the individual finds and settles into significant and meaningful places in which they feel comfortable, accepted, and effective. This model invites a sense of mastery over stigma, while not eradicating it. It also helps to reduce stigma by assuring that individuals laboring under a stigmatized identity 'show up and are counted' in the communities they choose for themselves so that others in the community develop familiarity with them and have opportunities to relate and potentially break down the stigma.

Future Directions

While mental illnesses, patients with them, clinicians who treat them, and clinics and communities that embrace them are highly stigmatized, we can understand some of the evolutionary, societal, and linguistic manifestations that perpetuate this negative bias. As we more clearly understand the internal, external, and structural barriers to acceptance, care, and help-seeking both in the military and veteran population and society at large, we can begin to address these barriers and offer a path toward greater acceptance of mental health care as routine health care.

The military and veteran population have the additional barrier of a culture of stoicism, mental and physical toughness, camaraderie, and mission-focus. These forces are antithetical to revealing any aspect on one's self that may be cause for rejection by the group. Mental illness, and the imputation that it might represent a vulnerability or make the person unreliable, is an especially important as a source of shame that may compel a service member to secrecy and avoidance of help-seeking. Stigma will persist without significant societal and cultural shifts in attitudes about the importance of maintaining health and fitness.

Health literacy is a critical and foundational element of any transformational change in attitudes and behaviors about mental illness. Transparency about psychological struggles by trusted and respected leaders will lift the cloak of shame and isolation about mental illness and demonstrate the value of help-seeking. Education about the prevalence of mental illnesses, their risk factors and protective factors, and the effectiveness of treatment may serve to demystify and normalize psychiatric care. Clear communication about the importance of primary prevention and health maintenance for the most important organ in our body can serve to normalize self-care and help-seeking for mental illnesses as routine health care.

Wellness principles present and opportunity to emphasize the importance of maintaining balance between our bio-psycho-socio-spiritual needs help to normalize discussions about the mind-body continuum. Emphasis should be given to integrating whole health approaches to all aspects of health care. Particularly useful is how these principles have a ready analogy within military culture. A soldier is expected to care for his weapon and equipment, perform individual level preventive maintenance, and identify when higher level specialized maintenance is required to ensure the equipment's peak performance. The principle of person-centered care aligns care with the values, motivations, and sense of purpose of the service member or veteran which can help to overcome internal barriers to care. And optimize prevention, treatment, and recovery using a full array of potential interventions that align best with the values of the person and the culture of their service and community.

References

1. Link BG, Stuart H. On revisiting some origins of the stigma concept as it applies to mental illnesses. In: Gaebel W, Rössler W, Sartorius N, editors. The stigma of mental illness – end of the story? New York, NY: Springer; 2017. p. 3–28.
2. Bennett S. Shame, stigma, and mental illness. In: Fink PJ, Tasman A, editors. Ancient Greece: in stigma and mental illness. Arlington, VA: American Psychiatric Association; 1992. p. 29–39.
3. Arboleda-Flórez J, Stuart H. From sin to science: fighting the stigmatization of mental illnesses. Can J Psychiatr. 2012;57(8):457–63. https://doi.org/10.1177/070674371205700803.
4. Mackay CS. The hammer of witches: a complete translation of the Malleus Maleficarum. Cambridge: Cambridge University Press; 2009.

5. Bourneville DM. Science et miracle: Louise Lateau, ou la stigmatisée belge. Paris: VA Delahaye; 1878.
6. Fabrega H. The culture and history of psychiatric stigma in early modern and modern western societies: a review of recent literature. Compr Psychiatry. 1992;32(2):97–119.
7. Lasalvia A, van Bortel T, Bonetto C, Jayaram G, et al. Cross-national variations in reported discrimination among people treated for major depression worldwide: the ASPEN/INDIGO international study. Br J Psychiatry. 2015;207:507–14.
8. Thornicroft G, Brohan E, Rose D, Sartorius N, et al. Global pattern of experienced and anticipated discrimination against people with schizophrenia: a cross-sectional survey. Lancet. 2009;373(9661):408–15. https://doi.org/10.1016/S0140-6736(08)61817-6.
9. Goffman E. Stigma: notes on the management of spoiled identity. Englewood Cliffs, NJ: Prentiss-Hall; 1963.
10. Miller CT, Major B. Coping with stigma and prejudice. In: Heatherton TF, Kleck RE, Hebl MR, Hull JG, editors. The social psychology of stigma. New York, NY: The Guilford Press; 2000.
11. Dovidio JF, Major B, Crocker J. Stigma: introduction and overview. In: Heatherton TF, Kleck RE, Hebl MR, Hull JG, editors. The social psychology of stigma. New York, NY: The Guilford Press; 2000. p. 1–28.
12. Crocker J, Major B, Steele C. Social stigma. In: Gilbert DT, Fiske ST, Lindzey G, editors. Handbook of social psychology, vol. 2. 4th ed. Boston, MA: McGraw-Hill; 1998.
13. Salzer MS, Burns-Lynch B. Peer facilitated community inclusion toolkit. Philadelphia, PA: Temple University Collaborative on Community Inclusion for Individuals with Psychiatric Disabilities; 2016. www.tucollaborative.org. Accessed 23 Jul 2021.
14. Snethen G, Jeffries V, Thomas E, Salzer M. Welcoming places: perspectives of individuals with mental illnesses. Am J Orthopsychiatry. 2021;91(1):76–85. https://doi.org/10.1037/ort0000519.
15. Oexle N, Waldmann T, Staiger T, Xu Z, Rusch N. Mental illness stigma and suicidality: the role of public and individual stigma. Epidemiol Psychiatric Sci. 2018;27(2):169–75. https://doi.org/10.1017/S2045796016000949.
16. McCauley C. Toward a psychology of humiliation in asymmetric conflict. Am Psychol. 2017;72(3):255–65. https://doi.org/10.1037/amp0000063.
17. Teplin LA, McClelland GM, Abram KM, Weiner DA. Crime victimization in adults with severe mental illness: comparison with the National Crime Victimization Survey. Arch Gen Psychiatry. 2005;62(8):911–21. https://doi.org/10.1001/archpsyc.62.8.911.
18. Maslow AH. A theory of human motivation. Psychol Rev. 1943;50(4):370–96. https://doi.org/10.1037/h0054346.
19. Foy DW. Treating PTSD: cognitive-behavioral strategies. New York, NY: Guilford Press; 1992.
20. McCann IL, Pearlman LA. Vicarious traumatization: a framework for understanding the psychological effects of working with victims. J Trauma Stress. 1990;3(1):131–49. https://doi.org/10.1007/BF00975140.
21. Janoff-Bulman R. Shattered assumptions: towards a new psychology of trauma. New York, NY: Free Press; 1992.
22. American Psychiatric Association. Diagnostic and statistical manual of mental disorders. 5th ed. Washington, DC: American Psychiatric Association; 2013.
23. Steadman HJ, Osher FC, Robbins PC, Case B, Samuels S. Prevalence of serious mental illness among jail inmates. Psychiatr Serv. 2009;60(6):761–5. https://doi.org/10.1176/ps.2009.60.6.761.
24. Torrey EF, Zdanowicz MT, Kennard AD, Lamb HR, et al. The treatment of persons with mental illness in prisons and jails: a state survey. Arlington, VA: Treatment Advocacy Center; 2014. https://nicic.gov/treatment-persons-mental-illness-prisons-and-jails-state-survey. Accessed 23 Jul 2021.
25. Hopper K, Jost J, Hay T, Welber S, Haugland G. Homelessness, severe mental illness, and the institutional circuit. Psychiatr Serv. 1997;48(5):659–65. https://doi.org/10.1176/ps.48.5.659.

26. Kuno E, Rothbard A, Averyt J, Culhane DP. Homelessness among persons with severe mental illness in an enhanced community-based mental health system. Psychiatr Serv. 2000;51(8):1012–6.
27. Corrigan PW, Kleinlein P. The impact of mental illness stigma. In: Corrigan PW, editor. On the stigma of mental illness: practical strategies for research and social change. Washington, DC: American Psychological Association; 2005. p. 11–44.
28. Hatzenbuehler ML. Structural stigma: research evidence and implications for psychological science. Am Psychol. 2016;71(8):742–51. https://doi.org/10.1037/amp0000068.
29. Corrigan PW, Watson AC. The paradox of self-stigma and mental illness. Clin Psychol Sci Pract. 2002;9(1):35–53. https://doi.org/10.1093/clipsy.9.1.35.
30. Jahn DR, Leith J, Muralidharan A, Brown CH, et al. The influence of experiences of stigma on recovery: mediating roles of internalized stigma, self-esteem, and self-efficacy. Psychiatric Rehabil J. 2020;43(2):97–105.
31. Major B, O'Brien LT. The social psychology of stigma. Annu Rev Psychol. 2005;56:393–421. https://doi.org/10.1146/annurev.psych.56.091103.070137.
32. Eriksson K. Self-stigma, bad faith and the experiential self. Hum Stud. 2019;42:391–405.
33. Corrigan PW, Rafacz J, Rüsch N. Examining a progressive model of self-stigma and its impact on people with serious mental illness. Psychiatry Res. 2011;189(3):339–43. https://doi.org/10.1016/j.psychres.2011.05.024.
34. Muñoz M, Sanz M, Pérez-Santos E, Quiroga M. Proposal of a socio-cognitive-behavioral structural equation model of internalized stigma in people with severe and persistent mental illness. Psychiatry Res. 2011;186(2–3):402–8. https://doi.org/10.1016/j.psychres.2010.06.019.
35. Watson AC, Corrigan P, Larson JE, Sells M. Self-stigma in people with mental illness. Schizophr Bull. 2007;33(6):1312–8. https://doi.org/10.1093/schbul/sbl076.
36. Corrigan PW. How stigma interferes with mental health care. Am Psychol. 2004;59(7):614–25. https://doi.org/10.1037/0003-066X.59.7.614.
37. Drapalski AL, Lucksted A, Perrin PB, Aakre JM, et al. A model of internalized stigma and its effects on people with mental illness. Psychiatr Serv. 2013;64(3):264–9. https://doi.org/10.1176/appi.ps.001322012.
38. Nowak L. Generic language and the stigma of mental illness. Philos Psychiatry Psychol. 2019;26(3):261–75.
39. Cantlie S. A request to move away from stigmatising language. Lancet Psychiatry. 2021;8(3):e10. https://doi.org/10.1016/S2215-0366(21)00007-9.
40. Flynn S, Gask L, Shaw J. Newspaper reporting of homicide-suicide and mental illness. BJPsych Bull. 2015;39(6):268–72. https://doi.org/10.1192/pb.bp.114.049676.
41. Corrigan PW. Language and stigma. Psychiatr Serv. 2006;57(8):1218. https://doi.org/10.1176/appi.ps.57.8.1218.
42. Tranulis C, Lecomte T, El-Khoury B, Lavarenne A, Brodeur-Côté D. Changing the name of schizophrenia: patient perspectives and implications for DSM-V. PLoS One. 2013;8(2):e55998. https://doi.org/10.1371/journal.pone.0055998.
43. Ashford RD, Brown AM, Ashford A, Curtis B. Recovery dialects: a pilot study of stigmatizing and nonstigmatizing label use by individuals in recovery from substance use disorders. Exp Clin Psychopharmacol. 2019;27(6):530–5. https://doi.org/10.1037/pha0000286.
44. Corrigan PW. The stigma effect: unintended consequences of mental health campaigns. New York, NY: Columbia University Press; 2018.
45. McGinty E, Pescosolido B, Kennedy-Hendricks A, Barry CL. Communication strategies to counter stigma and improve mental illness and substance use disorder policy. Psychiatr Serv. 2018;69(2):136–46. https://doi.org/10.1176/appi.ps.201700076.
46. McSween JL. The role of group interest, identity, and stigma in determining mental health policy preferences. J Health Polit Policy Law. 2002;27:773–800.
47. Kennedy-Hendricks A, Barry CL, Gollust SE, Ensminger ME, et al. Social stigma toward persons with prescription opioid use disorder: associations with public support for punitive and public health-oriented policies. Psychiatr Serv. 2017;68(5):462–9. https://doi.org/10.1176/appi.ps.201600056.

48. Burkhardt A. Euphemisms and truth. In: Burkhart A, Nerlich B, editors. Tropical truth(s): the epistemology of metaphor and other tropes. Berlin; New York, NY: Walter de Gruyter; 2010. p. 335–72.
49. Radulović M. Euphemisms through time: the rhetorical power of palliation. Facta Univ Ser Linguist Liter. 2016;14(2):173–87.
50. McGlone MS, Batchelor J. Looking out for number one: euphemism and face. J Commun. 2003;53(2):251–64.
51. Morris N. Maybe we should call psychiatry something else. Sci Am. 2016. https://blogs.scientificamerican.com/mind-guest-blog/maybe-we-should-call-psychiatry-something-else/. Accessed 23 Jul 2021.
52. Sato M. Renaming schizophrenia: a Japanese perspective. World Psychiatry. 2006;5(1):53–5.
53. Frankel FH. What's in a name? The "mental health" euphemism and the consequences of denial. Hosp Community Psychiatry. 1975;26(2):104–6. https://doi.org/10.1176/ps.26.2.104.
54. Gernsbacher MA, Raimond AR, Balinghasay MT, Boston JS. "Special needs" is an ineffective euphemism. Cogn Res Princip Impl. 2016;1(1):29. https://doi.org/10.1186/s41235-016-0025-4.
55. Pinker S. The game of the name. The New York Times. 1994:21, Section A.
56. American Psychiatric Association. DSM history. Washington, DC: American Psychiatric Association; 2021. www.psychiatry.org/psychiatrists/practice/dsm/history-of-the-dsm. Accessed 24 Jul 2021.
57. Surís A, Holliday R, North CS. The evolution of the classification of psychiatric disorders. Behav Sci. 2016;6(1):5. https://doi.org/10.3390/bs6010005.
58. Fischer BA. A review of American psychiatry through its diagnoses: the history and development of the Diagnostic and Statistical Manual of Mental Disorders. J Nerv Ment Dis. 2012;200(12):1022–30. https://doi.org/10.1097/NMD.0b013e318275cf19.
59. Cosgrove L, Krimsky S. A comparison of DSM-IV and DSM-5 panel members' financial associations with industry: a pernicious problem persists. PLoS Med. 2012;9(3):e1001190. https://doi.org/10.1371/journal.pmed.1001190.
60. Kawa S, Giordano J. A brief historicity of the Diagnostic and statistical manual of mental disorders: issues and implications for the future of psychiatric canon and practice. Philosophy Ethics Humanit Med. 2012;7:2.
61. Luciano M, Sampogna G, Del Vecchio V, De Rosa C, et al. Critiche e prospettive degli attuali sistemi di classificazione in psichiatria: il caso del DSM-5 [Critical evaluation of current diagnostic classification systems in psychiatry: the case of DSM-5]. Riv Psichiatr. 2016;51(3):116–121. https://doi.org/10.1708/2304.24798.
62. Clark LA, Cuthbert B, Lewis-Fernandez R, Narrow WE, Reed GM. Three approaches to understanding and classifying mental disorder: ICD-11, DSM-5, and the National Institute of Mental Health's Research Domain Criteria (RDoC). Psychol Sci Public Interest. 2017;18(2):72–145. https://doi.org/10.1177/1529100617727266.
63. Lewis HB. Shame and guilt in neurosis. New York, NY: International Universities Press; 1971.
64. Herman JL, Hirschman L. Father-daughter incest. Boston, MA: Harvard University Press; 1981.
65. Herman J. Trauma and recovery. New York, NY: Basic Books; 2015.
66. Kaufman G. The psychology of shame: theory and treatment of shame-based syndromes. New York, NY: Springer; 1989.
67. Yanos PT. Written off: mental health stigma and the loss of human potential. Cambridge: Cambridge University Press; 2018.
68. Wurmser L. The superego as herald of resentment. Psychoanal Inq. 2009;29(5):386–410.
69. Lazare A. Shame and humiliation in the medical encounter. Arch Intern Med. 1987;147(9):1653–8.
70. Kulesza M, Pedersen E, Corrigan P, Marshall G. Help-seeking stigma and mental health treatment seeking among young adult veterans. Mil Behav Health. 2015;3(4):230–9. https://doi.org/10.1080/21635781.2015.1055866.
71. Vogel DL, Wade NG. Stigma and help-seeking. The Psychologist. 2009;22:20–3.

72. Glowacki NA. Gender and veteran demographics: findings from 2019 annual averages, current population survey. Washington, DC: Veterans' Employment and Training Service: United States Department of Labor; 2019. https://www.dol.gov/sites/dolgov/files/VETS/files/2019-Gender-and-Veteran-Demographics-Slides.pptx. Accessed 23 Jul 2021.
73. Department of Veterans Affairs. VA utilization profile FY 2017. Washington, DC: Department of Veterans Affairs National Center for Veterans Analysis and Statistics; 2020. https://www.va.gov/vetdata/docs/Quickfacts/VA_Utilization_Profile_2017.pdf. Accessed 24 Jul 2021.
74. Adams RE, Hu Y, Figley CR, Urosevich, et al. Risk and protective factors associated with mental health among female military veterans: results from the veterans' health study. BMC Womens Health. 2021;21(1):55. https://doi.org/10.1186/s12905-021-01181-z.
75. Vogt D. Research on women, trauma, and PTSD. Washington, DC: US Department of Veteran Affairs: PTSD: National Center for PTSD; 2021. https://www.ptsd.va.gov/professional/treat/specific/ptsd_research_women.asp. Accessed 23 Jul 2021.
76. Kimerling R, Ouimette P, Wolfe J. Gender and PTSD. New York, NY: Guilford Press; 2002.
77. Macfarlane MM, Knudson-Martin C. How to avoid gender bias in mental health treatment. J Fam Psychother. 2013;14(3):45–66.
78. Evans-Lacko S, Brohan E, Mojtabai R, Thornicroft G. Association between public views of mental illness and self-stigma among individuals with mental illness in 14 European countries. Psychol Med. 2012;42(8):1741–52. https://doi.org/10.1017/S0033291711002558.
79. Miller CT, Grover KW, Bunn JY, Solomon SE. Community norms about suppression of AIDS-related prejudice and perceptions of stigma by people with HIV or AIDS. Psychol Sci. 2011;22(5):579–83. https://doi.org/10.1177/0956797611404898.
80. Pachankis JE, Hatzenbuehler ML, Hickson F, Weatherburn P, et al. Hidden from health: structural stigma, sexual orientation concealment, and HIV across 38 countries in the European MSM Internet Survey. AIDS. 2015;29(10):1239–46. https://doi.org/10.1097/QAD.0000000000000724.
81. McNamara KA, Lucas CL, Goldbach JT, Castro CA, Holloway IV. "Even if the policy changes, the culture remains the same": a mixed methods analysis of LGBT service members' outness patterns. Armed Forces Soc. 2020;47(3):505–29. https://doi.org/10.1177/0095327X20952136.
82. Hatzenbuehler ML, Link BG. Introduction to the special issue on structural stigma and health. Soc Sci Med. 2014;103:1–6. https://doi.org/10.1016/j.socscimed.2013.12.017.
83. Peris TS, Teachman BA, Nosek BA. Implicit and explicit stigma of mental illness: links to clinical care. J Nerv Ment Dis. 2008;196(10):752–60. https://doi.org/10.1097/NMD.0b013e3181879dfd.
84. Schulze B. Stigma and mental health professionals: a review of the evidence on an intricate relationship. Int Rev Psychiatry. 2007;19(2):137–55. https://doi.org/10.1080/09540260701278929. PMID: 17464792.
85. Wahl O, Aroesty-Cohen E. Attitudes of mental health professionals about mental illness: a review of the recent literature. J Commu Psychol. 2010;38:49–62. https://doi.org/10.1002/jcop.20351.
86. Maguen S, Litz BT. Predictors of barriers to mental health treatment for Kosovo and Bosnia peacekeepers: a preliminary report. Mil Med. 2006;171(5):454–8. https://doi.org/10.7205/milmed.171.5.454.
87. Sharp ML, Fear NT, Rona RJ, Wessely S, et al. Stigma as a barrier to seeking health care among military personnel with mental health problems. Epidemiol Rev. 2015;37:144–62. https://doi.org/10.1093/epirev/mxu012.
88. Cerully JL, Acosta JD, Sloan J. Mental health stigma and its effects on treatment-related outcomes: a narrative review. Mil Med. 2018;183(11–12):e427–37. https://doi.org/10.1093/milmed/usx219.
89. Rowan AB, Campise RL. A multisite study of Air Force outpatient behavioral health treatment-seeking patterns and career impact. Mil Med. 2006;171(11):1123–7. https://doi.org/10.7205/milmed.171.11.1123.

90. Britt TW, Sipos ML, Klinefelter Z, Adler AB. Determinants of mental and physical health treatment-seeking among military personnel. Br J Psychiatry. 2020;217(2):420–6. https://doi.org/10.1192/bjp.2019.155.
91. Britt TW, Wright KM, Moore D. Leadership as a predictor of stigma and practical barriers toward receiving mental health treatment: a multilevel approach. Psychol Serv. 2012;9(1):26–37. https://doi.org/10.1037/a0026412.
92. Kelley CL, Britt TW, Adler AB, Bliese PD. Perceived organizational support, posttraumatic stress disorder symptoms, and stigma in soldiers returning from combat. Psychol Serv. 2014;11(2):229–34. https://doi.org/10.1037/a0034892.
93. Barnes JB, Nickerson A, Adler AB, Litz BT. Perceived military organizational support and peacekeeper distress: a longitudinal investigation. Psychol Serv. 2013;10(2):177–85. https://doi.org/10.1037/a0032607.
94. Hoyt GB. Integrated mental health within operational units: opportunities and challenges. Mil Psychol. 2006;18(4):309–20.
95. Britt TW, Jennings KS, Cheung JH, Pury CL, Zinzow HM. The role of different stigma perceptions in treatment seeking and dropout among active duty military personnel. Psychiatric Rehabil J. 2015;38(2):142–9. https://doi.org/10.1037/prj0000120.
96. Hoge CW, Castro CA, Messer SC, McGurk D, Cotting DI, Koffman RL. Combat duty in Iraq and Afghanistan, mental health problems, and barriers to care. N Engl J Med. 2004;351(1):13–22. https://doi.org/10.1056/NEJMoa040603.
97. Hoge CW, Grossman SH, Auchterlonie JL, Riviere LA, Milliken CS, Wilk JE. PTSD treatment for soldiers after combat deployment: low utilization of mental health care and reasons for dropout. Psychiatr Serv. 2014;65(8):997–1004. https://doi.org/10.1176/appi.ps.201300307.
98. Government Accountability Office. GAO-16-404 Human Capital: additional actions needed to enhance DOD's efforts to address mental health care stigma. Washington, DC: Government Accountability Office; 2016. https://www.gao.gov/products/gao-16-404/. Accessed 31 May 2021.
99. Salmon TW. The care and treatment of mental diseases and war neuroses ("shell shock") in the British Army. National Committee for Mental Hygiene. Washington, DC: USUHS; 1917.
100. Flink P. Invisible disabilities, stigma, and student veterans: contextualizing the transition to higher education. J Veteran Stud. 2017;2(2):110–20.
101. Rodrigues S, Bokhour B, Mueller N, Dell N, et al. Impact of stigma on Veteran treatment seeking for depression. Am J Psychiatr Rehabil. 2014;17(2):128–46. https://doi.org/10.1080/15487768.2014.903875.
102. Hough S. Compassionate veteran care: embracing respect for the individual. Harvard Health Blog. 2015. https://www.health.harvard.edu/blog/compassionate-Veteran-care-embracing-respect-for-the-individual-201511118618. Accessed 23 Jul 2021.
103. Dickstein BD, Vogt DS, Handa S, Litz BT. Targeting self-stigma in returning military personnel and veterans: a review of intervention strategies. Mil Psychol. 2010;22(2):224–36.
104. Mittal D, Sullivan G, Chekuri L, Allee E, Corrigan PW. Empirical studies of self-stigma reduction strategies: a critical review of the literature. Psychiatr Serv. 2012;63(10):974–81. https://doi.org/10.1176/appi.ps.201100459.
105. Lincoln A. Second inaugural address [Speech transcript]. Abraham Lincoln papers at the Library of Congress, Manuscript Division. 1865. http://hdl.loc.gov/loc.mss/ms000001.mss30189a.4361300. Accessed 22 Jul 2021.
106. Department of Veterans Affairs. History. Washington, DC: Department of Veterans Affairs (VA); 2021. https://www.va.gov/HISTORY/VA_History/Overview.asp. Accessed 25 Jul 2021.
107. Falloon IRH, Boyd JL, McGill CW. Behavioral family therapy for schizophrenia. In: Curran JP, Monti P, editors. Social skills training. New York, NY: Guilford Press; 1982.
108. Anthony WA. Recovery from mental illness: the guiding vision of the mental health service system in the 1990s. Psychosoc Rehabil J. 1993;16(4):11–23. https://doi.org/10.1037/h0095655.

109. American Psychiatric Association. Diagnostic and statistical manual of mental disorders. 3rd ed. Washington, DC: American Psychiatric Association; 1980.
110. Vento CS. Treatment of war related psychiatric injuries post-World War II. Tampa, FL: Defense Media Network. Faircount Media Group; 2015.
111. Maguen S, Schumm JA, Norris RL, Taft C, et al. Predictors of mental and physical health service utilization among Vietnam veterans. Psychol Serv. 2007;4(3):168–80. https://doi.org/10.1037/1541-1559.4.3.168.
112. Rosenheck R, Fontana A. Do Vietnam-era veterans who suffer from posttraumatic stress disorder avoid VA mental health services? Mil Med. 1995;160(3):136–42.
113. New Freedom Commission on Mental Health. Achieving the promise: transforming mental health care in America. Report No. SMA-03-3832. Washington, DC: The US Department of Health and Human Services; 2003. https://govinfo.library.unt.edu/mentalhealthcommission/reports/FinalReport/InsideCover.htm. Accessed 25 Jul 2021.
114. Bellack AS, Mueser KT, Gingerich S, Agresta J. Social skills training for schizophrenia: a step-by-step guide. 2nd ed. New York, NY: The Guilford Press; 1997.
115. Gingerich S, Mueser K. Illness management and recovery: personalized skills and strategies for those with mental health disorders. Center City, MN: Hazelden; 2012.
116. Gronholm PC, Henderson C, Deb T, Thornicroft G. Interventions to reduce discrimination and stigma: the state of the art. Soc Psychiatry Psychiatr Epidemiol. 2017;52(3):249–58. https://doi.org/10.1007/s00127-017-1341-9.
117. Corrigan PW, River LP, Lundin RK, Penn DL, et al. Three strategies for changing attributions about severe mental illness. Schizophr Bull. 2001;27(2):187–95. https://doi.org/10.1093/oxfordjournals.schbul.a006865.
118. Harris JI, Leskela J, Hoffman-Konn L. Provider lived experience and stigma. Am J Orthopsychiatry. 2016;86(6):604–9. https://doi.org/10.1037/ort0000179.
119. Corrigan PW, Morris SB, Michaels PJ, Rafacz JD, Rush N. Challenging the public stigma of mental illness: a meta-analysis of outcome studies. Psychiatr Serv. 2012;63(10):963–73. https://doi.org/10.1176/appi.ps.201100529.
120. Evans J, Romaniuk M, Theal R. Evaluation of mental health first aid training for family members of military veterans with a mental health condition. BMC Psychiatry. 2021;21(1):128. https://doi.org/10.1186/s12888-021-03139-9.
121. Violeau L, Valery KM, Fournier T, Prouteau A. How continuum beliefs can reduce stigma of schizophrenia: the role of perceived similarities. Schizophr Res. 2020;220:46–53. https://doi.org/10.1016/j.schres.2020.04.014.
122. Yanos PT, Lucksted A, Drapalski AL, Roe D, Lysaker P. Interventions targeting mental health self-stigma: a review and comparison. Psychiatric Rehabil J. 2015;38(2):171–8. https://doi.org/10.1037/prj0000100.
123. Fung KM, Tsang HW, Cheung WM. Randomized controlled trial of the self-stigma reduction program among individuals with schizophrenia. Psychiatry Res. 2011;189(2):208–14. https://doi.org/10.1016/j.psychres.2011.02.013.
124. Yanos PT, Roe D, Lysaker PH. Narrative enhancement and cognitive therapy: a new group-based treatment for internalized stigma among persons with severe mental illness. Int J Group Psychother. 2011;61(4):577–95. https://doi.org/10.1521/ijgp.2011.61.4.576.
125. Corrigan PW, Kosyluk KA, Rusch N. Reducing self-stigma by coming out proud. Am J Public Health. 2013;103(5):794–800. https://doi.org/10.2105/AJPH.2012.301037.
126. Kranke D, Weiss EL, Gin J, Der-Martirosian C, et al. A "culture of compassionate bad asses": a qualitative study of combat Veterans engaging in peer-led disaster relief and utilizing cognitive restructuring to mitigate mental health stigma. Best Pract Ment Health. 2017;13(1):20–33.
127. Krafft J, Ferrell J, Levin ME, Twohig MP. Psychological inflexibility and stigma: a meta-analytic review. J Contextual Behav Sci. 2018;7:15–28.
128. Heath PJ, Brenner RE, Lannin DG, Vogel DL. Self-compassion moderates the relationship of perceived public and anticipated self-stigma of seeking help. Stigma Health. 2018;3(1):65–8.

129. Peters E, Klein W, Kaufman A, Meilleur L, Dixon A. More is not always better: intuitions about effective public policy can lead to unintended consequences. Soc Issues Policy Rev. 2013;7(1):114–48. https://doi.org/10.1111/j.1751-2409.2012.01045.x.
130. Kim H. The indirect effect of source information on psychological reactance against anti-smoking messages through perceived bias. Health Commun. 2017;32(5):650–6. https://doi.org/10.1080/10410236.2016.1160320.
131. Cabrera NL, Matias CE, Montoya R. Activism or slacktivism? The potential and pitfalls of social media in contemporary student activism. J Divers High Educ. 2017;10(4):400–15.
132. Kirkwood AD, Stamm BH. A social marketing approach to challenging stigma. Prof Psychol Res Pract. 2006;37(5):472–6.
133. Corrigan PW. Where is the evidence supporting public service announcements to eliminate mental illness stigma? Psychiatr Serv. 2012;63(1):79–82. https://doi.org/10.1176/appi.ps.201100460.
134. Engel GL. The need for a new medical model: a challenge for biomedicine. Science. 1977;196(4286):129–36. https://doi.org/10.1126/science.847460. PMID: 847460.
135. Sarris J, Logan AC, Akbaraly TN, Amminger GP, et al. Nutritional medicine as mainstream in psychiatry. Lancet Psychiatry. 2015;2:271–4.
136. Schuch FB, Vancampfort D, Rosenbaum S, Richards J, et al. Exercise improves physical and psychological quality of life in people with depression: a meta-analysis including the evaluation of control group response. Psychiatry Res. 2016;241:47–54. https://doi.org/10.1016/j.psychres.2016.04.054.
137. Levy CE, Spooner H, Lee JB, Sonke J, et al. Telehealth-based creative arts therapy: transforming mental health and rehabilitation care for rural veterans. Arts Psychother. 2018;57:20–6. https://doi.org/10.1016/j.aip.2017.08.010.
138. Seppälä EM, Nitschke JB, Tudorascu DL, Hayes A, et al. Breathing-based meditation decreases posttraumatic stress disorder symptoms in U.S. military veterans: a randomized controlled longitudinal study. J Trauma Stress. 2014;27(4):397–405. https://doi.org/10.1002/jts.21936.
139. Mori DL, Smidt K, Brown L, Pless Kaiser A, et al. Acceptability of a wellness group program for veterans with symptoms of posttraumatic stress disorder. Glob Adv Health Med. 2019;8:2164956119867048. https://doi.org/10.1177/2164956119867048.
140. Vitale A, Byma L, Sun S, Podolak E, et al. Effectiveness of complementary and integrative approaches in promoting engagement and overall wellness toward suicide prevention in veterans. J Altern Complement Med. 2021;27(S1):S14–27. https://doi.org/10.1089/acm.2020.0245.
141. Drapalski AL, Lucksted A, Brown CH, Fang LJ. Outcomes of ending self-stigma, a group intervention to reduce internalized stigma, among individuals with serious mental illness. Psychiatr Serv. 2021;72(2):136–42. https://doi.org/10.1176/appi.ps.201900296.
142. Hall KS, Morey MC, Beckham JC, Bosworth HB, et al. Warrior wellness: a randomized controlled pilot trial of the effects of exercise on physical function and clinical health risk factors in older military veterans with PTSD. J Gerontol A Biol Sci Med Sci. 2020;75(11):2130–8. https://doi.org/10.1093/gerona/glz255.
143. Department of Veterans Affairs. National strategy for preventing veteran suicide: 2018–2028. Washington, DC: US Department of Veterans Affairs Office of Mental Health and Suicide Prevention; 2018.
144. Saeri AK, Cruwys T, Barlow FK, Stronge S, Sibley CG. Social connectedness improves public mental health: investigating bidirectional relationships in the New Zealand attitudes and values survey. Aust N Z J Psychiatry. 2018;52(4):365–74. https://doi.org/10.1177/0004867417723990.
145. Sun Y, Shi L, Bao Y, Sun Y, Shi J, Lu L. The bidirectional relationship between sleep duration and depression in community-dwelling middle-aged and elderly individuals: evidence from a longitudinal study. Sleep Med. 2018;52:221–9. https://doi.org/10.1016/j.sleep.2018.03.011.
146. Rolin D, Fox I, Jain R, Cole SP, et al. Wellness interventions in psychiatrically ill patients: impact of WILD 5 wellness, a five-domain mental health wellness intervention on depression,

anxiety, and wellness. J Am Psychiatric Nurs Assoc. 2020;26(5):493–502. https://doi.org/10.1177/1078390319886883.
147. Swarbrick M. A wellness approach. Psychiatric Rehabil J. 2006;29(4):311–4. https://doi.org/10.2975/29.2006.311.314.
148. Gagne C, White W, Anthony WA. Recovery: a common vision for the fields of mental health and addictions. Psychiatric Rehabil J. 2007;31(1):32–7. https://doi.org/10.2975/31.1.2007.32.37.
149. Wong YL, Stanton MC, Sasnds RG. Rethinking social inclusion: experiences of persons in recovery from mental illness. Am J Orthopsychiatry. 2014;84(6):685–95. https://doi.org/10.1037/ort0000034.
150. Mueser KT, Glynn SM. Behavioral family therapy for schizophrenia. Prog Behav Modif. 1990;26:122–49.
151. Burns JC, Paul DP, Paz SR. Participatory asset mapping. In: Bonilla T, Cooke D, Farris T, editors. A community asset map toolkit. Los Angeles, CA: Health City Advancement Project; 2012.

The Deployment Experience

5

Chris A. Alfonzo

When discussing military deployments, the term "deployment" typically describes the physical movement of military personnel to an area of operations in support of various duties—e.g., contingency missions, humanitarian assistance, disaster relief. Areas of operations may include combat zones. Whatever technical term may be used to describe movement of military personnel to away sites, be it "show of force," "carrier cruise" and so forth, the intent of this chapter is to describe inherent commonalities of these diverse experiences and help the reader better understand and serve their veteran patient population.

Following the tragic events of September 11th, 2001, the average deployment experience changed significantly and became more unpredictable in terms of frequency, length and mission sets across the United States Armed Forces. In the new century, America has conducted military operations in the Middle East, Southwest Asia and other hotspots, continuing its global projection of forward presence and force in regions with vacillating degrees of politico-social stability. In turn, deployments became more dynamic to meet evolving mission needs as America shifted its overall military strategy from Cold War operations to Operations Other Than War (OOTW) and the Global War on Terror (GWOT). Major Combat Operations have given way in part to Stability Operations but American doctrine and policies remain poised for future engagement in Major Combat Operations with emerging global superpowers. The military continuously plans, trains and prepares for future large-scale action whilst actively engaging in OOTW and Stability Operations and consequently, the scale and scope of modern military deployments are progressively diversified.

In today's military, the majority of active-duty members will participate in at least one deployment during the course of their career; certain military occupational specialties and career length affect the likelihood of multiple deployments. Although each branch of the armed forces and the total military population have traditionally

C. A. Alfonzo (✉)
Great Plains Health Psychiatric Services, North Platte, NE, USA

C. H. Warner, C. A. Castro (eds.), *Veteran and Military Mental Health*,
https://doi.org/10.1007/978-3-031-18009-5_5

been made up mostly of young single males, much of the deployed population in today's military is comprised of young families with children [1]. To clarify, the term "deployed population" refers to those military members who have participated in at least one deployment. The deployed population includes all genders and ethnic backgrounds as well as social and service circumstances such as single parents and members of part-time components such as the National Guard and Reserve forces. Women represent the fastest growing group of veterans and the number of women deploying has steadily increased. Military family members currently outnumber active-duty service members [2]. Any effort to understand and describe the deployment experience in toto must include consideration of how family members may affect, and be affected by, the member's deployment.

To understand the potential impacts of the experience, it is important to consider the full range of deployment settings. Be it a combat mission by an Army armor regiment or an undersea patrol by a Navy fast attack submarine, a member's experience may be unique in contrast to other military branches as well as amongst their own service community. To wit, a Sailor aboard a frigate will have a different experience to that of a Sailor deployed on an aircraft carrier, just as a Marine in a ground combat element will have a different deployment compared to serving in an aviation squadron. The U.S. Armed Forces perform operations across all domains that include ground, air, sea, undersea, space, and cyberspace. Military deployments range in mission type from combat action to regional security activities to counter-drug operations to humanitarian assistance and more.

For the purpose of this chapter, consideration should also be given to military families whose service members serve at an away location but are not technically deployed. Often referred to as a "geo-bachelor" tour, this type of assignment may require the service member to be stationed apart from their family and may last from a period of months to years; the distance apart varies depending on the circumstance. A member's duty orders may necessitate a "geo-bachelor" tour as seen with unaccompanied duty (i.e., family members are not permitted to follow the service member to the assigned location). Reasons for the unaccompanied duty stipulation include safety and security factors, host-nation restrictions, and family members' special needs or inability to obtain overseas clearance. In other "geo-bachelor" circumstances, a family may elect to remain in place away from the service member assigned elsewhere. The decision for such may rest on the intent to minimize disruption to spouse employment, family educational or medical needs, or may even stem from unfortunate circumstances such as marital or family discord.

It is an onerous task to create an all-encompassing description of the deployment experience—not only in terms of today's military population and culture, but across veteran populations of prior-century military service as well. In dismissing the notion of any universal characterization, there remain common factors to acknowledge such as the stages of deployments. Deployments are routinely defined by three stages: pre-deployment, deployment, and post-deployment. How these stages are experienced vary broadly due to myriad factors. Each deployment experience, and any acute- and long-term consequences of such, may be influenced by individual, social, and occupational factors.

Individual factors include age, gender, religion, cultural identity and traditions, personality traits, resiliency, mindset, maturity, physical and mental health conditions, marital and family status, past experiences (personal and deployment-related), financial situation, and geographical location. Recent or ongoing stressors can impact an individual's ability and capacity to handle the unique challenges encountered during any phase of deployment.

Social factors include family members' military backgrounds (e.g., "military brats" versus "married into the military"), length of relationship/marriage, foreign spouse, age and developmental stage of children, dependent employment status (i.e., unemployed, part-time, full-time), health and special needs, available support resources and networks, dysfunctional relationships, past deployment experiences and attitudes, and pets. Broader social elements such as community support, national will, and popular opinion may also influence the deployment experience.

Examples of occupational factors include service-specific community and culture, member's rank, role and specialty, the deploying unit's mission and training, deployment frequency, each deployment's length and location, and command support and communication.

Inestimable combinations of vast and varied factors ultimately determine the quality of a deployment experience. Any mental health provider privileged to work with military members and their family would be better suited in that role to realize the diverse nature of deployment experiences. The provider's efforts and ability to appreciate the wide-ranging factors that influence each stage of deployment will foster identification of potential acute- and long-term consequences, and better guide interventions for timely definitive care. This chapter's reflection on experiences across the three stages of deployment includes illustrative vignettes with follow-on discussions. The intent of this chapter is to help mental health providers better understand and relate to the deployed population and their family members, thereby enhancing rapport and the provision of therapeutic services.

Pre-deployment Stage

I knew that I would deploy at some point during my career but it still felt surreal when I received orders for my first tour in Iraq. I had checked in to my unit shortly after its return from the last deployment. Everyone knew it was only a matter of time before the unit would be up for its next rotation to "the sandbox." The unit's state-side time was really spent training for that next deployment.

I had been married to Lee for eight years and we often discussed what my first deployment would be like for the family. Our children were too young to understand any talk of a deployment so Lee and I mostly discussed that privately. After getting my orders, we occasionally mentioned to the kids I would be going away for a while like some of the other Army parents. We were careful to say I was going to help others and I'd be back before Christmas. We tried to put a positive spin on things. Lee would describe me as a hero-of-sorts to them, promising that I would come back as soon as possible.

Now and then the children would ask questions that seemed silly or sad—"Can we go with Daddy?" "Will Daddy die?" "Will you bring me back a toy?" The whole concept may have been too abstract for them. They usually got bored with our answers and would change the topic to more important matters, like their favorite cartoons and games.

As the departure date got closer, I wondered more and more how I would bear the deployment and being away from my family for so long. Part of me hoped I would handle it in stride and be excited about the opportunity to serve my country. But another part of me secretly wished I would never have to leave my family. I felt ashamed every time I indulged in that fantasy, like I was fraud to wear the uniform. It didn't help when Lee openly yearned for the same. I really did want to prove my worth to my unit and nation. (Army Captain)

There is an Emotional Cycle of Deployment (ECOD) experienced by military families across the stages of deployment that was originally described by Kathleen Logan in her article published in the February 1987 edition of Proceedings—a monthly magazine by the U.S. Naval Institute that is one of the oldest running magazine publications in the United States [3]. While noting there exist concurrent cycles of cognitive, physical, behavioral and existential changes throughout the deployment phases which are highlighted in part throughout this chapter, the ECOD serves as a relevant means to frame understanding of the broader aspects of deployment. Originally developed for Navy spouses, the ECOD has been utilized by other military branches, governmental agencies, and several allied nations. The ECOD has demonstrated applicability not only for military spouses but deployed members as well. It is a multi-stage model defined by stage-specific emotional phenomena. Its stages include: Anticipation of Loss; Detachment and Withdrawal; Emotional Disorganization; Recovery and Stabilization; Anticipation of Homecoming; Renegotiation of the Marriage Contract; and Reintegration and Stabilization. The first couple ECOD stages—Anticipation of Loss, and Detachment and Withdrawal—occur during pre-deployment. Anticipation of Loss may begin when deployment orders arrive, which may be months in advance of the actual deployment, but is more pronounced in the 4–6 week time frame before actual departure. During this stage, the military family encounters a wide array of emotions along with denial and anxiety. The stress of the unknown may exacerbate feelings of helplessness and frustration. Tensions increase within the family and home environment as members deal with new responsibilities and projects to prepare for the deployment. Irritability, agitation, sadness and other symptoms may manifest, along with guilt that stems from either a sense of helplessness or self-attribution for the family's current hardships.

During the pre-deployment stage, military families face an ever-growing list of tasks with ever-less time to complete them. The service member must see to preparation of Family Care Plans, legal documents (e.g., Power of Attorney), procuring necessary gear and uniforms for the deployment, taking care of pre-deployment physical examinations and vaccinations, and other needs. Training requirements entail longer work-hours and even periods of separation before the actual departure. Prepared families will anticipate what responsibilities the family members will need to assume but may have never handled before, such as filing taxes, house payments, assorted bills, car maintenance, work and school obligations.

In the final days leading up to the deployment, the family will experience the ECOD stage of Detachment and Withdrawal. There are moments during this time frame that typify the "hurry up and wait" experience which is a too-common fact of military life. Family time together becomes limited and various types of fatigue (i.e., physical, mental, emotional, spiritual) from preparation for the deployment takes a toll. Emotional distance increases between the member and family. Intimacy can be affected and couples may feel ambivalent about sexual relations. It becomes difficult for couples to maintain intimacy as they subconsciously separate on an emotional level to handle the eventual physical separation. For sensitive individuals, this may be interpreted as rejection which adds to emotional turmoil. There is also the commonly described phenomenon of "the fight before the night" the service member deploys. Such instances of functional arguments may superficially make the early separation seem more tolerable but significant discord may have lingering consequences with negative effects. In particularly vulnerable relationships, a hurtful argument on the eve of separation may foster uneasiness or suspicions of infidelity. The last days before the deployment are commonly described as the most difficult.

Compared to "deployment-naive" families, those who have experienced previous deployments or come from a military upbringing (e.g., "military brats") may possess more resiliency and emotional readiness to handle pre-deployment stressors. Practical readiness is also a consideration. Whether noting the member's personal preparation, family arrangements, the unit's mission readiness (i.e., training, supplies, et cetera), or other factors critical to deployment, how well these tasks are accomplished can affect the manner in which this stage is experienced. Poor stress tolerance, financial concerns, relational discord, pregnancy, pending divorce, job dissatisfaction, special family needs, and other items can complicate the pre-deployment stage. In turn, there may be subsequent lasting effects upon the actual deployment and its aftermath.

An individual's mindset and attitude can determine how the deployment stages are ultimately experienced. Is the deployment seen as an opportunity to embrace challenge and achieve growth? Is it something that is dreaded? A positive attitude and realistic outlook during the pre-deployment phase portends a better deployment experience.

Deployment Stage

This was my third cruise, my second aboard "Abe" (USS Abraham Lincoln). Before we left port, my wife Darlene threw a huge going away party. She got a taco truck, bouncy castle, and a bunch of other fun things. We live in enlisted housing and all the neighbors came by ... probably for the free food more than to say goodbye, right? The event was fun but we could have used that money towards a second car.

Two months into my deployment, I received some emails from friends back home saying Darlene was going out to bars and clubs. Another Sailor that lived on our street was seen spending time at our house. I checked in with our babysitter and learned that the babysitter was watching our kids almost every Friday and Saturday night. The babysitter told me that she ended up staying overnight on a few occasions because Darlene didn't make it back until the next morning. The babysitter didn't mind though because Darlene always apologized and paid her extra.

> *That news was a punch to the heart. I was already trying to deal with my dumbass Chief who had it out for me. He told me I had to stand watch during our next port visit, which was going to be Singapore. I had always wanted to see Singapore but Chief screwed me out of that. I was hoping to buy some local treats to send back home to my kids. On top of that, I work in the Engineering Department. We drill all the time and work insane hours trying to keep systems up.*
>
> *When I tried to confront Darlene to find out what the hell was going on, she started crying and hung up on me. After that, I wasn't able to reach her again. I sent tons of emails and letters but ... nothing. She would never answer when I called the house. I didn't know if my kids got any of the letters I sent them. I couldn't get anywhere with my friends back home. How was I supposed to do my job with all that crap going on? (Navy Petty Officer Second Class)*

The actual deployment is overlapped by the next three stages of the ECOD: Emotional Disorganization; Recovery and Stabilization; and Anticipation of Homecoming. Emotional Disorganization may last for up to 6 weeks following the member's departure. The military member may arrive to a new and uncertain environment fraught with stressors and experiences previously never encountered. Some of the most challenging, and dangerous, times during a deployment are the first and last months when individual and unit vulnerabilities are more salient during transitional phases. Adapting to new roles and routines in a demanding setting can be overwhelming until familiarity and confidence attenuate the natural stress. Family members face the void left in the member's absence with a sense of uncertainty and perhaps aimlessness. Common experiences include problems with sleep, indecisiveness, feelings of resentment, confusion, and fears of infidelity. Depending on the family situation and its members, there may be difficulty moving past the Emotional Disorganization stage.

Successful mastery of Emotional Disorganization though permits advancement to Recovery and Stabilization. As new routines are established and people adapt to the responsibilities and demands of the deployment, a sense of independence is gained that is coupled with confidence in one's ability to function amidst many challenges. Determination and morale improve with each challenge successfully handled. That sense of accomplishment increases personal pride and independence.

For the service member, the deployment is a profound experience that is challenging to prepare for sans any previous deployments. Each day brings reminders of sacrificed freedoms and comforts many civilians take for granted. Daily attire is largely limited to prescribed uniforms. Individual expression afforded by personal wardrobes, accessories, and make-up are restricted. Outside of duty hours, members may be limited to regulation physical training ("PT") clothing for comfort attire. Amenities, conveniences, and choices are narrowed under the reality of the situation—military bases and ships do not have capacity to provide expansive choices for dining, shopping, and recreation. Food choices are limited to whatever is on the menu at the base dining facility or ship's galley, available for purchase at the local exchange (military store), or whichever Meal Ready to Eat (MRE) was acquired. Deployed troops have relied on MREs for daily nutrition for extended periods of time. Although creative "field chefs" may find ways to make MREs more palatable when no other food options are available, to live off of MREs more than a day is a stressor in itself.

Environmental stressors include exposure to harsh weather conditions, temperature extremes, noises, smells, predatory bugs and animals, and other difficulties. Whether exposed to an oppressive desert sun or biting cold winds, suffocating sand storms or stinging winter rains, physical and mental endurance are drained. Continuous noise from weapons, machinery, vehicles, and public address system announcements, invade all aspects of living. Smells common to military sites like fuels, oil, paints, propellants, and expended ammunitions, follow a person throughout the deployment and permeate their hair, skin, and attire. There is poor escape from pungent smells on deployment, unlike back home where one can return to living spaces with more pleasant aromas from air freshener products, scented candles, fresh flowers, and home cooking. The chemical or industrial smells that fill ship spaces may sometimes seem suffocating and can drown out any smell of the saltwater outside. The recycled air in a submarine has a piquant scent of its own. Acrid smells not usually encountered back home are particularly striking, such as the fetid stench of third-world sewage, burning of waste and feces, or even the peculiar stink of death. Memories are strongly tied to the olfactory senses and certain smells may cause aversive memories and emotions to surface. Conversely, particular smells that pervade a person's time in service may trigger pleasant nostalgia. It is not uncommon for active-duty members and veterans to happen upon a whiff of gunpowder, jet fuel, saltwater or such, and enjoy a pleasurable remembrance.

Long hours and the repetition of mundane duty schedules strain a member's ability to maintain focus and motivation. Privacy and personal space are lost when living in cramped tents, barracks and ship berthing. There is no proper escape from work or peers (including any antagonists) after finishing a duty shift. A sense of confinement abounds when daily life and any free time are limited to only the base (i.e., living "inside the wire") or aboard a ship at sea. Hygiene becomes a luxury when time or access to shower facilities is not readily available. When showers are not accessible or the ship's water systems are down, "baby wipe" products may be the best alternative.

Communication and entertainment resources are limited which can add to frustration and a sense of helplessness or hopelessness. Any member who has ever had a phone call or video-chat session interrupted by communications going down will attest to the severe irritation they suffered. Periods of restricted communication are a loathed, but often necessary, fact of deployment. Many families have shared the experience of talking with the deployed member only to hear an alarm or commotion in the background, followed by an abrupt break in communication. Stranded with no understanding of what happened, the family's stress increases as minutes, hours, or even days go by before they are able to next speak with the deployed member. The unknown is peppered with catastrophic thoughts, which leads to miserable dread until the family can ultimately confirm their loved one is okay.

On deployment, exposure to danger and trauma is a fact of life. Working in perilous conditions is a daily hazard—be it combat, carrier flight deck operations, heavy machinery and military vehicles, or other threats. Risk of infection, accidents, injury, and death are increased by fatigue from stress and difficulty maintaining optimal hygiene, nutrition, hydration and sleep. Acute and lasting consequences can stem from traumatic exposures to combat, casualties, disaster sites, and other horrors many civilians may never experience nor understand. A deployed member may witness first-hand injuries, gore and death. Seeing casualties of war and disaster that involve women, children, and animals can be especially traumatic. Of note, deployed military medical personnel may be more affected by exposure to high-magnitude medical stressors than combat stressors [4]. The habitants of other countries may demonstrate their enmity towards outside forces with protests, sabotage, and actual violence. Members may face their own mortality during deployment. They may also be confronted with unpleasant truths about the realities of life and left with a sense of institutional betrayal.

On the home front, the family deals with daily reminders of their deployed member's absence. A partner's bed may seem empty or too big, mail arrives with the deployed member's name, the member's car remains where last parked. The partner becomes a single parent-of-sorts who must not only find a way to cope with their own anxiety and sadness but also maintain an outward appearance of "happy stoicism" for the children. Partners often find themselves doing the same during communication with the military member, lest any hint of struggle add further strain upon the deployed loved one who may be overstressed and unable to help from afar. Depending on the family, the children may thrive or suffer with a parent away on deployment. Recent studies demonstrated that older children experienced a greater number of problems during a deployment, and girls reported having more challenges than boys [5]. The at-home parent must find a way to help those who are struggling without the immediate or full support of the deployed member. One of the most distressing circumstances is that of a first-time mother handling pregnancy, birth, and early motherhood without her loved one present to share the experience and provide support. Pets may be confused by the member's absence and exhibit new behaviors. The family may encounter a sense of vulnerability without the member around for reassurance or security (e.g., unexpected nighttime noises seem more sinister). Dealing with limited information and updates from the member's command is challenging, especially when exposed to media and rumors that convey vexing news. Coping with responsibilities that the deployed member previously managed (e.g., taxes, bills) and handling unanticipated emergencies can be overwhelming. However, each issue mastered can lead to personal accomplishment and self-growth.

The next ECOD stage—Anticipation of Return—occurs during the 6 weeks antecedent to the member's return. This is usually a positive time in which service members and their family members look forward to the reunion. A metaphorical finish line is in sight and individuals feel invigorated with optimism for the future. Along with a sense of renewed energy and spirit, there may also be apprehension. Planning and efforts begin for families to make room for each other in their lives again. This may lead to tension and anxiety over what roles and responsibilities may be sacrificed upon the reunion. There is worry about whether others can accept certain changes that have occurred during their time apart, not only in routines and lifestyle but in the individuals themselves. As these concerns persist amongst preparations for an ideal homecoming, individuals may feel overwhelmed and restless.

The overall stage of deployment and how it is experienced emotionally may be affected by the family's location and circumstance. National Guard or Reserve members typically have part-time commitments to military service and the members with their families may live away from regions with military communities and resources. These families may be unfamiliar with military support systems and have difficulty accessing such. This may occur with active-duty military families as well (e.g., those that reside away from military bases and communities). A family stationed in a foreign country, living off-base and apart from other military families, may feel estranged and unsupported during a deployment. Overseas families may not have the social support that extended family could provide more readily stateside. It is not uncommon for extended family to help affected relatives during a deployment; in some circumstances, relatives may even serve as "proxy parents" [6].

Communication during deployment is an important factor to consider. Although it is beneficial when there is ready communication, it is also stressful when communication is compromised. Today's deployed population enjoys better communication resources than any other time in history; via hand-written letters, telephone calls, emails, text messages, video-chat with webcams, et cetera. Communication is an important protective factor across all stages of deployment when families are able to develop positive communication skills that are consistently applied [7]. Convenient communications may help individuals manage the challenges of deployment and separation, but communications can also have a negative impact. Aside from any disquiet due to discussion of stressful topics or sensitive matters, the frequency of communication (too little, too much) may also lead to tension or distress [8].

There are positive consequences for those able to manage deployment stressors which include increased family bonding, autonomy, self-worth, skills, maturity, and resiliency. For those unable to handle deployment in a mature and healthy manner, there may negative consequences like infidelity, personal or professional misconduct, financial troubles, family dysfunction, and other dilemmas.

Extended families, friends, and other acquaintances of the deployed population may have difficulty understanding the stressors the military family has faced. They may also have trouble discerning or accepting any changes in the military family's members. Contrarily, the deployed population may feel annoyed when those without similar experience act as though they fully understand and can directly relate to them.

Post-deployment Stage

After Anthony went to Iraq, our seven year-old son spent the first couple weeks mostly under his bed. I remember lifting up the bed skirt to slide him snacks. I would read him stories while I lied there on the bedroom floor. Our six year-old daughter seemed to handle things better but sometimes I would find her favorite stuffed toy damp from tears she was hiding.

It was hard to wear a smile around our children when I was going through a box of Kleenex almost every day and crying myself to sleep most nights. Things got a bit better once I was able to hear his voice again on the phone. Our time apart was tough but we made it through. Any time I felt overwhelmed and was ready to fall apart, I thought of how tough things probably were for Anthony. I knew I had to be strong not only for the children, but for Anthony as well.

The toughest part was the last couple months before his return. We had reached the halfway point a month or so earlier and the daily countdown to Anthony's return was in the double-digits. It seemed like the clock was moving slower and the days were getting longer. I came up with a plan for fun activities to help us pass the time. The kids and I worked on a big banner and posters to welcome Daddy home. Our son had been through a difficult time with Daddy away and had become withdrawn and quiet. However, reunion preparations seemed to bring the boy I once knew back to us. Seeing him smile again and play with his sister made those final weeks much easier.

I can't describe how it felt when the day finally came and we met Anthony at the airport. I tried to look my best for him but I couldn't stop happy tears from ruining my make-up. I must have seemed such a selfish mother leaving the children standing to the side when I ran into his arms. I don't think the kids were bothered because they were all smiles when we had our first big family hug there. That moment was simply wonderful.

Although it was great having our Anthony home again, it was also awkward in some weird ways. Not in a bad sense. We just had to get used to being a whole family again. (Marine Spouse)

After reaching the post-deployment stage when the service member has redeployed to their home duty station and reunited with family members, the family will experience the final stages of the ECOD: Renegotiation of the Marriage Contract; and Reintegration and Stabilization. Renegotiation of the Marriage Contract typically spans the first 6 weeks following the family's reunion. Changes in the deployed individual and their family members may be welcomed or possibly lead to conflict. Although the family is reunited physically, there may linger an emotional distance until they have had adequate time and opportunity to reconnect, share their experiences, and get to know each other once more. Family members may worry that new roles and routines established during the deployment may be undone. They may also feel any independence gained could be threatened by a return to the pre-deployment family hierarchy and practices. Service members may feel less-valued as other family assumed former responsibilities during their absence. Intimacy can seem awkward until sufficient time together permits healthy renewed acquaintance. Prominent changes that occurred during deployment, such as significant trauma exposure (perhaps with medical/psychiatric sequelae), birth of a child, and other critical events, may permanently alter family roles and dynamics.

There may be a feeling of overstimulation for the member during the first week or two upon return. Coming back from a deployed daily life visually defined by particular palettes such as desert browns or ocean blues, to days again filled with a brighter and broader spectrum of colors, may be pleasant but likewise stunning at first. After living with limited selections in consumer products, clothing, entertainment and activities, the member faces an abundance of options once more. Many troops relish having access anew to ample television channels, especially after months of maybe only eight channels provided via the Armed Forces Network

(AFN). Returned troops often experience initial difficulty sleeping in a more comfortable bed and without the "white noise" of the deployed setting. Some couples may struggle adjusting to a shared bed once again.

For the deployed member who was living in more primal environments, uncensored language was likely the norm and that way of life was often defined by action before words. Returning home means relearning etiquette, unwritten social norms and using words before actions as appropriate. During the initial weeks or months of the reunion, family members may see the member as surly, prone to profanity, seeming distant, and self-absorbed in pastimes like violent video games or "adrenaline activities;" possibly forfeiting time that could otherwise be spent with loved ones.

Members may experience paradigm shifts during deployment and return with broadened worldviews. Their first-hand exposure to life beyond America and any potent personal experiences may lead to existential crises, shifts in self-identity, and disillusionment with previous values and perspectives (i.e., community, religious, political, et cetera). Large-scale disasters and mass casualties are rarer occurrences in America but exist as a common fact in many other regions. Deployments often take military members to impoverished countries with little-to-nil infrastructure and resources which are exposed to frequent natural disasters, incessant conflict and other tumultuous events. The underside of global reality that was otherwise camouflaged by first-world distractions or only experienced vicariously through media then becomes a part of the deployed member's life. The consequences of those experiences will ultimately depend upon the individual.

As the reunited family moves into the next ECOD stage—Reintegration and Stabilization—the process of readjusting to the member's return continues for everyone. This process commonly lasts up to 6 months or more. During that time frame, a new baseline is established as the family becomes more secure and accepting of altered roles and routines. A healthy reintegration is evidenced by a shift in family language from personal to plural possessive adjectives and pronouns (i.e., from "my …" and "mine," to "our …" and "ours").

There are positive consequences of deployment (acute- and long-term) that include increased family closeness, improved resiliency, occupational advancement, and financial gain (associated with special duty pay/allowances). There are also potential negative consequences that include separation/divorce, inability to adjust to new roles or changes, and occupational discord. Family members may inadvertently engage in a "Who Had It Worst?" competition that can harm relationships. Also, the member and the spouse may both assert personal entitlement to respite after the deployment and inability to reach a compromise may lead to toxic discord.

Each deployment experience and the culmination of such will in kind influence how future deployments are experienced and whether the sum effects upon the family as a whole, and each member, are considered helpful or hurtful. While some service members and military families may speak negatively of deployment experiences or self-portray as victims-of-sorts, others may describe their experiences in positive terms that reflect their sense of duty, pride, and accomplishment [9]. Many experienced service members in the midst of their military careers may never fully reconnect with their families. The motive for such a schism may be consciously, or unconsciously, derived from a notion that the service member will be separated again from their family anyways. This type of behavior is a detrimental risk to the family's overall dynamic and welfare.

In summary, this chapter was intended to enlighten the reader to the countless factors and considerations that confound offering a simple illustration of the deployment experience. In discussing pre-deployment, deployment, and post-deployment in association with the ECOD, the common phenomena encountered across the three stages were highlighted to help the reader better anticipate the stressors and process of adjustment. These discussion points may also bolster the reader's ability to anticipate possible problems that a service member and family members may encounter. For providers working with military members and families, this information should be applied to their assessment and understanding of patient cases to afford more comprehensive and individualized care. Coupled with sincere respect, professional modesty, and a genuine interest in each individual and family's circumstance, the provider can use the information in this chapter to optimize rapport and therapeutic services for any patients with deployment experience.

References

1. Wenger JW, O'Connell C, Cottrell L. Examination of recent deployment experience across the services and components. Santa Monica, CA: RAND Corporation; 2018. https://www.rand.org/pubs/research_reports/RR1928.html.
2. U.S. Department of Defense (DoD). 2017 Demographics profile of the military community. Arlington, VA: Office of the Deputy Assistant Secretary of Defense for Military Community and Family Policy (ODASD(MC&FP)); 2017. https://download.militaryonesource.mil/12038/MOS/Reports/2017-demographics-report.pdf.
3. Logan KV. The emotional cycle of deployment. Proceedings. 1987;113(2):1008.
4. Peterson AL, Baker MT, Moore BA, et al. Deployed military medical personnel: impact of combat and healthcare trauma exposure. Mil Med. 2018;184(1):e133–43.
5. Chandra A, Lara-Cinisomo S, Jaycox LH, et al. Children on the homefront: the experiences of children from military families. Pediatrics. 2010;25(1):13–25.
6. Huebner AJ, Mancini JA, Wade KE, et al. Resilience and vulnerability: the deployment experiences of youth in military families. 2010. https://www.researchgate.net/publication/228534218_Resilience_and_vulnerability_The_deployment_experiences_of_youth_in_military_families.
7. Creech SK, Hadley W, Borsari B. The impact of military deployment and reintegration on children and parenting: a systematic review. Prof Psychol Res Pr. 2014;45(6):452–64.
8. Houston JB, Pfefferbaum B, Sherman MD, et al. Family communication across the military deployment experience: child and spouse report of communication frequency and quality and associated emotions, behaviors, and reactions. J Loss Trauma Int Perspect Stress Coping. 2012;18(2):103–19.
9. O'Neal CW, Lucier-Greer M, Duncan JM, et al. Vulnerability and resilience within military families: deployment experiences, reintegration, and family functioning. J Child Fam Stud. 2018;27(2):3250–61.

6 Understanding the Experience and Mental Health Challenges of National Guard and Reserve Service Members

Sara Kintzle, Justin Jaesung Lee, and Airy Ramirez

Vignette: David

David is a 26-year-old male Corporal in the Marine Reserves who is 3 months post a 7-month deployment to Kuwait. Along with his service in the Marines, David works as an assistant manager at a sporting goods store. David is married to Maddie, who is 23-years old and works as a nursing assistant. The couple has been struggling to adjust after David's return. David blames these issues on his difficulty at work. He has reported reduced hours and responsibilities since his return, as well as the denial of an expected promotion to manager. These changes are frustrating for David as he feels it is a direct result of his time away. The reduced hours have also caused financial strain as the couple is no longer receiving the active duty pay earned during David's deployment.

Maddie feels there is more going on beyond the work and financial stress. She has noticed David having a shorter temper than usual and that he doesn't discuss his feelings about his deployment or return with Maddie. She was surprised David didn't receive much in terms of reintegration support from the Marines. She has encouraged David to spend time with their friends and family but he has resisted, saying he just doesn't feel like it. Maddie suggested throwing a barbeque for his Reserve buddies who he deployed with, but realized the distance between them would make such an event difficult. When she confronts David about how he is feeling, he responds that she doesn't understand, that no one does.

David hasn't shared much of what he is struggling with since his return from deployment. He feels a bit like a stranger in his own life. Just 3 months ago he was

S. Kintzle (✉) · J. J. Lee
University of Southern California, Los Angeles, CA, USA
e-mail: kintzle@usc.edu

A. Ramirez
California Army National Guard, Los Angeles, CA, USA

C. H. Warner, C. A. Castro (eds.), *Veteran and Military Mental Health*,
https://doi.org/10.1007/978-3-031-18009-5_6

serving his country in Kuwait, and now he's back like nothing has changed. David knows his deployment has changed him, but has resisted taking the time to understand and process that change. He wasn't prepared for these feelings and is having trouble finding his way back. David also feels guilty for having these difficulties. He knows Marines who deployed to more dangerous places who experienced severe injuries and losses in their unit. Although stressful, David's unit deployed without any major incidents. He doesn't understand why he can't adjust back and feels weak for not being able to do so.

When Maddie finally suggested counseling, it took time to get David on board as he was worried about how getting help might impact his career in the Marines. He didn't want people to know he was getting help. It also took time to find someone who could help. David's insurance switched back to TRICARE after his deployment, and Maddie struggled finding a provider in their city. The first provider she called didn't seem to know much about the military or the experience of a Reservist. Maddie knew that would be a red flag for David. After a continued search, she found a suitable provider and booked an appointment.

Introduction to National Guard and Reserve Service Members

The National Guard and Reserve are unique components of the U.S. military. The National Guard (NG) is an element of the U.S military that consists of the Army National Guard and the Air Force's Air National Guard. Composed of civilians who joined the military to primarily serve in part-time roles, the NG has a home in each state in the U.S and the following territories: District of Columbia (DC), Guam, Virgin Islands, and Puerto Rico. The NG serves a unique dual role by standing ready to be activated by the President of the United States or mobilized by state governors through their state Adjutant Generals [1]. On the other hand, the U.S Military's Reservists are divided by each branch of the military. The Reserve's purpose is to train and maintain reservist service members that are qualified and ready to support the active duty units and their efforts [2]. The most common responsibility of the Reserves is to fill in for stateside active duty units when they are deployed overseas. Similar to the NG, the majority of the Reserves are in uniform part-time but can be activated to serve either stateside or internationally on full-time status.

Throughout literature and research, it is not uncommon to observe a discrepancy in the language used to refer to NG and Reserve service members. Often, "National Guard" and "Reserve" are used interchangeably, leading to a confusion and blending of the two components. While the distinction between the two components may be evident for service members, it can add to the already confusing terminology for civilians working with service members. The NG and Reserves together form the "Reserve component (RC)" [3]. The RC is comprised of the Army National Guard, Air National Guard, Army Reserve, Air Force Reserve, Navy Reserve, Marine Corps Reserve, and Coast Guard Reserves. Together, the collective seven components have supported and stood beside their active duty counterparts, representing 38% of the total United States Armed Forces [4]. With all five military branches possessing a reserve force, training and operations are often conducted at major military installations, joint Reserve bases, airfields, armories, and Reserve centers within the U.S and across the Nation [5]. Professionals that work with service members within the RC need to be competent not only on the overall military culture as a whole, but also the unique subcultures, languages, and operational structures within the seven components.

As of 2019 more than 800,000 selected RC members make up the NG/Reserves, with approximately 440,000 in the NG and 360,000 in the Reserves [6]. Of the seven components of the selected reserve, the Army National Guard and Army Reserve are responsible for roughly 65% of the entire force. Similar to the active duty component, the selected reserve consists of 83.5% enlisted and 16.5% officers [7]. Although the gender representation in the military has steadily increased towards a more diverse force, the selected reserve members are predominantly 80% male and 20% female. Racial and ethnic minorities are not evenly represented across the military as racial minorities makes up 26.4% of this component, with the remaining 73.6% being white. Whereas nearly 90% of officers have obtained a bachelor's degree or higher, only 12% of the enlisted possessed at least a bachelor's degree. While 81% of the selected reserve members are age 40 years or younger and 19% are age 41 years or older, only 43.7% are reported as being married.

In the NG/Reserves, service members typically sign contracts to perform inactive duty for training (drill) for a weekend each month and 2 weeks of active duty training (annual training) [8]. It is important to note however, that the commitment to NG/R often goes beyond the drill and 2 weeks training initially outlined. Weekend drill can turn into 4 days due to extra training, members may be called to drill two weekends in a row, or be required to attend extra weeklong training. The RC does produce Active Guard Reservists (AGR) that serve full-time while enjoying the same pay and benefits as active duty members. On top of fulfilling the original duties one weekend a month and 2 extended weeks as selected reserve members, AGRs fill critical billets within NG and Reserve units that require full-time staff to adequately support the ongoing missions and tasks at hand. As a result, many AGRs often find themselves working longer hours and having more responsibilities than their active duty counterparts. AGR positions are slotted as commitments that can last from 180 days up to 3 years and are exclusive to the Army National Guard, Army Reserve, Air National Guard, and Air Force Reserve [9]. A key difference however between AGRs in the National Guard and the Reserves is that an AGR in the NG will generally be stationed in their home state in which they are serving whereas an AGR in the Reserves will be subject to possibly being stationed to an entirely different state or country.

Service members in the NG/R can be activated to full-time status through two different U.S. Codes: Title 10 and Title 32 [10]. Title 10 orders are issued by the President or Secretary of Defense and obligate service members to full-time duty to primarily support federal missions. Title 32 orders on the other hand, allow governors of each state to activate their service members and still have jurisdiction over them as they are mobilized within their home states to respond to emergencies. While some activations onto full-time status can involve deployments overseas for combat missions and humanitarian missions, examples of stateside activations include natural disaster support, counterdrug efforts, or civil disturbances. As these two types of orders simply require activation periods that are 30 days or longer, the duration as to how long the service members are mobilized can vary. It is important to note that while activated on federally funded, the selected reserve members receive or can accrue the exact benefits that active duty members do such as tuition assistance and full health care coverage [11].

The RCs role and involvement have dramatically shifted and intensified since the attacks on September 11, 2001. Immediately after the attacks, the U.S. government at the time launched a campaign called the Global War on Terrorism which has heavily impacted the NG/R and their roles the past two decades. NG/R have since been activated and deployed in unprecedented numbers and they continue to serve as key components of the total forces overseas [12]. Many NG/R members have found themselves activating more than once in order to meet wartime demands. Although the military initially found justification in the increased activations of the RC in support of overseas missions, the frequency of deployments eventually became a large concern. Whenever NG/R members deployed, their families and full-time employers were heavily impacted and affected the members' willingness to continue serving beyond their original obligations [13]. Secondly, leadership within the military quickly identified that a large proportion of reserve units were underprepared and needed additional substantial training to effectively work alongside their active duty counterparts.

While there was overall roughly 150,000 service members deployed to Iraq during the beginning years of the Global War on Terrorism in 2004, there is less than 5000 maintaining a presence in the same country today [14]. Despite the RC members' large reductions to those deployment numbers over the past few years, the rate as to which they are being activated and mobilized domestically continue to maintain volatile and high levels. In 2020 and 2021, over 50,000 NG/R members were activated across the nation to respond to the COVID-19 pandemic and support efforts in combating and mitigating its devastating impact [15]. Prior to addressing the COVID-19 pandemic, many RC members were mobilized to fight ravaging fires in the west coast and will continue to be relied on whenever natural disasters impact the nation. Most recently, many U.S. governors activated their states' NGs to ramp up security at their state capitols after the U.S. Capitol was attacked on January 6, 2021 [16]. While federal mobilizations for overseas support have decreased, this federal and state reliance on NG continues to increase.

Unique Features of NG/R Service Members

In order for practitioners to understand the vulnerabilities to challenges NG/R may face, it is important to recognize their unique experience. The most distinctive feature of NG/R are their dual roles as civilians and service members. Unlike their active duty counterparts, NG/R have civilian jobs and live in civilian communities. The service member uniform comes on and off, requiring NG/R to balance life between two very different worlds, while at the same time being prepared to be quickly activated or deployed in times of need. This duality creates unique occupational stress for NG/R members. Challenges include difficulty finding and sustaining employment and stress on relationships with employers, finding understanding within a civilian community, access to competent care, frequent disruptions to civilian life, and added stress on the family, who unlike active duty families are not part of the military community their loved one serves in. These stressors have become more prevalent as the military commitments required of NG/R have increased.

NG and Reserve service members wear the same uniform and comply to the same rank and pay structure [17]. When conducting training, members of the RC often train with units that are established within their own communities. However, if availability is limited, it is not uncommon for service members to require driving several hours to their training locations. This is a significant cultural and geographical counter experience than an active duty service member who lives on or significantly near military posts or installations [18]. Additionally, whereas active duty service members are reassigned to a new duty station every 3–5 years, NG and Reserve members take a more active role in choosing their duty stations, electing to be chosen by units 50, 75, 100 or more miles away from their home of record.

It is a common misconception that NG and Reserve service members rarely deploy or deploy less often than active duty components. While the RC typically spend less time engaging in military training and service, they are eligible for deployment, representing one third of all deployed personnel [4]. It is now common practice that the RC receive more notice prior to being mobilized, which allows them to get their personal and professional lives in order [3]. Previous policy did not require a time limit of which to give notice and thus lead to various issues with pre-deployment and re-integration adjustment. There are several challenges that the RC faces during a deployment, especially in comparison to active service members. Members of the RC are not accustomed to being engulfed into the military lifestyle on a full-time basis and are much less likely to access or accept aid from support programs and mental health services [4, 18]. Family members of reserve families are often geographically isolated from their duty stations, leading to a discrepancy in the access of social support and mental health resources during a deployment. This could contribute to the difficulty in reintegrating that NG and Reserve service members have with their families and civilian lives upon return. Whereas active-duty service members return to their full-time military jobs and a military community that understands the unique challenges service in the military may create, service members within the RC return to their civilian lives, civilian jobs, civilian community and part-time military careers.

While there are legal implications for civilian employers who choose to reprimand or discriminate against deploying service members, these laws are filled with loopholes and there are still many issues with income loss during the service member's deployment and financial issues upon resuming their civilian jobs post deployment. This is additionally informed by the unstable schedules of part-time service members that come with activations, drill, trainings, military schools, and mobilizations. Thus, it is not uncommon to see an inconsistency or a reduction of work hours assigned prior to deployment, and a difficult reintegration process for the service member at their civilian jobs as employers value consistency. This can lead to a loss of income, increased economic instability, and distress about finding a new job. Thus, it comes to no surprise that young NG and Reserve service members are more likely to be unemployed than civilians of the same age [3]. This is further exacerbated by the fact that employers who hire veterans are eligible for the Work Opportunity Tax Credit (WOTC) [19]. This is not applicable for hiring Guardsmen that have not been deployed, regardless of their participation in state emergencies or 2-week training deployments.

NG components alone represent the world's 11th largest army and fifth largest Air Force [20]. On average, NG service members are older and more likely to have a family than active duty service members [21]. This can have implications for how professionals understand, prepare, and implement interventions that are appropriate to the service member. Understanding the culture and environment in which they are submerged and how it can be affected by the service members age, identity, culture, and beliefs can be essential to better understand the service member's influences, and stressors.

The NG is well regarded as a community-based organization that primarily serves local communities and its respective states [22]. Though it responds when called to action on a global level, its main focus remains domestic, integrated within their respective communities and in close relationship with civilian agencies, law enforcement, and other emergency responders due to its community-based knowledge and integration, geographically and financially [22]. Due to this unique relationship, communities more often identify with Guardsmen than any other component due to their accessibility. Most civilians never see an active duty service member in person, as they do the guardsmen that support their community in times of crisis and uncertainty.

The Reserves are commanded by the President to be mobilized for Federal missions of the Nation [18]. One of the biggest responsibilities of reservists is filling in for active duty positions in times of war or national emergencies, serving as drill sergeants, instructors, and security personnel [23]. This is a unique responsibility to Reserve service members, and as such, reservists often travel around the world more often than Guardsmen. Reservists have deployed to every major combat zone and fought in various wars such as WWI, WWII, the Cold War, the Korean War, the Vietnam War, and the Persian Gulf War [24]. Unlike the NG, Reservists do not have a state mission, and thus cannot be called to respond to state emergencies such as floods and hurricanes [25]. This leads to a different relationship and perceptions from community members towards reservists in comparison to Guardsmen.

The military culture as a whole is a strong dominating identity that can often feel more prominent among a service members many identities. Service members of different components become exposed to multiple subcultures based on their job, duty station, position, and even their disability status. Due to the dramatic differences among active duty and the RC's level of integration with the military lifestyle, there are cultural differences and perceptions that have often caused a divide. Although NG, Reserve, and active duty service members all receive the same initial training into the armed forces together, there is a long history of negative perceptions from the active components towards the RC [26]. This cultural divide can be dated back as far as the Vietnam War, where it is argued that the feud initially began [3]. During the Vietnam War, President Lyndon Johnson received advice from his joint Chiefs of staff to mobilize the RC, however his advice was ignored as the president refused to activate them. This led to the active component's negative perception and loss of respect for the RC, which was further exacerbated by the fact that young men began to join the NG and Reserves as a refuge from the War. Later during the Gulf War, many NG infantry units were not activated to assist in the fight. This caused the already existing friction to increase between the active component and the RC. Active-duty service members felt that guardsmen were "amateurs" and lazy [26]. As a result, the divide between the active-duty component and the RC has been measured in levels of readiness to deploy and commitment to the armed forces, all of which significantly influence the military subcultures and the service member's identities and their perception of self.

One of the most consequential differences between active duty and NG/R service members are the access to benefits after service. Benefit eligibility is a complex issue, what is important for practitioners to know is that NG/R veterans are not always eligible for the same benefits (e.g. healthcare, education, disability compensation, etc.) as their active duty counterparts. In general, the distinction in eligibility is defined by whether a NG/R service member served in a full-time capacity. For Reservists, this most often requires unit deployment. For the NG, this requires activation by the federal government. This could include a deployment or responding to national emergencies. NG service in response to activation by state Governors does not count towards benefit eligibility.

Mental Health Challenges of NG/R

Although the mental health experiences of service members and veterans are well documented within the literature, limited research explores mental health in those serving or with prior service in the NG/R. The following describes what we do know empirically about the mental health challenges of NG/R service members and veterans.

Deployment

The majority of the research that does exist on NG/R examines mental health challenges around combat and deployment, and were conducted at the height of NG/R deployments in the conflicts in Iraq and Afghanistan. In general, research has found NG/R service members to be vulnerable to mental health issues during and post deployment. These include posttraumatic stress disorder, depression, anxiety as well as issues that impact overall well-being such as increases in substance use, chronic pain, readjustment challenges, engagement in aggressive and risky behaviors, and relationship issues [27–29]. While mental health concerns have been reported in NG/R immediately following deployment, research has demonstrated significant increases in mental health challenges 3–6 months post return [27, 28]. This indicates the importance of assessing mental health status beyond the initial post deployment screen.

Some research has found NG/Rs to be at higher risk for mental health issues after deployment than their active duty counterparts [27]. While the literature on this comparison is mixed, what is important for practitioners to recognize is how the unique features of NG/R service may create vulnerability for challenges after deployment. The first factor is deployment preparedness. NG/R are often less prepared for the occupational stressors associated with deployment. Historically, NG/R receive less training than active duty military personnel. Additionally, information regarding upcoming deployments can be vague, with little certainty until close to the leave date. While active duty populations are prepared for this, NG/R have civilian obligations to sort out. Lower levels of deployment preparedness have been associated with increased likelihood of PTSD, depression, and drinking problems in NG/R [29].

A second unique factor related to NG/R vulnerability after deployment is their community. This is an important factor as research has found high perceived social support and having a large and diverse social network to be significantly associated with lower likelihood of mental health conditions in NG/R [30]. Unlike their active duty counterparts, NG and Reserve service members return to civilian communities. They are not embedded within a community and culture where people have had similar experiences and where there is a shared understanding of and support for readjustment needs. This dynamic creates many vulnerabilities for NG/R, including a sudden shift to civilian life, limited contact with the social network development during deployment, feelings of isolation, lack of access to military culturally competent care, and a lack of adjustment resources most often found on military installations. NG/R return home from mobilizations and deployments abruptly, often without the numerous support services (decompression, reintegration) provided by military installations. While some states have worked to provide resources, a nationally coordinated approach to demobilization for NG/R does not exist.

Finally, unlike active duty personnel, NG/R service members have civilian circumstances (family, jobs), that are less-suited for the prolonged absence of a deployment [31]. Most NG/R have civilian careers that may be severely impacted by a long absence. NG/R families have less support during deployments, are more isolated than active duty military families, and live in civilian communities with little understanding of military deployments. These issues can cause additional stress during and following deployments.

NG/R Suicide

While risk for suicide continues to be a major concern in all military and veteran populations, some recent reports have highlighted rates of suicide in NG members. The Defense Department Annual Suicide Report for calendar year 2018 showed rates of suicide to be the highest in the NG [32]. However, the 2019 report saw a significant decrease in the rates of suicide for NG service members [33] and found suicide to be most frequent in the active component. Generally, the RC has the lowest rates of suicide. While trends in rates may fluctuate, what practitioners must recognize is the unique stress NG/R may experience due to factors described above. In addition to what has been previously discussed, literature has described additional risk factors for suicide in NG/R. Financial stress and income instability can be contributors to depression and suicide ideation. It has been established that NG/R are often unemployed or underemployed, and experience employment difficulties related to their military service. Financial difficulties also can create barriers to receiving mental health care [34]. Barriers to mental health care, discussed in more detail below, also create risk for NG/R. Lastly, data has suggested that NG/R suicide is most likely to happen while members on are not on active duty. Unlike active duty service members, NG/R do not have frequent interactions with their military leaders and co-workers, thus limiting peer's ability to recognize behaviors that may indicate risk [34]. This lack of military community can also create isolation, an additional risk for suicide. Lastly, NG/R face challenges that are local to their own communities. This variability creates difficulty in developing service wide prevention and intervention strategies.

NG/R Mental Health Care Utilization

Although limited, research available suggest NG/R utilize mental health care at similar rates as active duty service members and report similar barriers (stigma, concern over career impact, difficulty scheduling and time off work, not knowing where to get help, handling issues on their own) [35, 36]. Kehle et al. [21] examined mental health care utilization in NG service members who spent 16 months in Iraq. Over half of service members who screened positive for a mental health problem were not engaged with mental health treatment. Authors found NG who had positive attitudes about mental health treatment, were injured during deployment, had an illness-based need, and received mental health treatment during deployment were more likely to have received treatment.

There are some mental health care barriers that are specific to the population of NG/R. While these service members are eligible for TRICARE insurance coverage, access and affordability remain concerns. TRICARE requires premiums, deductibles and cost shares when receiving care and finding mental health care providers who participate in the network can be challenging, particularly in rural areas [34]. Cost sharing for mental health services to out-of-network may be too expensive for many NG/R. These service members may also have challenges finding health care providers who are culturally competent in the experience of military populations. NG/R often report feeling civilian providers are not prepared to handle their concerns.

NG/R Mental Health Post Service

Those who previously served as NG/R service members are most often represented in the literature on mental health of veterans in general. It is hard to explore unique mental health challenges in NG/R veterans as most research doesn't separate results based on those who served active duty and those who served as NG/R. One study examining trends and risk factors for mental health diagnoses in Iraq and Afghanistan veterans utilizing VA healthcare from 2002 to 2008, found higher rates of PTSD, depression and all other mental health diagnoses in NG/R veterans seeking care when compared with active duty veterans [37]. In general, it is important for practitioners to recognize NG/R veterans are at risk for experiencing mental health issues post service. What may make NG/R particularly vulnerable to these challenges are the access to care and benefits issues described above. This makes ensuring NG/R veterans have military culturally competent options for care outside of the VA especially important.

Impact of Events of COVID-19 Pandemic and Civil Unrest

It is essential to note that we can expect the NG to be impacted by the occupational stress of the events of 2020 and beyond. NG members were deployed at record rates to deal with the COVID-19 pandemic, civil unrest, and the events related to the Jan. 6th insurrection. The year 2020 was described as unprecedented and the "year of the Guard" due to the high levels of mobilization and is expected to continue through 2021. Practitioners should be prepared to recognize the potential impacts of these events, including increases in mental health challenges and suicidal behaviors.

Vignette: Jacky

Jacky is a 25 year old female serving part time as a proud Private First Class in the National Guard. She is also completing the last year of her dual graduate school program that includes a 20 h a week internship. Recently, Jacky filed for divorce and is adjusting to a single income household. She has two kids, a 2-year-old boy and 8-month-old baby boy. She is a full time single parent, lives alone with the boys, and works multiple part time jobs.

As a National Guard service member, Jacky attends drills once a month. Drill length is often inconsistent, ranging from 2 to 4 days. Once a year, Jacky must attend a 2-week annual training. While for the most part she has ample time to plan to be away for drill, it has become more difficult now as a single parent to find childcare for 3–4 days. Her closest relative, a younger brother, lives 40 min away. Jacky relies on her friends or an overnight day care facility for childcare when she needs to be gone for more than 2 days. The day care charges are expensive, and her National Guard commitment has required her to need the service more frequently, causing financial strain.

When Jacky shows up to drill, the schedule is often unpredictable. She never knows what time she will be home or when she will have a break. This can be particularly stressful on days when she needs to complete important school work. As a result, when her fellow battle buddies are resting or sleeping, she uses any spare moment to tackle to study or write papers while at drill.

Jacky has a history of anxiety that has become more frequent in recent months. She has also experienced several panic attacks and trouble sleeping. This becomes more prominent when she feels the stress of school and work pile up. She has also noticed increased anxiety as many of her National Guard peers have become activated responding to the pandemic and civil unrest. Jacky worries about how she would manage a month or longer activation. What would she do with the kids? Would her professors understand? What if she can't complete the program? She knows her anxiety is becoming too much to handle but doesn't want to get help. Jacky is frequently encouraging her National Guard peers to get care when it is needed and works to push back against the stigma of mental health care in her unit. However, when it comes to her own mental health care, she can't seem to overcome her internal dialogue telling her she should handle it on her own.

Conclusion

NG/R service members represent a unique and vital subpopulation within the military. Although there is much more to be learned about the experience of NG/R, outlined throughout this chapter is the information practitioners can use to provide culturally competent care to NG/R. Practitioners should take the time to understand what differentiates NG/R service members and veterans from their active duty counterparts, recognize the unique stressors and vulnerabilities NG/R service members and veterans may experience and develop ways to incorporate this knowledge into work with NG/R. As our country continues to depend heavily on the service of NG/R, our commitment to their care must match the commitment National Guard and Reservists have made to all of us.

Clinical Pearls

- NG/R are service members who serve in a part time status. These service members typically sign contracts to perform inactive duty for training (drill) for a weekend each month and 2 weeks of active-duty training (annual training).
- It is important to note commitment to NG/R goes beyond drill and training and often includes additional trainings, mobilizations and deployments. The use of NG/R at the state and federal level has significantly increased over the last 20 years.
- NG/R are unique in that they have dual roles as service members and civilians. The service member uniform comes on and off, requiring NG/R to balance life between two very different worlds, while at the same time being prepared to be quickly activated or deployed in times of need, creating unique occupational stress.

- Challenges NG/R experience include difficulty finding and sustaining employment and stress on relationships with employers, finding understanding within a civilian community, access to competent care, frequent disruptions to civilian life, and added stress on the family.
- Unlike their active-duty counterparts who live on or near military installations, NG/R live in civilian communities which limits their access to supportive services as well as a shared military community.
- NG/R service members and veterans are not always eligible for the same benefits (e.g. healthcare, education, disability compensation, etc.) as their active duty counterparts.
- NG/R are vulnerable to challenges after deployment, including posttraumatic stress disorder, depression, anxiety as well as issues that impact overall well-being such as increases in substance use, chronic pain, readjustment challenges, engagement in aggressive and risky behaviors, and relationship issues.
- The unique stressors of NG/R service may create vulnerability for risk for suicide.
- NG/R report similar barriers to care as active-duty service members (stigma, concern over career impact, difficulty scheduling and time off work, not knowing where to get help, handling issues on their own) but also experience unique barriers, such as eligibility for care, access to providers and affordability.

References

1. United States National Guard. Army national guard. https://www.nationalguard.com/guard-faqs. Accessed 13 Jul 2021.
2. U.S. Department of Veterans Affairs. Active duty vs. reserve or national guard. 2015. https://www.va.gov/vetsinworkplace/docs/em_activeReserve.asp. Accessed 13 Jul 2021.
3. Nagl J, Sharp T, Sullivan G. An Indispensable Force: Investing in America's National Guard and Reserves. Washington. DC: Center for a New American Security; 2010.
4. Anderson-Goodell EM, Homish DL, Homish GG. Characteristics of US Army Reserve and National Guard couples who use family readiness programs. Mil Behav Health. 2019;7(2):185–97.
5. Assistant Secretary of Defense for Reserve Affairs. The reserve components of the national guard. Fort Belvoir, VA: DTIC; 1996. https://apps.dtic.mil/dtic/tr/fulltext/u2/a315871.pdf. Accessed 13 Jul 2021.
6. Congressional Research Service. Defense primer: reserve forces. Washington, DC: FAS; 2021. https://fas.org/sgp/crs/natsec/IF10540.pdf. Accessed 13 Jul 2021.
7. Military One Source. 2019 Demographics profile of the military community. 2020. https://download.militaryonesource.mil/12038/MOS/Reports/2019-demographics-report.pdf. Accessed 13 Jul 2021.
8. Army News Service. Army reserve full-time AGR positions. The Balance Careers. 2019. https://www.thebalancecareers.com/army-reserves-open-more-full-time-agr-positions-3332673. Accessed 13 Jul 2021.
9. U.S. Army Reserve. Ways to serve: active guard reserve (AGR). https://www.usar.army.mil/AGR/#:%7E:text=Active%20Guard%20Reserve%20(AGR)%20Soldiers,20%20years%20of%20active%20service. Accessed 13 Jul 2021.

10. National Guard and Reserve. VA.gov. Veterans Affairs. U.S. Department of Veterans Affairs. 2020. https://www.benefits.va.gov/guardreserve/active-reserve.asp. Accessed 13 Jul 2021.
11. Military Officers Association of America. Your benefits: title 10 vs. title 32 vs. the state. 2020. https://www.moaa.org/content/publications-and-media/moaa-blog/your-benefits-title-10-vs.title-32-vs.-the-state/#:%7E:text=Federal%20authority%20over%20servicemembers%20falls,duty%20for%20federal%2Dlevel%20missions.&text=Federal%20authority%20over%20National%20Guard,32%20of%20the%20U.S.%20Code. Accessed 13 Jul 2021.
12. U.S. Department of Defense. Report of the Eleventh Quadrennial review of military compensation: main report. United States Government. 2021. https://militarypay.defense.gov/Portals/3/Documents/Reports/SR17_Chapter_14.pdf. Accessed 12 Jul 2021.
13. Defense Science Board Task Force. Deployment of members of the national guard and reserve in the global war on terrorism. Washington, DC: Office of the Under Secretary of Defense; 2007. https://dsb.cto.mil/reports/2000s/ADA478163.pdf. Accessed 13 Jul 2021.
14. Berger M. Invaders, allies, occupiers, guests: a brief history of U.S. military involvement in Iraq. Washington Post. 2020. https://www.washingtonpost.com/world/2020/01/11/invaders-allies-occupiers-guests-brief-history-us-military-involvement-iraq/. Accessed 13 Jul 2021.
15. National Conference of State Legislatures. National guard assists response to the COVID-19 pandemic. 2020. https://www.ncsl.org/research/military-and-veterans-affairs/national-guard-activation-in-every-state-assisting-response-to-the-covid-19-pandemic.aspx. Accessed 13 Jul 2021.
16. Military Times. States begin activating National Guard after FBI warns of armed protests at capitols. Military Times. 2021. https://www.militarytimes.com/news/your-military/2021/01/13/states-begin-activating-national-guard-after-fbi-warns-of-armed-protests-at-capitols/. Accessed 13 Jul 2021.
17. Joyner J. National guard vs. reserves. 2018. https://work.chron.com/national-guard-vs-reserves-19508.html. Accessed 13 Jul 2021.
18. Halvorson A. Understanding the military: the institution, the culture, and the people. 2010. https://www.samhsa.gov/sites/default/files/military_white_paper_final.pdf. Accessed 13 Jul 2021.
19. International Revenue Service. Work opportunity tax credit. 2020. https://www.irs.gov/businesses/small-businesses-self-employed/work-opportunity-tax-credit. Accessed 13 Jul 2021.
20. Give An Hour. Facts about US Reserve components. 2020. https://giveanhour.org/wp-content/uploads/RCP-Fact-Sheet-2017-a.pdf. Accessed 13 Jul 2021.
21. Kehle SM, Polusny MA, Murdoch M, et al. Early mental health treatment-seeking among US National Guard soldiers deployed to Iraq. J Trauma Stress. 2011;23(1):33–40.
22. Schuurmans TE. Should army national guard force structure be based on the federal warfight mission for the emerging home land security mission. Carlisle Barracks, PA: US Army War College; 2002.
23. GoArmy. Army reserve. 2020. https://www.goarmy.com/reserve/role.html. Accessed 13 Jul 2021.
24. USO. Historical facts about the Army Reserve. 2019. https://www.uso.org/stories/2350-11-historical-trivia-facts-about-the-army-reserve-for-its-111th-anniversary. Accessed 13 Jul 2021.
25. Molina D, Morse A. Military-connected undergraduates: exploring differences between National Guard, reserve, active duty, and veterans in higher education. 2015. https://www.acenet.edu/Documents/Military-Connected-Undergraduates.pdf. Accessed 13 Jul 2021.
26. Harris BC. Relevance of Army National Guard infantry units in the force structure and their role in combat. Carlisle Barracks, PA: US Army War College; 2004.
27. Milliken CS, Auchterlonie JL, Hoge CW. Longitudinal assessment of mental health problems among active and RC soldiers returning from the Iraq war. JAMA. 2007;298(18):2141–8.
28. Thomas JL, Wilk JE, Riviere LA, et al. Prevalence of mental health problems and functional impairment among active component and National Guard soldiers 3 and 12 months following combat in Iraq. Arch Gen Psychiatry. 2010;67(6):614–23.

29. Ursano RJ, Wang J, Fullerton CS, et al. Post-deployment mental health in Reserve and National Guard service members: deploying with or without one's unit and deployment preparedness. Mil Med. 2018;183(1–2):e51–8.
30. Sripada RK, Bohnert ASB, Teo AR, et al. Social networks, mental health problems, and mental health service utilization in OEF/OIF National Guard veterans. Soc Psychiatry Psychiatr Epidemiol. 2015;50:1367–78.
31. Erbes CR, Kaler ME, Schult T, et al. Mental health diagnosis and occupational functioning in National Guard/Reserve veterans returning from Iraq. J Rehabil Res Dev. 2011;48(10):1159–70.
32. Department of Defense. Annual suicide report calendar year 2018. Arlington, VA: Department of Defense; 2019. https://www.dspo.mil/Portals/113/2018%20DoD%20Annual%20Suicide%20Report_FINAL_25%20SEP%2019_508c.pdf. Accessed 13 Jul 2021.
33. Department of Defense. Annual suicide report calendar year 2019. Arlington, VA: Department of Defense; 2020. https://www.dspo.mil/Portals/113/Documents/CY2019%20Suicide%20Report/DoD%20Calendar%20Year%20CY%202019%20Annual%20Suicide%20Report.pdf?ver=YOA4IZVcVA9mzwtsfdO5Ew%3d%3d. Accessed 13 Jul 2021.
34. Kamarck KN, Mendez BHP, Arriage XL. Suicide rates and risk factors for the National Guard. Congressional Research Service. 2019. https://www.everycrsreport.com/files/20190909_IN11164_44de6298db642aca0da3810b65f989da4f40d8a7.pdf. Accessed 13 Jul 2021.
35. Gorman LA, Blow AJ, Ames BD, Reed PL. National Guard families after combat: mental health, use of mental health services, and perceived treatment barriers. Psychiatr Serv. 2011;62(1):28–34.
36. Pietrzak RH, Johnson DC, Goldstein MB, et al. Perceived stigma and barriers to mental health care utilization among OEF-OIF veterans. Psychiatr Serv. 2009;60(8):1118–22.
37. Seal KH, Metzler TJ, Gima KS, et al. Trends and risk factors for mental health diagnoses among Iraq and Afghanistan veterans using Department of Veterans Affairs health care, 2002–2008. Am J Public Health. 2009;99(9):1651–8.

Part II

The Veteran and Military Mental Health System

7 Medical and Community Resources for Veterans and Military Personnel

Kelly M. DeSousa, Kelly-Lynne Ward, and Christopher H. Warner

Vignette

Tom is a 27 year old male who served for 4 years in the Marine Corps before being honorably discharged upon completion of his enlistment. During his time in the Marines he twice deployed to Iraq where he served in the Anbar province. His deployments were marked with significant combat exposure and a number of Marines from his platoon were killed or severely wounded.

Tom himself sustained minor injuries from an improvised explosive device but was able to continue to perform his duties and complete his tour of duty and subsequent term of enlistment without follow on medical care requirements. Tom received a Purple Heart due to his combat injury. While he was screened on multiple occasions for potential mental health issues and did meet once with a military mental health professional. He chose not to report the intrusive memories he had of his deployment, the negative changes in his mood, or the changes in his physical and emotional reactions because he felt that asking for help would make him look weak in the eyes of his fellow Marines.

Upon completion of his service, Tom returned to his hometown in Montana where he was able to find work in a gun shop. Since his departure from military service he has had minimal contact with members of his former unit and he does not talk with his family about his military experiences as he feels they do not understand since he is the only one in his family to serve. The nearest VA clinic is over 2 h away and Tom has not sought any support or services through the VA. Outside of work,

K. M. DeSousa · K.-L. Ward
Providence VA Healthcare System, Providence, RI, USA
e-mail: Kelly.desousa@va.gov; Kelly-lynne.ward@va.gov

C. H. Warner (✉)
Department of Psychiatry, Uniformed Services University of the Health Sciences, Bethesda, MD, USA

C. H. Warner, C. A. Castro (eds.), *Veteran and Military Mental Health*,
https://doi.org/10.1007/978-3-031-18009-5_7

Tom is not engaging in any activities and while he previously enjoyed running and hiking, he has not been actively doing either activity.

Until the last 2 weeks, Tom was attending work without problem but recently he has become more isolative and has noted a worsening in his symptoms which have been present since the time of his service. After discussing with his primary care physician, he is referred to a local mental health clinic where he is diagnosed with posttraumatic stress disorder and treatment is started.

Introduction

Tom's case is very representative of a large portion of veterans from the Global War on Terror. Many of them completed their service, left the military, and are now integrating back into our communities. They carry with them the burdens of the trauma and exposure that they experienced. As outlined in greater detail in the stigma chapter, both the Department of Defense and Veterans Affairs health systems have enacted numerous programs to reduce stigma and barriers to care. However, stigma towards seeking mental health care remains and can serve as a barrier to seeking help. As military personnel transition back to civilian service, some will go on to attend college using their GI Bill benefits while others seek employment. As outlined in the transition chapter of this book, the quality and experience of that transition can have significant impact on veterans such as Tom.

Additionally, while veterans like Tom are eligible for care through the VA's health system, it is not uncommon that eligible veterans may not take advantage of available resources, especially if they are receiving health care benefits/insurance coverage through other employer provided programs or there are not nearby VA health system resources. Providers who care for military service members and veterans should be familiar with what Military Health System and VA services exist as they may be resources they can tap their patients into. Additionally, as providers and mental health teams develop their treatment plans, it is important to not only consider the medications and therapies required to treat these conditions but also the tailored social support resources and networks that may be available for this population.

Multiple studies in veteran populations have shown the positive impact of social support on posttraumatic stress disorder, depression, and suicidal ideations [1–5]. However, the concept of social support is not well defined and varies between family, friends, significant others, and co-workers. Additionally, these studies all focused specifically on mental health outcomes but not other factors such as financial support/need or other challenges. There are numerous resources available for military and veteran personnel designed to increase access to care, provide assistance for specific situations, and to enhance their social connectedness.

This chapter aims to provide some awareness of both the general medical services available to this population through the Departments of Defense and Veterans Affairs, as well as, emphasize military and veteran specific community resources and how they can be integrated into treatment plans for this specific patient population. The resources identified and listed within this chapter (Fig. 7.1) are not meant

- www.tricare.mil – Overview of the Military Health System Benefits and Resources
- www.va.gov/health-care/ - Overview of the VA Health System Benefits and Resources
- www.mentalhealth.va.gov –Overview of VA provided mental health services and veteran information
- www.vetcenter.va.gov – Specific information about and locations of VA Vet Centers
- www.militaryonesource.mil – DoD resource and counseling program for military service and family members
- militarybenefits.info/state-veterans -affairs -office -directory/ - Provides overview of the various state veteran's offices and benefits
- www.defense.gov/Resources/Veteran-Support -Organizations/ - List of DoD recognized Veteran Support Organizations
- www.va.gov/vso/vso-directory.pdf - List of VA recognized Veteran Support Organization

Fig. 7.1 Key website for veteran medical and mental health resources

to be an all-encompassing list nor a recommendation or endorsement of any specific program but rather they are highlighted to increase awareness that such programs exist and to encourage mental health providers to become aware of what programs may be available within their area.

Department of Defense

The Military Health System provides medical care to 9.6 million military service members, family members, and military retirees. This care is provided through two systems. The first is the direct care delivered by the more than 50 military hospitals and 425 ambulatory health clinics at military installations around the world [6]. While these facilities have the primary responsibility to support active duty military service members and their families, they also support other beneficiaries that live within 50 miles of the facilities.

Most all of these facilities provide at a minimum outpatient mental health services and larger facilities will include sub-specialty mental health services, inpatient mental health capability, and in some cases, residential treatment facilities. Military treatment facilities will include a mix of active duty military and Department of Defense Civilian psychiatrists, psychologists, and licensed clinical social workers capable of treating both acute and chronic conditions with pharmacology and psychotherapeutic interventions. All installations will also have personnel specifically trained in substance abuse and family advocacy (military equivalent of child protective services). Select installations have specific centers affiliated with the National intrepid Center of Excellence to provide specialized treatment for those with both posttraumatic stress disorder and traumatic brain injury.

These military treatment facilities also support the various mental health screening initiatives that are conducted by the Department of Defense. This includes pre- and post-deployment health screenings that seek to identify potential exposures, medical ailments, and mental health issues that may be present at the time. In the terms of pre-deployment screening the emphasis is to ensure that injured and ill service members are not deploying or if they are deployable, have the necessary medical resources and capabilities [7]. Post-deployment efforts have increased in frequency and more recently all US military personnel now complete an annual screening separate from deployment called the periodic health assessment. These screens are focused on the early identification of depression, posttraumatic stress disorder, alcohol disorders, and risk factors for suicide and domestic violence and linking those service members for care [8]. Separately, the Military Health System introduced depression and posttraumatic stress disorder screening to each service member primary care encounter [8]. Unfortunately, these processes are limited by the willingness to self report and the lack of anonymity in the process leads to service member under-reporting [9].

Additionally, Military Health System beneficiaries have the ability to access civilian medical services around the world through the purchased care network using their selected TRICARE plan. Of note, National Guard and Reserve service members have limited health coverage under these programs unless on an activated status. This is covered in further detail in Chap. 6.

Beyond the Military Health System capabilities, there are several other mental health services that are available for military service members to help reduce barriers to seeking care. Some military installations offer Military Family Life Consultants which are mental health providers who are working throughout the military community to educate service members and their family members about potential mental health challenges and services available. These consultants are not permitted to enter into a therapeutic relationship but do have the ability to coordinate mental health care if needed. In contrast, the Military One Source program provides free, short-term, confidential, non-medial counseling for a wide range of issues including marital conflicts, stress management, and coping with grief and deployment transitions. Military One Source providers are not able to make a clinical diagnosis nor are they able to provide medication or specialized therapies. However, they can coordinate and transfer care to a TRICARE provider if necessary. Despite these limitations, both of these services are used frequently due to the confidential nature.

It is also important to understand community resources that are available to military service and family members through the Department of Defense. As highlighted in the military culture chapter, military installations are cities within themselves with their own churches, in some case schools, and community resources. Additionally, most all military installations have morale and welfare resources on the installations to encourage recreation (golf course, bowling alley, swimming pool, outdoor areas) and social gathering of individuals with like interests (gyms, auto skills shop, woodworking and art studios, etc.). As highlighted several times in this book, one group that can have a difficult and challenging transition within the military are the junior enlisted service members, those who are unmarried and recently entered the military. Most military installations have activity programs in place for single service members to encourage them to socialize, interact with each other, and take advantage of recreation and education activities within the area of their installation. For example installations in Texas might organize a trip to attend a rodeo or those in Florida might take a weekend trip to one of the many amusement parks in Orlando. These types of activities not only get the service members some time away from their duties but also the opportunity to establish social networks within their community.

In the case of Tom, he was screened for mental health concerns and educated about available services as part of his post-deployment health assessments and annually as part of his periodic health assessments. Additionally, he would have received periodic screenings for depression and posttraumatic stress disorder as part of his engagements with his military primary care providers. But, these processes all require that Tom would want to get help and self report his symptoms. In this case, Tom chose not to do that because of stigma concerns. The result was that Tom did not receive any treatment while in the Military Health System and was not considered for potential associated disability due to the condition or coordination of care with the VA health care system.

Department of Veterans Affairs

Generally, veterans qualify for VA health care depending on income or disability rating. Further, these factors determine the cost of VA health care services. The VA is committed to providing free health care for conditions related to military service, or Veterans with catastrophic disabilities and disability ratings of at least 50%, as well as for those who cannot afford to pay for care. Additionally, the VA offers free health care related to readjustment counseling and mental health services, care and counseling related to military sexual trauma, exams to determine future risk of health problems linked to military service, care related to combat service for Veterans that served in a theater of combat operations after 11/11/1998, VA claims exams, care related to a VA-rated service-connected disability, and individual or group programs to help you quit smoking or lose weight [10].

In the absence of VA disability compensation or pension payments or special eligibility factors (like receiving the Medal of Honor, Purple Heart, or former Prisoner of War), the VA will ask for information about income as part of the health care enrollment process. It is required by law and is called an income assessment or financial assessment (formerly known as means test). Gross household income for the previous year is requested and if the information provided shows that the Veteran's income is below current limits and qualifies for free VA health care, medications, or both, the VA is required by law to verify the information. This is done by confirming the information provided with the Internal Revenue Service (IRS) and the Social Security Administration (SSA). Veterans do not have to provide financial information if they agree to co-payments for care. However, without this information, the VA will not be able to consider eligibility for free medications or beneficiary travel.

With more than nine million enrolled veterans, the VA is home to one of the United States' largest integrated health care systems providing care at nearly 1300 health care facilities around the United States include over 170 medical centers and more than 1100 outpatient clinics of varying capacity [10]. VA medical facilities provide a wide range of services including traditional hospital-based services, primary care, and most medical centers offer additional specialty services. Specific to mental health, the VA has an integrated system of care that offers inpatient, intensive outpatient, and comprehensive outpatient mental health services. To address the potential barrier to care of travel to the nearest VA clinic, VA mental health services have been in the forefront in the area of tele-mental health care.

The VA also offers mental health intensive case management for veterans with severe and persistent mental illness, opioid treatment programs, and collaborative addiction recovery services to help those veterans who are struggling with substance use disorders. For those who have significant polytrauma, the VA offers multiple polytrauma centers that focus in providing the highest quality of care for both those visible and invisible wounds of war. Additionally, there are countless other programs throughout the VA to support veterans with mental health disorders ranging from those specific to military sexual trauma, veterans who are victims of intimate partner violence, and those who are facing criminal justice issues related to their mental health disorder. If you have a veteran patient who may benefit from these services or you would like to learn more about the specific services offered, reach out to the social work services section of the local VA in your area.

The VA also offers some financial and support assistance that may be beneficial for patients including financial hardship assistance for those have accrued outstanding balances for co-payments related to VA care or medications and beneficiary travel support to potentially reimburse the veteran's travel necessary to get to and from the appointment. Additionally, multiple specialized case management programs exist based on the specialized care or veteran group which can help connect the veteran to the necessary resources depending on their case complexity or needs. Lastly, the VA also offers a caregiver support program that provides resources, education, and supportive counseling to caregivers of Veterans. This program offers text support, self-care courses, telephone support line, peer-support mentoring, and resources for health and stress management.

Outside of the VA medical facilities, the VA has community based counseling centers called Vet Centers that provide a wide range of social and psychological services. The counselors and staff of these facilities, many who are veterans themselves, offer individual, group, marriage, and family counseling to support a successful transition to civilian life or after a traumatic event experienced in the military.

It is important to recognize that the Veteran Health Administration is only one portion of the benefits and resources that the VA provides to veterans. These benefits can include disability compensation, veteran's pension programs, education programs, housing and home loan guarantees, job training, business loans, and cemetery services. A separate chapter in this book talks about disability benefits provided by both the military and VA.

Of note, the majority of veterans leave the military under honorable conditions. However, a certain few may receive dishonorable or bad conduct discharges which may bar VA benefits. If you are caring for a veteran who has received one of these discharge statuses, there are two ways to try and qualify for VA benefits: a discharge upgrade or a VA character of discharge review.

While Tom did not seek care for his conditions while in the military and has not engaged the VA for support to date, he may still be eligible for both VA health care and disability benefits. As noted, he lives a significant distance from the nearest VA but this may be overcome through the use of tele-mental health capabilities or through financial support for beneficiary travel.

State and City Supported Benefits

Most states and some large cities have established veteran's offices and provide unique benefits to their veteran residents. Some of these may be additional health care assistance either through state funded care or coordination with veteran support organizations in the area. Other resources may include counseling services, housing assistance, and food assistance. Homelessness in the veteran population is a significant issue and is addressed in greater detail in a chapter in this book as well as some of the services available in those situations.

States and cities also tend to offer educational, financial, and other benefits specific to veterans beyond health care. For example, Texas offers veterans who have received certain military awards and decorations specialized license plates that allow them to travel toll free on all state roads. Other states like Hawaii offer real estate tax exemption and discounted motor vehicle registration fees. While these types of benefits may be outside the scope of the treatment plan, it is important to encourage a veteran to get educated about their available benefits to help their situation.

Specific to health care, many states offer connections for those seeking mental health assistance to veteran support organizations who can arrange affordable or free mental health treatment. Additionally, most all states have one or more Veterans homes which provide independent living, assisted living, or nursing assistance to elderly veterans who either have low income or desire to spend their last years with their comrades.

As a resident of the State of Montana, Tom is encouraged to seek potential state resources. While there are no specific health resources available, he does learn about potential tuition and education assistance opportunities that would allow him to pursue some of his future goals. Additionally, he has now engaged with the VA and is undergoing evaluation for potential disability. This may make him eligible for state tax exemptions and reduced or no fee vehicle registration. These financial benefits may significantly reduce Tom's financial stress.

Veteran Service and Community Organizations

When discussing veteran service organizations, it is important to recognize that this is a non-specific term that encompasses a large group of organizations. The Department of Defense provides a list on their defense.gov website of organizations based only on the criteria that they are designed to support military service members, their families, or veterans; are a non-profit organization; do not represent or endorse partisan, hateful, or anti-American positions; and have received favorable vetting by at least two charity evaluators. The Department of Veterans Affairs provides a list on their va.gov website of recognized organizations sorted by whether they are congressionally chartered and if they are officially recognized by the VA to prepare, present, and prosecute claims on veteran's behalf.

Some organizations, such as large charitable entities like Salvation Army or national mental illness advocacy groups, have larger missions but have dedicated specific efforts targeting veterans or military personnel. In contrast, veteran service organizations generally have a primary mission focused on supporting the military and veteran population. Some of these organizations provide mental health counseling or will provide financial support for services. Many others provide referral services for mental health counseling. Before recommending any particular organization that does provide or coordinate care, ensure that you research what evidence based interventions they support or endorse. Other groups provide adjunct support such as retreats or service dogs. Some organizations are focused on specific groups either by injury, ethnicity, race, period of service, or rank of service. Many of these organizations also provide advocacy for their specific population through various avenues.

More importantly, these organizations can provide a mechanism for social networks and connectedness with individuals who have had shared experiences. Gold Star families are those who have lost a service member in combat. An organization specifically focused on supporting that group will not only create contacts between those who have recently lost loved ones but also a broader family of those who have experienced this loss from previous wars. One gold star wife whose spouse was killed in Afghanistan in 2012 noted that one of the most powerful and influential conversations she had was with a gold star wife whose husband was killed in the Korean War. She noted how that discussion more than any helped her find a direction for her life after the loss and helped her anticipate some of the challenges that lay ahead. These types of peer support connections can be very influential and supportive.

Additionally, some organizations may have a fairly sizeable local presence that helps promote this type of connectedness through activities such as running, hiking, etc. or through local gatherings. These organizations generally seek to have activities within the community such as supporting military and veteran holiday services or community service that also helps the members of their organization become more connected to their broader community, helping support their long term transition.

In the case of Tom, he is now back in his home town and has become increasingly isolated. Not many of the individuals that he grew up with chose to enter the military and he does not have a large veteran presence within his family. Yet, within his town there are two veteran service organizations that maintain activity halls and have frequent gatherings and a separate group that conducts weekly runs in honor of the fallen. He could be connected to these organizations that could promote him getting back into activities he previously enjoyed while also meeting other veterans from both his and prior generations who have shared experiences. It is important to note that there are no scientific studies that show what level of benefit that involvement with veteran service organizations provide, but as noted in the beginning of this chapter, there are clear benefits of increased social connectedness and support.

As previously noted, this section has predominantly focused on veteran service organizations. These are all organizations specifically dedicated to and focused on veterans. However, there remain many other organizations within communities that while may focus on larger national and community challenges, also provide services to veterans. For example, the United Way has a special program called Mission United which focuses on helping veterans and their families acclimate back into civilian life and the Salvation Army has efforts specifically targeting veteran homelessness. As stated previously, when supporting a military or veteran patient, it is important to be aware of what resources are specifically available in your area or have contacts who are adept at accessing and are knowledgeable about these resources.

Tom remained frustrated about the travel distance to the nearest VA and disengaged from his care with them. As part of his biopsychosocial treatment plan, he was recommended to engage with the Veteran Service Organizations that operated within his town. The first organization focused on addressing veterans who were suffering from mental health conditions. They were able to assist Tom in finding a nearby therapist that he felt comfortable with and understood veteran specific mental health issues. He remained engaged in treatment and was notably improving. A second group maintained a social gathering site in town and Tom was encouraged to visit. He attended two events and began to establish a friendship with a Vietnam veteran who himself had struggled with his own experiences and his return from military service. Based on Tom's prior enjoyment of distance running, his provider recommended that he participate in weekly run that a veteran service organization hosted honoring the fallen service members. Tom began participating and found that he enjoyed the people that he met at the events and the fellowship from the event while also feeling like he was honoring and remembering his friends that he lost through his participation. He began developing friendships and relationships that he had not had since his departure from military service.

Future Direction

The Military Health System and Veterans Health Administration will continue to evolve and develop capabilities to care for our nation's military personnel and veterans. However, due to stigma, barriers to care, and the broad dispersal of veterans throughout our nation, they will never be able to meet all of the needs of this population. States, cities, and Veteran Service Organizations will continue to be needed to support these individuals and their families who have sacrificed for our country.

As providers caring for this patient population develop their treatment plans, it is important to consider the aspects of social support and the resources that may be available within their community. Studies have shown positive impacts of social relationships, but the benefit of community provided social support is unclear. Future research should look to assess the impact of these organizations, clubs, and activities to more thoroughly address the full biopsychosocial needs of veterans.

Clinical Pearls

- The Military Health System provides medical and mental health services for military service members, their families, and retirees through both their direct care system and an international network of providers who accept TRICARE.
- To combat stigma concerns, Department of Defense provides non-medical, confidential counseling services to their beneficiaries to support transitions, grief, adjustments, and trauma.
- The VA provides the largest integrated health system to meet the medical and mental health needs of America's veterans. This is delivered through a large network of medical centers and health clinics throughout the United States.
- Most states and select cities provide specific veteran benefits and services to aid in transition to civilian life and deal with the consequences of military deployments and combat exposure.
- Multiple studies in veteran populations have shown the positive impact of social support on posttraumatic stress disorder, depression, and suicidal ideations.
- There are a large number of Veteran Support Organizations that provide varying services and support. Some are focused towards specific veteran sub-groups while others are focused on specific types of injuries.
- Depending on their aim, Veteran Support Organizations can provide medical, financial, and social support and should be considered for veterans in need.

References

1. Adams RE, Urosevich TG, Hoffman SN, et al. Social support, help-seeking, and mental health outcomes among veterans in non-VA facilities: results from the Veterans' Health Study. Mil Behav Health. 2017;5:393–405.
2. DeBeer BB, Kimrbel NA, Meyer EC, et al. Combined PTSD and depressive symptoms interact with post-deployment social support to predict suicidal ideation in Operation Enduring Freedom and Operation Iraqi Freedom veterans. Psychiatry Res. 2014;216:357–62.
3. Gradus JL, Smith BN, Vogt D. Family support, family stress, and suicidal ideation in a combat-exposed sample of Operation Enduring Freedom/Operation Iraqi Freedom veterans. Anxiety Stress Coping. 2015;28:706–15.
4. Pietrzak RH, Goldstein MB, Malley JC, et al. Risk and protective factors associated with suicidal ideation in veterans of Operations Enduring Freedom and Iraqi Freedom. J Affect Disord. 2010;123:102–7.
5. Price M, Lancaster CL, Gros DF, et al. An examination of social support and PTSD treatment response during prolonged exposure. Psychiatry. 2018;81(3):258–70.
6. Office of the Assistant Secretary of Defense for Health Affairs. TRICARE annual report: 2020 evaluation of the TRICARE Program: fiscal year 2020 report to congress. 2020. https://www.health.mil/Reference-Center/Reports/2020/06/29/Evaluation-of-the-TRICARE-Program-Fiscal-Year-2020-Report-to-Congress. Accessed 7 Jul 2021.

7. Warner CH, Appenzeller GN, Parker JR, et al. Effectiveness of mental health screening and coordination of in-theater care prior to deployment to Iraq: a cohort study. Am J Psychiatry. 2011b;168:378–85.
8. Hoge CW, Ivany CG, Brusher EA, et al. Transformation of mental health care for U.S. Soldiers and Families During the Iraq and Afghanistan wars: where science and politics intersect. Am J Psychiatry. 2016;173:334–43.
9. Warner CH, Appenzeller GN, Grieger T, et al. Importance of anonymity to encourage honest reporting in mental health screening after combat deployment. Arch Gen Psychiatry. 2011a;68:1065–71.
10. Panangala SV, Sussman JS. Introduction to veterans health care. Congressional Research Service. 2019. https://crsreports.congress.gov/product/pdf/IF/IF10555. Accessed 7 Jul 2021.

Defining the Limits of Medical Privacy Within the US Departments of Defense and Veterans Affairs

8

David E. Johnson and David M. Benedek

The expectation of confidentiality for one's medical information is widely recognized in the United States. At its core, confidentiality is a component of the belief held by our society in a basic right to privacy—although such a right is never specifically articulated in the U.S. Constitution or its amendments. In the practice of medicine, the physician's obligation to maintain confidentiality is derived from principles initially articulated in the Hippocratic Oath and then reiterated though years of published codes of medical ethics [1].

At times, healthcare providers must struggle with practice challenges arising from competing ethical principles. When a patient is permitted to decline recommended treatment, the physician acknowledges that the ethical principle of respect for autonomy supersedes the clinician's competing obligation for beneficence. If a healthcare institution quarantines a person with a highly contagious disease over the patient's objections, respect for autonomy is deferred to prevent greater harm to others. Perhaps even more than in traditional medical settings the military clinician must grapple with ethical conflicts arising from dual agency—the clinician's simultaneous obligation to both the patient and to the military organization and mission. Considerable attention has been paid to addressing the challenges of dual agency in military healthcare [2–4]. Still, striking the appropriate balance between competing patient expectations, ethical principles and mission imperatives is not always straightforward.

In the area of behavioral health care in particular, existing professional ethical guidelines articulate the need to maintain patient confidentiality in the treatment

D. E. Johnson
Center for Forensic Behavioral Sciences, Uniformed Services University of Health Sciences, Bethesda, MD, USA

D. M. Benedek (✉)
Department of Psychiatry, Uniformed Services University of Health Sciences, Bethesda, MD, USA

C. H. Warner, C. A. Castro (eds.), *Veteran and Military Mental Health*,
https://doi.org/10.1007/978-3-031-18009-5_8

setting [5–7]. However, there are situations where other legal or ethical obligations—or both—mandate reporting clinical findings to third parties (e.g., child abuse reporting, warning others against imminently dangerous behavior). Federal law, military regulation and policy all define circumstances where a patient's protected health information (PHI) may—or in some cases must—be shared with third parties [8]. The Veterans Health Administration (VHA) health system, part of the Department of Veterans Affairs (DVA), generally mirrors the policies and practices of the civilian sector with regard to information sharing. However, in the active duty military community, demands such as deployment readiness, mission capability, and the requirement for ready access to weapons place additional constraints on the degree to which confidentiality may be maintained. These circumstances and the laws, policies and regulations defining them create greater limits to the patient's medical privacy in U.S. Military health care setting. Although service members presenting for evaluation and treatment at military facilities are required to sign disclosure documents acknowledging that they have read and understand the reasons for which their health information may be released, patients often do not adequately understand—or even read--such documents [9]. Moreover, uniformed care providers may not fully comprehend the laws, policies and regulations defining the limits of what they should or should not hold in confidence.

Ethics committees or hospital counsel may offer assistance in interpreting regulations and policies at times when care providers or patients become uncomfortable with a request for release of medical information. However any disclosure over a patient's objection—even if legally required—represents a compromise between competing interests and values. In these situations, the ethical "best practice" may be to ensure that confidentiality is maintained to the fullest extent possible (see "minimum necessary" below). Equally important—and consistent with the ethical principle of truthfulness—is insuring that patients are made aware of the limits to confidentiality that may be imposed by the context in which they serve and in which they seek care. With adequate discussion of these limits, service members can enter into the therapeutic relationship more freely, having consented to treatment with knowledge of the circumstances in which their health information may be shared with others [4]. This chapter explains the limits of confidentiality defined by current military policy, regulation and law. With greater knowledge of these parameters health care providers may be able to more fully engage their patients in frank discussions about the implications of their treatment decisions, and may be more confident that any information they release is shared in a manner consistent with the expressed limits.

Two key terms related to the concept of privacy that are often confused are *confidentiality* and *privilege*. Confidentiality refers to the general concept that medical personnel should not release patient information in any other (i.e., non-treatment) setting, i.e. to third parties, except as allowed by laws and policies. Privilege relates to the legal prohibition against release of specific patient information, *privileged communications*, in a legal setting such as a trial, investigation, or administrative hearing.

Confidentiality

Prior to 1996, the practice of medical confidentiality by health care providers and institutions was governed by the Hippocratic Oath, varying statutory policies in different states, the ethical guidelines of professional and state licensing bodies, and occasional precedent-setting court decisions. While the Privacy Act of 1974 [10] codified confidentiality for all personal information handled by U.S. federal employees, whether on active duty status or in the VHA, this law was not specific to medical confidentiality. No national Federal statutory language referred specifically to health care institutions prior to the enactment of the Health Insurance Portability and Accountability Act of 1996 [11]. HIPAA's "Privacy Rule" created national standards for the confidentiality of medical information as part of an effort to facilitate health insurance coverage when individuals change jobs. . . HIPAA only applies to providers known as "covered entities" who transmit medical information in certain defined electronic transactions, such as for billing purposes, not merely an email to another colleague [12].

HIPAA established the term Protected Health Information (PHI), which refers to any "individually identifiable health information" which could be used to identify an individual. PHI consists of medical/psychiatric conditions, provision of healthcare, and payment for provision of healthcare, whether in the past, present, or future that qualifies for HIPAA protection. VHA and DOD medical facilities qualify as "covered entities" under HIPAA. The language of HIPAA articulated the minimum standard to which "covered entities" are to be held with regard to safeguarding PII in terms of protective measures as well as reporting requirements and penalties for identified breaches. More stringent privacy laws may trump HIPAA if enacted by individual states, but HIPAA establishes the federal minimum which applies to both VHA and DoD. However, the language of HIPAA itself carves out exceptions to this law specifically for the DoD. The armed forces exception is found in Title 45, Code of Federal Regulations (CFR), Section (§) 164.512(k) and these exceptions are discussed in detail below.

In the US military, Department of Defense (DOD) Manual 6025.18 [13] implements HIPAA for the military services, except for prisoners in correctional facilities. Each service currently maintains their own branch regulations concerning the confidentiality of PHI and rules for disclosing such information, which are Army Regulation 40-66 for the Army, NAVMED MANMED 15-6 for the Navy and Marines, and AFI 41-200 for the Air Force. However, the ongoing realignment of all military medical services under the Defense Health Agency (DHA) may eventually result in a proposed DHA-level privacy regulation. In the meantime, the current version of DOD Manual 6025.18 assigns ultimate responsibility for HIPAA oversight to the Director of the DHA.

Within the VHA, VHA Directive 1605.01 [14] governs all healthcare-related privacy rules and lists pertinent privacy-related VHA statutes. The Privacy Act, rather than HIPAA, applies to PHI transmitted to the non-VHA components of the Department of Veterans Affairs (DVA), including the disability-processing Veterans Benefits Administration (VBA) [15].

Both the military and the VHA are integrated with their respective medical disability operations, as well as a joint Integrated Disability Evaluation System (IDES). The HIPAA Privacy Rule and the Federal Privacy Act apply to any and all patient information handled within those systems.

Privilege

PHI may be important in administrative, civil, or criminal proceedings as the presence or absence of a claimed illness may either support or refute a presumption of innocence or serve to mitigate or otherwise explain alleged misconduct. In some circumstances, individuals may wish to withhold such personal information as part of their Fifth Amendment right to silence. For example, a psychiatrist may treat a service member who expresses feelings of guilt or shame due to alcohol intoxication only to learn later that the service member is under investigation for hitting a pedestrian while driving drunk. Alternatively, a sexual assault victim way wish to stop her assailant's defense attorney from obtaining the victim's psychiatric records in order to find history or symptoms that could cast doubt on her memory, truthfulness, or perception of the alleged offense. Within the military, the patient does hold the right to exert a psychotherapist-patient privilege, i.e., to prevent the admission of his or her medical PHI into evidence at court-martial, as defined by Military Rule of Evidence 513 [16]. It is important to note the patient-psychotherapist privilege is held by the patient, not the clinician, although the clinician may invoke this right on behalf of the patient until the patient's wishes are clarified. This exercise may be important in the event that legal authorities request medical information directly from clinician or health care agency. Regardless of who initiates the exercise of privilege, significant exceptions to the rule exist. Requests for all types of medical records would generally be processed by each medical treatment facility in accordance with their service-specific privacy/confidentiality regulation. For VHA patients, local state laws regarding privilege would apply to their PHI. Within the federal court system, the existence of the psychotherapist-patient privilege, but not a general medical privilege, was upheld in the case decision [17]. This has been interpreted to apply to attempts to subpoena VHA or military medical records.

Exceptions to Confidentiality and Privilege

HIPAA allows for several exceptions under which the military and the VHA may disclose PHI without permission of the patient [11]. These generally take the form of complying with court orders, law enforcement requests, matters of national security. DOD and military regulations on confidentiality generally include a number of exceptions under which medical providers should or must break confidentiality. HIPAA established that determining the degree of PHI disclosure required should follow a "minimum necessary" standard. In general, providers for both the military and the VHA should consult with supervisors before disclosing any PHI to third parties, in order to assure the proper identification of the requestor and how much PHI must be disclosed. For the VHA, an additional factor is whether local State law has stricter privacy statutes which would trump HIPAA. Specific situations regarding disclosure of different types of information are described below.

Situations Requiring Notification of Military Commanders

Many military behavioral health providers have experienced pressure from commanders, sometimes transmitted through their MTF chain of command, to reveal more information about patient(s) than they feel comfortable doing. One common version of this involves active duty members on psychotropic medications who may be experiencing a side effect such as sedation. Commanders may complain about service members "falling asleep at formation" or oversleeping their alarm clock, causing extra work for other members of the unit such as efforts to find the service member, write up the incident, and make phone calls to determine if this is a legitimate medical situation, a case of deliberate work avoidance, or exaggerating a medical situation for other secondary gain. Commanders may tell the service members or clinicians within their command that they need to know everyone who is on a medication which could in any way compromise activities ranging from equipment operation (e.g. machinery, vehicles, or technical devices), physical fitness, field training activities, or deployments to combat zones. Service members, like their civilian counterparts may prefer that details regarding their medical treatment, particularly any behavioral health treatment, not be provided to their "employer"--their chain of command. Their desire for privacy may lead them to seek care outside the military health system, or to seek care through other DOD programs that technically exist outside of the military health system and thus are not subject to the DOD regulations described in this chapter. These would include the Military Family Life Consultants (MFLCs) and the OneSource website and phone line, both of which have The RAND Corporation assessed in regards to quality [18]. Alternatively, privacy concerns might lead some service members to avoid seeking what might otherwise be beneficial or lifesaving care altogether.

DODI 6490.08 [19] "provides guidance for balance between patient confidentiality rights and the commander's right to know for operation and risk management decisions." This regulation states that care providers should have a "presumption" to not contact a commander just because the service member is seeking mental health care services, unless a specific exception is met. Those exceptions are presented in Table 8.1. Specific examples of exceptions are also articulated in service specific regulations, such as Army Regulation 40-66 [20]. However, each of these Army exceptions can be slotted into one of the nine categories in DODI 6490.08. For example, behavioral health treatment may be released for purposes of disability determination, health oversight activities, preventative medicine purposes, incident investigations, and Line of Duty determinations in the event of attempted or completed suicidal behavior or harm to others. Interpretations of the exceptions can be far-ranging depending on who is being asked. "Harm to mission" may be defined by

Table 8.1 Situations that mandate the breaking of confidentiality in the military

Harm to self
Harm to others (includes child abuse and domestic violence)
Harm to mission
Special personnel (e.g. Personnel Reliability Program)
Inpatient care
Acute medical conditions interfering with duty
Substance abuse treatment program
Command-directed mental health evaluation
Other special circumstances (determined on a case by case basis by an O-6 level, or equivalent, provider or commander)

some as any service member behavior which results in a negative local news story, thus creating negative public image for the military and perhaps creating increased friction or roadblocks for future military activities, however benign they may be. Providers should ask themselves questions such as could the lives of others depend on this Service member serving a critical role as a weapon operator, a vehicle or flight mechanic, or through work requiring a high-level security clearance.

Patients reporting past crimes may or may not reach the threshold at which a provider fears for future harm to mission. Some crimes, such as child abuse and viewing of child pornography, represent a mandatory reporting situation for all military and VHA facilities [21]. Crimes involving spousal abuse must be reported in military facilities [22] but varies in VHA facilities according to local state laws [23]. Patient reports of crimes committed in the past such as theft, physical altercations with strangers, or remote drug abuse could conceivably be viewed as behavior that is no longer active. On the other hand, such past behavior might comprise a general picture of someone with an ongoing, evolving personality disorder or psychiatric condition. It is difficult to refute the idea that any past behavior might flare up in the future and compromise a unit's mission in some way. Providers are left to determine their own comfort with their ability to predict possible future maladaptive behavior and what level of probability could require command notification. Additionally, notification to the commander might still be made in a "minimum necessary" format, without specific description of the past crimes that were revealed in treatment session. Past crimes involving violations of the law of war are addressed later in this chapter.

Command-directed mental health evaluations, more simply called command-directed evaluations (CDEs), deserve special mention as they represent a significant activity at all military treatment facilities and have limited confidentiality by their very nature [24]. DODI 6490.04 [25] authorizes commanders to mandate a service member's evaluation by the local military mental health clinic, generally due to command identified concern about safety or a psychiatric condition which could compromise the unit's mission. The mental health clinic is required to provide the minimum necessary information to address the commander's concerns. CDEs sometimes result in inpatient hospitalization of the service member, but, regardless of the initiating reason, DODI 6490.04 requires transmission of "sufficient clinical information and recommendations to allow the commander or supervisor to understand service member's condition and make reasoned decisions about the Service member's safety, duties, and medical care requirements."

Duty to Protect

Mental health providers often reference "*Tarasoff*" when describing a duty to break confidentiality if they believe their patient may harm a third party. The *Tarasoff* case has holding power only in the state of California, where it was litigated [26], although most states and the District of Columbia have enacted *Tarasoff*-like legislation describing the clinician's obligation to either notify others or take reasonable precautions to protect third parties from harm [27]. Thus, there is a *Tarasoff*-like exception to confidentiality in VHA facilities as defined by the state-specific statute for the given facility.

In the military, DODI 6490.04, paragraph 6, does indeed contain such a provision, which states, "in any case in which a Service member has communicated to a privileged healthcare provider an explicit threat to kill or seriously injure a clearly identified or reasonably identifiable person, or to destroy property under the circumstances likely to lead to serious bodily injury or death, and the Service member has the apparent intent and ability to carry out the threat, the responsible healthcare provider will make a good faith effort to take precautions against the threatened injury." The provision goes on to describe the required notification of a third party, either a commander, supervisor, or law enforcement officer. Law enforcement must be informed of specifically named targets of violence, and any previous such targets must also be informed if the patient is being released from an inpatient psychiatric ward.

Providers may feel uncertain how to proceed when a threat is semi-explicit or the patient does not appear to have the means to carry out the threat. Consultation with a supervisor or other providers would assist. Hospitalizing such a patient could be justified in an analysis of the potential risks if the violent act were carried out, and the hospitalization alone would then justify notification of the command that some sort of psychiatric crisis is occurring.

Military and VHA providers may also be subject to local state laws, some of which require reporting of patients who have been involuntarily committed to a psychiatric ward. Guidance on this subject is best gleaned from the general counsel at the local facility. If required the reporting of this status, may have significant implications such as loss of the right to carry or purchase a firearm in that state. The report may also lead to placement on a similar federal list known as the National Instant Criminal Background Check System (NICS) created via the Gun Control Act of 1968 as modified by the Brady Handgun Violence Prevention Act of 1993 [28]. While patients may be advised to voluntarily self-enroll on the federal list by signing a form in the presence of their medical provider, they must be warned that the process is irreversible. The NICS self-selection form is available by contacting the Federal Bureau of Investigation (FBI) directly.

Substance Abuse

DODI 1010.04 [29] provides guidance for the screening and enrollment of service members at all levels of treatment for Substance Use Disorders (SUDs). Notification of commanders is still in accordance with DODI 6490.08, which states that commanders must be notified when medical personnel enroll or discharge Service members from outpatient or inpatient SUD treatment. However, a mere referral for substance education, without treatment, would not trigger a requirement to notify a patient's commander. Additionally, DHA-PI 6025.15 [30] clearly states that "routine outpatient treatment" would not automatically trigger a reporting requirement. Each military service maintains its own substance abuse treatment program, which require command notification even when Service members self-refer.

In 2009, the Army established a Confidential Alcohol Treatment and Education Pilot (CATEP) to allow treatment without mandatory command notification. Reports about the program in popular media have been positive and limited available information from academic sources has also been encouraging [31]. Although expansion of the pilot Army-wide and DOD-wide has been recommended by some commentators, at present the program only exists on some Army installations. Regulatory guidance regarding SUD treatment by DHA-PI 6025.15 in 2019 makes no mention of CATEP or similar concepts.

Within the VHA, besides HIPAA, 38 U.S.C. 7332 [32] provides federal guidance for the confidentiality of alcohol and drug treatment records. The Secretary of Veterans Affairs may allow the release of such records to medical professionals in the event of a bona fide medical emergency, for health and hospital care outside of the VHA, for internal quality review, for research purposes using de-identified data, to local state controlled substance monitoring programs, and for billing for treatment of non-service connected disabilities. State and federal courts may also subpoena such records if a judge rules that the public interest, i.e. the pursuit of justice, outweighs the privacy concerns. VHA and military health records may be viewed in both domains via current electronic means ("HAIMS") and the future joint electronic health record known as Genesis, a development that only occurred in the context of record-sharing struggles during the wars in Afghanistan and Iraq.

Psychiatric Medical Records and "Psychotherapy Notes"

HIPAA includes a provision for additional privacy protection for psychotherapy notes, which are generally considered separate from the medical record and for the psychotherapist's reference during in the course of therapy. Electronic health records in the military and VHA further blurred the concept of the definition of psychotherapy notes. HIPAA and clinical practice allow for the concept that certain written treatment content could be harmful to a patient if released to them. Considering that patient requests for records generally go through a Military Treatment Facility's (MTF) records department, rather than directly through a mental health department, a protocol should exist for providers to redact records that could be harmful, or portions that might constitute “psychotherapy notes.” A sometimes confusing aspect of such requests are that service members may move through multiple duty stations in their career. Should the service member then send record requests to every MTF he/she has ever gone to, or can the most current provider conduct a screen of all of the combined records and authorize release? Common sense is best applied here, based on the note content, the patient’s diagnosis, and behavioral profile. The most current provider might inform the patient to send a request to previous MTFs if the provider cannot make an informed decision concerning certain notes from that previous MTF. Similar quandaries may exist in the VHA, if patients have been seen in multiple VHA locations. VHA generally does not release active duty medical records even though they may be accessed through the joint electronic health record. Patients are referred to the National Archives or else to their specific services for further information. Medical records are exempt from Freedom of Information Act (FOIA) requests due to the invasion of personal privacy [33].

Health Oversight Activities

Hospitals commonly use peer review as a method for checking on the quality of care by their providers as required by hospital according organizations such as The Joint Commission. Peer review may also occur when concern a hospital identifies other concern for the care provided by a provider as a result of complaints of adverse outcomes. DODI 6490.04 allows for Quality Management Case Review for any Service member that “commits an act resulting in suicide, homicide, serious injury, or significant violence.” For the VHA, 38 U.S.C. 5705 provides for the confidentiality of these quality assurance activities. In both VHA and DOD, whereas third parties may review these records for purposes of quality assurance, and presumably document evidence of deviation from practice standards in their reviews, the extent to which a patient may exert privilege over communications replicated in quality assurance documentation is not clarified by existing law or policy.

Sexual Assault

Sexual assault victims receive special administrative attention and protections in regards to their confidentiality [34]. Sexual assault victims may seek treatment for psychiatric sequelae through the local military mental health clinic but may also seek guidance from their provider concerning confidentiality of treatment. In the case where a service member has sexually assaulted a family member, mandatory reporting is required as per DODI 6400.01, “Family Advocacy Program (FAP)” [22]. However, if service members sexually assault a non-family member, then mental health providers are under no obligation to report the incident to command, at least when the information is gleaned via a victim. Although an argument could be made that an active duty assailant could represent a harm to mission exception, the right to confidentiality of the victim, who is a patient, must also be considered.

Victims have further treatment options than just going to their local military emergency room or primary care clinic. The DOD's Sexual Assault Prevention and Response Office (SAPRO) creates standard protocols for handling victim reports depending on the degree of confidentiality the victim desires [35]. A victim who first seeks care at a military mental health clinic should be referred to the Sexual Assault Response Coordinator (SARC) for that MTF. Victims may receive limited medical services from a Sexual Assault Forensic Examiner (SAFE) as well as contact with a Victim Advocate (VA), all without requiring notification of law enforcement or command. The combined expertise of the above professionals may help guide the victim toward making a decision about reporting to law enforcement, and/or may assist in providing treatment for physical and psychiatric trauma. Of note, in line with the previous discussion about Military Rule of Evidence (MRE) 513 privilege for patient-psychotherapist communications, the military also has enacted MRE 514 which creates a privilege for communications between victims and Victim Advocates [13].

One aspect of the SAPRO process not always apparent to mental health providers is that the electronic health records of a victim may be subpoenaed, and perhaps released to court members as either an exception to MRE 513 or an exception to MRE 412 which seeks to shield victim sexual history from being used as evidence at court-martial [13]. This remains true despite recent revision to the Uniform Code of Military Justice (UCMJ) by the President which noted that disclosure of PHI was no longer required even in circumstances previously identified as "constitutionally required" (i.e., the accused's sixth Amendment right to confront witnesses). Items of potential relevance to a defense attorney of a service member accused of sexual assault would notably include a victim's psychiatric diagnoses, prescribed medications and side effects, their report of the sexual assault, their sexual history, substance abuse, and any evidence of inconsistent statements about these topics from one note to the next. Providers are advised to avoid certain topics and/or avoid documenting certain facts if their discovery in court might prove damaging to the victim's credibility. Providers should also note that even without writing a note, they could be called to testify under oath as to their memory of a session.

VHA settings maintain confidentiality in a manner similar to the above, but are also subject to local state law. Some states have "rape shield laws" similar to MRE 412, while others do not. Thus, providers should still maintain caution in the event that a victim's mental health records are subpoenaed and, ensure that an exception to privilege has been appropriately granted by the appropriate judicial authority.

Violations of the Law of War

Anecdotal experiences reveals that some healthcare providers in military treatment facilities, which include substantial numbers of civilian DOD personnel, are unclear about whether they have a legal duty to report possible war crimes revealed during treatment sessions. The current status of DOD regulations contributes to that ambiguity, as described in detail by two former Army attorneys [36]. Department of Defense Directive (DODD) 2311.01E, "DOD Law of War Program," states in paragraph 6.3 that "all military and U.S. civilian employees [and contractors] ... shall report reportable incidents through their chain of command" [37]. DODD 2311.01E was last "certified current" on February 22, 2011. However, DODI 6490.08, published on August 17, 2011, seems to reduce this requirement for mental health providers.

DODI 6490.08 provides a list of nine situations in which a military mental health provider "shall notify the commander" and thus break confidentiality. The list does not specifically state violations of the law of war. However, the list could allow for reporting if certain qualities are met. For example, if a patient appears at risk for harming other in the future, including via war crimes, then that could qualify for reporting. The rationale would include the general duty to protect others from harm, but also that such actions could harm the overall mission of his/her unit should such war crimes become known. The ninth category on the list "Other special circumstances," allows for a weighing of whether "proper execution of the military mission outweighs the interests served by avoiding notification" by an O-6 level health care provider or equivalent.

To summarize, DODI 6490.08 appears to allow mental health providers to break confidentiality and report violations of the law of war by their patients, but only if legitimate concern exists that future such acts might occur and/or those acts could harm a military mission. This potential harm may include indirect means such as public outcry in host countries or within the U.S. Although a review by an O-6 level provider to authorize reporting is an option, DODI 6490.08 appears to only require such review when the provider does not believe clear harm to others or harm to mission exists. Unless DODD 2311.01E is modified at a future date, DODI 6490.08 appears to present more precise and more recent guidance to mental health providers.

R.C.M. 706 Sanity Board Evaluations

Sanity Boards are psychiatric evaluations ordered by a Convening Authority via a Military Judge's request [38]. Though they are commonly performed in military mental health clinics, no information or written reports generated from the evaluation should be loaded into the military electronic health record, i.e. AHLTA or Genesis. The reason is that these evaluations are not medical treatment sessions, are not covered by Tricare, and are performed under attorney-client privilege, not psychotherapist-patient privilege. For purposes of generating credit for workload, a note could be created stating that the RCM 706 evaluation occurred, but no resulting reports, whether the full version or the abbreviated version, should be uploaded, nor any free-text description of observations and findings from the evaluation. Failure to do so might result in a breach of the accused's privilege and derailment of the time-sensitive court-martial process.

Dependent Children of Active Duty Service Members

Child dependents of Service members sometimes seek to join the military in adulthood. Once accessioned to active duty, some services allow merging of their dependent record with their new active duty record, as both exist on the same electronic health record. It remains an open question as to whether this is consistently explained as part of informed consent at child and adolescent clinics or described in clinic limits of confidentiality disclosure forms. At the least, providers in such clinics should have awareness of the issue. Of note, the relevant DOD regulation on accession procedures states that all recruits must consent to release all past medical records to DOD [39]. One could interpret this to mean that the military would have the authority to gain access to the records regardless. However, it also imposes greater scrutiny on military dependents, as non-dependents' past records may not be as easily obtained from civilian institutions, may be kept secret or may not be preserved. At present, DOD has not issued any instruction disallowing the use of merged medical records for service members that are former dependents.

Other Exceptions: Medical Evaluation Boards, Screenings, and Other Mandatory Evaluations

A large number of other DOD administrative processes may require mandatory mental health evaluation with the "minimum necessary" findings transmitted to non-medical commanders and/or decision makers. Military providers have an obligation to their service to recommend Service members to the Integrated Disability Evaluation Service (IDES) via a Medical Evaluation Board when they believe the Service member is permanently unfit for service due to a qualifying psychiatric condition. Service members have no ability to block such an action should they disagree with their provider.

Many military training programs and administrative functions require medical and psychiatric screening. Service members generally have no ability to prevent disclosure of results of these screenings. They include: (1) Service school screening such as for recruiters, drill sergeants, snipers, long range surveillance operators, and Special Forces operators; (2) Administrative separation screening for PTSD, mTBI, or other conditions that may have affected the circumstances leading to separation; (3) Personnel Reliability Program screening, such as for personnel handling nuclear, chemical, or biological weapons; (4) Flight status screening; (5) Security clearance screening; and (6) Treatment planning meetings for Warrior Transition Units (WTUs).

One final category involves deployment-related screening, especially when the Service member is under treatment for a psychiatric disorder and/or is prescribed a psychotropic medication. These patients may require a CENTCOM-approved waiver before they can enter that theater. Situations requiring a waiver are listed under MOD 14—Tab A, can be found online [40]. More detailed guidance on mental health conditions and specific medications may be procured through military medical channels. Mandatory post-deployment screening, which occurs in two iterations, may also generate information that might need sharing with command, though historically Service members tend not to reveal much psychiatric information in such screenings.

Handling Unauthorized Breaches of HIPAA

Complex rules govern how military and VHA facilities handle inappropriate disclosures of PHI. Breaches are handled at the highest level by the Office for Civil Rights (OCR) of HHS in accordance with the HIPAA Enforcement Rule [12]. Not all violations result in penalties, but OCR may work with the Department of Justice (DOJ) if necessary, including for the pursuit of criminal charges for intentional violations. However, some HIPAA violations may be handled at a local level. The military and VHA generally require their providers to inform their local privacy officer when they discover a possible HIPAA violation. Responsibility for reporting the breach falls upon the organization. If military providers believe an unauthorized breach of PHI confidentiality has occurred, DODI 5400.11, "DOD Privacy and Civil Liberties Programs," paragraph 3.1.d. [41], states that all such instances are handled by the Defense Health Agency Privacy and Civil Liberties Office, in accordance with DOD regulation [16]. Both military and VHA facilities are reliant on staff to report HIPAA breaches for appropriate handling. If, for instance, a patient reports a breach to OCR and the subsequent investigation finds the facility did not appropriately investigate in the incident, then that facility may face substantial monetary fines. Employees in both systems are advised to ensure they are aware of the reporting requirements of their facility to avoid adverse action for failure to follow organizational rules.

Future Directions

While HIPAA applies to both VHA and DOD healthcare facilities and the care providers who work within these institutions, the laws, military regulations and policies superimposed upon the "federal minimum standard" for privacy articulated in HIPAA add considerable limitations to these protections—particularly for active duty members. Although the sponsors of HIPAA recognized the additional needs for information exchange the broad language of its military exception, others have since challenged the range of exceptions it has been interpreted to permit. Social scientists and legal authorities, keenly aware of the barrier to care imposed by stigma, argue that weakened confidentiality limits make it more difficult for military members to seek the mental health care they need, noting that military members accurately perceive that seeking treatment can harm their careers [42]. Others point to the lack of evidence that limits actually improve military readiness or function and to the fact that military service members are entitled to nearly the same levels of privacy protection for communications with chaplains and attorneys as are civilians [43]. Some believe that the institution of more stringent civilian standards for confidentiality will encourage service members to seek needed care, noting that regulations governing command-directed evaluations will allow for feedback to the commander in situations where a commander's concern about a service member's fitness for duty or safety prompts an involuntary command directed evaluation [44].

As the military continues to search for effective programs and policies to address the alarming increase in military suicide rates noted over the last 15 years, leaders and legislators will no doubt consider the role of stigma as they continue to refine medical privacy regulations. At the same time military and civilian scientists continue to expand and integrate existing military medical, legal, training and administrative databases and develop Automated Intelligence (AI) algorithms combining these to identify risk profiles for suicide and other negative behavioral health outcomes [45, 46]. Commanders call for "health-risk dashboards" that might provide increased visibility on perceived health threats to mission readiness. The extent to which commanders may ultimately gain access to AI generated measures of risk from information contained in medical and other databases is not clear. Thus, while law and regulatory guidance may evolve to either strengthen or even potentially weaken privacy protections for service member health information, the limits will continue to reflect a balance of competing interests. Regardless of the individual provider's personal beliefs, awareness of the current status of the law and policy best serves our patients.

References

1. Higgins GL. The history of confidentiality in medicine. Can Fam Physician. 1989;35(914):921–6.
2. Johnson WB, Grasso I, Maslowski K. Conflicts between ethics and law for military mental health providers. Mil Med. 2010;175:548–53.
3. Kennedy CH, Johnson WB. Mixed agency in military psychology: applying the American Psychological Association ethics code. Psychol Serv. 2009;6:22–31.
4. Warner CH, Appenzeller GN, Grieger T, et al. Ethical considerations in military psychiatry. Psychiatr Clin N Am. 2009;32:271–81.
5. American Psychological Association. Ethical principles of psychologists and code of conduct. Am Psychol. 2002;57:1060–73.
6. American Psychological Association. 2010 Amendments to the 2002 "Ethical principles of psychologists and code of conduct". Am Psychol. 2010;65:493.
7. American Psychiatric Association. The principles of medical ethics with annotations especially applicable to psychiatry. 2013th ed. Arlington, VA: American Psychiatric Association; 2013.
8. Hoyt T. Limits to confidentiality in U.S. army treatment settings. Mil Psychol. 2013;25(1):46–56.
9. Krumholz HM. Informed consent to promote patient-centered care. JAMA. 2010;303:1190–1.
10. Privacy Act of 1974. 5 U.S.C. ch. 5 § 552a; 1974.
11. Health Insurance Portability and Accountability Act of 1996. 45 C.F.R. § 164.502-512; 1996.
12. HHS.gov. HIPAA for Professionals. https://www.hhs.gov/hipaa/for-professionals/index.html. Accessed 28 Jan 2020.
13. Department of Defense. Manual for courts-martial. 2019d. https://jsc.defense.gov/Portals/99/Documents/2019%20MCM%20(Final)%20(20190108).pdf?ver=2019-01-11-115724-610. Accessed 21 Jan 21 2020.
14. Department of Veterans Affairs. Privacy and release of information (VHA Directive 1605.01). Washington, DC: Government Printing Office; 2016. https://www.va.gov/vhapublications/ViewPublication.asp?pub_ID=3233/. Accessed 22 Jan 2020.

15. Department of Veterans Affairs. Health insurance portability and accountability act applicability in VBA (Memorandum ADV 3-2003). 2003. https://jsc.defense.gov/Portals/99/Documents/2019%20MCM%20(Final)%20(20190108).pdf?ver=2019-01-11-115724-610. Accessed 21 Jan 2020.
16. Department of Defense. Implementation of the health insurance portability and accountability act (HIPAA) privacy rule in DOD health care programs (DOD Manual 6025.18). Washington, DC: Government Printing Office; 2019c.
17. Jaffee v. Redmond. 518 U.S. 1; 1996.
18. Trail TE, Martin LT, Burgette LF, et al. An evaluation of U.S. military non-medical counseling programs. Rand Health Q. 2012;8(2):6.
19. Department of Defense. Command notification requirements to dispel stigma in providing mental health care to service members (DOD Instruction 6490.08). Washington, DC: Government Printing Office; 2011a.
20. Department of the Army. Medical record administration and healthcare documentation (AR 40-66). Washington, DC: Government Printing Office; 2010.
21. Victims of Child Abuse Act of 1990. 42 U.S.C. 13031; 1990.
22. Department of Defense. Family advocacy program (FAP) (DOD Instruction 6400.01). Washington, DC: Government Printing Office; 2019b.
23. Department of Veterans Affairs. Reporting cases of abuse and neglect (VHA Directive 1199). Washington, DC: Government Printing Office; 2017. https://www.va.gov/vhapublications/ViewPublication.asp?pub_ID=5624. Accessed 24 Jan 2020.
24. Warner CH, Appenzeller GN, Breitbach JE, et al. Psychiatric consultation to command. In: Ritchie EC, editor. Combat and operational behavioral health. Fort Sam Houston, TX: Office of the Surgeon General; 2014. p. 182–4.
25. Department of Defense. Mental health evaluations of members of the military services (DOD Instruction 6490.04). Washington, DC: Government Printing Office; 2013.
26. Tarasoff v. The Regents of the University of California. 17 Cal. 3d 425; 1976.
27. Kachigan C, Felthous AR. Court responses to Tarasoff statutes. J Am Acad Psychiatry Law. 2004;32:263–73.
28. Gun Control Act of 1968. 18 U.S.C. 922; 1968.
29. Department of Defense. Problematic substance use by DOD personnel (DOD Instruction 1010.04). Washington, DC: Government Printing Office, 2014.
30. Defense Health Agency. Management of problematic substance use by DOD personnel (DHA-PI 6025.15). Washington, DC: Government Printing Office; 2019.
31. O'Brien CP, Oster M, Morden E. Committee on prevention, diagnosis, treatment, and management of substance use disorders in the US Armed Forces, Board on the Health of Select Populations & Institute of Medicine. In: Oster M, Morden E, editors. Substance use disorders in the U.S. armed forces. National Academies Press; 2013.
32. 38 U.S.C. 7332 ("Confidentiality of Certain Medical Records). https://www.law.cornell.edu/uscode/text/38/7332. Accessed 13 Jul 2021.
33. FOIA.gov. https://www.foia.gov/faq.html. Accessed 28 Jan 2020.
34. Johnson DE, Yeaw J. Military sexual assault. In: Robert LW, Warner CH, editors. Military and veteran mental health. New York: Springer; 2018.
35. Department of Defense. Sexual assault prevention and response (SAPR) program procedures (DOD Instruction 6495.02). Washington, DC: Government Printing Office; 2017.
36. Topinka JB, Caspari MW. In: Ritchie EC, editor. Legal overview of confidentiality and reporting of military behavioral health records. Fort Sam Houston, TX: Office of the Surgeon General; 2014. p. 13–9.
37. Department of Defense. DOD Law of war program (DOD Directive 2311.01E). Washington, DC: Government Printing Office; 2011b.
38. Montalbano P. Sanity board evaluations. In: Ritchie EC, editor. Forensic and ethical issues in military behavioral health. Fort Sam Houston, TX: Office of the Surgeon General; 2014.

39. Department of Defense. Medical standards for appointment, enlistment, or induction into the military services (DOD Instruction 6130.03). Washington, DC: Government Printing Office; 2018.
40. MOD 14. PPG-Tab A, Amplification of the minimal standards of fitness for deployment to the CENTCOM AOR; to accompany MOD fourteen to USCENTCOM individual protection and individual/unit deployment policy. https://www.health.mil/Reference-Center/Publications/2019/11/19/PPG-Tab-A. Accessed 22 Jan 2020.
41. Department of Defense. DOD privacy and civil liberties programs (DOD Instruction 5400.11). Washington, DC: Government Printing Office; 2019a.
42. Neuhauser JA. Lives of quiet desperation: the conflict between military necessity and confidentiality. Creighton Law Rev. 2011;44:1003–44.
43. Engel C. Compromised confidentiality in the military is harmful. Psychiatric Times. 2014. https://www.rand.org/blog/2014/10/compromised-confidentiality-in-the-military-is-harmful.html. Accessed 13 Jul 2021.
44. Engel C. Suicide, mental disorders, and the US military: time to focus on mental health service delivery. JAMA. 2013;310(5):484–5.
45. Kessler RC, Stein MB, Petukhova MV, et al. Predicting suicides after outpatient mental health visits in the Army Study to Assess Risk and Resilience in Service-members (Army STARRS). Mol Psychiatry. 2017;22:544–51.
46. Rosellini A, Monahan J, Street A, et al. Predicting non-familial major physical violent crime perpetration in the US Army from administrative data. Psychol Med. 2016;46(2):303–16.

Mental Health Care During Military Deployment

9

Christopher H. Warner and Teresa D. Murray

Vignette

Sergeant S is a 24 year old U.S Army Non-Commissioned Officer in an airborne infantry brigade who is on month seven of his second combat deployment. He spends on average 50–60 h per week "outside the wire" leading his squad of eight to ten soldiers in stability and security operations interacting with the local leaders and populace in ongoing efforts to restore essential services (water, power, etc.) for the village. His squad has encountered numerous improvised explosive devices during their operations and on multiple occasions have engaged in direct engagements with insurgent forces who sought to ambush them. One week ago, one of Sergeant S' soldiers was killed by an improvised explosive device and two others wounded while they were coming back from one of their missions. Since that time, Sergeant S has noted increased anger, irritability, difficulty sleeping, and has frequently been playing back the events of that mission in his head questioning if he made all of the correct choices.

Introduction

The presence of mental health providers on the battlefield directly coincides with the emergence of modern psychiatry. Prior review of medical casualty data from the United States Civil War identified that it was very rare for a service member to be given a mental health diagnosis (3 per every 1000 Union Soldiers) even though battlefield physicians were describing conditions such as nostalgia and Soldier's

C. H. Warner (✉)
Department of Psychiatry, Uniformed Services University of the Health Sciences, Bethesda, MD, USA

T. D. Murray
Army College of Social Work, University of Kentucky, San Antonio, TX, USA

C. H. Warner, C. A. Castro (eds.), *Veteran and Military Mental Health*,
https://doi.org/10.1007/978-3-031-18009-5_9

Heart [1]. However, by the turn of the century, multiple nations were becoming increasingly aware of the impact of combat and operational stress. This led to the development of the first formal battlefield mental health treatments initially by the Russian military medical team and subsequently by the Russian Red Cross during the Russo-Japanese War. These lessons learned, coupled with the emergence of a new condition known as "shell shock" early in World War I, led to all major military participants initiating trial and error battlefield mental health treatment [2, 3].

As the United States Army prepared to potentially enter World War I, the Army Medical Department enhanced their mental health capabilities within the United States and Dr. Thomas Salmon established the first deployable mental health capabilities for the United States military. Under Salmon's leadership, the first successful battlefield mental health system was implemented incorporating treatment, prevention, and consultation. Many of the principles that guide the current approach to combat and operational stress casualties were outlined by this team [4].

In the aftermath of World War I, much of the military mental health effort focused on mechanisms for screening out mental health disorders with an expectation that if screening was successful, the battlefield capabilities would not be necessary. However, by the North African campaign of 1943, it was evident that battlefield mental health capabilities would be a necessity and have been deploying with United States military personnel since that time [2, 3]. While the conditions treated and mechanisms for delivery have changed over the years with the United States Army developing Combat and Operational Stress Control teams during the Korea and Vietnam wars to provide more area support versus unit specific support and the United States Marine Corps implementing their Operational Stress Control and Readiness program, the need to provide battlefield mental health has remained [5].

Changing Nature of Demands

While the mental health impacts of war have long been recognized and are documented both in historical accounts and classical literature, the medical community did not begin to recognize the effects sustained from combat until the mid-eighteen century. Auenbrugger coined the diagnosis of nostalgia in 1761 to describe the condition of French soldiers losing hope and becoming sad, isolative, inattentive, and apathetic in the aftermath of combat [6]. Subsequently, during the United States Civil War a new condition identified as DaCosta's Syndrome or sometimes referred to as Soldier's Heart was identified for an anxiety condition characterized by fatigue upon exertion, shortness of breath, palpitations, sweating, and chest pain with a normal physical exam [7]. As warfare evolved into the twentieth century and the destructive capabilities of military forces fueled by the industrial revolution expanded, physicians began identifying service members presenting with symptoms ranging from panic attacks to near catatonia after periods of intense combat, especially those involving field artillery shelling. This new condition was termed, shell shock [8]. The discovery of these conditions led not only to the employment of mental health professionals on the battlefield but also to changes in the treatments provided. Prior to World War I, those identified with a mental health condition were evacuated off the battlefield and many times out of the theater of war [9]. However, the presence of mental health professionals established the implementation of forward treatment principles and battlefield mental health professionals identified that the optimal window for treatment was within a few hours after combat exposure. Over the course of the subsequent decades, these conditions were later referred to as war neuroses and then as combat operational stress. The specific treatment principles for combat operational stress are outlined in greater detail in this book in the chapter on combat operational stress.

As the presence of mental health professionals on the battlefield continued to evolve, so did an understanding of the factors impacting combat and operational stress. Analysis of World War II data showed that while combat exposure was a significant driver of combat operational stress citing a strong correlation between combat stress casualties and the intensity of combat and total number of wounded personnel; it did also identify other key factors including deployment length, unit cohesion and morale, and unit leadership effectiveness [10]. This led to an expansion of the roles and responsibilities of the deployed mental health capabilities. During the Korean and Vietnam Wars, the United States military began deploying area support mental health capabilities that began employing not only treatment capabilities but for the first time, preventive focused capabilities focused on assessment and consultative services to enhance resiliency [2].

The most recent prolonged United States conflicts in Iraq and Afghanistan have identified new mental health challenges. These wars presented the first major test for the all-volunteer military force which dictated new military employment and deployment strategies and has led to a large number of military personnel being deployed multiple times into the combat theater. Additionally, the advances in our mental health treatment capabilities including safety profiles and transportability of medications and the interconnectedness of our world has had a significant impact both in care delivery and the stressors that our deployed service members face.

During the Persian Gulf War in 1990–1991, service members who were suffering from depression and/or anxiety were still dominantly being treated with tri-cyclic antidepressants and would not be capable of deploying. Those who did deploy, would wait for weeks to months before receiving letters from their loved ones and may have an occasional opportunity to make a brief phone call home. Over the next 10 years, the introduction of the internet, the propagation of cellular phone technology, and medical advances including the expansion and increased understanding of Selective Serotonin Reuptake Inhibitors brought dramatic change. A 2005 utilization review of one Division Mental Health unit deployed to Iraq found that nearly 6% of deployed personnel sought care for mental health conditions that existed prior to the deployment including Major Depressive Disorder and Generalized Anxiety Disorder. That same review identified that the most prominent causative factors for combat operational stress reactions was not combat exposure, but rather home front stressors such as failing relationships and financial problems [11]. These changes drove significant changes to battlefield mental health delivery.

Evolving Role of Treatments

Prior to World War I, the majority of mental health casualties were evacuated from the battlefield and most often out of the theater of war. World War I brought the introduction of the forward psychiatry principles that provided not only treatment near the front lines but also established an expectancy that service members would be returning to the fight. These principles, outlined in greater detail in the chapter on Combat and Operational Stress, served as the cornerstone of battlefield mental health intervention for nearly the next century. It is important to note, that in persistent, high intensity combat, these principles would remain the bedrock of care, and likely only measure that could be delivered without evacuation. However, as theaters of war mature, battle lines become more established, and/or phases of war transition into stability operations, modern psychiatry has additional resources which can serve as additional interventions.

Psychotherapy in Theater

Due to the mission-oriented nature of the combat environment, therapy while deployed centers on meeting immediate psychological and emotional needs in order to enhance combat readiness for both the individual service member and the unit. These encounters must be time-limited, brief interventions as the high operational tempo and geographic placement of units and their behavioral health providers may not allow for regularly scheduled sessions [12, 13]. Therapy sessions in theater often look quite different compared to those in garrison as they may take place at unconventional times to accommodate for unit mission schedules and in unusual locations, such as in shipping containers that have been converted into work spaces or supply closets in the unit aid station.

Thanks to advances in battlefield communications, therapy sessions, risk assessments, and intake assessments may also take place over virtual means using telebehavioral health capabilities through either computer-based video chatting or over the telephone in the event of technological difficulties. This capability can be especially helpful when conditions limit travel to or from the location of the patient or the behavioral health provider, or for those far forward outposts that may not receive routine visits by a behavioral health provider [14]. Because of the possibility for high-risk situations where a patient's safety may be in question, it is critical that these sessions are held in close coordination with the medical personnel on the ground with the patient as these individuals will be crucial in responding to any potential safety concerns that may be disclosed during the therapy session [15]. Command consultation may also be critical in these situations to ensure appropriate measures are taken to ensure patient safety. Privacy is another important consideration when using tele-behavioral health to conduct therapy sessions. A private space must be established for tele-behavioral health services so that service members will feel comfortable participating in the session and so that the conversation will not be overheard by others.

As previously mentioned, therapy in the deployed environment must provide some immediate relief or reduction in distress that will allow service members to remain ready for upcoming missions. The focus of therapy sessions in theater may often include education on coping skills, relaxation techniques, and other measures to help reduce physiological and psychological arousal that is common among service members while deployed [16]. Service members in the combat environment are frequently exposed to dangerous situations and may find themselves in a sustained high level of vigilance that can make it difficult to relax or rest between missions. As a result, therapy sessions that include education on relaxation techniques, such as diaphragmatic breathing, progressive muscle relaxation, and guided imagery can help service members decompress between missions when they have the opportunity [17]. This education also helps to teach service members about the link between their physiological and their psychological states and can help them to become more effective in future anxiety-provoking situations.

Additional psychoeducation and coaching focused on the importance of healthy eating, physical activity, and sleep routines can give service members a way to combat anxiety and control factors that they can control within the constraints of the combat environment [16]. Of course, even these areas can be difficult to control while deployed due to unpredictable work-rest cycles, lack of access to regular healthy meals on remote bases, shared living quarters, austere conditions that are not conducive to restful sleep, and the prevalence of caffeine and nicotine use among many service members.

In addition to education on relaxation techniques, therapy provided downrange often focuses on adjustment disorders, relationship difficulties, anxiety, depression, post-traumatic stress, combat operational stress, grief, occupational problems, and insomnia [18]. Although most of these are topics that frequently emerge in the garrison environment, treatment interventions for these conditions in the deployed setting must be approached in unique ways. Therapy must always be focused on individual readiness as it relates to mission success, and must be scheduled around the service member's mission requirements. Behavioral health providers should use time-limited, brief therapies that can produce tangible benefits in a short period of time, such as solution-focused brief therapy, cognitive behavioral therapy, and psychoeducation, among others [19]. These modalities may be especially helpful as they can provide instant reframing and challenging of cognitive distortions, a focus on strengths and resilience, and practical skills that can be implemented outside the session. Additionally, these brief interventions are important because the unpredictable nature of the combat mission may make it difficult to schedule future sessions. Mission requirements, hectic schedules, and a lack of privacy may make homework or out of session work impractical or impossible, so practical exercises and assignments may have to be completed in the therapy session with the provider. However, for those service members whose jobs primarily keep them inside the wire of the base and who are co-located with their behavioral health provider, regularly occurring therapy sessions with homework outside the session may be feasible.

Treatment using manualized approaches, such as prolonged exposure therapy and cognitive processing therapy for post-traumatic stress disorder, can be challenging in the context of the combat deployment [20]. As previously stated, it can be difficult, if not impossible, to schedule regularly occurring therapy sessions due to the operational tempo and time constraints; however, providers have had success with truncated or shortened versions of these modalities [21]. The homework assignments that often accompany these modalities may not be feasible due to environmental and time constraints. It may also be unrealistic to challenge irrational beliefs associated with previous traumatic events when the service member is still being exposed to new potentially traumatizing events. The vigilance and arousal a service member exhibits while on a mission serve a very real and important purpose as they are realistically facing dangerous threats on a regular basis [22]. Therefore, the behavioral health provider should practice caution when deeming certain thoughts to be maladaptive or irrational as healthy behaviors and thoughts held on deployment may differ significantly from those considered to be healthy in garrison.

Advances in technology, including wireless internet, cell phones, laptops, and gaming consoles, allow service members in a combat zone to remain connected to their family members despite being thousands of miles away. Although this connectedness can certainly facilitate communication and strengthen relationships, it can also lead to service members with one foot in the combat zone and one foot back at home, potentially distracted while on mission by a stressful situation that is happening on the home front.

Medication Management

Before the United States Global War on Terror operations in Iraq and Afghanistan, the use of psychotropic medication was limited to emergent use and was frequently accompanied with evacuation from theater [23]. Due to the improved safety of psychotropic medications, Iraq and Afghanistan brought about a change in attitude towards the deployment of service members on psychotropic medications and the prescribing of those medications in a deployed environment. The new guidance recommended using medications when appropriate, emphasizing the importance of considering side effects, limited availability of laboratory monitoring, and continued application of the forward psychiatry principles [5].

While the United States military provides policy guidance on medication management of mental health conditions in the deployed environment, it is ultimately the psychiatrist who will have to make decisions regarding the extent of services they can safely and effectively provide based on patient and unit safety, the deployed environment and military situation, and supply and monitoring capabilities.

When considering prescribing psychotropic medications in a deployed environment, psychiatrists must consider several factors including the ability to provide follow up care and availability of medication re-supply. In general, providers will prescribe Selective Serotonin Reuptake Inhibitors and/or Selective Serotonin/

Norepinephrine Reuptake Inhibitors as well as some Atypical Antidepressants for treatment of depression, anxiety, and trauma related conditions. The use of atypical antipsychotics, benzodiazepines, and stimulant medications is less common and requires a case by case evaluation. The treatment of conditions such as acute psychosis and/or mania would receive immediate treatment with appropriate medication interventions but will generally be followed by a rapid evacuation from theater and should not managed for prolonged periods of time or in a maintenance period in a deployed environment [5].

For those who are preparing to deploy and are already prescribed a psychotropic medication, their unit medical screening process will review their requirements and apply the current Department of Defense minimum mental health standards for deployment [24]. These requirements emphasize a need for medication stabilization prior to deployment consideration of storage and monitoring requirements, as well as, resupply capabilities. For example, a service member prescribed a Selective Serotonin Reuptake Inhibitor within 1 month of deployment may be delayed in their deployment until their condition stabilizes and they are not exhibiting significant side effects, but will be able to subsequently deploy. In contrast, a service member on lithium even at a maintenance dose is unlikely to be cleared for deployment because of the inability to continue laboratory monitoring and the environmental risks to the service member while taking the medication. Of note, one study showed that establishing a continuity of care plan for deploying service members reduced the risk of worsening symptoms, mental health evacuations, and serious events for the duration of the deployment [25].

Restoration and Disposition from Theater

Patient disposition options in a deployed environment are limited with the majority of resources available being outpatient settings. Theater level hospitals may have a small inpatient psychiatric holding capacity specifically designed to manage an acutely psychotic, manic, or suicidal patient who is receiving acute treatment and pending evacuation from theater. Within the deployed environment, the majority of service members are treated locally at the mental health unit. If there is a requirement to have them spend a night away from their unit to ensure accessibility to resources or services, this generally can be accomplished at the nearest aid station. Service members who present a safety risk concern will be placed on a "unit watch". Service members who symptoms persist for 72 h or are more significant can be sent to a restoration center. These centers, located within the theater of operations but generally further away from the front lines, can provide focused, intensive, outpatient treatment for up to 7 days. The majority of service members seen and treated at the restoration center recover and return to duty; however, those whose symptoms worsen or do not resolve within the 7 days are evacuated from theater [5].

Prevention

The role of psychiatrists in the deployed environment began transitioning solely from treatment and disposition to prevention in the latter years of World War II with the establishment of command consultation and the development of mental hygiene training programs [26]. The effectiveness of these programs was highlighted in the Group for the Advancement of Psychiatry's 1960 report that cited preventive military mental health care allowed for early recognition and prompt outpatient treatment of emotional difficulties thus reducing combat ineffectiveness [27]. More recently, prevention has expanded to include pre/post deployment mental health screening. The challenge to military mental health providers is balancing the available time to conduct prevention work with the demands of identified mental health patients. Additionally, providers must commit time to building relationships with the unit leaders to maintain credibility, to garner support for their recommendations, and to ensure that they have situational awareness and understanding of the ongoing mission to help shape their recommendations.

From a primary prevention standpoint, there are two measures that deployed psychiatrists can implement to encourage the development of adaptive stress responses and resiliency: health promotion/mental health education and battlefield circulation.

Psychoeducation can be conducted prior to and during deployments and should be tailored in product and delivery to match the audience, setting, and military situation. These efforts should focus on recognition of key stressors associated with these situations, recognizing service member's strengths, and teaching service members how to develop resiliency [28]. Further discussion on resiliency development and these tools can be found in a separate chapter of this book.

Vignette

During a unit's repeated deployment to Afghanistan, mental health and unit leaders were concerned about how to promote adaptive stress responses. The combat stress detachment and unit behavioral health personnel including psychologists, social workers, behavioral health technicians, chaplains, and chaplains' assistants, we planned and executed a full-day stress management education event that was centrally located on the forward operating base. The event was conducted at a central location near the dining facility which allowed large groups of service members for participation. The event included brief psychoeducational classes on stress management, healthy coping skills, relaxation techniques, and other helpful subjects that were deemed appropriate based on previous presenting difficulties that the mental health professional encountered during the deployment. The event also incorporated games, yoga classes, and free giveaways of snacks, toiletries, and other desirable items that served as non-stigmatizing ways for mental health professionals to interact with the service members and to provide them information about who they were and the services they could provide if needed in the future. Additionally, they provided attending service members with psychoeducational pamphlets and audio recordings that service members could take with them and read in their free time.

Battlefield circulation, sometimes referred to as therapy by walking around or walkabouts, describes time spent traveling around the battlefield visiting with service members and leaders to develop a better understanding of the overall situation and the needs of subordinate commanders and service members. These interactions allow psychiatrists to educate, counsel and advise junior leaders and service members on applicable mental health topics and coping strategies. During these visits, psychiatrists sometimes meet individually or with a group of service members and junior leaders to assess unit climate, morale, and cohesion and to provide psychoeducation on relevant topics such as sleep hygiene, dealing with loss, and anger management. Additionally, this circulation provides opportunities to advise unit leaders on actions they can take which may impact the mental hygiene of the organization to include potential improvements to operational and environmental factors such as living conditions, work/rest cycles, etc. [29].

Vignette

During a recent deployment to Afghanistan, a unit mental health team (consisting of a psychologist or licensed clinical social worker and a mental health technician) frequently included walking around the internal perimeter of their forward operating base with the sergeant of the guard in their routine. This action allowed the mental health team to interact and check in with the service members assigned to guard tower duties. Guard tower duty tends to be an isolative task that involves long shifts for multiple days in a row. Additionally, those service members assigned to these duties might have limited accessibility to medical and mental health services. These circulations were coordinated ahead of time through the unit who owned the base security mission to ensure that they were conducted in a way that would not detract from that mission. At each guard post, the sergeant of the guard would take over the guard mission so that the assigned guards would be able to take a break and speak with the mental health team while not leaving their guard posts vacant. As the team visited with the service members, they offered cold drinks and snacks, introduced themselves and provided the service members with information about the available mental health services and where we were located on the base. As part of this visit, the team engaged in casual conversation with the service member developing a rapport and gathering information about potential stressors that not only the individual service member was facing but the unit as well and taught the service member about basic relaxation and stress management techniques. In summary, these encounters developed low-threat opportunities to educate service members about available services and how to access them, while also providing an opportunity to gain helpful information about soldier concerns, unit trends, and other factors that might be impacting service member well-being and unit readiness.

Commonly employed secondary prevention measures include mechanisms for early identification of those at risk of developing mental health problems and employing interventions to prevent worsening of or development of symptoms after exposure. These include individual and unit level screenings, as well as, traumatic event management.

The United States military implemented post-deployment physical and mental health screening in the late 1990s to identify all of those service members who may have had potential environmental, physical, or mental health exposures [30]. This screening initially included only a few questions but with lessons learned from Iraq and Afghanistan expanded to included objective scales for Posttraumatic Stress Disorder, Depression, Substance Use Disorders, and Domestic Violence. Additionally, the frequency and timing was expanded to include multiple iterations [28]. Later, a pre-deployment screen was implemented to identify whether a service member should be deployed or if they were and had a mental health condition, included a care plan for ensuring their continuation of care [25]. While these tools have a number of limitations to include a reliance on self-reporting and a lack of such reporting due to the lack anonymity, they provide key touchpoints for both education on resources available and how to access them, as well as, for psychoeducation on tools that service members can implement. One key aspect to these screenings being successful is the coordination of care between the screening team and either the unit mental health team or the home station mental health team to ensure that those who are identified receive further evaluation and treatment. The deployed mental health team plays a key role in this process both when they are conducting screenings for returning service members and when they are receiving those who are arriving to theater who will require continuation of care. This communication is accomplished through multiple mechanisms including the world wide electronic medical record, secure communications, and coordination with unit leaders.

Within the deployed environment, military mental health providers may be asked to assess the mental health and welfare of a unit. These teams are equipped with service developed assessment tools and also have psychologists on their teams capable of developing specific screening and assessment tools based on the needs of the unit. The mental health team can conduct interviews, surveys, or other assessment and provide recommendations to unit leaders on actions they can take to improve unit resiliency, morale, cohesion, and quality of life. These are all factors which can not only enhance a unit's effectiveness in combat, but also reduce the rate of combat operational stress reactions during the deployment [28].

Another frequently used prevention mechanism is traumatic event management. Traumatic event management is an intervention that occurs after exposure to a potentially life threatening or deadly event. These interventions are meant to decrease the effect of the event and prevent long term mental health complications from them. Of note, traumatic event management is a process that includes consulting with the onsite leaders, conducting a needs assessment for the unit/organization, and subsequently employing appropriate interventions. These interventions serve as an opportunity to reduce stigma and barriers to mental health care by showing that the leaders recognize and support mental health assistance in response to these events and also provide education to those impacted on resources available [5]. However, some interventions may be more specific.

One such intervention is the use of psychological debriefings. Over the past 20 years, there has been significant debate about the risk/benefit of debriefings with the World Health Organization issuing a strong recommendation that single session debriefing after a traumatic event not be conducted due to evidence that not only does it not prevent the emergence of post-traumatic mental health conditions, but may potentially increase the development of Posttraumatic Stress Disorder [31]. Despite these concerns, debriefings remain a technique that the United States military continues to use in the deployed environment [5]. Current United States military doctrine leaves the decision of whether to conduct a psychological debriefing and what method to use up to the deployed mental health provider [13]. These types of findings show the importance of continued research and study to ensure that our understanding, treatments, and interventions evolve.

Challenges in Deployed Mental Health Care

Up to this point, this chapter has focused on the mechanisms for delivering mental health care in a deployed environment; however, we would be remiss if we did not also highlight a number of the unique challenges to the provider operating in this environment. It is important to recognize these challenges as they impact both the therapeutic alliance and the patient's perception of the care that they received. This section will focus specifically on deployment related issues as a number of the broader ethical challenges such as confidentiality and dual agency are covered in other chapters.

Safety

The mental health provider on the battlefield has a unique role that will require, at times, a level of personal risk beyond that experienced by most providers in a non-combat setting. It is not uncommon for providers to be asked to travel into areas that may be subject to enemy fire or improvised explosive devices. Additionally, providers must consider safety measures beyond those encountered in a routine setting in the United States. First, due to the fact that they are in a combat zone and need to be prepared to respond to potential enemy attack, service members are armed with automatic weapons and ammunition at all times, including the mental health provider. While access to weapons increases the potential risk for self harm or harm to others, restricting access to weapons must be balanced with providing the service member with the ability to defend themselves and their unit. If weapons restriction is required such as in cases of patients who are dangerous or have impulse control issues, then providers should consider evacuating the service member to a safer location. Other possible interventions include temporarily confiscating the service members weapon or removing their firing pin.

It should be clarified that mental health providers do not have direct authority over service members' mission status, but rather makes recommendations to commanders. Providers do not remove, stockpile or store suicidal patients' weapons. Instead, mental health providers must engage and ally with the unit to keep service members safe. In making their recommendations, however, providers can work with unit leaders to help them maintain an appropriate balance of limits and support. Providers must also manage the fact that leaders themselves may need clinical support.

For patients who require inpatient psychiatry, other solutions need to be found. Inpatient psychiatry in a deployed environment is not the same as in the United States. Inpatient psychiatric beds, of which there are few, are beds in a medical ward with a sitter; there is no therapeutic milieu. Restoration programs provide a therapeutic milieu in a day-treatment, or partial hospitalization setting with service members living at the facility, but not typically in a fully-supervised or locked setting. Service members with suicidal or homicidal thoughts that are not resolved by being temporarily removed from the immediate situation and setting require urgent evacuation.

Boundaries

A deployed environment can be similar to operating in a small community. Providers will likely live amongst their patients and encounter their patients in non-clinical settings such as mess halls, gymnasiums, and even in shower stalls. While providers want to avoid establishing social relationships with current or potentially future patients, they must also develop their own social support network. It is recommended that they choose stable, resilient service members for their social circles. Perhaps the most challenging request a deployed provider may face is when a previous non-patient, such as a tent mate, exercise partner, or friend comes to need mental health care. If there is no other mental health provider to whom to refer, then the social relationship changes which can be awkward and isolating for a provider and for the new patient as well.

Furthermore, with some regularity, senior officers and supervisors of the mental health provider, request treatment. Depending on the situation, there may be no other provider to whom to refer, and providing treatment is not only in the senior officer's best interest, but the entire unit's. In cases of potential dual relationship, boundaries must be clearly discussed at the outset of treatment, separating the treatment from the professional relationship and establishing expectations on both sides.

Lastly, deployed environments do not always permit a traditional office type setting for a mental health encounter. Deployed mental health providers should whenever possible arrange a specific time and place for therapy even if they are not in an office setting or during traditional office hours to ensure that the service member knows it is a therapeutic encounter. This emphasizes the importance of differentiating therapeutic from social encounters. At the beginning of treatment, the provider should discuss with the service member how both parties will handle daily interactions such as seeing each other at the dining facility, the gym, or in the general living area. Key areas to be discussed include whether and how each party would like to be recognized and greeted in a non-clinical setting and appropriate times to approach with non-emergent questions or concerns. If not discussed, these boundaries can negatively impact the therapeutic alliance between the service member and the military mental health provider.

Detainee Care

The role of deployed mental health providers in the care of detainees is generally limited to providing assessments and care when a detainee is displaying odd behavior or there is concern about suicidal or homicidal thoughts. In these cases, the provider will conduct a safety assessment and determine if appropriate measures are being taken and necessary facilities and equipment are available at that location to safely care for the detainee and if not, clearly state the necessary safety requirements so the detainee can be transferred to an appropriate facility. These evaluations can be very difficult as there are likely to be language barriers requiring evaluations to be conducted through an interpreter. Furthermore, there will be cultural barriers and generally a lack of trust by both the provider and the detainee [32].

In some instances, deployed military mental health providers will serve in hospitals where their primary mission is to care for the medical needs of the detainee. Prior to this assignment, the provider will be given specialized training on interacting and caring for detainees [32]. An additional challenge in these settings is caring for the service members who serve as guards. Working as a guard can be very stressful, and it is imperative that the mental health providers assigned to detention centers help the service members develop adaptive responses [33]. This development is accomplished not only through ensuring that readily accessible care is provided, but also through frequent circulation throughout the unit's area to help identify detention facility guards and other personnel who may be developing a combat operational stress reaction [32].

Lastly, many non-medical personnel may not be aware of the scope, capabilities, and limitations of a deployed mental health provider. At times, the provider may be asked to participate in or review an interrogation to provide insight or asked to provide information from a patient encounter with a detainee so that the information can be used during an interrogation. In these instances, the provider should reject this request and set very clear boundaries. They need to be sure that their mental health staff and the leadership understand that providers cannot be involved in these activities at any level.

Future Directions

Despite the changing nature of war, the scientific advances of medicine and pharmacology, and the increasing impact of technology, mental health providers will continue to play an instrumental role in the deployed environment. Continued research will be required to determine the most effective treatments and methods of delivery, but the requirement to provide direct care to patients in a high stress environment and to provide consultation towards the prevention of psychological casualties will remain paramount.

Clinical Pearls

- The bedrock of deployment mental health care in persistent, high intensity combat are the combat operational stress control principles.
- As theaters of war mature, battle lines become more established, and/or phases of war transition into stability operations, modern psychiatric resources including select pharmacotherapy and limited psychotherapy can be employed.
- When considering prescribing psychotropic medications in either a deployed environment or to a service member preparing to deploy, psychiatrists must consider several factors including the ability to provide/access follow up care, availability of medication re-supply, and potential inability to access lab or special storage resources.
- Telehealth capabilities are expanding the ability to deliver mental health services to forward deployed locations.
- Military mental health professionals employ multiple methods to promote adaptive stress responses to the combat and operational stressors service members face during deployments including battlefield circulation, health promotion, psychoeducation, early identification screening, and traumatic event management.
- Deployed mental health providers should anticipate some specific challenges for which they need to mentally prepare for how they will handle including considering that in a deployed environment all mental health providers and their patients are armed with deadly force, boundaries will be challenged when the provider may be living and operating in close physical proximity to their current and potential patients, and mental health providers may be asked to evaluate and provide care for enemy prisoners of war and other detainees.

References

1. Deutsch A. Military psychiatry: the civil war 1861-65. In: Hall JK, Zilboorg G, Bunker HA, editors. One hundred years of American psychiatry: 1844-1944. New York: Columbia University Press; 1944. p. 367–84.
2. Rock NL, Stokes JW, Koshes RJ, et al. US Army combat psychiatry. In: Jones FD, Sparacino LR, Wilcox VL, Rothberg JM, Stokes JW, editors. War psychiatry. Washington, DC: Department of the Army, Office of The Surgeon General, Borden Institute; 1995. p. 149–75.
3. Warner CH, Appenzeller GN, Yosick T, et al. The division psychiatrist and brigade behavioral health officers. In: Ritchie EC, editor. Combat and operational behavioral health. Washington, DC: Department of the Army, Office of The Surgeon General, Borden Institute; 2011b. p. 89–105.
4. Bailey P, Williams FE, Komora PA, et al. Neuropsychiatry. In: The medical department of the United States Army in the world war. Washington, DC: Department of the Army, Office of The Surgeon General; 1929. p. 303–10.
5. West JC, Warner CH. Combat and operational stress control. In: O'Connor FG, Schoomaker EB, Smith DC, editors. Fundamentals of military medicine. Fort Sam Houston, TX: Department of the Army, Office of The Surgeon General, Borden Institute; 2019. p. 573–84.
6. Rosen G. Nostalgia: a "forgotten" psychological disorder. Psychol Med. 1975;5:340–54.
7. Engel CC. Post-war syndromes: illustrating the impact of the social psyche on notions of risk, responsibility, reason, and remedy. J Am Acad Psychoanal Dyn Psychiatry. 2004;32:321–43.

8. Jones FD. Psychiatric lessons of war. In: Jones FD, Sparacino LR, Wilcox VL, Rothberg JM, Stokes JW, editors. War psychiatry. Washington, DC: Office of the Surgeon General – Borden Institute; 1995. p. 1–33.
9. Jones E, Wessely S. Forward psychiatry in the military: its origins and effectiveness. J Trauma Stress. 2003;16:411–9.
10. Glass AJ. Lessons learned. In: Anderson RS, Glass AJ, Bernucci RJ, editors. Neuropsychiatry in World War II. Vol I. Zone of the interior. Washington, DC: Government Printing Office; 1966. p. 735–59.
11. Warner CH, Breitbach JE, Appenzeller GN, et al. Division mental health in the new brigade combat team structure: part I. Predeployment and deployment. Mil Med. 2007;172:907–11.
12. Glass AJ. Psychotherapy in the combat zone. Am J Psychiatry. 1954;110:725–31.
13. United States Department of the Army. Field manual 4-02.51 combat and operational stress control. Washington, DC: Department of the Army; 2006.
14. Dailey JI, Stanfa-Brew MR. Telebehavioral health in Afghanistan. Mil Med. 2014;179:708–10.
15. Pelton D, Wangelin B, Tuerk P. Utilizing telehealth to support treatment of acute stress disorder in a theater of war: Prolonged exposure via clinical videoconferencing. Telemed E-Health. 2015;21:382–7.
16. Bryan CJ, Kanzler KE, Durham TL, West CL, Greene E. Challenges and considerations for managing suicide risk in combat zones. Mil Med. 2010;175:713–8.
17. Schell TL, Marshall GN, Jaycox LH. All symptoms are not created equal: the prominent role of hyperarousal in the natural course of posttraumatic psychological distress. J Abnorm Psychol. 2004;113:189–97.
18. Schmitz KJ, Schmied EA, Webb-Murphy JA, Hammer PS, Larson GE, Conway TL, Galarneau MR, Boucher WC, Edwards NK, Johnson DC. Psychiatric diagnoses and treatment of U.S. military personnel while deployed to Iraq. Mil Med. 2012;177:380–9.
19. Mattila AM, Crandall BD, Goldman SB. U.S. Army combat operational stress control throughout the deployment cycle: a case study. Cancer Biomark. 2011;38:13–8.
20. Toukolehto OT, Waits WM, Preece DM, Samsey KM. Accelerated resolution therapy-based intervention in the treatment of acute stress reactions during deployed military operations. Mil Med. 2020;185:356–62.
21. Cigrang JA, Peterson AL, Schobitz RP. Three American troops in Iraq: evaluation of a brief exposure therapy treatment for the secondary prevention of combat-related PTSD. Pragmat Case Stud Psychother. 2005;1:1–25.
22. Wangelin BC, Tuerk PW. PTSD in active combat soldiers: to treat or not to treat. J Law Med Ethics. 2014;42:161–70.
23. Schneider BH, Bradley JC, Warner CH, Benedek DM. Psychiatric medications in military operations. In: Ritchie EC, editor. Combat and operational behavioral health. Washington, DC: Department of the Army, Office of The Surgeon General, Borden Institute; 2011. p. 151–62.
24. United States Department of Defense. Department of Defense instruction 6490.07 deployment-limiting medical conditions for service members and DoD civilian employees. Washington, DC: Department of Defense; 2010.
25. Warner CH, Appenzeller GN, Parker JR, et al. Effectiveness of mental health screening and coordination of in-theater care prior to deployment to Iraq: a cohort study. Am J Psychiatry. 2011a;168:378–85.
26. Appel JW. Preventive psychiatry in neuropsychiatry. In: Glass AJ, Bernucci RJ, editors. World War II. Washington, DC: Office of the Surgeon General; 1966. p. 373–416.
27. Group for the Advancement of Psychiatry. Preventive psychiatry in the armed forces: with some implications for civilian use (Report 47). New York: Group for the Advancement of Psychiatry; 1960.
28. Warner CH, Appenzeller GN, Breitbach JE, Lange J, et al. Psychiatric consultation to command. In: Ritchie EC, editor. Combat and operational behavioral health. Washington, DC: Department of the Army, Office of The Surgeon General, Borden Institute; 2011c. p. 171–88.
29. Warner CH, Appenzeller GN, Breitbach JE, Mobbs A, et al. The CARE framework: the broadening of mental health services in a deployed environment. In: Adler AB, Bliese PD, Castro

CA, editors. Deployment psychology: evidence based strategies to promote mental health in the military. Washington, DC: American Psychological Association; 2011d. p. 35–68.
30. Hyams KC, Riddle J, Trump DH, Wallace MR. Protecting the health of United States military forces in Afghanistan: applying lessons learned since the Gulf War. Clin Infect Dis. 2002;15:S208–14.
31. World Health Organization. Psychological debriefing in people exposed to a recent traumatic event [WHO Website]. 2012. https://www.who.int/mental_health/mhgap/evidence/other_disorders/q5/en/. Accessed 27 Mar 2021.
32. Toye R, Smith M. Behavioral health issues and detained individuals in military operations. In: Ritchie EC, editor. Combat and operational behavioral health. Washington, DC: Department of the Army, Office of The Surgeon General, Borden Institute; 2011. p. 645–56.
33. Campbell JS, Thurston AJ, Koffman RL. Detainee operations guards in Iraq and Afghanistan reported elevated risk for posttraumatic stress disorder during deployment. Traumatology. 2019;25:41–50.

The Military and Veteran Disability System

10

Christian C. Schrader and Christopher H. Warner

Vignette

The service member sitting in front of the military psychiatrist was not your average American young man. At age 25, he had successfully completed 3 combat tours as an infantryman in both Iraq and Afghanistan. On his last deployment he sustained serious injury to his left lower leg when he was involved in a roadside bombing attack on his convoy and has undergone multiple surgeries to save the limb and heal the complex injury. Unfortunately, 1 year out from the treatment he has limited mobility in his left leg and moderate to severe chronic pain which limits his daily performance of duties. Since his return he has had continued difficulties with insomnia, recurrent combat related nightmares, depressive symptoms and heightened senses of anxiety especially when in public areas that are crowded which has led to a diagnosis of and treatment for post-traumatic stress disorder. Today his physician is discussing the need for the initiation of a medical evaluation board, since he will not be likely to continue performing his service member duties given his physical and behavioral health conditions which limit his performance in both the social and occupational settings.

C. C. Schrader
US Army Psychiatry Residency Program, Carl R Darnall Army Medical Center, Fort Hood, TX, USA
e-mail: christian.c.schrader.mil@mail.mil

C. H. Warner (✉)
Department of Psychiatry, Uniformed Services University of the Health Sciences, Bethesda, MD, USA

C. H. Warner, C. A. Castro (eds.), *Veteran and Military Mental Health*,
https://doi.org/10.1007/978-3-031-18009-5_10

Introduction

To the vast majority of athletic men and women within our country the thought of becoming permanently disabled at the age of 25 is unthinkable. The military is perhaps the only organization that places our citizenry in extremely hazardous areas around the world to perform life threatening duties on a daily basis. For those individuals injured within the bounds of their service in the military, in conjunction with the Department of Veterans Affairs strives to employ a system to ensure service members are taken care of as quickly as possible.

Prior to 2007, the Department of Defense and Veteran's Affairs conducted separate disability evaluation processes. This frequently led to service members medically separating or retiring from the military without coordination for follow on Veteran's Affairs medical services or disability benefits being put in place resulting in delays in care and benefits gaps leading to financial hardship. From 2007 to 2009, the two departments began the Integrated Disability Evaluation System. The Integrated Disability Evaluation System was intended to resolve those issues by providing a unified, less complex system that provided consistent evaluations and ratings, and most importantly ensured that disabled service members leaving the military were linked into the Veteran Affairs and receiving benefits [1].

This focus on ensuring veterans are connected to available resources has resulted in post 9/11 veterans having a 43% chance of having a service connected disability which was significantly higher than prior eras [2]. However, post 9/11 veterans do no represent the overwhelming majority of the veterans in our population and even then, there are many who are entitled and needing of disability support who have not been connected. For example, a 2017 Government Accountability Office assessment found that 62% of the 91,764 service members separated for misconduct from the military between 2011 and 2015 were subsequently diagnosed with posttraumatic stress disorder within 2 years of separation [3]. Therefore, while the Integrated Disability Evaluation System helps service members such as our young man in the vignette above, there are many others who may have left the military prior to 2007 or left the military through mechanisms other than a medical separation or retirement that still may be eligible for Veteran's Affairs medical and disability benefits. As such, it is important that all providers who are delivering care to military and veteran patients understand these systems and processes to ensure that the patients are taking advantage of the full scope of benefits afforded them. This chapter will provide an overview of the initial steps taken within the military after injury for recovery and rehabilitation, outline the Integrated Disability Evaluation System, provide information on how to seek out and determine eligibility for Veteran's Affairs services for those who were not medically retired or separated from the military, and dispel some of the common myths about the military and Veterans Affairs disability system.

Initial Injury and Rehabilitation

All providers within the military medical system work to heal our service members in order to return them to training or to return them to the fight. Whenever an injury or illness halts a service member from being able to train or fight the treating provider does two things: render appropriate medical care, and communicate to command any limitations to duty that are required to allow healing to occur quickly. For example, should one of our many airborne infantry men perform a training jump from an airplane and twist his ankle on landing (a common enough occurrence given the amount of weight of the military gear) the provider would do the examination, obtain radiographs if indicated, treat the injury, and prescribe any medications that may be needed. But that is only the first step in recovery, and there is a third party that is interested in the service member's recovery as well—his commanding officer. Per military doctrine and federal law, the Commanding Officer may be provided specific and limited medical information on any injured or ill service member [4, 5]. This does not represent a HIPPA violation so long as the provider adheres to the boundaries set and reports on only the Diagnosis (What happened), Prognosis (How long until better), Treatment Plan (How will he/she get better), and the Limitations to Duty (What things shouldn't the service member do, and how long shouldn't they do them). This is communicated in a document called the Military Medical Profile, and it allows the Commanding Officer to make decisions about the service members such as: Should they jump out of an airplane tomorrow? Probably not.

So, in the ankle sprain example described above the provider treats the service member, and then sits with them and discuss exactly what is going to be written in the profile, or better yet, write the profile while they are in the office and show it to them. Transparent. No surprises. In plain language. The provider might write something like: "Sprained ankle, 4 weeks until full recovery is expected. Treatment of rest, intermittent icing, ankle wrapping, and elevation for 1 week, with light duty for the full 4-week period. Service member may run at own pace as tolerated. No jumping, airborne duties, or high impact exercises/work details for 4 weeks and then may return to full duty status." This profile is temporary, 4 weeks in duration, and communicates everything in plain language in a way the service member and their commander understand it. The goal is to prevent re-injury during the period of healing, to return the service member to full duty quickly, and to avoid a more complex injury from occurring—one that might warrant medical separation from service. Should the provider desire a more comprehensive understanding on medical profiling, they are encouraged to review the service specific guidance as the specific processes vary for the Army, Navy/Marines, and Air Force.

While some service members desire to continue serving after serious injury or illness, often their sense of duty and patriotism is unable to overcome the injuries that they have sustained. Specifically, if they will not be able to perform their essential military duties and functions within a year they will be referred into the Integrated Disability Evaluation System to determine if they may continue serving or if they will need to undergo a medical separation or retirement. This decision point about whether a service member will be able to return to full duties within a year is known as the Medical Retention Determination Point. Figure 10.1 outlines how this begins the disability evaluation process.

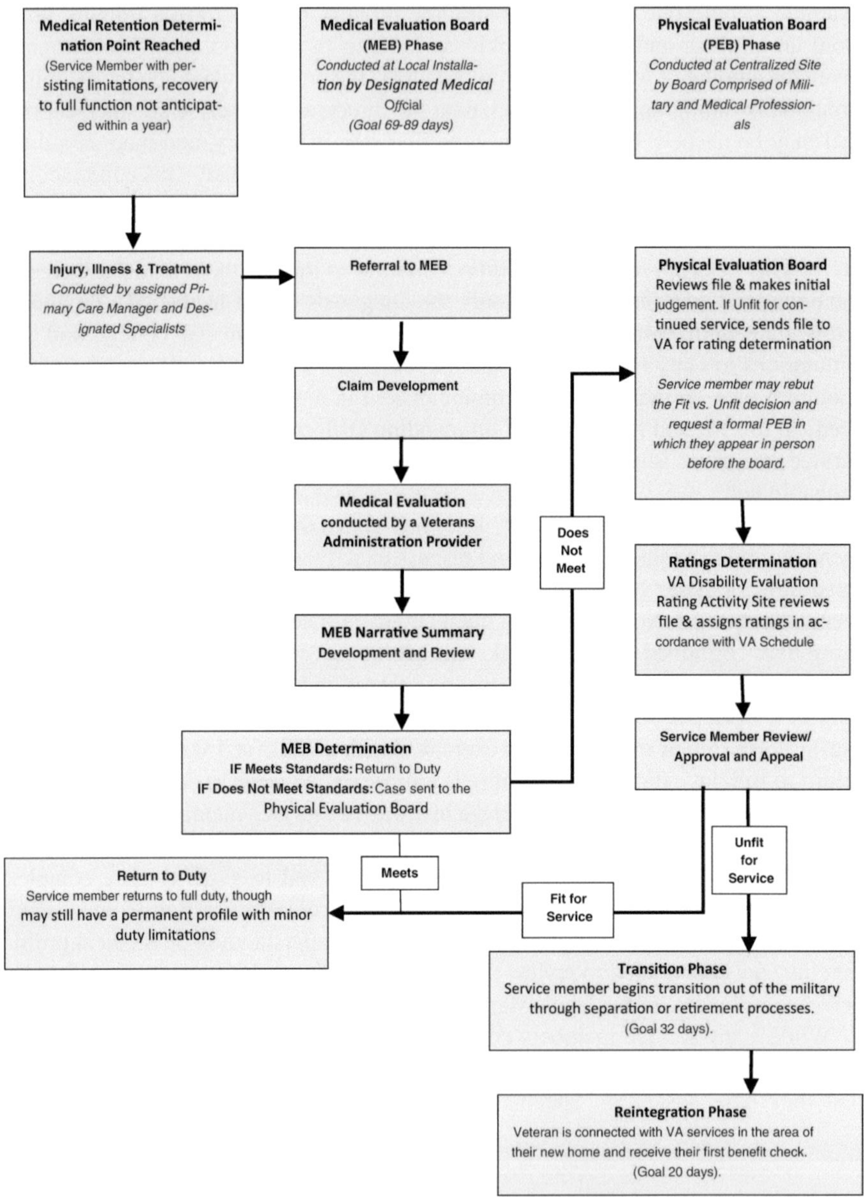

Fig. 10.1 Overview of VA/DoD integrated disability evaluation system

It is important to note that mental health conditions fall into these categories in the same manner as other illness and injuries. Service members with conditions such as depression, posttraumatic stress disorder, substance use disorders, and adjustment disorders may be placed on limited duties while they initially undergo treatments or start new medications but may return to full responsibilities while on maintenance or long-term management and not require a referral to the disability system unless their condition remains refractory to treatment. In contrast, certain conditions such as Bipolar Disorder or Psychotic Disorders will result in permanent military restrictions as those service members who carry these diagnoses are not able to participate in overseas deployments. As such, those individuals do not need to wait a year before being referred to the disability process, but rather just a stabilization of any acute exacerbation [5].

In order to conceptualize the decision point, let us take our wounded service member from earlier and go through the decision-making process up through Medical Retention Determination Point. For the sake of brevity, we can say that the service member has undergone multiple surgeries and the surgeons have placed their assertion in the medical record that the service member has reached maximum benefit from medical care for his leg injury. He has seen both his primary care manager and a pain management specialist for care for his chronic pain and they too have documented the service member reaching maximum benefit from the care delivered. Pain remains, and it limits his activities but is moderately controlled with the medications and complimentary alternative medicine approaches. His behavioral health provider in this visit has noted as that the service member has done well in therapy and completed an evidence supported treatment such as prolonged exposure therapy, but that symptoms which are limiting his social and occupational function do remain and which still meet diagnostic criteria for PTSD.

Integrated Disability Evaluation System

Once a service member reaches the Medical Retention Determination Point, they are referred to the Integrated Disability Evaluation System. This four-phase process, outlined in Fig. 10.1, is the military's mechanism for determining a service member's fitness for continued service while ensuring the timeliness of Veterans Affairs disability benefits when applicable. The process is expected to take approximately 6 months to complete the four phases but may be extended due to several factors [6, 7].

Medical Evaluation Board (MEB)

The first phase of the Integrated Disability Evaluation System is the Medical Evaluation Board. This phase is accomplished at the local military installation medical facility by designated and specially trained medical providers. Upon referral, the service member is assigned a liaison officer who supports the service member through process, assemble the service member's case file, and gathers all necessary documents to include medical records and a non-medical assessment from the service member's commanding officer.

Once the service member's claim is assembled including a list of all potential medical conditions which require evaluation for potential disability, then the service member undergoes a thorough medical evaluation by both general and specialty providers. This exam is specifically performed by Department of Veterans Affairs providers. These providers will review the service member's medical records and conduct independent evaluation. It is important to note, that if there are discrepancies between the Veterans Affairs and prior military provider's diagnoses and or limitations, the Veterans Affairs exam is the one that will be used for determination of duty limitations and disability ratings. This exam is generally completed at the nearest Veterans Affairs facility. Several military installations have Veterans Affairs clinics located on site; however, this practice varies from site to site.

Upon completion of the medical exam, the findings and evaluation are returned to the local military health system Integrated Disability Evaluation System team where the exam is reviewed by the Medical Evaluation Board physician. The physician reviews all the diagnoses, limitations, and conditions and applies military regulations to determine whether the service member meets medical retention standards [8]. If they do meet medical retention standards, then the medical evaluation board can be terminated at this time and the service member returned to duty. These findings are summarized by the Medical Evaluation Board physician in a document called the Narrative Summary. If it is determined that the service member does not meet the medical retention standards then the Medical Evaluation Board physician must comment in the narrative summary on whether the condition existed prior to military service, if it was service aggravated, and whether the service member has been compliant with treatment recommendations and protocols. These three areas can all have an impact on the disability rating that is awarded by the Department of Veterans Affairs for a condition.

Prior to moving on to the next phase, the service member is given the opportunity to review the narrative summary and may appeal the findings and recommendations. As part of this system, the service member has access to legal counsel familiar with this process who can provide counsel and recommendations. Upon either service member approval or disposition of the appeal, the narrative summary is forwarded to the Physical Evaluation Board. This completes the medical evaluation board phase. The goal is to complete this phase in approximately 69–89 days; however, that timeline can vary. The factors which most influence the timeline for completion is the scheduling of the Veterans Affairs physical, any appeals to the narrative summary, and if the service member has some ongoing disciplinary action.

Physical Evaluation Board (PEB)

The Physical Evaluation Board occurs in one of a few centralized locations. This phase begins when the narrative summary is forwarded by the local medical evaluation board team to the physical evaluation board. The physical evaluation board will review the service member's narrative summary, medical records, Veterans Affairs evaluation, and the Commander's statement about the service member's performance and will determine if they meet fitness for duty standards. This process is completed at the centralized site without the service member present. One of the most influential documents in this review process is the Commander's statement as they provide important information about how the duty limitations and medical condition impact the service member's ability to perform their individual tasks and the unit's ability to complete their mission. In this statement, the service member's unit leader will provide feedback on how the injury or illness has impacted their occupational performance and ability to serve. A statement which talks positively about how the individual has overcome those challenges and continues to be able to perform key roles and responsibilities may influence the board to consider a determination of fit for service. In contrast, a statement that the service member's condition prevents them from being able to perform necessary duties needed for future service greatly influences the decision towards an unfit for continued service determination.

If the Physical Evaluation Board determines that all of the service member's condition is fit for continued duty, then the process is complete, and the service member is returned to duty. However, if any of their medical conditions are determined to not meet fitness for duty standards, then the service member's case is forwarded to the VA where it is sent to the Veterans Affairs Disability Evaluation System Rating Activity Site (D-RAS). This site applies the VA Schedule for Rating Disability (VASRD) to assign a disability rating for each condition [9]. It is important to note that ratings are impacted based on when the condition began (i.e., existed prior to service), if it was the direct result of combat service, and if the condition was aggravated during military service. Ratings can range from 0% to 100% and rise in increments of tens. Once D-RAS assigns the ratings, they are forwarded back to the Physical Evaluation Board which makes final determination on whether the service member will be medically retired or separated because of their conditions.

Separation without benefits occurs when the unfitting condition existed prior to service and was not aggravated by the individual's military service. This can only occur for those who served less than 8 years in the military. Separation with severance pay occurs for a service member who has served less than 20 years and is determined to have a less than 30% disability rating. The severance pay is based on a formula dependent upon the number of years served in the military. Medical retirement occurs for those who have served in the military for 20 or more years or are determined to have a disability rating of 30% or higher. These individuals will receive an enduring monthly retirement stipend dependent upon their base pay, years of service, and level of disability. Of note, while the VA assigns the rating levels, the military will only use the disability ratings assigned for those conditions found to be unfitting for continued service in their calculations to determine separation versus retirement. Additionally, it is important to note that the disability ratings do not combine in a simple addition formula. Both the VA and veteran advocacy sites have available calculators for determining the expected level of disability and associated benefits based on the assigned ratings, as well as other factors including the veteran's marital status and number of dependents.

When this process is complete, the results are forwarded by the Physical Evaluation Board to the service member's Physical Evaluation Board Liaison Officer. The service member will review and can appeal. As before, the service member is afforded counsel with a lawyer if they desire. This stage ends when the service member approves their Physical Evaluation Board findings and ratings or has exhausted their appeals.

In our case, the service member suffered his injury while on active duty, during a combat deployment. His conditions were caused because he was performing his military duties and were not present before signing up for the military. The Physical Evaluation Board in review of his file notes his inability to perform his duties due to the chronic pain, limitations in the mobility of the damaged limb, and due to PTSD. As such, his case is handed to the VA Disability Rating Activity Site which reviews each condition and proposes a disability rating (from 0% to 100%) for each condition. The Physical Evaluation Board then uses the proposed disability ratings to determine whether a service member is Separated from service (disability rated as 0%, 10%, or 20%) with severance pay, or medical Retirement (disability rated at 30% or higher) which will give retirement pay and benefits. Our sergeant receives 50% for his limb damage, 30% for chronic pain, and 70% due to the severity of the PTSD, all conditions which were deemed to be unfitting for continued military service. His combined total rating is judged to be 90% (in accordance with VA Disability formulas).

Transition Phase

After concurring with the Physical Evaluation Board findings and Veterans Affairs disability ratings, the service member enters the transition phase. During this process, the service member either undergoes military retirement or separation. The local installation will generate the appropriate orders and the service member begins the process of clearing the installation and preparing for departure from the military including returning all required equipment, closing out evaluations, clearing housing, shipping household goods, etc. This phase is completed when the service member is officially out of the military.

Reintegration Phase

Upon departure from the military, the goal of the Integrated Disability Evaluation system is to ensure that the service member is a Veterans Affairs beneficiary within 1 month. This includes receiving their Veterans Affairs disability check and integrated into the Veterans Affairs medical system for ongoing medical care. The liaison officer along with Veterans Affairs coordinators are integral to the success of this phase as they will ensure appointments are established with the local Veterans Affairs medical facility that services wherever the service member chooses to locate after departing the military.

It is important to note that some conditions may be deemed temporary versus permanently disabling. A designation of temporary may both the medical retirement and the disability rating as they may require reassessment to determine if the condition has stabilized, improved, or worsened which could result in a re-adjudication of the decision. Specifically, for those veterans who were separated for a mental disorder due to traumatic stress resulting in a disability rating of 50% or higher, they are required to have a reevaluation 6 months after discharge from the military to assess whether a change in evaluation is warranted [9].

Eligibility for Veterans Affairs Services and Disability Benefits

As previously mentioned, the majority of service members will leave the military through channels other than a medical separation or retirement. The overwhelming majority will leave with an honorable discharge upon completion of their contracted term of service. These veterans may still be eligible for healthcare and benefits through the Department of Veterans Affairs. In general, anyone who has served honorably for 24 continuous months on active duty since late 1980 or served in Vietnam between 1962 and 1975 is eligible for Veterans Affairs health benefits. More specific eligibility requirements can be found on the Department of Veterans Affairs website [10].

Additionally, veterans may have health conditions that present or worsen after they leave the military that are connected to their military service which may make them eligible for Veterans Affairs disability benefits. For example, those who had environmental exposures during Vietnam or the Persian Gulf War that were not realized to be toxic until years later or a veteran whose significant symptoms of PTSD did not present until after departure from the service. If a provider is caring for a veteran that is not linked in with the Department of Veterans Affairs, they are encouraged to refer the patient to the Veterans Affairs website to apply for health benefits and, if indicated, disability benefits. The web site provides the documentation requirements, necessary forms, and offers assistance services for completion. Access to these resources is not intended to replace other services or divert a patient's healthcare back in the Veterans Administration but rather to ensure that the full complement of benefits, services, and resources are available to patients. Additionally, there are disability resources available for a veteran's spouse and children which should may be of assistance to the family.

Key Considerations and Concerns

Clear, Concise Documentation

Along with documenting any duty limitations due to the medical condition, the provider must understand that the medical record is the document that is used to review all cases for determination of medical suitability and for decisions of disability. It is imperative that all providers use clinical language, in a clear and concise manner, to convey a patient's condition and prospects for recovery using objective data coupled to subjective symptom report. Symptoms, injuries, and data such as radiographs or other tests should support the diagnosis and drive a treatment plan that is appropriate over time.

> One example that meets the above criteria might be: "Patient with 5 weeks depressed mood, loss of desire for enjoyable activities (anhedonia), with sleep onset insomnia with multiple awakenings through the night most nights total sleep time 3–4 h on average. Additional symptoms of poor concentration with failure to achieve work deadlines, poor energy with missed workdays, and recurrent suicidal thinking without plan or intent to harm self. Symptoms occur daily, impair work completion, and have caused strain in his family relationships. Reports 2 negative military counselling statements over past week due to failure to complete service member duties on time or to standard, previously high performing with early promotion rate. Denies delusions, hallucinations, paranoia. Denies history of depression..."

The above subjective note portion clearly states symptoms and impact to function. When combined with the appropriate physical and mental exam results (objective), the full diagnosis (Major Depression, Single Episode, Severe, without psychotic features) and the treatment plan, they give anyone reading and reviewing the documentation much later an understanding of what that provider evaluated, and what was done to treat the condition. While viewed serially over time, these notes would accurately explain what diagnosis was treated, how those treatment affected the condition, and exactly what impact the condition had on the patient over time.

So, it is not just a good note that matters, it is good documentation consistently that is needed. Failure of clear and consistent medical documentation over the entirety of the treatment time is always the weakest link in the Disability Evaluation System, and often what causes a service member to be "in" the Disability Evaluation System process longer than should be needed. When any diagnosis is not properly supported by the symptoms in the note, it causes the Medical Evaluation Board evaluators to either guess at what you meant or downgrade your diagnosis. In the example above, if the provider only stated: "patient depressed for last 5 weeks, is sad, low energy" in the subjective portion it would not meet the diagnostic criteria for a major depressive episode and creates ambiguity and room for assumptions. Those in turn create more work for the provider to elaborate after the fact, more work for the Medical Evaluation Board physician attempting to search for data points due to inadequacies in the charting and usually increased wait time for the patient.

Chronic conditions that had their start while in military service but that were not captured in a disability evaluation will require a referral back to the Department of Veterans Affairs for determination of disability. For conditions such as this, clear documentation of the time of onset and chronicity of symptomology over time including functional limitations which have waxed or waned is extremely helpful to the veteran as they gather their medical records for submission to the Department of Veterans Affairs for a disability review. In these cases the veteran can apply for benefits and disability evaluation through the Veterans Affairs website or by visiting their local Veterans Affairs treatment center.

Fitness for Duty Standards

As previously mentioned, ultimately the decision on whether a service member is deemed medically capable of continuing to serve in the military is based on a determination of fitness for duty by a medical evaluation board and subsequently a physical evaluation board. This process starts when a service member's medical care reaches the medical retention determination point. To assist in both identifying this determination point and making the fitness for duty determination, the Department of Defense publishes the Department of Defense Instruction 6130.03, Volume 2—Medical Standards for Military Service: Retention [8]. This document outlines which conditions are not compatible with continued military service.

Specifically, for mental health disorders diagnosed using the fifth edition of the Diagnostics and Statistics Manual of Mental Disorders, the majority are evaluated on a case-by-case assessment of the persistent duty modifications required to reduce psychological stressors or enhance safety and the degree to which the condition impairs function to satisfactorily perform military duties commensurate with the service members rank and/or position. However, primary psychotic disorders and Bipolar I Disorder are immediate indicators for referral to the disability evaluation system.

Disability Ratings

As previously mentioned, disability ratings are issued by the Veterans Affairs Disability Evaluation System Rating Activity Site (D-RAS) applying the Veterans Affairs Schedule for Rating Disability (VASRD). These rating are impacted based on when the condition began (i.e., existed prior to service), if the condition was aggravated during military service, the ability of the service member to perform their military duties (level of occupational dysfunction), and the stability of the disabling condition. The ratings are not specific to any one diagnosis, but rather to the degree of disability that results from the condition and the origin of the disability [9].

One common misnomer is that a diagnosis of posttraumatic stress disorder is specifically needed to get a higher rating. This is generated by the requirement in the disability rating scale to assign a rating of not less than 50% for those who develop a mental disorder while in service as a result of a highly stressful event that is severe enough to bring about the veteran's release from active military service (i.e. deemed to be an unfitting condition). The confusion arises that many interpret the highly stressful event to be a requirement for PTSD. In reality, any condition that resulted from a highly stressful event such as combat exposure including chronic adjustment disorder, depression, anxiety disorders, or PTSD will receive a minimum of 50% disability; however, if the service member has a diagnosis of PTSD associated with a traumatic event that occurred prior to military service or was not deemed to be an unfitting condition, then their disability percentage will be determined like all other mental health conditions based on the level of social and occupational dysfunction occurring from the condition [9].

System Design Concerns

The discussion of disability ratings leads to another recurrent issue for providers to be aware of. Certain medical conditions, including mental health disorders, may be reassessed by both the Department of Defense and the Department of Veterans Affairs at varying intervals. These evaluations may occur both with the military if they were placed on a temporary retirement status or with the VA if their condition was not determined to be permanent and required reassessment. This process incentivizes the patient to remain in the sick role and to not improve their medical condition. This has led to some criticisms of the current processes to imply that the increase in service members and veterans applying for disability is somehow abusing or taking advantage of the system [11]. While there is no evidence to support large-scale fraud or abuse, it does highlight this structural disadvantage and has led to a call by some, to include Department of Veterans Affairs leadership, to consider systematic changes that would focus on enhancing wellness [12]. In the interim, providers should believe service members and veterans unless they have specific reason to doubt. Future revisions and enhancements to the system will ideally look at how to address this concern.

In conclusion, the military and veteran disability systems can be complicated and frustrating, but they offer access to medical resources and benefits that can be vital to the support of our patients. Consider, in another chapter in this book there is a whole discussion about the challenges of homelessness in the veteran population and it includes multiple resources that are available to Veterans Affairs beneficiaries that a provider might include in their treatment plan. Therefore, it is essential when treating a military or veteran patient to understand this process and assess what avenues the patient has already pursued or should pursue. In addition, it is important that providers keep in perspective the importance of their documentation to include the clear, concise documentation of not only the condition, its origins and relation to military service, but also the limitations it places on the patient.

Clinical Pearls

- Veteran patients who have conditions that either developed as a result of their military service or were worsened in association with their military service may be eligible for Veterans Affairs disability benefits.
- The disability process is complex, occurring both in the military service and the Veterans Affairs systems concurrently. Encourage patients who are going through this process to take advantage of support resources including military provided legal advice and services provided by veteran service organizations.
- The goal for completion of the disability evaluation and separation from active service is 180 days, although the process often endures longer (as long as 1 year).
- Clear and concise documentation of symptomology which meets diagnostic criteria for the disorder, and discussion of functional limitations is very important for determination of disability status.
- Clear documentation of a timeline of onset of symptoms, and impact to function over time will assist a veteran in seeking disability evaluation for their condition from the Veterans Affairs if that did not occur during their active service time.

References

1. U.S. Congress. Senate: Committee on Veterans Affairs. Seamless transition: review of the integrated disability evaluation system. 112th Cong., 2nd sess., May 23, 2012.
2. Vespa JE. Those who served: America's veterans from World War II to the war on terror, ACS-43, American Community Survey Reports. Washington, DC: U.S. Census Bureau; 2020.
3. U.S. Government Accountability Office. DoD health: actions needed to ensure post-traumatic stress disorder and traumatic brain injury are considered in misconduct separations. GAO-17-260. Washington, DC. 2017. http://www.gao.gov/assets/GAO-17-260.pdf. Accessed 12 Mar 2021.
4. U.S. Department of Defense. Department of Defense Directive 5124.02: under secretary of defense for personnel and readiness. Washington, DC: Department of Defense; 2008.
5. U.S. Department of Defense. Department of Defense instruction 6490.07: deployment-limiting medical conditions for service members and DoD civilian employees. Washington, DC: Department of Defense; 2010.
6. Military Health System. Integrated disability evaluation system [Health.mil web site]. 2015. https://www.health.mil/Military-Health-Topics/Conditions-and-Treatments/Physical-Disability/Disability-Evaluation/Integrated-Evaluation-System. Accessed 12 Mar 2021.
7. U.S. Department of Defense. Department of Defense instruction 1332.18: disability evaluation system. Washington, DC: Department of Defense; 2018.
8. U.S. Department of Defense. Department of Defense instruction 6130.03, Vol. 2: medical standards for military service: retention. Washington, DC: Department of Defense; 2020.
9. U.S. Department of Veterans Affairs. 38 CFR Book C, schedule for rating disabilities—web automated reference material system (VA web site). 2015. https://www.benefits.va.gov/WARMS/bookc.asp. Accessed 12 Mar 2021.
10. U.S. Department of Veterans Affairs. Veterans affairs benefits (VA web site). 2021. https://www.benefits.va.gov. Accessed 23 Mar 2021.
11. Zarembo A. Disability system for veterans strays far from its official purpose. Los Angeles Times. 2014. https://www.latimes.com/nation/la-me-adv-disability-politics-20141116-story.html. Accessed 24 Mar 2021.
12. Jowers K. VA Chief: "Time to rethink disability system: current setup 'not sustainable.'" Military Times. 2017. https://www.militarytimes.com/veterans/2017/06/23/va-chief-time-to-rethink-disability-system-current-setup-not-sustainable/. Accessed 24 Mar 2021.

Part III

Unique Aspects, Conditions, and Situations in Veteran and Military Mental Health

Combat and Operational Stress

11

Jeffrey Millegan, Eileen Delaney, and Robert Gerardi

Vignette

A 23-year-old active duty service member (SM), married, rank of E-3 (Seaman) in the US Navy is deployed on the aircraft carrier, USS Ronald Reagan. The service member has completed 6 months of a 9-month deployment, and had experienced several difficult events. A few months into his deployment, one of his sisters passed away in a car accident. He was able to return home for the funeral; however, his mother was very distraught and did not want him to return to his ship saying she could not bear the thought of losing a son as well. After he returned to the ship, the service member remained shaken by the loss of his sister and developed feelings of guilt for leaving his mother. Several weeks later he witnessed one of his friends getting medically evacuated after being struck by the turning propeller of an aircraft on the flight deck and started having frequent flashbacks of his friend being injured. Additionally, his sleep has been significantly affected, and he feels extremely anxious at the thought of going onto the flight deck [1].

J. Millegan
Uniformed Services University of Health Sciences, Bethesda, MD, USA

E. Delaney (✉) · R. Gerardi
Naval Center for Combat & Operational Stress Control, San Diego, CA, USA
e-mail: Eileen.m.delaney2.ctr@mail.mil; Robert.d.gerardi3.ctr@mail.mil

C. H. Warner, C. A. Castro (eds.), *Veteran and Military Mental Health*,
https://doi.org/10.1007/978-3-031-18009-5_11

Combat and Operational Stress Control

Combat and operational stress control (COSC) programs in the US military are designed to prevent, identify, and manage adverse combat and operational stress as well as promote the resilience and psychological health of military units. These programs aim to optimize mission performance, maintain combat capability, and prevent or minimize the impact of combat and operational stress reactions (COSRs) on the physical, psychological, and spiritual well-being of military service members.

The purpose of this chapter is to define combat and operational stress and COSRs, provide a brief history of the conceptualization and management of COSRs, and describe the current military doctrines for addressing COSC. We also provide a case example of how an operational unit might treat a service member experiencing combat and operational stress as well as how a mental health provider outside of the unit might care for a patient who presents with a COSR.

It is important to emphasize three features of COSRs. First, COSRs are expected psychobiological reactions in response to combat and military operations. Second, a COSR is not a mental health disorder despite sharing common symptoms with psychiatric diagnoses (e.g., intrusive thoughts, anxiety), such as Acute Stress Disorder (ASD) and Posttraumatic Stress Disorder (PTSD). Third, a defining characteristic of COSRs is that they are limited to 72 hours or less than 4 days from the event [2].

Combat and Operational Stress

Stress is inherent in military settings because of demanding physical conditions, duration of operations, and warfighting. Combat and operational stress includes environmental, physical, cognitive, and emotional stressors encountered as a direct result of mission demands. See Table 11.1 for examples of combat and operational stressors.

Combat and operational stress is experienced by all service members in every type of military operation, whether serving in the infantry, providing health care, or

Table 11.1 Examples of combat and operational stress [3]

Environmental: Extreme weather conditions; constant noise; fumes, poisons, and chemicals; infectious agents; poor visibility; difficult terrain	**Cognitive**: Information (too much or too little); sensory overload or deprivation; ambiguity, uncertainty, and unpredictability; time pressure or waiting; difficult decisions; organizational dynamics and change; working beyond skill level, previous failures
Physical: Sleep deprivation; dehydration; malnutrition; poor hygiene; muscular fatigue; decreased immune system; illness or injury; sexual frustration	**Emotional**: Fear and anxiety-producing threats; grief-producing losses; resentment, anger, frustration and guilt; boredom (from inactivity); conflicting/divided motives and loyalties; spiritual/religious confrontation; interpersonal conflicts (peers, leader); home-front worries and homesickness; loss of privacy; victimization/harassment; loneliness (if in a new unit)

Table 11.2 Definitions of combat and operational stress [4]

Combat stress: Distressing events that are the direct result of using deadly force with an enemy	**Operational stress**: Distressing operational conditions associated with military operations
Examples: Attacks; personal injury; killing combatants; witnessing death and injury	Examples: Prolonged exposure to extreme environments (wear and tear); separation from family and community; austere living conditions; demanding work hours; sleep-wake cycle disruption; exposure to threatening environments; training accidents; military (non-combat) operations

giving logistical support. These operations include training, all phases of deployment, peacekeeping, humanitarian missions, stability and reconstruction, government support missions, and missions that may include weapons of mass destruction or chemical, biological, radiological, nuclear, and explosive weapons. Each service member continually faces the potential for deployment and combat, long and arduous training missions, and separation from family. Combat and operational stress continues after the mission is over as service members deal with the aftermath, whether they served in combat or support units, were prisoners of war, or experienced severe injuries. See Table 11.2 for definitions of combat and operational stress.

Adaptive Stress Reactions are positive responses that occur when stressors result in enhanced individual and unit performance and is often associated with effective leadership and good relationship with peers [5]. Maladaptive Stress Reactions are when adverse effects or stressors impact functioning. COSR refers to any maladaptive stress reaction in a military environment. According to Department of Defense (DoD) Directive 6490.05, a combat stress reaction is not a clinical disorder but instead is a consequence associated with prolonged exposure to high-demand environments or traumatic events.

The Evolution of Combat and Operational Stress Reactions

Classical literature proffers that psychological symptoms arising from extreme stress, such as war and battle, are a fundamental human experience. In the battle of Marathon (440 BC), Herodotus describes stress symptoms resulting from fear on the battlefield, and frightening battle dreams were noted by Hippocrates, the "Father of Medicine" [6].

World War I (WWI) marked the beginning of the study of combat stress. Although WWI started out as a war of movement where few stress casualties were observed, it transitioned to trench warfare with an unexplained phenomenon that impacted the combat effectiveness of service members [5]. The term "shell shock" was coined as a reaction to direct intense combat and bombardments, with symptoms of tinnitus, amnesia, startle affect, light-headedness, fear, panic, confusion, crying, and intrusions of memory. In 1916, the term "war neurosis" replaced shell shock as the number of stress casualties arose from different types of combat situations and in attempts to limit the number of individuals diagnosed with shell shock [6]. However, a diagnosis of war neurosis often inferred that those afflicted were malingering in attempts to be removed from the frontline. Consequently, service members suffering from war neurosis could be subjected to a Court Martial, with some being tried and executed for desertion and cowardice [6, 7].

During World War II (WWII), shell shock and war neurosis was replaced with "battle fatigue" and "combat exhaustion". These new terms had less of a negative connotation and made it easier for the medical corps to treat service members, often through rest and sleep [5]. In the Vietnam War, stress symptoms associated with military operations were referred to as "combat stress", and from the Gulf War until today common terms include "combat stress reaction", "combat operational stress", and "combat operational stress reactions" [5, 8].

History of Managing Combat and Operational Stress Reactions

"Forward psychiatry" was derived and introduced by the French during WWI due to concerns about the number of psychological cases being referred to base hospitals and ultimately lost to fighting units [9]. Military behavioral health was further influenced by lessons learned in the war by providing behavioral health interventions far forward on the battlefield. These practices allowed the military to take more of a proactive posture in managing the impact of combat stress [10].

By the onset of WWII, psychiatrists had been placed in most Army divisions, and the first trials of restoration care for Soldiers were implemented in "Training and Rehabilitation [T&R] Centers." Soldiers sent to T&R Centers practiced battle drills daily and maintained an exercise routine. It became well believed that allowing Soldiers experiencing stress reactions to "remain a part of their unit positively affected unit cohesion and prevented further deterioration of psychiatric functioning [9]."

Epidemiology

Historically, COSRs account for nearly half of all battle casualties [3]. Although rates of COSRs have remained high during the twenty-first century, losses due to COSRs have significantly decreased as a result of institutionalizing COSC into military operations, procedures, and policies. In today's military environment, leaders can expect to retain and return to duty (RTD) over 95% of service members who experience a COSR [10].

Most studies and surveillance of the mental health and well-being of service members have focused on diagnosable mental health disorder symptoms (e.g., PTSD) as opposed to more transient COSRs. In all, an estimated 20–30% of US military personnel returning from current combat operations report significant psychological symptoms [11]. Although COSRs are believed to be highly prevalent in military units during combat and operational missions, the rates of COSRs have not been sufficiently documented [12]. There is also a lack of data reporting on the rates of COSRs that develop into mental health disorders, such as ASD and PTSD. Though there is a consensus that having a COSR puts individuals at elevated risk for PTSD [2].

A New Perspective on Combat and Operational Stress Control

Today, the Army's combat stress control services operate under the doctrine established in *Field Manual (FM) 4-02.51*. The Navy and Marine Corps COSC initiative operates under MCWP 6-11C/NTTP 1-15M *Combat and Operational Stress Control*. Appendix denotes key terms of COSC. The Army, Navy, and Marine Corps COSC doctrines rely on many of the same principles. Their aims are to prevent, identify, and treat combat and operational stress injuries and COSRs within the military operational environment using organic assets. For the purpose of this chapter, we will describe in detail the use of COSC principles within the US Navy Fleet.

To address the shortcomings and social stigma of the twentieth century model, a new concept of COSC was developed in the Navy and Marine Corps. In 2007, a working group of Navy and Marine leaders, chaplains, and medical and mental health professionals developed a new COSC model that includes the *Stress Continuum Model, Five Core Leader Functions,* and *Combat and Operational Stress First Aid (COSFA)* [8].

Stress Continuum Model. A central tenet of this new COSC concept is the Stress Continuum Model that is —

- Unit leader oriented
- Multidisciplinary
- Integrated throughout the organization
- Without stigma
- Consistent with the warrior ethos
- Focused on wellness, prevention, and resilience

The Stress Continuum Model, outlined in Fig. 11.1, is the foundation for all COSC doctrine, training, surveillance, and interventions in the Navy and Marine Corps. The Stress Continuum Model recognizes the entire spectrum of stress responses and outcomes and includes, from left to right, adaptive coping and wellness (color coded Green as the "Ready" Zone), mild and reversible distress or loss of function (the Yellow "Reacting" Zone), more severe and persistent distress or loss of function (the Orange "Injured" Zone), and mental health disorders arising from unhealed stress injuries (the Red "Ill" Zone).

The fundamental idea behind the Stress Continuum Model is that stress tends to push individuals toward the Yellow, Orange, or Red Zones. The goal of COSC is to keep service members, units, and families in the Green "Ready" Zone as much as possible and to return them to that zone as quickly as possible if they leave it.

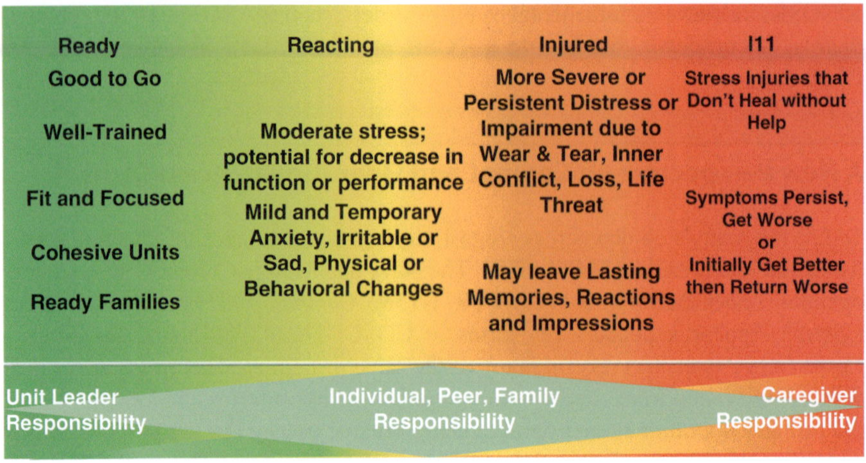

Fig. 11.1 Combat and operational stress continuum model

Monitoring and managing the stress responses of the unit is primarily the responsibility of unit leaders, but individual service members and their family members also bear responsibility for continuously monitoring and managing stress reactions for themselves, their peers, and their family.

Five Core Leader Functions

Although the Stress Continuum Model provides a framework for understanding and recognizing the spectrum of stress reactions, it does not by itself meet the COSC objectives of preserving force readiness and maintaining individual health and well-being. Toward those ends, the Navy and Marine Corps have established the following Five Core Leader Functions: Strengthen, Mitigate, Identify, Treat, and Reintegrate.

Strengthen

Strategies for strengthening service members and units fall into three main categories: (1) training, (2) social cohesion, and (3) leadership.

Training should be as realistic as possible so that unit members will have few surprises during deployment, and it should push unit members to develop new skills without making it so tough they fail to master training challenges or experience stress injuries. Training should also promote communication and trust both horizontally (peer to peer) and vertically (leader to unit member) through shared hardships and success.

Social cohesion is created in all groups in much the same way, whether that group is a ground combat fire team, the crew of a ship, health care professionals taking care of injured Marines and Sailors, or a family in the US. Cohesion develops gradually through the interaction of the following factors: Familiarity, communication, trust, respect, loyalty, and love.

Leadership is the most fundamental strategy for strengthening units as the other strategies (training, social cohesion) depend on it for their success. There can be no training or unit cohesion without the direct and continuous involvement of leaders. Also, leadership directly strengthens Sailors and Marines through discipline, modeling fortitude, clear communication, and the promotion of ethics.

Mitigate

Mitigation aims to keep unit members in the Green "Ready" Zone in the face of operational challenges. Optimal mitigation of stress requires the balancing of competing priorities: intentionally subjecting service members to stress to optimize training while reducing or eliminating stressors not essential to training or mission accomplishment and ensuring adequate sleep, rest, and restoration between periods of challenge.

Identify

Since even the best strengthening and mitigating efforts cannot eliminate all stress reactions, operational leaders must continually monitor stressors and know the individuals in their units. Leaders must recognize when individuals' confidence in themselves, peers, or leaders, or when units have lost cohesion because of casualties, changes in leadership, or challenges to the unit.

Treat (Engage)

The overall responsibility for ensuring that appropriate and timely care is delivered rests with unit leaders. Additional resources that may be utilized to provide intervention and support for stress reactions and injuries include Caregiver Occupational Stress Control (CgOSC) teams and Command Resilience Teams (CRTs), Family Support Centers, chaplains, and organic medical and mental health assets. Buddy care (i.e., peer to peer identification and intervention) is also an important tool for addressing COSC.

If a stress injury is properly treated, it will likely improve significantly or completely remit. Leaders must attack stigma in their units to increase the likelihood that care will be accepted by the individuals who need it.

Reintegrate

Unit leaders must continuously monitor and mentor service members to bring them back to full duty. Stigma must be constantly addressed in order to restore the confidence that stress-injured service members have for themselves as well as restore the confidence of their peers and leaders.

Combat and Operational Stress First Aid (COSFA)

COSFA is a tool for leaders to use when individual or units present in the yellow "Reacting" or orange "Injured" zone. Leaders can use COSFA as a flexible, multistep process for the timely assessment and pre-clinical care of COSC injuries in individuals or units. Similar to the aftermath of a physical injury, the primary goals are to provide "first aid": preserve life, prevent further harm, and promote recovery. Individuals who have recently experienced a traumatic event may have disruptions in sleep, nutrition, hygiene, and other necessities, and they may also have unmet needs for information about their current situation and the welfare of others [2]. Figure 11.2 outlines the COFSA process.

COSFA consists of *seven core actions* grouped on *three levels*:

- *Continuous Aid—Check* (assess and reassess) and *Coordinate* (inform others and refer if needed)
- *Primary Aid—Cover* (get to safety and keep safe) and *Calm* (reduce physiological and emotional arousal)
- *Secondary Aid—Connect* (restore social support from peers and family) and *Competence* (restore personal, occupational, and social self-efficacy) and *Confidence* (restore self-esteem and hope)

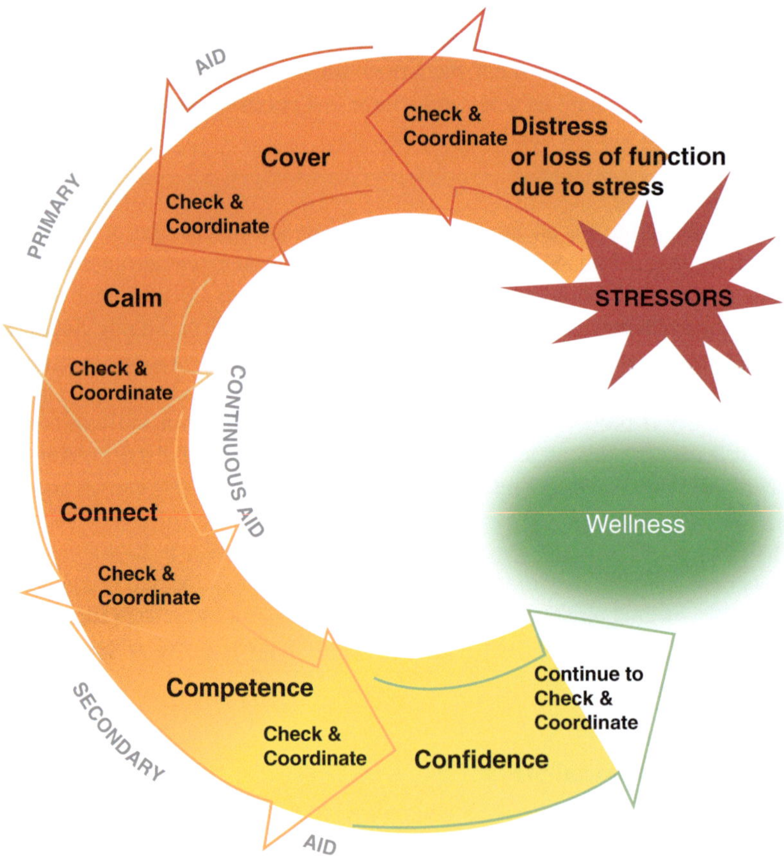

Fig. 11.2 Combat and Operational Stress First Aid (COFSA)

Prevention and Early Intervention

Practices performed by the military services to keep their service members healthy (in the "green/ready" zone) include pre-deployment preparation and training (in order to promote self-efficacy and unit cohesion), management of sleep-work cycles, provision of adequate nutrition and hydration, and continuous engagement with COSC resources (e.g., behavioral health personnel) [4].

The COSC program within each of the services aims to prevent and early identify COSRs before they result in chronic dysfunction. The management of COSRs within an operational environment is a multidimensional process that includes military leaders, service members, and behavioral health experts. Leaders and service members learn to recognize COSR symptoms in order to prevent or reduce their disruptive effects, and behavioral health experts help prevent stress-related impairment by providing further treatment should the need arise [3].

For individuals categorized as "reacting (yellow)" or "injured (orange)" per the stress continuum model, initial intervention ideally occurs within the unit and does not require medical intervention. However, when symptoms persist and become more severe ("orange" or "red" on the stress continuum), medical assessment is warranted either by organic medical personnel or by outside medical resources (e.g., local military hospital).

Vignette: Identifying a COSR Within the Operational Unit
SM's supervisor noticed that SM was having difficulty concentrating at work, was late on several occasions, and appeared more tired than usual. His supervisor pulled him aside one day, discussed his observations with the service member, and asked what stress zone he was currently in. Although SM was somewhat reluctant, he admitted that he was in the "yellow" zone for quite some time and might be moving into the "orange" zone. His supervisor recommended that he take the rest of the day off and try to get good rest that evening. When his supervisor checked in on SM the next morning, SM still seemed to be struggling so his supervisor referred him to the ship's psychologist.

Diagnosis and Assessment

COSRs can stem from any type of operational environment, not just in deployment settings. Additionally, COSRs may become noticeable immediately after a highly stressful event or may develop after days or weeks of prolonged exposure to the hardships of military operations (e.g., harsh and austere environments, disruptions in sleep-wake cycle) [4].

It is important to understand the difference between a COSR, ASD, and PTSD. A COSR, ASD, and PTSD can share symptoms in presentation, but a COSR *is not* the same as ASD or PTSD. A COSR is a negative adjustment from exposure to stress and traumatic events, classified as a sub-clinical diagnosis with a high percentage for recovery when appropriate interventions are provided. There is no threshold or

Table 11.3 Signs and symptoms of COSRs [4]

Physical: Exhaustion; inability to sleep; somatic signs (sweating, palpitations, nausea); trembling; numbness or tingling of extremities; total loss of function in limbs or body parts
Cognitive: Inability to make decisions or process information; difficulty concentrating; nightmares; memory loss; flashback; loss of reality testing/sense of what is real; self-doubt/loss of confidence; apathy
Emotional: Worry; nervousness; irritability; anger; sadness; fear; anxiety; loss of humor
Behavioral: Inability to complete tasks; decreased efficiency; distractibility; carelessness; recklessness; isolation; inappropriate aggression; hypervigilance; immobility; somatic complaints

severity of symptoms that establish the presence of a COSR [4]. Though a COSR is typically limited to 72 hours or less than 4 days post-incident. Due to its pre-clinical nature, a COSR is not included in the Diagnostic and Statistical Manual of Mental Disorders, Fifth Edition (DSM-5) and is classified as a Z-code (Z86.51) in the International Classification of Diseases—10th Revision—Clinical Modification (ICD-10-CM). It is only if the signs and symptoms of a COSR (Table 11.3) persist that it is further assessed to determine if it meets diagnostic criteria for a psychiatric disorder, such as ASD or PTSD.

The primary elements of an evaluation for a COSR include collecting information about stressors, current symptoms, and degree of impairment. This includes assessing for both acute (e.g., recent losses, injuries, traumatic events) and chronic (e.g., relationship, work, financial) stressors. It is also important to collect a medical and mental health history, including screening for serious mental illness, to determine if additional support or treatment is required. A safety assessment should be conducted for the self (e.g., suicidal ideation) and others (e.g., homicidal ideation) as well as if there is any potential harm to unit or mission (e.g., the patient is unable to perform military duties). The military places strong emphasis on a service member's ability to perform his/her duties since occupational impairment may put others within the unit at risk [4].

Vignette: COSC Assessment and Consultation in the Unit

COSC Assessment. The clinical psychologist assigned to the USS Ronald Reagan conducted a thorough assessment of SM's symptoms. SM felt extremely guilty about abandoning his mother, not helping his friend more when he was injured, and now, letting his unit down. Symptoms consisted of lack of sleep, extreme fatigue, and feeling hopeless. He did not have any feelings of harming himself or others. However, the culmination of stressors impeded his ability to perform his duties. The recent history of the events and acute onset of his symptoms warranted withholding a formal diagnosis, instead conceptualizing his symptoms as a COSR. The clinical psychologist determined that SM was temporarily unable to successfully perform his duties and required short-term treatment. If a brief course of treatment proved unsuccessful, then a formal psychiatric diagnosis would be considered.

COSC Consultation. With SM's consent, the psychologist met with his leadership to formulate strategies for a successful treatment plan and reintegration back to full duty. His leadership reported that SM has been an excellent Sailor but have seen him deteriorating in the last few weeks. The psychologist described the optimal COSC intervention, explaining that it was critical for leadership to not treat him as a "broken Sailor" in order to facilitate restoring the Sailor's competence and confidence, and maintain the expectation that, with appropriate support, he would recover and be able to continue the mission.

Treatment

When treating a service member presenting with a COSR, it is crucial that COSRs are seen as pre-clinical as opposed to clinical. Rather than identifying specific interventions or techniques to treat COSRs, the following approaches offer a general restorative model.

The Four R's Studies suggest COSRs respond well to what are known as the four (4) R's [13]:

- *Rest*: allow time for uninterrupted sleep far from enemy contact
- *Reassure*: that the individual will get better
- *Replenish*: food and water
- *Restore*: confidence in their warrior tasks/training
- The Army uses the 5 R's and includes *Return* (return to duty and reunite Soldier with his/her unit)

PIE and BICEPS Other similar frameworks used for treating combat stress reactions in deployed settings are the PIE and BICEPS principles. PIE was first documented in World War I and includes the following concepts [9]:

- *Proximity*: treat stress casualties close to the battle front
- *Immediacy*: treat without delay
- *Expectancy*: expectation of returning to the battle front

From lessons learned using the PIE approach, its principles were later expanded into BICEPS [14]:

- *Brevity*: treatment usually lasts less than 72 hours
- *Immediacy*: treat as soon as symptoms are evident
- *Centrality*: treat in a centralized Combat Stress Control (CSC) unit separate from but near a medical unit
- *Expectancy*: expect that casualties will recover and return to duty
- *Proximity*: treatment at or as near to the battle front as possible
- *Simplicity*: use of approaches such as rest, food, hygiene, and reassurance

Psychological First Aid Psychological First Aid (PFA) is a conceptual and practical framework that is evidence-informed for treating individuals in the early aftermath of traumatic stress. PFA includes a strong assessment and reassessment component to ensure the fundamental needs of the individual is being met. Further, since experiencing a COSR puts individuals at elevated risk for PTSD, follow-up monitoring and rescreening should occur for at least 6 months [2].

The following are the key elements of PFA:

- Contact and engagement
- Safety and comfort
- Stabilization (if needed)
- Information gathering
- Practice assistance
- Connection with social supports
- Information on coping
- Linkage to collaborative services (if needed)

The COSFA model described earlier is a modified approach to PFA that leverages the military's pre-existing social structures (e.g., clearly defined leadership, cohesive units, a network of available support) [2].

Adjunctive treatments Targeted pharmacological and psychological interventions may be beneficial and/or warranted to address and mange acute symptoms, such as sleep disturbances, pain, excessive arousal and irritability, panic attacks, and anger. Short-term medication regimens can help alleviate intense anxiety, agitation, or sleep disturbance in the immediate period following a COSR event [2]. Short-term benzodiazepines may be used adjunctively; though given the abuse potential of benzodiazepines some clinicians may prefer a low dose atypical antipsychotic [4]. (Note: the VA/DoD Clinical Practice Guidelines [15] recommend against the use of benzodiazepines and atypical antipsychotics for the treatment of PTSD due to low quality evidence.) In all cases that include medication management, it is critical to continuously assess the impact of psychiatric medication on military duties (e.g., guard duty, handling weapons) [4]. Psychological interventions that may be considered to help mitigate acute symptoms include relaxation training, meditation, sleep-hygiene strategies, and avoidance of caffeine [2].

Vignette: COSC Treatment Within the Unit

COSC Intervention. After the psychologist explained the treatment plan to both SM and his leadership, they all agreed to put SM on light duty. SM was removed from flight deck duties and temporarily assigned to hangar deck maintenance duties to minimize operational stressors as he worked toward a full recovery. SM began seeing the psychologist 3 days per week. During treatment, SM maintained a structured daily routine, attending command physical fitness and general military training sessions, and completing many of his assigned duties throughout the day. This structure allowed SM to maintain a military identity as opposed to that of a medical patient, aiding in the expectation that he would fully recover and return to duty. He effectively participated in treatment but had significant difficulty getting adequate rest due to intrusive and distressing thoughts and images. The psychologist referred SM to the Senior Medical Officer who prescribed a low dose of a medication to aid with sleep.

Counseling sessions with the psychologist focused on stress management and managing his conflicting thoughts. SM stated that he wanted to support his mother but still found it difficult given her distress and his feelings of guilt. Also, during these counseling sessions, he expressed losing his sense of purpose but not wanting to let his shipmates down. In addition to counseling, he also returned to his Senior Medical Officer for medication checks.

COSC Outcome. After 3 weeks of light duty and seeing the psychologist, SM began performing duties on the flight deck one day per week, eventually working back to a full duty status on the flight deck. As he reintegrated back into his unit, SM's confidence was restored in himself as well as in his shipmates and leaders. In consultation with the Senior Medical Officer, SM's medication was discontinued a few weeks later. The psychologist met with SM's leadership, and they all agreed that he was doing well and could return to full duty. In the end, it was SM's commitment to his shipmates that compelled him to push through his difficulties and stay committed to returning to his military duties. He completed his tour of duty and returned home with his unit. A year and a half after returning home, SM was promoted to the rank of Petty officer third class (E-4) and re-enlisted in the Navy.

Civilian Providers and COSRs

Today's military mental health care system is unable to meet the demands of all service members in need of care. There are also numerous instances in which service members are reluctant to seek care within the military health care system due to stigma and/or barriers to care [16]. Therefore it is common for service members to be treated by mental health providers outside of the military, especially when units are at their home station (i.e., not deployed). Since the late 1990s, in response to the increased demand for services, the military has been outsourcing care to local civilian providers. It is estimated that two-thirds of veterans receive care from outside Veterans Affairs (VA), and the majority of Reserve and Guard members get their care from civilian providers [17]. Accordingly, there are current initiatives to help civilian providers better understand the military environment and operations in order to provide culturally relevant care to military personnel.

Vignette: COSC Assessment and Treatment Outside of the Unit

Two years post-deployment, and shortly after moving to a new command on a guided missile destroyer, SM discovered a fellow shipmate in the ship's hangar bay who had died by a self-inflicted gunshot wound while the ship was in-port. After two nights of no sleep and multiple promptings by his wife, SM went to his Independent Duty Corpsman who recommended he go to the local military hospital, which then referred him to an "in-network" civilian psychiatrist.

The psychiatrist conducted an assessment of SM's symptoms and found that he was unable to sleep, was having flashbacks of finding his peer's body, and was experiencing feelings of anxiety and irritability. A safety assessment found that SM was not having thoughts of harming himself or others. After further assessing SM's work functioning, the psychiatrist determined that SM's military performance was not being significantly affected. Due to the recentness of the event, SM was not given a mental health diagnosis, and the short-term treatment plan was guided by a PFA framework.

The psychiatrist provided psychoeducation about trauma reactions, thereby normalizing SM's reaction, and discussed the importance of good nutrition, hydration, and rest for recovery. The psychiatrist also helped SM identify natural supports that he could use for both practical and emotional needs. In particular, he reported having a good friend from his previous deployment that he had been meaning to reach out to for several months. The service member was also encouraged to identify helpful ways he had coped with difficult situations in the past in order to re-establish his sense of self-efficacy. For the insomnia, a brief medication regimen was prescribed to provide some initial relief.

Returned for a 2-week follow up appointment. He had improvements in his sleep, had been eating better, and also started working out daily (something he found helpful in the past). He found that his daily workouts also decreased his anxiety and irritability. SM reached out to his friend from his last deployment which he found helpful because it reminded him that being in the military was not about only focusing on himself but that he also had a team that depended on him. He realized that if he wanted to be strong for his team, he needed to take care of himself. The psychiatrist discontinued the sleep medication and encouraged SM to continue his good nutrition and daily workouts as they help promote healthy sleep. SM was also taught deep breathing techniques that he could use at night to elicit a relaxing effect, further increasing his sense of self-efficacy. They scheduled another follow up appointment for 1 month, and the psychiatrist instructed SM to contact him if any of his symptoms re-emerged before their next appointment.

Future Directions

Moving into the future, the military services have been increasing their emphasis on building resilience to keep service members "in the green" and mission ready throughout the military life cycle. In 2009, after several years of sustained combat and operations, the Army launched their comprehensive soldier fitness (CSF) program to build resilience and enhance the performance of Army units. The vision of

CSF is to maintain "an Army of balanced, healthy, self-confident Soldiers, families and Army civilians whose resilience and total fitness enables them to thrive in an era of high operational tempo and persistent conflict [18]."

Mindfulness, a key ingredient to building resilience, is becoming the cornerstone for many military resilience initiatives. Mindfulness is a mental state achieved by focusing one's awareness on the present moment. In one paramount study, investigators implemented Mindfulness-Based Mind Fitness Training among infantry Marines undergoing pre-combat deployment training. Results showed that those Marines who participated in this training exhibited better self-regulation (e.g., enhanced recovery of heart rate) during training. These findings suggest that emphasizing mindfulness as a form of "mental fitness" may be a powerful strategy for management of stressful situations inherent to military operations [19].

In 2018, the Navy implemented a Warrior Toughness pilot program that introduces mindfulness, visualizations, and self-talk as a regular mental fitness practice during recruit training. After promising results, the Navy continues to explore ways to build on this introduction to mental fitness with complementary opportunities throughout military life. For example, Mind Body Resilience Training provides cognitive skills (e.g., psychological flexibility), energy management, strategies for regular recuperative sleep, and ways to build social connections to mindfulness practice in order to build the resilience and performance of military family members. Further discussion about the development of resiliency in service members is covered in a separate chapter in this book.

Conclusion

The goals of military COSC programs are to prevent, identify, and treat adverse effects of combat and operational stress with the long-term objectives of maintaining force readiness and promoting the health and well-being of service members and units. A COSR is not a clinical disorder but instead a consequence of being exposed to high stress situations. It is conceptualized as a normal and self-limited response to overwhelming experiences [2]. COSRs are managed by keeping affected service members close to their unit (when possible), using simple treatment methods (rest, nutrition, social contact), and having an expectation of reintegration and recovery.

Military service is filled with constant challenges and persistent adversity that must be faced, dealt with, and overcome. COSC has been instrumental in helping the military services identify stress injuries that can be readily treated to keep service members in the fight. Enhancing COSC through resilience initiatives has the capacity to further prepare military recruits, retain quality service members, and return contributing citizens to the civilian sector.

Clinical Pearls

- Combat and operational stress control (COSC) programs in the US military are designed to prevent, identify, and manage adverse combat and operational stress as well as promote the resilience and psychological health of military units.
- The objective of Combat and Operational Stress Control is the preservation and readiness maintenance of the military force and the long term well being and health of the individual service member.
- Historically, combat and operational stress reactions account for nearly half of all battle casualties but have significantly decreased with the institution of combat and operational stress control programs.
- The Stress Continuum Model recognizes the entire spectrum of stress responses and outcomes. The fundamental principle is that uncontrolled stress tends to push individuals from adaptive stress responses to distress and functional impairment.
- Monitoring and managing the stress responses of the unit is primarily the responsibility of unit leaders. This is accomplished through the Five Core Leader Functions: strengthen, mitigate, identify, treat, and reintegrate, and Combat and Operational Stress First Aid.
- It is important to understand the difference between a COSR, ASD, and PTSD. A COSR, ASD, and PTSD can share symptoms in presentation, but a COSR *is not* the same as ASD or PTSD. A COSR is a negative adjustment from exposure to stress and traumatic events, classified as a sub-clinical diagnosis with a high percentage for recovery when appropriate interventions are provided.
- When treating a service member presenting with a COSR, it is crucial that COSRs are seen as pre-clinical as opposed to clinical. Rather than identifying specific interventions or techniques to treat COSRs, several approaches offer a general restorative model, such as the 4 R's (Rest, Reassure, Replenish, Restore) and PIE (Proximity, Immediacy, Expectancy).

Appendix: Key Terms of Combat and Operational Stress and Operational Stress Control

Term/Definition

Combat and operational stress control: Leader actions and responsibilities to promote resilience and psychological health in military units and individuals, including families, exposed to the stress of combat or other military operations.

Combat stress: Changes in physical or mental functioning or behavior resulting from the experience of lethal force or its aftermath. These changes can be positive and adaptive or they can be negative, including distress or loss of normal functioning.

Combat and Operational Stress Reaction (COSR): The expected, predictable, emotional, intellectual, physical, and/or behavioral reactions of Service members who have been exposed to stressful events in combat or military operations other than war.

Mental health: The absence of significant distress or impairment due to mental illness. Mental health is a prerequisite for psychological health.

Operational (or occupational) stress control: Leader actions and responsibilities to promote resilience and psychological health in military units and individuals, including family members, exposed to the stress of routine or wartime military operations in noncombat environments.

Operational stress: Changes in physical or mental functioning or behavior resulting from the experience or consequences of military operations other than combat, during peacetime or war, and on land, at sea, or in the air.

Psychological health: Wellness in mind, body, and spirit.

Resilience: The process of preparing for, recovering from, and adjusting to life in the face of stress, adversity, trauma, or tragedy.

Stress Continuum Model: A paradigm that recognizes the entire spectrum of stress responses and outcomes and includes, adaptive coping and wellness (color coded Green as the “Ready” Zone), mild and reversible distress or loss of function (the Yellow “Reacting” Zone), more severe and persistent distress or loss of function (the Orange “Injured” Zone), and mental disorders arising from stress and unhealed stress injuries (the Red “Ill” Zone).

Stress illness: A diagnosable mental disorder resulting from an unhealed stress injury that worsens over time to cause significant disability in one or more spheres of life.

Stress injury: More severe and persistent distress or loss of functioning caused by disruptions to the integrity of the brain, mind, or spirit after exposure to overwhelming stressors. Stress injuries are invisible, but literal, wounds caused by stress, but, like more visible physical wounds, they usually heal, especially if given proper care.

Stressor: Any mental or physical challenge or set of challenges.

Stress reaction: The common, temporary, and often necessary experience of mild distress or changes in functioning due to stress from any cause.

References

1. Precin PJ, Mattila AM, Crandall BD, Goldman SB. U.S. Army combat operational stress control throughout the deployment cycle: a case study. Work. 2011;38:13–8.
2. Nash WP, Watson PJ. Review of VA/DoD Clinical Practice Guidelines on management of acute stress and interventions to prevent posttraumatic stress disorder. J Rehabil Res Dev. 2012;49:637–48.
3. Brusher EA. Combat and operational stress control. Int J Emerg Ment Health. 2007;9:111–22.
4. Benedeck D, Hamaoka D, West JC. Combat and operational stress reaction. In: Herman R, editors. UpToDate. 2018. https://www.uptodate.com/contents/combat-and-operational-stress-reaction. Accessed 10 Oct 2019.
5. Broadnax K. Combat and operational stress: minimizing its adverse effects on service members. School of Advanced Military Studies. United States Army Command and General Staff College. 2008. https://apps.dtic.mil/dtic/tr/fulltext/u2/a485474.pdf. Accessed 17 Jul 2001.

6. Crocq M, Crocq L. From shell shock and war neurosis to PTSD. Dialogues Clin Neurosci. 2000;2(1):47–55.
7. Shephard B. A war of nerves: soldiers and psychiatrists in the twentieth century. Boston, MA: Harvard University Press; 2003.
8. MCRP. 6-11 C/NTTP 1-15M: combat and operational stress control. Washington, DC: Department of the Navy; 2010.
9. Jones E, Wessely S. "Forward psychiatry" in the military: its origins and effectiveness. J Trauma Stress. 2003;16(4):411–9.
10. Jones FD. Psychiatric lessons of war. In: Jones FD, Sparacino LR, Wilcox VL, et al., editors. Textbook of military medicine. Washington, DC: Borden Institute; 1995. p. 1–34.
11. Dailey JI, James VL. Evolution of the combat and operational stress control detachment. US Army Med Dep J. 2014:8–13.
12. ATP 6-22.5: a leaders guide to soldier health and fitness. Washington, DC: Department of the Army; 2016. p. 7/1–7/20.
13. Potter AR, Baker MT, Sanders CS, Peterson AL. Combat stress reactions during military deployments: evaluation of the effectiveness of combat stress control treatment. J Ment Health Counsel. 2009;31:137–48.
14. DoD Directive 6490.5: combat stress control (CSC) programs. Washington, DC: Department of Defense; 1999.
15. Tschanz MP, Watts SA, Colburn MJA, Conlin PR, Pogach LM, Overview and Discussion of the 2017 VA/DoD Clinical Practice Guideline for the Management of Type 2 Diabetes Mellitus in Primary Care. Fed Pract. 2017;34(Suppl 8):S14–9. PMCID: PMC6375527, PMID: 30766312.
16. Delaney E, Webb-Murphy J, Bhakta J, et al. Barriers to mental health care in military settings: what we know and where to go from here. Mil Behav Health. 2019;7:1–3.
17. Meyer E. The importance of understanding military culture. Acad Psychiatry. 2015;39:416–8.
18. Millerrodgers M. Comprehensive soldier fitness marks change in army culture. 2010. https://www.army.mil/article/45723/comprehensive_soldier_fitness_marks_change_in_army-culture. Accessed 16 Oct 2019.
19. Johnson DC, Thom NJ, Stanley EA, et al. Modifying resilience mechanisms in at-risk individuals: a controlled study of mindfulness training in marines preparing for deployment. Am J Psychiatry. 2014;171(8):844–53.

PTSD in Military Service Members and Veterans

12

Johanna Thompson-Hollands, Lewina O. Lee, and Paula P. Schnurr

Vignette

George was drafted into the Army at age 19. He was deployed to Vietnam for 1 year, serving as a helicopter mechanic for his unit. He recalled encountering seriously wounded men on his first day in-country; the extent of their injuries was like nothing he had ever seen before. George reported that the most difficult experience of his deployment occurred midway through his tour; his unit was engaged in an intense firefight, including several helicopter missions to bring supplies to forces on the ground. One of the helicopters needed an urgent repair, but George was having difficulty due to a lack of appropriate supplies. As he was trying his best to make due with makeshift parts, he could hear reports coming through the radio from other soldiers who needed additional ammunition. He could tell that they were being gradually overpowered by the enemy forces. George was ultimately able to get the helicopter running, but more than half of the men on the ground were killed that day.

After George returned from his deployment and separated from the Army, he struggled to find his footing in civilian life. He felt resentful of the general public's attitude towards the Vietnam war, feeling that it did not honor the sacrifice and bravery of his fellow soldiers. At the same time, he felt unworthy of having survived the war as a relatively young man with no attachments. One of the men who was killed in the firefight was a Sergeant with a wife and child, and George asked himself,

J. Thompson-Hollands (✉) · L. O. Lee
Behavioral Science Division, National Center for PTSD, Boston, MA, USA

VA Boston Healthcare System, Boston, MA, USA

Boston University School of Medicine, Boston, MA, USA
e-mail: Johanna.thompson-hollands@va.gov; Lewina.lee@va.gov

P. P. Schnurr
Executive Division, National Center for PTSD, White River Junction, VT, USA

Geisel School of Medicine at Dartmouth, Hanover, NH, USA
e-mail: Paula.schnurr@va.gov

C. H. Warner, C. A. Castro (eds.), *Veteran and Military Mental Health*,
https://doi.org/10.1007/978-3-031-18009-5_12

"Why did I live, when he was a better man than me? Why should his family lose him, when I don't have anyone who depends on me?" He imagined his fellow soldiers brutally killed like the bodies he had seen on his first day of deployment.

George did not speak to anyone about his Vietnam service; he did not like to remember those days, and he did not believe that civilians could understand the realities of the war. He worked in a machine fabrication shop, but drank heavily on nights and weekends. Although he eventually married and had children, his family experienced him as emotionally withdrawn but occasionally volatile. He was especially irritable in crowds, complaining that "There's too many idiots moving around and getting in everyone's way!" He also had regular nightmares, and eventually he and his wife began sleeping separately. George's wife assumed that he had "seen some hard things" while deployed but thought it was best not to bring up the topic for fear of destabilizing him or causing him to be angry.

Introduction

Posttraumatic stress disorder (PTSD) first became a diagnostic entity in the Third Edition of the Diagnostic and Statistical Manual of Mental Disorders (*DSM-III*; [1]). However, the psychological sequelae of warfare involvement have been documented for centuries, such as Shakespeare's vivid account of Hotspur, a fierce soldier whose wife complained of "faint slumbers" in which he "murmur(s) tales of iron wars", startle, agitation ("beads of sweat… like bubbles in a late-disturbed stream"), "cursed melancholy", and self-isolation [2]; some writers have argued that the earliest depictions of PTSD can be found in writings from Mesopotamia (present-day Iraq) as long ago as 1300 BC [3]. In the early twentieth century, terms such as *battle fatigue*, *war neurosis*, and *shell shock* connoted psychological and physical symptoms thought to arise from combat environment and prevented soldiers from returning to front lines [4]. While current military personnel undergo routine screens for PTSD across their deployment cycle [5], many veterans of earlier conflicts lived with PTSD symptoms for decades without having an appropriate label for their condition and effective treatment, and many still lack an understanding of the nature of PTSD and how it has shaped their life trajectories. Practitioners working with military personnel and veterans must consider the diverse demographic, cultural, and contextual factors that influence how patients make sense of their symptoms and dealing with the condition [6]. To address these issues, we first provide an overview of the epidemiology of PTSD by eras of military service and summarize risk factors which increase susceptibility to PTSD onset and symptom maintenance. Next, we review evidence on comorbidity and quality of life in PTSD. We then turn to issues regarding screening, assessment, and treatment. Throughout the chapter, we use case vignettes to illustrate unique aspects of military and veteran PTSD; these vignettes are composite examples drawn from multiple different clinical cases.

Epidemiology of PTSD by Era of Military Service

Prevalence estimates of PTSD in any given war cohort vary as a function of the study design, sample, and assessment methods.

World War II (1941–1946) and Korean Conflict (1950–1955)

Prevalence estimates among WWII and Korean Conflict Veterans are typically based on small samples and inherently biased by survival effects, as it was impossible to assess PTSD among veterans who died before the diagnosis was formalized in 1980. For example, in a small sample of nonpsychiatric inpatients at a Department of Veterans Affairs (VA) hospital, 19% of WWII and 30% of Korean Conflict veterans scored above the PTSD cutoff on a self-report measure [7]. In the Medical Follow-Up Agency's longitudinal study of WWII and Korean Conflict prisoners of war (POWs), prevalence estimates for *DSM-III-R* [8] PTSD assessed via diagnostic interview were 12–19% for WWII POWs and 38% for Korean Conflict POWs, when their typical ages were 65–75 and 55–65, respectively [9].

Several contextual factors are useful in considering the experiences of WWII and Korean era veterans. For most of the twentieth century, psychiatrists and military officials commonly attributed "shell shock" or psychiatric difficulties in soldiers to stable individual vulnerability factors, cowardice, or malingering to seek repatriation [10]. Such beliefs likely reduced veterans' willingness to acknowledge psychiatric symptoms, despite shifts in popular opinions which only took place in their later lives. Other aspects of their military experience provided buffer against combat stressors, such as the use of "primary groups" or "buddy systems" which promoted group cohesion during lengthy deployments. Especially for WWII veterans, homecoming to a supportive community, a booming postwar economy, and GI Bill benefits for education and mortgages facilitated their long-term adaptation [10].

Vietnam Era (1961–1975)

In a large, nationally representative veteran sample, the National Vietnam Veterans Readjustment Study (NVVRS; [11]) estimated that among theater veterans (those who were deployed to Vietnam), 15% men and 8% women had current DSM-III-R PTSD in 1986–1988; lifetime prevalence was 31% for men and 27% for women. In a 25-year follow-up study of this cohort, current prevalence of DSM-5 [12] PTSD was 4.5% for men and 6.1% for women. Between the two occasions, self-reported PTSD symptoms remained high and increased modestly among theater veterans, whereas symptoms were low and stable among era veterans (those who were in the military during the Vietnam war but did not serve there) [13].

Combat and non-combat aspects of the Vietnam war influenced its psychiatric sequelae. For theater veterans, guerilla style warfare had no front line; base camps were under constant risk for guerilla attacks, and it was difficult to tell friend from foe. Soldiers faced significant unpredictability and threat daily. Because tours were limited to a year, soldiers arrived at and departed the war theater individually; such rotation schedules did not provide the sense of solidarity and social structure afforded by the earlier "buddy system" [14]. Both theater and era veterans faced an unwelcoming public at home who often opposed the war; many veterans were insulted for their war involvement, felt misunderstood about their difficulties, and had low desire to reintegrate into civilian culture [4]. Demographically, as the U.S. military transitioned to an all-volunteer force during this war (75% personnel enlisted), participation from Blacks and socioeconomically disadvantaged men increased compared to previous eras [15]. Vietnam veterans were younger on average than WWII Veterans (mean age: 19 vs. 26; [7]). As we discuss in the *Risk Factors* section below, it is useful to consider how these factors underlie cohort differences in susceptibility for psychiatric conditions.

Persian Gulf War (1990–1991)

Unlike the Vietnam War, the Persian Gulf War was an extremely brief, successful, and well-received military operation. However, shortly upon homecoming, some personnel reported symptoms that have come to be known as Gulf War Syndrome—fatigue, headaches, joint pain, cognitive and sleep disturbances, skin and respiratory conditions [16]. The unexplained symptoms are thought to be related to deployment-related environmental exposures, such as biological and chemical warfare agents, prophylactic medications, depleted uranium munitions, and pollutants including petroleum and fumes from oil-well fires. As for PTSD, a large epidemiologic survey estimated a population prevalence of 10.1% for current DSM-III-R PTSD assessed by survey in 1995–1997. Gulf War veterans had 2.6 times greater odds than their military counterparts not deployed to the Gulf to screen positive for PTSD [17]. Another large-scale survey reported similar estimates: 8.0% for active duty veterans and 9.3% for deployed reservists [18]. Of note, Gulf War troops differed from earlier cohorts in their large proportion of National Guards and Reservists (17%), and women (7%).

Operation Enduring Freedom and Operation Iraqi Freedom (OEF/OIF, 2001–2014)

OEF and OIF are U.S. military responses to the terrorist attacks on September 11, 2011 ("9/11"), and together they represent America's longest period of continuous combat operations. When assessed in 2011, OEF/OIF service members included more women compared to earlier cohorts (16% in OEF/OIF vs. 7% in Gulf War), and a significant proportion were married (53%) and had children (44%) [5, 19].

About one-third of the OEF/OIF and Persian Gulf cohorts were ethnic minorities, compared with approximately 10% in Vietnam War [19, 20]. As the size of the U.S. military declined steadily since the early 1990s, the number of military deployments per service member increased and there has been a greater reliance on Reservists and National Guards for frequent peacekeeping and humanitarian operations (28% in OEF/OIF; [20]).

While war fatalities have declined over time, more military personnel return home with severe war-related morbidities. Approximately 13–16% OEF/OIF Veterans were estimated to meet criteria for current DSM-IV-TR PTSD when assessed with anonymous surveys; estimates were similar when DSM-5 criteria were used [21, 22]. Suicide rates in the U.S. Army have increased sharply in recent years and are particularly high among younger OEF/OIF personnel [23]. Explosions account for nearly three-quarters of all OEF/OIF combat injuries [24], and nearly one-fifth of OEF/OIF personnel were estimated to have deployment-related traumatic brain injury (TBI; [25]).

Active Military Personnel

Fewer studies have evaluated the prevalence of psychological conditions among active military personnel relative to research on veterans. The Department of Defense (DoD) conducts periodic, anonymous Surveys of Health-Related Behaviors Among Active Duty Military Personnel (HRBS) to monitor lifestyle behaviors of service members and better understand how these behaviors relate to military readiness, health, and well-being. HRBS samples are representative of all active duty personnel. In the 2005 HRBS, prevalence of questionnaire-based DSM-IV PTSD was 6.7%. In the 2008 HRBS, PTSD prevalence increased to 12.4–13.3% among active duty personnel deployed to combat since 9/11, and to 8.2% among those not deployed post-9/11 [26]. These findings are consistent with the observation that PTSD rates tend to increase from assessments conducted shortly upon homecoming to longer-term follow-up conducted in subsequent years [27]. In a more recent study which also assessed PTSD anonymously via questionnaire among infantry soldiers, prevalence was 12% in the entire sample and 18% among those who had been deployed in Iraq or Afghanistan [22]. A slightly lower prevalence of 8.6% was reported in a study which collected personal identifiers [28]; work by Warner and colleagues has shown that when soldiers are allowed to report mental health issues (including PTSD) anonymously, rates are two- to fourfold higher compared to personally identifiable reports [29]. This work highlights the role of mental health stigma in screening and evaluating military personnel, particularly those in active duty.

Vignette

Andrea came from a military family; her father and older brother were both Marines, with her father having over 30 years of service prior to his retirement. Andrea eagerly enlisted in the Marines following her high school graduation. She felt motivated to emulate her father and brother's examples, and to serve her country. She also knew that the War on Terror was ongoing, and she was excited about defending American values overseas.

Andrea was quite familiar with "Marine culture" given her family environment. She was the only sister among four siblings, and identified as a tomboy and an athlete. She knew that basic training would be physically and emotionally exhausting but was excited to prove herself. As expected, her first weeks of basic training were grueling. One day while returning from the shower, she was cornered by 2 male Marines. Although she attempted to fight them off, they sexually assaulted her. During the incident, the men also taunted Andrea, alternately insinuating that she desired the attack and threatening her with slander or violence if she tried to report them. For portions of the event, Andrea felt as though she had left her body and was watching the scene from above.

Andrea did not report the attack. She did not want to jeopardize her standing as a new recruit. She felt ashamed for having been caught off-guard and for not having appropriate "situational awareness." She continued with her training, although it was extremely difficult to continue seeing the perpetrators around the base. She withdrew into herself and felt that she had become hardened towards others. Although previously she was outgoing and sociable, Andrea stopped keeping in touch with her old friends and would no longer attend parties or other events. She was not interested in dating, saying "Men just want to take advantage of you, they want to use you and then once they've gotten what they want they throw you away." She felt uncomfortable with any physical contact, including hugs from her family or being touched by a doctor during the course of an exam.

Risk Factors

A number of studies have examined factors associated with greater risks for developing PTSD or maintaining symptoms over time. Across cohorts, pre-trauma risk factors include female gender, ethnic minority status, younger age, lower socioeconomic status (SES), education, intellectual ability, psychiatric history, genetics, and prior stressor exposure including early adversity [30–33]. While some studies reported that women were more vulnerable to developing PTSD than men (e.g., [28]), gender differences in the type and severity of trauma exposure (e.g., interpersonal vs. combat), demographics (e.g., educated nurses in Vietnam War), psychosocial processes (e.g., familial concerns among deployed mothers) can at least partially explain the differential risks [34, 35]. It is also critical to note the changing roles of military women: from nurses in the Vietnam War, to military police and pilots in the Persian Gulf War, and being eligible for combat duties since 2013.

Military risk factors for PTSD include enlisted (vs. officer) status, lengthier and more frequent deployments, inadequate unit support, exposure to combat, atrocities or abusive violence, life-threatening situations, malevolent environments such as lack of shelter from weather, and peritraumatic dissociation [33, 36]. Post-military risk factors include inadequate post-deployment social support, psychological symptoms, and stressor exposure after homecoming [33, 37]. A growing literature has focused on identifying resilience factors, such as coping strategies, optimism, and locus of control, which protect against the development of PTSD [38].

Comorbidity

Military personnel and veterans with PTSD typically present with multiple comorbid neuropsychiatric and medical conditions. In the National Comorbidity Survey, PTSD was linked to 4–7 times greater odds of ever having a major depressive episode, 3–6 times greater odds of having Generalized Anxiety Disorder, and 2–4 times greater odds of having a substance use disorder [28]. PTSD is also related to greater risks of suicidal behaviors [39], TBI [25], and dementia [40]. In population-based veteran samples, comorbid physical health conditions include heart disease, obesity, migraine, chronic pain, arthritis and rheumatoid arthritis, osteoporosis, respiratory conditions, and sleep disorder [41, 42].

Quality of Life in PTSD

Quality of life refers to "physical, mental and social well-being" [43], and is increasingly recognized as an important aspect of health across many physical and mental health conditions. Quality of life can be thought of as consisting of material/social elements, functioning (role performance), and wellbeing or satisfaction [44, 45]. For example, individuals might be assessed in terms of their marital or employment status (material/social), interpersonal functioning (role performance), or overall life satisfaction (wellbeing). Studies have found that veterans and service members with PTSD are significantly impaired across all domains [46]. They generally have a higher likelihood of unemployment (e.g., [47]), impaired social and relationship functioning (e.g., [48–50]), and lower ratings of life satisfaction [51]. The bulk of research has focused on PTSD symptom severity predicting later quality of life outcomes, but a bidirectional relationship has been explored and supported in a smaller number of studies (e.g., [52]).

There is some evidence that OEF/OIF veterans show less impact of PTSD on various aspects of quality of life compared to what is seen among older veterans; for example, multiple studies among OEF/OIF veterans have failed to find a relationship between PTSD and unemployment status [50, 53]. However, it is possible that the "cohort advantage" observed in OEF/OIF veterans are due to the trends of increasing PTSD symptoms and declining social resources (e.g., social support) in the post-deployment years, combined with a longer lapse between homecoming and PTSD assessment among Gulf War veterans [54]. As discussed above (see "Epidemiology" section), recent veterans and current service members experience a unique military context that may serve to increase or decrease the impact of PTSD on their quality of life compared to earlier cohorts (e.g., greater awareness of PTSD and increased efforts to screen for symptoms, but also increased numbers of deployments and less time between them). Regardless, reintegration into society post-deployment or post-service can be challenging and may exacerbate symptoms of PTSD in some individuals. Military service provides a strong sense of routine and purpose, as well as structures for social interaction, and it may therefore be particularly important to attend to these factors as a way to promote robust quality of life among returning veterans.

Schnurr and Lunney [55] examined the question of what level of symptom reduction is associated with a meaningful improvement in quality of life among a sample of 235 female veterans and Army soldiers who underwent weekly PTSD treatment. At posttreatment the women were categorized into four mutually exclusive groups representing increasing levels of improvement: No Response, Response, Loss of Diagnosis, and Remission. Results showed that those who achieved Loss of Diagnosis also reached a good endpoint on all measures of quality of life, and the authors thus recommend the absence of a PTSD diagnosis as an optimal benchmark for clinical care.

Screening and Assessment

Proper assessment of PTSD is critical to providing high-quality clinical care, and therefore it is strongly recommended that patients be assessed before, during, and after treatment. Fortunately there are many validated measures of varying lengths and methods of administration (i.e., self-report versus clinician-administered) available, a selection of which are reviewed below.

Each assessment format has both strengths and weaknesses; for example, self-report measures are beneficial in environments where time is limited, but they necessarily entail fixed (and brief) item content and require respondents to display reasonable comprehension, insight, and honesty. In contrast, clinician-administered interviews allow for the judgment of a trained expert to be incorporated into the ratings but can take an hour or longer to complete. The selection of an assessment battery should be guided by the goals of the assessment, knowledge of the target population, and an appreciation for the limitations of the clinical environment [56]. The use of multiple measures is encouraged when possible, in order to reduce bias (Table 12.1).

Life Events Checklist (LEC-5; [57])

The LEC is a self-report measure that screens for exposure to potentially traumatic events across the lifespan. Sixteen specific categories are assessed (e.g., natural disasters, combat, sexual assault), and a final item captures "any other very stressful event or experience." Respondents indicate the type of exposure they have had to each event category, such as direct exposure, witnessing, learning about the event, or does not apply. The LEC may be used to identify an index event for more detailed symptom inquiry or can simply provide an overview of a patient's lifetime trauma load.

Table 12.1 Selected measures for the assessment of trauma and PTSD symptomatology

Measure	Purpose	Format	Length	Cut-score
Life Events Checklist (LEC-5)	Screening for exposure to potentially traumatic events across the lifespan	Self-report	Assesses 17 categories of potentially traumatic events	*N/A*
Primary Care for PTSD Screen for *DSM-5* (PC-PTSD-5)	Screening for PTSD	Self-report	5 items	3 or 4
PTSD Checklist for *DSM-5* (PCL-5)	Assessment of symptom severity and likely diagnosis	Self-report	20 items	33
Clinician-Administered PTSD Scale for *DSM-5* (CAPS-5)	Assessment of symptom severity and diagnosis	Clinician-rated	Items cover assessment of Criterion A, the 20 core PTSD symptoms, as well as distress/impairment and dissociative symptoms	*N/A*

All measures listed above are freely available through the National Center for PTSD website (www.ptsd.va.gov)

Primary Care PTSD Screen for DSM-5 (PC-PTSD-5; [58])

The PC-PTSD-5 is a 5-item screening tool for PTSD. The measure consists of dichotomous yes/no questions, including an initial prompt regarding exposure to potentially traumatic events and five subsequent questions regarding symptoms of nightmares, avoidance of thoughts/feelings, hypervigilance, numbness or detachment, and feelings of guilt or blame. Scores are calculated by summing the number of endorsed items. The measure has been validated among a sample of veterans in VA primary care, and either a three or a four was found to be an appropriate cut-score [58].

PTSD Checklist for DSM-5 (PCL-5; [59])

The PCL-5 is a questionnaire consisting of 20 items that correspond to the DSM-5 PTSD symptoms. The PCL is one of the most widely used and validated PTSD questionnaires available. Items are rated on a 0–4 scale (total score = 0–80), with higher scores indicating greater severity of symptoms. A cutoff score of 33 has been shown to indicate likely PTSD status among a clinical veteran sample [60], and 33/34 was the optimally efficient cutoff among an epidemiological sample of soldiers [22].

Clinician-Administered PTSD Scale for DSM-5 (CAPS-5; [61])

The CAPS-5 is a structured diagnostic interview for PTSD. Items are scored on a 0–4 scale that incorporates ratings of both intensity and frequency, and total scores for the measure range from 0 to 80. The CAPS-5 is considered the gold-standard measure for both symptom severity and diagnostic status and has been validated in a military sample [62].

Treatment Efficacy and Effectiveness

A meta-analysis examining randomized controlled trials demonstrated an effect size of $g = 1.26$ for cognitive behavioral treatments for PTSD (including Cognitive Processing Therapy and Prolonged Exposure) and $g = 1.01$ for Eye Movement Desensitization and Reprocessing, whereas antidepressant medications had an effect size of $g = 0.43$ [63]. Trauma-focused psychotherapies also maintain their impact for at least several months following the end of treatment, whereas medications have lower efficacy and must be maintained to show continued benefit [64]. Effectiveness studies of CPT and PE among veterans have shown that both treatments result in substantial symptom reductions (including secondary symptoms of depression and anxiety) when used in regular clinical care [65–67]. A study of veterans with comorbid PTSD and alcohol use disorder (current or past) showed that these dual-diagnosis patients also respond well to CPT [68]. Dropout from psychosocial treatments for PTSD is a concern, with reported rates from VA facilities ranging from approximately 35 to 50% (e.g., [69–71]). However, dropout from CBT for PTSD is comparable to and even lower than dropout from treatments for other mental disorders [72]. Encouragement from loved ones, particularly if the relationship in general is positive, appears to substantially decrease the risk of dropout from trauma-focused therapies [71].

Researchers continue to explore how to improve upon PTSD treatment. Recent studies have focused on how best to match patients to particular treatments (e.g., [73]), examining how providers modify treatments to fit their setting (e.g., [74]), and identifying ways to make treatment more efficient (e.g., [75, 76]).

Treatment Recommendations

The VA and the DoD jointly produce a practice guideline that can be used to inform the treatment of Veterans and Servicemembers with PTSD [77]. Some research suggests that military-related PTSD is associated with lesser treatment response relative to PTSD due to other factors (e.g., [63, 78]). However, many of the studies of treatments included in the VA/DoD guideline were conducted in individuals with military-related PTSD, so there is no reason to assume that effective treatments for PTSD in general should not be used to treat Veterans and Servicemembers. The

Table 12.2 Recommendations regarding specific treatments as outlined by the VA/DoD PTSD guideline

Intervention type	Recommended (first-line)	Suggested (weaker recommendation)	Do not recommend/ suggest against
Psychotherapy	Individual, manualized trauma-focused psychotherapy with a primary component of exposure and/or cognitive restructuring (e.g., Prolonged Exposure, Cognitive Processing Therapy, and Eye Movement Desensitization and Reprocessing)[a]	Stress Inoculation Therapy, Present-Centered Therapy, and Interpersonal Therapy	*None noted*
Medications	Sertraline, paroxetine, fluoxetine, and venlafaxine	Nefazodone, imipramine, and phenelzine	Divalproex, tiagabine, guanfacine, prazosin (for primary PTSD treatment), risperidone, benzodiazepines, D-cycloserine, hydrocortisone, and ketamine

[a]The guideline recommends individual trauma-focused psychotherapy as the initial treatment approach. If this treatment is not available or preferred, the guideline recommends one of the four recommended medications or the three suggested non-trauma-focused psychotherapies but does not prioritize one modality over the other

following text is based on the VA/DoD guideline, although it is consistent with recommendations in other PTSD guidelines [79, 80] (Table 12.2).

Regarding psychotherapy, the VA/DoD guideline recommends individual, manualized trauma focused psychotherapy that has a primary component of exposure and/or cognitive restructuring. The most well-studied of these trauma-focused treatments are Prolonged Exposure, Cognitive Processing Therapy, and Eye Movement Desensitization and Reprocessing. The guideline suggests—a weaker recommendation—several individual manualized non-trauma-focused psychotherapies as well: Stress Inoculation Therapy, Present-Centered Therapy, and Interpersonal Therapy. Recommended medications are sertraline, paroxetine, fluoxetine, and venlafaxine. Suggested medications are nefazodone, imipramine, and phenelzine. The guideline suggests group therapy over no treatment, but does not specify a type. The text notes that the evidence is strongest for group Cognitive Processing Therapy, but even that treatment appears to be more effective in individual format [81].

The evidence was judged insufficient for other types of psychotherapy, a number of medications, complementary and integrative treatments such as yoga and meditation, and somatic treatments such as repetitive transcranial magnetic stimulation and hyperbaric oxygen. Based on either demonstrated lack of efficacy and/or benefits relative to harms, the guideline recommends against divalproex, tiagabine, and guanfacine, and suggests against prazosin (for the primary treatment of PTSD), risperidone, benzodiazepines, D-cycloserine, hydrocortisone, and ketamine. Evidence on prazosin for treating nightmares was judged insufficient, and a large randomized clinical trial published after the guideline was finalized found that prazosin did not improve nightmares or PTSD in general [82].

The guideline recommends individual trauma-focused psychotherapy as the initial treatment approach. If individual trauma-focused therapy is not available, or not preferred, the guideline recommends one of the four recommended medications or the three suggested non-trauma-focused psychotherapies, but does not prioritize one modality over the other.

When using any guideline it is important to remember that it is just that—a guide to inform care, and not a mandate to prescribe care. Treatment should begin with a conversation about choice. The VA/DoD guideline's first recommendation is to engage in shared decision-making, in which the patient and clinician collaborate to help a patient to choose a preferred treatment [83, 84]. Elwyn et al. [83] summarize the process in three steps. First is *team talk*, supporting patients when they learn about choices and clarifying their goals. Next is *option talk*, to help them understand treatment options, and finally *decision talk*, to clarify the patient's preferences and values make a choice that is right for them. The National Center for PTSD [85] has developed a decision aid to help patients and providers engage in shared decision-making.

Vignette

"Casey" returned from his second deployment to Iraq in 2010. He was 25 years old and eager to get out of the Army and begin a new life. He used funds from the GI Bill to enroll in a community college, with hopes of eventually transferring to a 4-year institution and then going on to receive an MBA. However, he quickly found that focusing in the classroom was impossible for him. He struggled to follow the lectures ("The teacher sounds like the grown-ups in Peanuts – wah wah") and he was uncomfortable in the crowded classroom. He found his classmates to be unserious and would get visibly irritated by their joking or complaints about everyday hassles. At the same time, he was having frequent intrusive thoughts about his deployment experiences. His best friend Tom had been killed on a mission while they were in Iraq, and Casey was constantly bombarded by memories of Tom and his death. After failing his midterm exams, Casey withdrew from the two courses he had signed up for that semester. He began to feel helpless, and his previously passive suicidal ideation began to become more frequent and active.

During a routine appointment with his primary care doctor, Casey reported that he was experiencing frequent nightmares and had had to withdraw from school due to his concentration difficulties and irritability. His doctor asked more questions about Casey's nightmares, and Casey told the doctor about Tom's death. The doctor administered the PC-PTSD-5 and explained to Casey that he had screened positive for PTSD. This conversation helped Casey to make sense of his confusing mix of symptoms (feeling edgy and tense, but also shut down and numb), and he felt somewhat relieved to have a better understanding of what was happening with him. He agreed to accept a referral for treatment.

Soon afterwards, Casey began weekly individual trauma-focused therapy. The clinician talked with Casey about his goals for treatment and provided an overview of the recommended approaches. Casey thought that Prolonged Exposure felt like the right fit for him. Each week he and the therapist would walk through the day of Tom's death, including describing vivid details of the mission and of Casey holding Tom's body while he died. As his therapy "homework," the clinician had Casey listen to tapes of the session and also to engage in in vivo exposures such as attending a lecture and sitting in the front of the room, or going to a parade on Veterans' Day.

Treatment was not easy. Casey struggled with full engagement during the first several imaginal exposure sessions; he admitted to his clinician that he was holding back because he was afraid of letting himself genuinely experience his reaction. However, the clinician provided encouragement and with time Casey allowed the emotions to come. Gradually the in-session practice and homework exercises resulted in a reduced emotional response to reminders of Tom's death. Casey was able to process his grief, fear and anger. Although his PCL-5 score at the beginning of treatment was a 40, after 15 sessions of PE he scored a 20, well below the clinical cutoff. He had also re-started his college courses and was excited to be doing well. He reported, "I think I'm honoring Tom more this way, by remembering him but also moving forward in my life."

Clinical Pearls

- When working with service members and veterans with probable or confirmed PTSD, providers should take into account how their military experience (e.g., era of service, warzone exposure), demographic (e.g., age, education), contextual (e.g., social support, life stressors, treatment history), and health (e.g., comorbid conditions) may intersect to influence their symptomatology, as well as their awareness of and openness to endorsing the symptoms.
- Although military and veteran patients share a similar status, different cohorts across time have had quite varied experiences of their military service, their post-service reintegration into civilian society, and the level of cultural/systemic awareness with regards to PTSD.
- Military cultural competence [86] is a starting point for working with these patients, but an appreciation for the diversity of their experiences and trends over time are critical.
- Many service members and veterans have experienced both military- and non-military-related traumas [87, 88]. Women veterans who have experienced MST are particularly likely to have also experienced sexual traumas as children, or as adults in civilian life. PTSD symptoms may be related to one or more of the patient's lifetime traumatic events and understanding the patient's overall trauma load (perhaps via administration of the LEC), as well as how earlier traumatic experiences may be impacting the presentation of PTSD related to a later "index" trauma will be useful clinically.
- It may be beneficial to incorporate patients' family members or other loved ones into treatment in some way, whether by conducting a joint session to provide psychoeducation and address concerns or by sending materials home for family members to read.

- Recent evidence suggests that veterans who reported that their family members encouraged them to face distressing situations were twice as likely to persist in trauma-focused psychosocial treatment rather than dropping out [71]. Incorporating family members may help to bolster their support for treatment, and therefore increase patients' compliance and retention.

Acknowledgements Johanna Thompson-Hollands was supported by the U.S. Department of Veterans Affairs (Clinical Sciences Research and Development Service) under Career Development Award # IK2 CX001589. Lewina O. Lee was supported by funding from the National Institute on Aging (award number K08-AG048221). The views expressed in this chapter are those of the authors and do not necessarily reflect the position or policy of the U.S. Department of Veterans Affairs, the U.S. government, or the National Institutes of Health.

References

1. American Psychiatric Association. Diagnostic and statistical manual of mental disorders. 3rd ed. Washington, DC: Author; 1980.
2. Bennet G. Shakespeare and post-traumatic stress disorder. Br J Psychiatry. 2011;198:255. https://doi.org/10.1192/bjp.198.4.255.
3. Abdul-Hamid W, Hughes J. Nothing new under the sun: post-traumatic stress disorders in the ancient world. Early Sci Med. 2014;19:549–57. https://doi.org/10.1163/15733823-00196p02.
4. Oei TP, Lim B, Hennessy B. Psychological dysfunction in battle: combat stress reactions and posttraumatic stress disorder. Clin Psychol Rev. 1990;10:355–88. https://doi.org/10.1016/0272-7358(90)90066-J.
5. Institute of Medicine. Preventing psychological disorders in service members and their families: an assessment of programs. Washington, DC: The National Academies Press; 2014.
6. Knight B, Lee L. Contextual adult lifespan theory for adapting psychotherapy. In: Laidlaw K, Knight B, editors. Handbook of emotional disorders in later life: assessment and treatment. New York, NY: Oxford University Press; 2008. https://www.oxfordclinicalpsych.com/view/10.1093/med:psych/9780198569459.001.0001/med-9780198569459-chapter-3.
7. Blake DD, Keane TM, Wine PR, Mora C, Taylor KL, Lyons JA. Prevalence of PTSD symptoms in combat veterans seeking medical treatment. J Trauma Stress. 1990;3:15–27. https://doi.org/10.1002/jts.2490030103.
8. American Psychiatric Association. Diagnostic and statistical manual of mental disorders. 3rd ed., revised. Washington, DC: Author; 1987.
9. Page WF. The health of former prisoners of war results from the medical examination survey of former POWs of World War II and the Korean conflict. Washington, DC: National Academy Press; 1992.
10. Pols H, Oak S. War & military mental health: the US psychiatric response in the 20th century. Am J Public Health. 2007;97:2132–42. https://doi.org/10.2105/AJPH.2006.090910.
11. Kulka RA, Schlenger WE, Fairbank JA, Hough RL, Jordan BK, Marmar CR, Weiss DS. Trauma and the Vietnam War generation: report of findings from the National Vietnam Veterans Readjustment Study. New York, NY: Brunner/Mazel Publishers; 1990.
12. American Psychiatric Association. Diagnostic and statistical manual of mental disorders. 5th ed. Washington, DC: Author; 2013.
13. Marmar CR, Schlenger W, Henn-Haase C, Qian M, Purchia E, Li M, et al. Course of posttraumatic stress disorder 40 years after the Vietnam War: findings from the National Vietnam Veterans Longitudinal Study. JAMA Psychiatry. 2015;72:875–81. https://doi.org/10.1001/jamapsychiatry.2015.0803.

14. Bourne PG. Military psychiatry and the Vietnam experience. Am J Psychiatry. 1970;127:481–8. https://doi.org/10.1176/ajp.127.4.481.
15. Segal D, Burns T, Falk W, Silver M, Sharda B. The all-volunteer force in the 1970s. Soc Sci Q. 1998;79:390–411.
16. Haley RW, Kurt TL, Hom J. Is there a Gulf War syndrome? Searching for syndromes by factor analysis of symptoms. J Am Med Assoc. 1997;277:215–22. https://doi.org/10.1001/jama.277.3.215.
17. Kang HK, Natelson BH, Mahan CM, Lee KY, Murphy FM. Post-traumatic stress disorder and chronic fatigue syndrome-like illness among Gulf War veterans: a population-based survey of 30,000 veterans. Am J Epidemiol. 2003;157:141–8. https://doi.org/10.1093/aje/kwf187.
18. Stretch RH, Marlowe DH, Wright KM, Bliese PD, Knudson KH, Hoover CH. Post-traumatic stress disorder symptoms among Gulf War veterans. Mil Med. 1996;161:407–10. https://doi.org/10.1093/milmed/161.7.407.
19. U.S. Department of Veterans Affairs. Gulf War era veterans report: Pre-9/11. 2011. https://www.va.gov/vetdata/docs/SpecialReports/GW_Pre911_report.pdf.
20. Institute of Medicine. Returning home from Iraq and Afghanistan: preliminary assessment of readjustment needs of veterans, service members, and their families. Washington, DC: The National Academies Press; 2010.
21. Dursa EK, Reinhard MJ, Barth SK, Schneiderman AI. Prevalence of a positive screen for PTSD among OEF/OIF and OEF/IOF-era veterans in a large population-based cohort. J Trauma Stress. 2014;27:542–9. https://doi.org/10.1002/jts.21956.
22. Hoge CW, Riviere LA, Wilk JE, Herrell RK, Weathers FW. The prevalence of post-traumatic stress disorder (PTSD) in US combat soldiers: a head-to-head comparison of DSM-5 versus DSM-IV-TR symptom criteria with the PTSD Checklist. Lancet Psychiatry. 2014;1:269–77. https://doi.org/10.1016/S2215-0366(14)70235-4.
23. Ursano RJ, Kessler RC, Stein MB, Naifeh JA, Aliaga PA, Fullerton CS, et al. Suicide attempts in the US army during the wars in Afghanistan and Iraq, 2004 to 2009. JAMA Psychiatry. 2015;72:917–26. https://doi.org/10.1001/jamapsychiatry.2015.0987.
24. Greer N, Sayer N, Kramer M, Koeller E, Velasquez T. Prevalence and epidemiology of combat blast injuries from the military cohort 2001-2014. Washington, DC: Department of Veterans Affairs (US); 2016.
25. Lindquist LK, Love HC, Elbogen EB. Traumatic brain injury in Iraq and Afghanistan veterans: new results from a national random sample study. J Neuropsychiatry Clin Neurosci. 2017;29:254–9. https://doi.org/10.1176/appi.neuropsych.16050100.
26. Bray RM, Pemberton MR, Lane ME, Hourani LL, Mattiko MJ, Babeu LA. Substance use and mental health trends among U.S. military active duty personnel: key findings from the 2008 DOD health behavior survey. Mil Med. 2010;175:390–9. https://doi.org/10.7205/MILMED-D-09-00132.
27. Friedman MJ. Acknowledging the psychiatric cost of war. N Engl J Med. 2004;351:75–7. https://doi.org/10.1056/NEJMe048129.
28. Kessler RC, Sonnega A, Bromet E, Hughes M, Nelson CB. Posttraumatic stress disorder in the National Comorbidity Survey. Arch Gen Psychiatry. 1995;52:1048–60. https://doi.org/10.1001/archpsyc.1995.03950240066012.
29. Warner CH, Appenzeller GN, Grieger T, Belenkiy J, Breitbach J, Parker J, et al. Importance of anonymity to encourage honest reporting in mental health screening after combat deployment. Arch Gen Psychiatry. 2011;68:1065–71. https://doi.org/10.1001/archgenpsychiatry.2011.112.
30. Blosnich JR, Dichter ME, Cerulli C, Batten SV, Bossarte RM. Disparities in adverse childhood experiences among individuals with a history of military service. J Am Med Assoc Psychiatry. 2014;71:1041–8. https://doi.org/10.1001/jamapsychiatry.2014.724.
31. Brewin CR, Andrews B, Valentine JD. Meta-analysis of risk factors for posttraumatic stress disorder in trauma-exposed adults. J Consult Clin Psychol. 2000;68:748–66. https://doi.org/10.1037/0022-006X.68.5.748.
32. Duncan LE, Cooper BN, Shen H. Robust findings from 25 years of PTSD genetics research. Curr Psychiatry Rep. 2018;20:115. https://doi.org/10.1007/s11920-018-0980-1.

33. Schnurr PP, Lunney CA, Sengupta A. Risk factors for the development versus maintenance of posttraumatic stress disorder. J Trauma Stress. 2004;17:85–95. https://doi.org/10.1023/B:JOTS.0000022614.21794.f4.
34. Crum-Cianflone NF, Jacobson I. Gender differences of postdeployment post-traumatic stress disorder among service members and veterans of the Iraq and Afghanistan conflicts. Epidemiol Rev. 2014;36:5–18. https://doi.org/10.1093/epirev/mxt005.
35. Vogt D, Smith B, Elwy R, Martin J, Schultz M, Drainoni M-L, Eisen S. Predeployment, deployment, and postdeployment risk factors for posttraumatic stress symptomatology in female and male OEF/OIF veterans. J Abnorm Psychol. 2011;120:819–31. https://doi.org/10.1037/a0024457.
36. Xue C, Ge Y, Tang B, Liu Y, Kang P, Wang M, Zhang L. A meta-analysis of risk factors for combat-related PTSD among military personnel and veterans. Public Libr Sci One. 2015;10(3):e0120270. https://doi.org/10.1371/journal.pone.0120270.
37. Koenen KC, Stellman JM, Stellman SD, Sommer JF. Risk factors for course of posttraumatic stress disorder among Vietnam veterans: a 14-year follow-up of American Legionnaires. J Consult Clin Psychol. 2003;71:980–6. https://doi.org/10.1037/0022-006X.71.6.980.
38. Hoge EA, Austin ED, Pollack MH. Resilience: research evidence and conceptual considerations for posttraumatic stress disorder. Depress Anxiety. 2007;24:139–52. https://doi.org/10.1002/da.20175.
39. Pompili M, Sher L, Serafini G, Forte A, Innamorati M, Dominici G, et al. Posttraumatic stress disorder and suicide risk among veterans: a literature review. J Nerv Ment Dis. 2013;201:802–12. https://doi.org/10.1097/NMD.0b013e3182a21458.
40. Yaffe K, Vittinghoff E, Lindquist K, Barnes D, Covinsky KE, Neylan T, et al. Posttraumatic stress disorder and risk of dementia among US veterans. Arch Gen Psychiatry. 2010;67:608–13. https://doi.org/10.1001/archgenpsychiatry.2010.61.
41. El-Gabalawy R, Blaney C, Tsai J, Sumner JA, Pietrzak RH. Physical health conditions associated with full and subthreshold PTSD in U.S. military veterans: results from the National Health and Resilience in Veterans Study. J Affect Disord. 2018;227:849–53. https://doi.org/10.1016/j.jad.2017.11.058.
42. Kubzansky LD, Bordelois P, Jun HJ, Roberts AL, Cerda M, Bluestone N, Koenen KC. The weight of traumatic stress: a prospective study of posttraumatic stress disorder symptoms and weight status in women. JAMA Psychiatry. 2014;71:44–51. https://doi.org/10.1001/jamapsychiatry.2013.2798.
43. World Health Organization. Constitution of the World Health Organization. Geneva: World Health Organization; 1948.
44. Gladis MM, Gosch EA, Dishuk NM, Crits-Christoph P. Quality of life: expanding the scope of clinical significance. J Consult Clin Psychol. 1999;67:320–31. https://doi.org/10.1037/0022-006X.67.3.320.
45. Schnurr PP, Lunney CA, Bovin MJ, Marx BP. Posttraumatic stress disorder and quality of life: extension of findings to veterans of the wars in Iraq and Afghanistan. Clin Psychol Rev. 2009;29:727–35. https://doi.org/10.1016/j.cpr.2009.08.006.
46. Olatunji BO, Cisler JM, Tolin DF. Quality of life in the anxiety disorders: a meta-analytic review. Clin Psychol Rev. 2007;27:572–81. https://doi.org/10.1016/j.cpr.2007.01.015.
47. Savoca E, Rosenheck R. The civilian labor market experiences of Vietnam-era veterans: the influence of psychiatric disorders. J Ment Health Policy Econ. 2000;3:199–207. https://doi.org/10.1002/mhp.102.
48. Kehle SM, Reddy MK, Ferrier-Auerbach AG, Erbes CR, Arbisi PA, Polusny MA. Psychiatric diagnoses, comorbidity, and functioning in national guard troops deployed to Iraq. J Psychiatr Res. 2011;45:126–32. https://doi.org/10.1016/j.jpsychires.2010.05.013.
49. Norman SB, Stein MB, Davidson JR. Profiling posttraumatic functional impairment. J Nerv Ment Dis. 2007;195:48–53. https://doi.org/10.1097/01.nmd.0000252135.25114.02.
50. Vogt D, Smith BN, Fox AB, Amoroso T, Taverna E, Schnurr PP. Consequences of PTSD for the work and family quality of life of female and male U.S. Afghanistan and Iraq War

veterans. Soc Psychiatry Psychiatr Epidemiol. 2017;52:341–52. https://doi.org/10.1007/s00127-016-1321-5.

51. Lapierre CB, Schwegler AF, Labauve BJ. Posttraumatic stress and depression symptoms in soldiers returning from combat operations in Iraq and Afghanistan. J Trauma Stress. 2007;20:933–43. https://doi.org/10.1002/jts.20278.
52. Vasterling JJ, Schumm J, Proctor SP, Gentry E, King DW, King LA. Posttraumatic stress disorder and health functioning in a non-treatment-seeking sample of Iraq War veterans: a prospective analysis. J Rehabil Res Dev. 2008;45:347–58. https://doi.org/10.1682/JRRD.2007.05.0077.
53. Schnurr PP, Lunney CA. Work-related quality of life and posttraumatic stress disorder symptoms among female veterans. Womens Health Issues. 2011;21:S169–75. https://doi.org/10.1016/j.whi.2011.04.013.
54. Fontana A, Rosenheck R. Treatment-seeking veterans of Iraq and Afghanistan: comparison with veterans of previous wars. J Nerv Ment Dis. 2008;196:513–21. https://doi.org/10.1097/NMD.0b013e31817cf6e6.
55. Schnurr PP, Lunney CA. Symptom benchmarks of improved quality of life in PTSD. Depress Anxiety. 2016;33:247–55.
56. Weathers FW, Keane TM, Foa EB. Assessment and diagnosis of adults. In: Foa EB, Keane TM, Friedman MJ, Cohen JA, editors. Effective treatments for PTSD: practice guidelines from The International Society for Traumatic Stress Studies. 2nd ed. New York, NY: Guilford Press; 2009. p. 23–61.
57. Weathers FW, Litz BT, Keane TM, Palmieri PA, Marx BP, Schnurr PP. The life events checklist for DSM-5 (LEC-5). Boston, MA: National Center for PTSD; 2013. www.ptsd.va.gov.
58. Prins A, Bovin MJ, Smolenski DJ, Marx BP, Kimerling R, Jenkins-Guarnieri MA, et al. The Primary Care PTSD screen for DSM-5 (PC-PTSD-5): development and evaluation within a veteran primary care sample. J Gen Intern Med. 2016;31:1206–11. https://doi.org/10.1007/s11606-016-3703-5.
59. Weathers FW, Litz BT, Keane TM, Palmieri PA, Marx BP, Schnurr PP. The PTSD checklist for DSM-5 (PCL-5). Boston, MA: National Center for PTSD; 2013. www.ptsd.va.gov.
60. Bovin MJ, Marx BP, Weathers FW, Gallagher MW, Rodriguez P, Schnurr PP, Keane TM. Psychometric properties of the PTSD Checklist for Diagnostic and Statistical Manual of Mental Disorders-Fifth Edition (PCL-5) in veterans. Psychol Assess. 2016;28:1379–91. https://doi.org/10.1037/pas0000254.
61. Weathers FW, Blake DD, Schnurr PP, Kaloupek DG, Marx BP, Keane TM. The clinician-administered PTSD Scale for DSM-5 (CAPS-5). 2013. www.ptsd.va.gov.
62. Weathers FW, Bovin MJ, Lee DJ, Sloan DM, Schnurr PP, Kaloupek DG, et al. The Clinician-Administered PTSD Scale for DSM-5 (CAPS-5): development and initial psychometric evaluation in military veterans. Psychol Assess. 2018;30:383–95. https://doi.org/10.1037/pas0000486.
63. Watts BV, Schnurr PP, Mayo L, Young-Xu Y, Weeks WB, Friedman MJ. Meta-analysis of the efficacy of treatments for posttraumatic stress disorder. J Clin Psychiatry. 2013;74:e541–50. https://doi.org/10.4088/JCP.12r08225.
64. Lee D, Schnitzlein C, Wolf J, Vythilingam M, Rasmusson A, Hoge C. Psychotherapy versus pharmocotherapy for posttraumatic stress disorder: systemic review and meta-analyses to determine first-line treatments. Depress Anxiety. 2016;33:792–806. https://doi.org/10.1002/da.22511.
65. Alvarez J, McLean C, Harris A, Rosen C, Ruzek J, Kimerling R. The comparative effectiveness of Cognitive Processing Therapy for male veterans treated in a VHA Posttraumatic Stress Disorder Residential Rehabilitation Program. J Consult Clin Psychol. 2011;79:590–9. https://doi.org/10.1037/a0024466.
66. Eftekhari A, Ruzek J, Crowley J, Rosen C, Greenbaum M, Karlin B. Effectiveness of national implementation of prolonged exposure therapy in Veterans Affairs care. JAMA Psychiatry. 2013;70:949–55. https://doi.org/10.1001/jamapsychiatry.2013.36.
67. Forbes D, Lloyd D, Nixon RD, Elliott P, Varker T, Perry D, et al. A multisite randomized controlled effectiveness trial of Cognitive Processing Therapy for military-related

posttraumatic stress disorder. J Anxiety Disord. 2012;26:442–52. https://doi.org/10.1016/j.janxdis.2012.01.006.
68. Kaysen D, Schumm J, Pedersen ER, Seim RW, Bedard-Gilligan M, Chard K. Cognitive Processing Therapy for veterans with comorbid PTSD and alcohol use disorders. Addict Behav. 2014;39:420–7. https://doi.org/10.1016/j.addbeh.2013.08.016.
69. Chard K, Schumm J, Owens G, Cottingham S. A comparison of OEF and OIF veterans and Vietnam veterans receiving Cognitive Processing Therapy. J Trauma Stress. 2010;23:25–32. https://doi.org/10.1002/jts.20500.
70. Kehle-Forbes S, Meis L, Spoont M, Polusny M. Treatment initiation and dropout from prolonged exposure and Cognitive Processing Therapy in a VA Outpatient Clinic. Psychol Trauma Theory Res Pract Policy. 2016;8:107–14. https://doi.org/10.1037/tra0000065.
71. Meis LA, Noorbaloochi S, Hagel Campbell EM, Erbes CR, Polusny MA, Velasquez TL, et al. Sticking it out in trauma-focused treatment for PTSD: it takes a village. J Consult Clin Psychol. 2019;87:246–56. https://doi.org/10.1037/ccp0000386.
72. Fernandez E, Salem D, Swift J, Ramtahal N. Meta-analysis of dropout from cognitive behavioral therapy: magnitude, timing, and moderators. J Consult Clin Psychol. 2015;83:1108–22. https://doi.org/10.1037/ccp0000044.
73. Schnurr PP, Chard KM, Ruzek JI, Chow BK, Shih M-C, Resick PA, et al. Design of VA Cooperative Study #591: CERV-PTSD, comparative effectiveness research in veterans with PTSD. Contemp Clin Trials. 2015;41:75–84. https://doi.org/10.1016/j.cct.2014.11.017.
74. Stirman SW, Gamarra J, Bartlett B, Calloway A, Gutner C. Empirical examinations of modifications and adaptations to evidence-based psychotherapies: methodologies, impact, and future directions. Clin Psychol Sci Pract. 2017;24:396–420. https://doi.org/10.1111/cpsp.12218.
75. Foa EB, McLean CP, Zang Y, Rosenfield D, Yadin E, Yarvis JS, et al. Effect of Prolonged Exposure Therapy delivered over 2 weeks vs 8 weeks vs Present-Centered Therapy on PTSD symptom severity in military personnel: a randomized clinical trial. JAMA. 2018;319:354–64. https://doi.org/10.1001/jama.2017.21242.
76. Sloan DM, Marx BP, Lee DJ, Resick PA. A brief exposure-based treatment vs Cognitive Processing Therapy for posttraumatic stress disorder: a randomized noninferiority trial. JAMA Psychiatry. 2018;75:233–9. https://doi.org/10.1001/jamapsychiatry.2017.4249.
77. U.S. Department of Veterans Affairs & U.S. Department of Defense (VA/DoD). VA/DoD clinical practice guideline for the management of posttraumatic stress disorder and acute stress disorder. 2017. https://www.healthquality.va.gov/guidelines/MH/PTSD/VADoDPTSDCPGFinal.pdf.
78. Steenkamp MM, Litz BT, Hoge CW, Marmar CR. Psychotherapy for military-related PTSD: a review of randomized clinical trials. J Am Med Assoc. 2015;314:489–500. https://doi.org/10.1001/jama.2015.8370.
79. American Psychiatric Association. Clinical practice guideline for the treatment of the posttraumatic stress disorder (PTSD) in adults. 2017. https://www.apa.org/ptsd-guideline/ptsd.pdf.
80. International Society for Traumatic Stress Studies. Posttraumatic stress disorder prevention and treatment guidelines: methodology and recommendations. 2019. http://www.istss.org/getattachment/Treating-Trauma/New-ISTSS-Prevention-and-Treatment-Guidelines/ISTSS_PreventionTreatmentGuidelines_FNL-March-19-2019.pdf.aspx.
81. Resick PA, Wachen JS, Dondanville KA, Pruiksma KE, Yarvis JS, Peterson AL, et al. Effect of group vs individual Cognitive Processing Therapy in active-duty military seeking treatment for posttraumatic stress disorder: a randomized clinical trial. JAMA Psychiatry. 2017;74:28–36. https://doi.org/10.1001/jamapsychiatry.2016.2729.
82. Raskind MA, Peskind ER, Chow B, Harris C, Davis-Karim A, Holmes HA, et al. Trial of prazosin for post-traumatic stress disorder in military veterans. N Engl J Med. 2018;378:507–17. https://doi.org/10.1056/NEJMoa1507598.
83. Elwyn G, Frosch D, Thomson R, Joseph-Williams N, Lloyd A, Kinnersley P, et al. Shared decision making: a model for clinical practice. J Gen Intern Med. 2012;27:1361–7. https://doi.org/10.1007/s11606-012-2077-6.

84. Langer DA, Mooney TK, Wills CE. Shared decision-making for treatment planning in mental health care: theory, evidence, and tools. Oxford Handbooks Online. 2015. https://www.oxfordhandbooks.com/view/10.1093/oxfordhb/9780199935291.001.0001/oxfordhb-9780199935291-e-7.
85. National Center for PTSD. National Center for PTSD treatment decision aid: the choice is yours. 2019. https://www.ptsd.va.gov/apps/decisionaid/.
86. Meyer EG, Writer BW, Brim W. The importance of military cultural competence. Curr Psychiatry Rep. 2016;18:26. https://doi.org/10.1007/s11920-016-0662-9.
87. Lapp KG, Bosworth HB, Strauss JL, Stechuchak KM, Horner RD, Calhoun PS, et al. Lifetime sexual and physical victimization among male veterans with combat-related post-traumatic stress disorder. Mil Med. 2005;170:787–90. https://doi.org/10.7205/MILMED.170.9.787.
88. Maguen S, Turcotte DM, Peterson AL, Dremsa TL, Garb HN, McNally RJ, Litz BT. Description of risk and resilience factors among military medical personnel before deployment to Iraq. Mil Med. 2008;173:1–9. https://doi.org/10.7205/MILMED.173.1.1.

Traumatic Brain Injury 13

Rachel Sayko Adams, Diana P. Brostow, and Lisa A. Brenner

Vignette

Sam is a 37-year old Veteran who served in the Army, and was deployed to Iraq three times. While overseas, he was exposed to multiple blasts, one of which was particularly memorable. In this incident, Sam was a passenger in a High Mobility Multipurpose Wheeled Vehicle (HMMWV; Humvee) that drove over an improvised

---

R. S. Adams (✉)
VHA Rocky Mountain Mental Illness Research Education and Clinical Center, Aurora, CO, USA

Department of Health Law, Policy and Management, Boston University School of Public Health, Boston, MA, USA
e-mail: adamsr@bu.edu

D. P. Brostow
VHA Rocky Mountain Mental Illness Research Education and Clinical Center, Aurora, CO, USA

Department of Physical Medicine and Rehabilitation, University of Colorado Anschutz Medical Campus, Aurora, CO, USA

Department of Psychiatry, University of Colorado Anschutz Medical Campus, Aurora, CO, USA
e-mail: Dianna.brostow@va.gov

L. A. Brenner
VHA Rocky Mountain Mental Illness Research Education and Clinical Center, Aurora, CO, USA

Department of Physical Medicine and Rehabilitation, University of Colorado Anschutz Medical Campus, Aurora, CO, USA

Department of Psychiatry, University of Colorado Anschutz Medical Campus, Aurora, CO, USA

Department of Neurology, University of Colorado Anschutz Medical Campus, Aurora, CO, USA
e-mail: Lisa.brenner@va.gov

C. H. Warner, C. A. Castro (eds.), *Veteran and Military Mental Health*,
https://doi.org/10.1007/978-3-031-18009-5_13

explosive device (IED). Both the Humvee driver and a friend of Sam's were killed. His last memory prior to the explosion was driving down the road. He then recalled "waking up" and seeing his friend "slumped over." Soldiers from other vehicles in the convoy were already surrounding the damaged Humvee to assist. Sam recalled feeling "out of it" for several days after the incident: "I had the worst headache of my life." As the TBI was sustained early in the conflicts in Iraq, prior to the recognition that some individuals were incurring long-term effects from blast injuries, Sam proceeded in completing his duties without taking a break. "Other guys were way more hurt than I was. My buddy was killed." During his military service, Sam continued to have headaches, but he always pushed through. At times, he had trouble thinking as quickly as he was used to, but the structure of the military and support of his buddies were helpful, and he was able to compensate. After his last deployment, he did not apply for a military disability rating or associated benefits related to his TBI. Once home, Sam began having post traumatic symptoms (e.g., hypervigilance, nightmares). The chronic headaches continued and Sam began drinking to dull the pain. After receiving a DUI, he started substance use treatment at a local VA. He is also trying to find the right doctor to help him with his headache pain, as well as assistance with submitting a claim for veterans affairs (VA) service connection.

Introduction

Traumatic brain injury (TBI) is a common neurological condition, defined as a disruption to brain functioning caused by a blow, bump, jolt to the head, or a penetrating head injury [1]. The damage caused by the primary insult is exacerbated by the secondary injury (e.g., metabolic changes, cranial bleeding, swelling) [2]. Injury severity is graded as mild, moderate, or severe according to a number of factors, including duration of loss of consciousness, length of amnesia, level of responsiveness, and/or structural imaging results [3]. Military members, including those who have deployed in Operation Enduring Freedom, Operation Iraqi Freedom and/or Operation New Dawn (OEF/OIF/OND), have faced an increased risk for experiencing a TBI compared to civilian populations [4].

Mild TBI (mTBI), herein considered synonymous with concussion, is commonly referred to as one of the signature injuries of the military conflicts in Afghanistan and Iraq [5]. This is in part related to the use of improvised explosive devices (IED), resulting in blast-related injuries [6]. In addition, advancements in military body armor, battlefield medical care, and medical evacuations have improved survival rates for military members, as compared to those in previous conflicts, where brain injuries from blasts, flying debris, or other physical shocks were more likely to be fatal [7–9]. While these improvements in military medicine have reduced mortality, they have also dramatically increased the number of military members returning home from deployment with combat-related injuries, primarily TBI, musculoskeletal injuries, chronic pain, and mental health problems, collectively referred to as *polytrauma* [10–12].

In this chapter, the authors will discuss the epidemiology and etiology of TBI and associated comorbidities among military members and Veterans, and will describe challenges and considerations for treatment. Instructive vignettes will be used to outline evidence-based best practices for TBI and mental health comorbidities, as well as the management of symptoms.

Vignette

Carlos is a 25-year old Army Veteran who served in Afghanistan as a military bomb technician. His work while overseas was primarily comprised of improvised explosive device disposal (IEDD). Sometimes he and his teammates would be called in after IEDs had partially exploded. The scenes could be "messy." After returning home from deployment, Carlos was involved a motor vehicle accident in which he was hit head-on by a drunk driver at 60 miles per hour. Carlos remembers leaving his house that day and then "waking up" 10 days later in the hospital. He sustained a severe TBI, as well as a broken pelvis and left arm. Sequelae associated with the TBI included cognitive impairments, including problems with attention, memory, and problem-solving. After a prolonged period of inpatient rehabilitation, he was discharged from the military on Permanent Disability Retirement. His injuries were rated as 100% Service Connected by the VA. Returning home, he found himself without a job or a support system. Carlos became increasingly depressed and at times thought about ending his own life with a gun he had purchased prior to being injured. He is seeing a counselor at his local VA in the Mental Health Community-Based Outpatient Clinic (CBOC). As he lives in a rural community, the closest TBI specialty team is over 150 miles from his home. As no local TBI community providers were identified, Carlos's family drives him to see the polytrauma team at the Regional VA Medical Center.

Etiology and Epidemiology

Since 2000, the Defense and Veterans Brain Injury Center (DVBIC) has been maintaining a database to record incident TBI diagnoses among military members. Since then, nearly 384,000 incident TBI cases have been documented among military members [13, 14]. Approximately 82% of all TBI cases recorded by DVBIC have been mTBIs [13, 14]. Nearly 10% of cases were classified as moderate; characterized by a confused state lasting more than 24 hours, a longer duration of loss of consciousness (LOC), and the presence of posttraumatic amnesia (PTA—see Table 13.1). Over 1% (approximately 4000 cases) were classified as severe TBI, in which LOC, disorientation, and PTA extend for a longer period of time. 1.4% (approximately 5200 cases) were classified as penetrating TBI, in which there was an open head injury penetrating through the scalp, skull, and outer layer of the meninges, and the remaining 5.4% of cases had incomplete information to determine severity, and were deemed "not classifiable" [13, 14].

Table 13.1 TBI severity classification

Criteria	Mild	Moderate	Severe
Structural imaging	Normal	Normal or abnormal	Normal or abnormal
Alteration of consciousness/mental state (AOC)[a]	Up to 24 h	>24 h. Severity based on other criteria	>24 h. Severity based on other criteria
Loss of consciousness (LOC)	0–30 min	>30 min and <24 h	>24 h
Posttraumatic amnesia (PTA)	0–24 h	>24 h and < 7 days	>7 days
Glasgow coma scale (GCS) (best available score in first 24 h)	13–15	9–12	<9

Table adapted from Veterans Affairs/Department of Defense Clinical Practice Guideline for the Management of Concussion-mTBI [3]

[a] AOC must be immediately following the injury event. Symptoms may include: feeling dazed, confusion, difficulty thinking clearly or responding appropriately, and being unable to describe events immediately before or after the injury event

It is crucial to bear in mind that the above stated incidence rates alone do not adequately convey the disease burden of TBI in military and Veteran populations. According to alternate sources, TBI prevalence estimates among military members and Veterans of the Afghanistan/Iraq conflicts range from 7% to 23% [15, 16]. This wide degree of variation is due to several factors. Reporting injuries sustained during deployment can be logistically difficult, more so when an injury is "invisible" like a TBI. At times, reporting may be perceived as being discouraged, as stoicism and self-reliance are highly valued among those in the military. This was especially true during the earlier years of the Afghanistan/Iraq conflicts, before awareness grew regarding the long-term effects of TBI [17, 18]. Additionally, there has been a lack of consistency in both the measures used to screen for TBI [15, 16, 19] and the clinical symptom profiles used to diagnose TBI (see Sequelae and Symptoms below). Further, reliance on self-report and/or witness reports in a combat setting may have been particularly problematic when attempting to estimate the severity of a given injury [4].

Blast-related injuries, including blasts co-occurring with blunt trauma, are the most common mechanism of TBI during the Afghanistan/Iraq conflicts, stemming largely from the pervasive use of IEDs [20]. Contrary to public perception, however, the vast majority of incident TBI diagnoses among military members since 2000 have occurred in *non*-combat settings where the U.S. military maintains bases (e.g., Western Europe, Japan) or at a home station in the U.S. The leading mechanisms of non-combat related TBI are similar to those observed in civilian populations [21, 22], namely accidents (e.g., motor vehicle crashes, falls, strikes by/against objects), intentional assaults (e.g., fights), and sports or other recreational activities [23]. Additional risk factors for TBIs during non-combat periods specific to military culture include physically demanding operational and training activities, high rates of risky behaviors (e.g., binge drinking), and a largely male, younger (aged 18–24) population [24, 25].

Little is known about the lifetime history of TBI among military members and Veterans beyond what is captured by the Department of Defense (DoD) and the Department of Veterans Affairs (VA), which predominantly screen for TBIs that occurred during the Afghanistan/Iraq conflicts (DoD and VA). One recent study used the Ohio State University TBI Identification Method [26], a structured, validated clinical interview which was used to establish the lifetime history of TBI among soldiers following return from an Afghanistan/Iraq deployment [27]. Over half of soldiers who did not report a TBI on their most recent deployment *did* report at least one prior TBI that occurred either during military service or prior to military service, and the median number of lifetime TBIs was 2 [27]. These data suggest that only assessing for recent deployment-acquired TBIs does not capture the full lifetime burden of TBI.

Sequelae and Symptoms

Most individuals with one mTBI report returning to baseline functioning within 1 year, however, as many as 15%, report experiencing persistent post-concussive symptoms (PCS) [28, 29]. Less is known about recovery after multiple mTBIs, particularly among those with co-occurring mental health conditions. This will be discussed further below. While the definition of persistent PCS has varied, it is commonly accepted that it includes specific symptoms (usually three or more; see Table 13.2) that occur shortly after the TBI, which last at least 3 months post-injury, and which present functional challenges for those living with such injuries [31].

Psychological Sequelae

It is important to note that mTBIs that occur in combat settings, particularly blast-related mTBIs, may have distinct features that complicate recovery. Such exposures may result in sensory and physical impairments [6, 25]. Recovery may also be further complicated by the presence of mental health comorbidities such as posttraumatic stress disorder (PTSD), depression, anxiety, substance use problems, and chronic pain [30, 32–34]. A particular challenge associated with diagnosing and treating combat-related mTBI is that many of the signs and symptoms associated with such injuries overlap with those frequently associated with PTSD (e.g., trouble concentrating, insomnia, irritability) [35]. While such diagnostic and treatment

Table 13.2 Common symptoms of post-concussion syndrome

Physical symptoms	Cognitive symptoms	Behavior/emotional symptoms
Headache, dizziness, imbalance, nausea, incoordination, vomiting, blurred vision, sensitivity to light, hearing difficulties/loss, tinnitus, sensitivity to noise, numbness, tingling	Problems with attention, concentration, memory, speed of processing, judgment, executive control	Depression, anxiety, posttraumatic stress disorder, agitation, irritability, impulsivity, aggression, fatigue, insomnia

Table adapted from [3, 30, 31]

challenges have been a focus of research and practice following the most recent conflicts, similar co-morbidities were surely present among those who served in previous conflicts (e.g., "shell shock" in World War I) [36].

Moderate to Severe TBI Symptoms and Psychological Sequelae

While less common than mTBI, moderate and severe TBIs are often associated with more significant post-injury sequelae. In addition to the physical, cognitive, and psychological impairments associated with mTBI, military members and Veterans with moderate and severe TBIs also contend with additional, often lifelong conditions that can adversely impact their reintegration into civilian life. Moreover, it is estimated that only approximately 20% of individuals with a moderate or severe TBI report a return to baseline functioning [37], and it can take years (two or more) to experience improvements in symptoms and function [38].

Currently, there are no methods for predicting whether a Veteran with moderate or severe TBI will fully recover functional independence [39]. Individual predictors of worse functional outcomes, however, include increasing age [39], lower educational attainment [40], minority race [41, 42], and a TBI in which the injury resulted in penetration of the skull [43]. It is unclear whether sex influences moderate or severe TBI outcomes, with evidence both for and against female sex as a protective factor [39, 44].

Among many, much of the symptom burden in Veterans with moderate or severe TBI, and therefore most treatment efforts, relate to cognitive dysfunction. Specifically, moderate or severe TBI can affect both complex processes such as attention, judgment, and insight, as well as simpler processes, such as completing daily tasks or keeping track of appointments [38]. Neurocognitive deficits may also manifest as behavioral changes, most notably, disinhibition, impulsivity, and verbal or physical aggression, all of which can interfere with rehabilitation care [45], psychosocial functioning, and community reintegration. Estimates vary between populations, but up to a third of patients with a moderate or severe TBI may exhibit such significant behavioral changes [46, 47].

In the long term, up to 20% of moderate or severe TBI survivors will experience seizures related to posttraumatic epilepsy [48], which may manifest early in the recovery process, or years post-injury [49]. Additionally, emerging evidence suggest that patients with moderate or severe TBI experience increased risk of developing dementia in later life compared to people without such a TBI [50]. There is also evidence to suggest that patients with a hereditary predisposition to Alzheimer's disease experience poorer functional outcomes after a TBI [51].

Screening in the DoD and VA

Routine post-deployment screening for mTBI began in 2008 with the implementation of the DoD's updated post-deployment health surveillance program. The program for the first time included screening for TBI using a 4-item questionnaire modified from the Brief Traumatic Brain Injury Screen [17], and assessed for TBI that occurred on the *most recent deployment* only. Generally, those who sustained more severe injuries were medically evacuated, and therefore did not participate in post-deployment screening (such injuries were therefore likely identified in the context of medical care received). A positive screen for possible TBI is defined as report of: (1) an injury event (e.g., blast, motor vehicle accident) followed by (2) an alteration of consciousness or LOC. Positive screens suggest that further clinical evaluation may be indicated. In 2007, the Veterans Health Administration (VHA) also implemented a systematic screening program for Veterans who had deployed to the Afghanistan/Iraq conflicts, and included the same 4-item questionnaire. Since then, upon entrance to the VHA, Veterans who deployed in the Afghanistan/Iraq conflicts are screened for possible TBI that occurred *during any OEF/OIF/OND deployment.* Veteran's who reported immediate and ongoing post-concussive symptoms following the injury event and AOC/LOC met criteria for a positive screen, which the VHA triggers further clinical evaluation.

Screening and Evaluation of Lifetime History of TBI

Because the DoD and the VA TBI screening instruments only assess for TBIs that occurred during an OEF/OIF/OND deployment, military members or Veterans presenting for care in a civilian setting may have a history of TBI that was not previously documented in the DoD or VA or recognized by the individual. The Ohio State University Traumatic Brain Injury Identification Method (OSU TBI-ID) is structured clinical procedure for eliciting a person's lifetime history of TBI in a 3–5 min structured interview [26, 52]. The OSU TBI-ID is based on Centers for Disease Control and Prevention recommendations for TBI surveillance, uses validated injury recall methods, and captures information about presence, severity (e.g., worst), nature of alteration of loss of consciousness, and age of injuries [26, 52, 53]. If clinicians do not have the training or time to do a full evaluation for lifetime history of TBI with the OSU TBI-ID, the OSU TBI-ID—Short Form Screening Items could be used to assess for probable history of lifetime TBI relatively quickly. The first five questions of the OSU TBI-ID can be used to assess whether a patient has experienced a lifetime TBI (see Table 13.3), and if it occurred in a particular setting (e.g., military service, motor vehicle accident, etc.) [54]. While the fifth item specifically screens for military-related TBIs and mentions blasts/explosions, it does not solicit information specific to hitting one's head on tank doors or other common types of military-specific injuries. An affirmative response to any of the five questions should prompt further assessment using the full OSU TBI-ID [26].

The TBI-4 was developed as a brief screening based on the OSU-TBI-ID for inclusion in the mental health assessment process for Veterans entering the VHA [55]. On the TBI-4, a "yes" response to any of the questions is indicative of a possible TBI history (see Table 13.4). A positive response to question 2 is a more reliable indicator of possible TBI. If an individual answers "no" to all of the TBI-4 questions, a comprehensive assessment is likely not warranted, however, this does not mean that a TBI has not occurred, nor that full recovery has taken place.

Table 13.3 OSU TBI-ID short form screening items

1. In your lifetime, have you ever been hospitalized or treated in an emergency room following an injury to your head or neck? Think about any childhood injuries you remember or were told about.	Y/N
2. In your lifetime, have you ever injured your head or neck in a car accident or from crashing some other moving vehicle like a bicycle, motorcycle, or ATV?	Y/N
3. In your lifetime, have you ever injured your head or neck in a fall or from being hit by something (for example, falling from a bike or horse, rollerblading, falling on ice, being hit by a rock?) Have you ever injured your head or neck playing sports or on the playground?	Y/N
4. In your lifetime, have you ever injured your head or neck in a fight, from being hit by someone, or from being shaken violently? Have you ever been shot in the head?	Y/N
5. In your lifetime, have you ever been nearby when an explosion or a blast occurred? If you served in the military, think about any combat-or training-related incidents.	Y/N

Table 13.4 TBI-4 screening items

1. Have you ever been hospitalized or treated in an emergency room following a head or neck injury?	Y/N
2. Have you ever been knocked out or unconscious following an accident or injury?	Y/N
3. Have you ever injured your head or neck in a car accident or from some other moving vehicle accident?	Y/N
4. Have you ever injured your head or neck in a fight or fall?	Y/N

In the first vignette, Sam experienced a LOC due to the IED blast. Post-exposure he also noted feeling "out of it." His blast injury would be classified as an mTBI using the severity classification presented in Table 13.1. Sam's injury is typical of that experienced by deployed military members who served during the earlier years of combat operations in Afghanistan and Iraq. This was before the DoD and VA implemented policies and programs to improve awareness, diagnosis, treatment, and research, as well as to attempt to reduce stigma [56]. Given that he did not undergo screening or treatment for TBI during his military service, Sam's TBI would have gone undetected until he was evaluated by a primary care physician or mental health care provider in a non-military setting. This may not have happened for years post-injury. Additionally, although he was obtaining care for his substance use disorder in the VA, he was seeking care for his TBI-related headaches from his non-VA primary care provider, potentially contributing to less integrated and coordinated care. Accurate assessment of his symptoms (e.g., cognitive complaints) were also complicated by pain medications which impacted his ability to concentrate. Veterans with TBI and/or pain have been more likely to receive prescription opioids [57, 58], and thus, the lack of coordinated care may increase risk of negative opioid-related outcomes. Further, substance use treatment practices may require modifications to address the cognitive and neurobehavioral sequelae of TBI [59–61], yet it remains unclear how comfortable or knowledgeable substance use providers are regarding assessing for or providing accommodations for treating patients with a history of TBI.

For Carlos in the second vignette, his severe TBI diagnosis was well documented in his VA health record, yet his ability to access VA polytrauma transitional rehabilitation services was logistically difficult because he lived so far away from one of the VA polytrauma system of care locations [62]. Carlos has been accessing local VA services for depression treatment. In providing depression care, his provider should consider modifications to evidence-based psychotherapies that may be required to facilitate treatment uptake (see Accommodating the Symptoms of TBI [63]). Moreover, there is some evidence to suggest that those with moderate to severe TBI also benefit from antidepressants [64]. His providers should also consider that TBI has been associated with elevated risk for death by suicide among Veterans, and of further concern, moderate/severe TBI is associated with an increased risk of death by firearm among decedents [65]. Carlos's therapist should incorporate conversations about lethal means safety since Carlos owns a firearm, has expertise using a firearm from military training, and has already struggled with suicidal thoughts since his TBI injury (see https://www.mirecc.va.gov/lethalmeanssafety/—[66]).

Evaluation of Sequelae and Function

Once TBI history and severity have been established, a thorough evaluation of sequelae, as well as functioning is recommended. See Table 13.5 for a selection of instruments that can be used to augment standard clinical interviews. Many of the measures are highlighted in the VA/DoD Clinical Practice Guidelines for the Management of Concussion–mild Traumatic Brain Injury and co-occurring conditions [3]. For further information about comorbidities of mTBI see the chapter by Brenner et al. [28].

Even though Sam in the first vignette is receiving treatment for his unhealthy alcohol use, his history of witnessing his friend's death, subsequent minimization of this trauma ("Other guys were way more hurt than I was"), and ensuing nightmares and hypervigilance all indicate he should be evaluated for PTSD (PCL-5). Additionally, Sam's report that he has "trouble thinking as quickly as he used to" and his frequent headaches warrant an assessment of PCS, perhaps using the NIS. Lastly, his service history suggests that he was able to draw upon a strong social support system while deployed, but that he may not have a supportive social network now that he is reintegrating into civilian life. Evaluation of his psychosocial quality of life is also likely warranted (WHOQOL-BREF).

After deployment, Carlos from the second vignette began to experience depression and suicidal ideation, and reported having purchased a firearm. The severe TBI he sustained in the motor vehicle accident further complicated his situation, and he continues to experience cognitive difficulties after completing rehabilitation. Like Sam in Vignette #1, Carlos would benefit from an assessment of his psychological symptoms, depression (PHQ-9), and overall quality of life (WHOQOL-BREF). Social isolation and unemployment are additional stressors for Carlos, and it is also likely that he has some persistent post-traumatic stress related to his work disposing of IEDs in "messy" combat settings (PCL-5). More importantly, as Carlos reports

Table 13.5 Psychometrically sounds measures of PCS severity, mental health symptoms, or function/disability/quality of life/participation

Symptom	Comorbid with mTBI	Measure	# of items	Time to administer (min)
Anxiety	17–31%	Neurobehavioral Symptom Checklist (NSC)	5	30
		Beck Anxiety Inventory (BAI)	21	5–10
		General Anxiety Disorder—7 Item (GAD-7)	7	5–10
		Traumatic Brain Injury Quality of Life (TBI-QOL)	20	5–10
Depression	31–50%	Beck Depression Inventory (BDI-II)	21	5–10
		Patient Health Questionnaire—9 (PHQ-9)	9	5–10
		TBI-QOL	20	5–10
Post-traumatic stress	63–77%	PTSD Checklist for DSM-5 (PCL-5)	20	5–10
At-risk substance use	4–19%	AUDIT Alcohol Consumption Questions (AUDIT-C)	3	5
		Drug Abuse Screening Test (DAST-10)	10	5–10
Post-concussive symptoms	15%	Neuro-behavioral Symptom Inventory (NSI)	22	15
Functioning/ disability/quality of life/participation	N/A	Craig Handicap Assessment and Reporting Technique Short For (CHART)	19	15
		World Health Organization Quality of Life (WHOQOL-BREF)	26	15
		TBI-QOL	20	5–10
		Daily Living Activities—20 (DLA-20)	20	Completed by provider
		Participation Assessment with Recombined Tools-Objective (PART-O)—17	17	10–15
Suicide risk	0.5% (suicide attempts)	Columbia-Suicide Severity Rating Scale Screener (C-SSRS-Screener)	6	5
		Beck Scale for Suicide Ideation (BSS)	19	5–10

Citations for table: [28, 67, 68]

having access to lethal means, it is crucial that he undergo continued assessment of his suicidal symptoms (CSSRS-Screener). While he is receiving polytrauma care at a VA outpatient clinic, he may benefit from psychiatric/psychological treatment via telehealth. Safety planning, a brief intervention to reduce suicide risk, should be initiated [69]. As Carlos has difficulty with his memory, educating his family members about the Safety Plan is also indicated.

Intervention and Management

Mild TBI

It is important to note that the majority of individuals who experience a mTBI recover fully [29], and providing Veterans with an expectation of full recovery, particularly if their injury was recently sustained, may help to alleviate fears. However, for many, symptoms do persist. While mTBI symptoms may resolve without intervention, the length of time until resolution can vary, ranging from days to months [70, 71]. Treatment, therefore, is focused on symptom management and a return to activities (e.g., work, play). For individuals with an mTBI who do not return to baseline function within a year, Clinical Practice Guidelines suggest non-pharmacological therapies as a first line of intervention [3]. Management of persistent headaches may include medication for acute pain, but principally focuses on education for avoiding exacerbating substances (e.g., caffeine, tobacco, alcohol), and minimizing environmental exposures that may promote headache (e.g., noisy environments, strong scents). Sleep disturbances are also common after mTBI [72], and interventions often entail education on topics such as avoiding stimulants and developing consistent sleep habits (i.e., sleep hygiene). For sleeplessness, interventions may include cognitive behavioral therapy tailored for insomnia (CBTi), relaxation strategies, dietary modification, and physical activity, among others [3]. Finally, for cognitive difficulties or behavioral concerns, cognitive-behavioral interventions, psychoeducation, and supportive stress management may be used and adapted for patients' individual treatment goals. Given that some patients with a TBI struggle with executive functioning (e.g., planning/organization, impulsivity), providers should be prepared to adapt treatments to accommodate such limitations. It is recommended that patients are only referred for neuropsychological assessment with a specialist if the symptoms do not improve or resolve after 90 days [3]. In most cases, research also supports employing evidence-based practices (medications, psychotherapy) among those with TBI and co-occurring mental health conditions [28].

Moderate to Severe TBI

For military members and Veterans who have experienced a moderate or severe TBI in deployed or non-deployed settings, TBI treatment is often provided through the Polytrauma System of Care (PSC), a national network of providers and specialized clinics distributed across VA medical centers [73]. These interdisciplinary teams address both psychological and physical issues faced by Veterans. Of note, for Veterans living in sparsely populated or rural areas, particularly Veterans with moderate to severe TBIs like Carlos, accessing care in the VA's PSC can be difficult. VA Points of Contact are sometimes available in smaller clinics, but they function primarily as care coordination and case management for injured Veterans. In Carlos's case, his family drives him to a Regional VA Medical Center for his TBI rehabilitation services. That being said, he may be able to receive some of his polytrauma care via telehealth. Either way, his polytrauma and mental health providers should work collaboratively to address current symptoms (depression), decrease suicide risk (e.g., Safety Planning), and increase function (e.g., identify avocational activities of interest and help Carlos engage in such activities).

Prevention

After the first several years of combat operations in Afghanistan and Iraq, significant concern emerged about the acute and long-term health effects for military members with deployment-acquired TBI, and the DoD and VA began improving assessment and prevention efforts. In 2010, the DoD began implementing an incident-based policy to improve identification of potentially concussive events in theater as close to the point of injury as possible, which required that following all potentially concussive incidents, military members must receive a medical evaluation before being cleared to return to duty [74]. By relieving military members from duty until fully recovered, this reduced the likelihood of sustaining a *second* head injury while the brain is still recovering from metabolic abnormalities associated with the initial injury, and therefore, reduced risk for long term neurologic injury [20].

Evaluations of the success of the incident-based policy have reported mixed results. As of 2018, it was estimated that, depending on the service branch, TBI reporting among active duty military members increased by approximately 50–250% [75]. Much of this variation was due to inconsistencies in how widely the policy was disseminated and communicated [14]. Increases in reporting also coincided with increases in TBI-related medical evaluations, primarily CT scans, mental health evaluations, and physical therapy assessments [76], however, it remains unknown if there was a corresponding increase in injured military members being relieved from duty or given adequate time to recover. Crucially, among military members who experience a non-combat-related mTBI, up to 40% initially seek care in private purchased care settings. In such cases, the military member may not report the TBI to commanding officers or military clinicians, making civilian settings the only point of contact for TBI treatment. Clinicians in civilian settings should be aware of this possibility when treating military members. For military members and Veterans alike, particularly those who have a history of TBI, clinicians should encourage helmet use and recommend protective gear suited to specific activities, such as motorcycling and bicycling.

Conclusion

Civilian clinicians and mental health providers should be encouraged to screen their patients for prior military service, with the understanding that patients with a history of military service may be more likely to have a history of TBI and its associated comorbidities. Using the OSU TBI-ID short form is recommended for evaluating an individual's lifetime history of TBI. In addition, augmenting traditional clinical interviews with psychometrically sound tools (e.g., depression, post traumatic symptoms) is indicated. Training civilian clinicians to screen for lifetime history of TBI and its associated co-occurring conditions and symptoms will be invaluable to improve the health and wellbeing of our nation's military members and Veterans. In addition, providers with less experience working with military members or Veterans are encouraged to become familiar with military culture (see https://psycharmor.org/courses/15-things-veterans-want-you-to-know/—[77]). The acute and potentially lasting effects of TBI on physical and mental health, functioning, and overall quality of life necessitate ongoing research into the pathophysiology of head injury, as well as continued improvement in rehabilitation and treatment methods.

Clinical Pearls

- Mild TBI (mTBI), herein considered synonymous with concussion, is commonly referred to as one of the signature injuries of the military conflicts in Afghanistan and Iraq
- Most individuals with one mTBI report returning to baseline functioning within 1 year, however, as many as 15%, report experiencing persistent post-concussive symptoms
- A particular challenge associated with diagnosing and treating combat-related mTBI is that many of the signs and symptoms associated with such injuries overlap with those frequently associated with PTSD (e.g., trouble concentrating, insomnia, irritability)
- While less common than mTBI, moderate and severe TBIs are often associated with more significant post-injury sequelae. In addition to the physical, cognitive, and psychological impairments associated with mTBI, military members and Veterans with moderate and severe TBIs also contend with additional, often lifelong conditions that can adversely impact their reintegration into civilian life.
- TBI treatment is often provided through the Polytrauma System of Care (PSC), a national network of providers and specialized clinics distributed across VA medical centers [73]. These interdisciplinary teams address both psychological and physical issues faced by Veterans.

Acknowledgements and Disclosures The opinions and assertions herein are those of the authors and do not necessarily reflect the official views of the Veterans Health Administration.

References

1. Centers for Disease Control and Prevention. Traumatic Brain Injury & Concussion. 2019. https://www.cdc.gov/traumaticbraininjury/index.html.
2. Kochanek PM, Clark RS, Jenkins LW. TBI: pathobiology. Brain injury medicine. New York, NY: Demos Medical Publishing; 2007. p. 81–92.
3. Department of Veterans Affairs and Department of Defense. VA/DoD clinical practice guideline for management of concussion/mild traumatic brain injury. 2016. http://www.healthquality.va.gov/management_of_concussion_mtbi.asp.
4. Chapman JC, Diaz-Arrastia R. Military traumatic brain injury: a review. Alzheimers Dement. 2014;10(3):S97–S104.
5. Okie S. Traumatic brain injury in the war zone. N Engl J Med. 2005;352(20):2043–7.
6. French LM. Military traumatic brain injury: an examination of important differences. Ann N Y Acad Sci. 2010;1208(1):38–45.
7. Belmont PJ, Schoenfeld AJ, Goodman G. Epidemiology of combat wounds in Operation Iraqi Freedom and Operation Enduring Freedom: orthopaedic burden of disease. J Surg Orthop Adv. 2010;19(1):2–7.
8. Clark ME, Bair MJ, Buckenmaier CC III, Gironda RJ, Walker RL. Pain and combat injuries in soldiers returning from Operations Enduring Freedom and Iraqi Freedom: implications for research and practice. J Rehabil Res Dev. 2007;44(2):179–94.
9. Gawande A. Casualties of war -- military care for the wounded from Iraq and Afghanistan. N Engl J Med. 2004;351(24):2471–5.
10. Department of Veterans Affairs - Veterans Health Administration. Polytrauma system of care (VHA Handbook 1172.01). Washington, DC; 2013. https://www.va.gov/optometry/docs/vha_handbook_1172_01_polytrauma_system_of_care.pdf.
11. Holtkamp MD, Grimes J, Ling G. Concussion in the military: an evidence-base review of mTBI in US military personnel focused on posttraumatic headache. Curr Pain Headache Rep. 2016;20(6):37.
12. Kulas JF, Rosenheck RA. A comparison of veterans with post-traumatic stress disorder, with mild traumatic brain injury and with both disorders: understanding multimorbidity. Mil Med. 2017;183(3–4):e114–22.
13. Defense and Veterans Brain Injury Center. DoD worldwide numbers for TBI. Silver Spring, MD: Defense and Veterans Brain Injury Center; 2018.
14. Defense and Veterans Brain Injury Center. Identification of brain injuries in deployed environment surged after enactment of DoD policies. 2018. https://health.mil/News/Articles/2018/03/27/Identification-of-brain-injuries-in-deployed-environment-surged-following-enactment-of-DoD-policies?type=Policies.
15. Hendricks AM, Amara J, Baker E, Charns MP, Gardner JA, Iverson KM, et al. Screening for mild traumatic brain injury in OEF-OIF deployed US military: an empirical assessment of VHA's experience. Brain Inj. 2013;27(2):125–34. https://doi.org/10.3109/02699052.2012.729284.
16. Vasterling JJ, Aslan M, Lee LO, Proctor SP, Ko J, Jacob S, Concato J. Longitudinal associations among posttraumatic stress disorder symptoms, traumatic brain injury, and neurocognitive functioning in army soldiers deployed to the Iraq war. J Int Neuropsychol Soc. 2018;24(4):311–23. https://doi.org/10.1017/S1355617717001059.
17. Schwab KA, Ivins B, Cramer G, Johnson W, Sluss-Tiller M, Kiley K, et al. Screening for traumatic brain injury in troops returning from deployment in Afghanistan and Iraq: initial investigation of the usefulness of a short screening tool for traumatic brain injury. J Head Trauma Rehabil. 2007;22(6):377–89.
18. Tanielian T, Haycox LH, Schell TL, Marshall GN, Burnam MA, Eibner C, et al. Invisible wounds of war. Summary and recommendations for addressing psychological and cognitive injuries. Santa Monica: RAND Corporation; 2008.
19. Terrio H, Brenner LA, Ivins BJ, Cho JM, Helmick K, Schwab K, et al. Traumatic brain injury screening: preliminary findings in a US Army Brigade Combat Team. J Head Trauma Rehabil. 2009;24(1):14–23.

20. Helmick KM, Spells CA, Malik SZ, Davies CA, Marion DW, Hinds SR. Traumatic brain injury in the US military: epidemiology and key clinical and research programs. Brain Imaging Behav. 2015;9(3):358–66.
21. Corrigan JD, Selassie AW, Orman JA. The epidemiology of traumatic brain injury. J Head Trauma Rehabil. 2010;25(2):72–80. https://doi.org/10.1097/HTR.0b013e3181ccc8b4.
22. Langlois J, Rutland-Brown W, Wald M. The epidemiology and impact of traumatic brain injury: a brief overview. J Head Trauma Rehabil. 2006;21(5):375–8.
23. Williams VF, Stahlman S, Hunt DJ, O'Donnell FL. Diagnoses of traumatic brain injury not clearly associated with deployment, active component, US Armed Forces, 2001-2016. MSMR. 2017;24(3):2–8.
24. Adams RS, Larson MJ, Corrigan JD, Horgan CM, Williams TV. Frequent binge drinking after combat-acquired traumatic brain injury among active duty military personnel with a past year combat deployment. J Head Trauma Rehabil. 2012;27(5):349–60. https://doi.org/10.1097/HTR.0b013e318268db94. PMCID: PMC3633079.
25. Armistead-Jehle P, Soble JR, Cooper DB, Belanger HG. Unique aspects of traumatic brain injury in military and veteran populations. Phys Med Rehabil Clin. 2017;28(2):323–37. https://doi.org/10.1016/j.pmr.2016.12.008.
26. Corrigan JD, Bogner J. Initial reliability and validity of the Ohio State University TBI identification method. J Head Trauma Rehabil. 2007;22(6):318–29. https://doi.org/10.1097/01.HTR.0000300227.67748.77.
27. Betthauser LM, Adams RS, Hostetter TA, Scher AI, Schwab K, Brenner LA. Characterization of lifetime TBIs in a cohort of recently deployed soldiers: the warrior strong study. Rehabil Psychol. 2019;64:398–406.
28. Brenner LA, Otis J, Grassmeyer RP, Adams RS, Laker SR, Filley CM. Assessment and management of psychiatric symptoms among adults with mild traumatic brain injury. In: Eapen BC, Cifu DX, editors. Concussion: assessment, management and rehabilitation. Amsterdam: Elsevier; 2020. p. 47–58.
29. Katz DI, Cohen SI, Alexander MP. Mild traumatic brain injury. In: Handbook of clinical neurology, vol. 127. Amsterdam: Elsevier; 2015. p. 131–56.
30. IOM (Institute of Medicine). Gulf war and health, volume 7: long-term consequences of traumatic brain injury. Washington, DC; 2008.
31. Walker WC, Lacey RW. Postconcussive syndrome (PCS). In: Eapen BC, Cifu DX, editors. Concussion: assessment, management and rehabilitation. Amsterdam: Elsevier; 2020. p. 37–46.
32. Cifu DX, Scholten J, Campbell EH. Traumatic brain injury, posttraumatic stress disorder, and pain diagnoses in OIF/OEF/OND veterans. J Rehabil Res Dev. 2013;50(9):1169–76.
33. Hoge CW, McGurk D, Thomas JL, Cox AL, Engel CC, Castro CA. Mild traumatic brain Injury in U.S. soldiers returning from Iraq. N Engl J Med. 2008;358(5):453–63.
34. Spira JL, Lathan CE, Bleiberg J, Tsao JW. The impact of multiple concussions on emotional distress, post-concussive symptoms, and neurocognitive functioning in active duty United States marines independent of combat exposure or emotional distress. J Neurotrauma. 2014;31(22):1823–34. https://doi.org/10.1089/neu.2014.3363.
35. Stein MB, McAllister TW. Exploring the convergence of posttraumatic stress disorder and mild traumatic brain injury. Am J Psychiatr. 2009;166(7):768–76.
36. Jones E, Fear NT, Wessely S. Shell shock and mild traumatic brain injury: a historical review. Am J Psychiatr. 2007;164(11):1641–5.
37. Thornhill S, Teasdale GM, Murray GD, McEwen J, Roy CW, Penny KI. Disability in young people and adults one year after head injury: prospective cohort study. Br Med J. 2000;320(7250):1631–5.
38. Centers for Disease Control and Prevention, U.S. Department of Health and Human Services, Department of Defense, and VA Leadership Panel. Report to congress on traumatic brain injury in the United States: epidemiology and rehabilitation. Atlanta, GA. 2015. https://www.sciencedirect.com/science/article/pii/S000399931500547X.

39. Mushkudiani NA, Engel DC, Steyerberg EW, Butcher I, Lu J, Marmarou A, et al. Prognostic value of demographic characteristics in traumatic brain injury: results from the IMPACT study. J Neurotrauma. 2007;24(2):259–69. https://doi.org/10.1089/neu.2006.0028.
40. Gollaher K, High W, Sherer M, Bergloff P, Boake C, Young ME, Ivanhoe C. Prediction of employment outcome one to three years following traumatic brain injury (TBI). Brain Inj. 1998;12(4):255–63. https://doi.org/10.1080/026990598122557.
41. Berry C, Ley EJ, Mirocha J, Salim A. Race affects mortality after moderate to severe traumatic brain injury 1. J Surg Res. 2010;163(2):303–8. https://doi.org/10.1016/j.jss.2010.03.018.
42. Gary KW, Arango-Lasprilla JC, Ketchum JM, Kreutzer JS, Copolillo A, Novack TA, Jha A. Racial differences in employment outcome after traumatic brain injury at 1, 2, and 5 years postinjury. Arch Phys Med Rehabil. 2009;90(10):1699–707. https://doi.org/10.1016/j.apmr.2009.04.014.
43. Wertheimer JC, Hanks RA, Hasenau DL. Comparing functional status and community integration in severe penetrating and motor vehicle–related brain injuries. Arch Phys Med Rehabil. 2008;89(10):1983–90. https://doi.org/10.1016/j.apmr.2008.04.010.
44. Slewa-Younan S, Mond JM, Bussion E, Melkonian M, Mohammad Y, Dover H. Psychological trauma and help seeking behaviour amongst resettled Iraqi refugees in attending English tuition classes in Australia. Int J Ment Health Syst. 2015;9:5. https://doi.org/10.1186/1752-4458-9-5.
45. Rao V, Rosenberg P, Bertrand M, Salehinia S, Spiro J, Vaishnavi S, et al. Aggression after traumatic brain injury: prevalence and correlates. J Neuropsychiatry Clin Neurosci. 2009;21(4):420–9. https://doi.org/10.1176/appi.neuropsych.21.4.420.
46. Kim E, Lauterbach EC, Reeve A, Arciniegas DB, Coburn KL, Mendez MF, et al. Neuropsychiatric complications of traumatic brain injury: a critical review of the literature (a report by the ANPA Committee on Research). J Neuropsychiatry Clin Neurosci. 2007;19(2):106–27. https://doi.org/10.1176/appi.neuropsych.19.2.106.
47. Tateno A, Jorge RE, Robinson RG. Clinical correlates of aggressive behavior after traumatic brain injury. J Neuropsychiatry Clin Neurosci. 2003;15(2):155–60. https://doi.org/10.1176/jnp.15.2.155.
48. Englander J, Bushnik T, Duong TT, Cifu DX, Zafonte R, Wright J, et al. Analyzing risk factors for late posttraumatic seizures: a prospective, multicenter investigation. Arch Phys Med Rehabil. 2003;84(3):365–73. https://doi.org/10.1053/apmr.2003.50022.
49. Annegers JF, Hauser WA, Coan SP, Rocca WA. A population-based study of seizures after traumatic brain injuries. N Engl J Med. 1998;338(1):20–4. https://doi.org/10.1056/NEJM199801013380104.
50. Shively S, Scher AI, Perl DP, Diaz-Arrastia R. Dementia resulting from traumatic brain injury: what is the pathology? Arch Neurol. 2012;69(10):1245–51. https://doi.org/10.1001/archneurol.2011.3747.
51. Wilson M, Montgomery H. Impact of genetic factors on outcome from brain injury. Br J Anaesth. 2007;99(1):43–8. https://doi.org/10.1093/bja/aem142.
52. Bogner J, Corrigan JD. Reliability and predictive validity of the Ohio State University TBI identification method with prisoners. J Head Trauma Rehabil. 2009;24(4):279–91. https://doi.org/10.1097/HTR.0b013e3181a66356.
53. Corrigan JD, Bogner J, Mellick D, Bushnik T, Dams-O'Connor K, Hammond FM, et al. Prior history of traumatic brain injury among persons in the traumatic brain injury model systems National Database. Arch Phys Med Rehabil. 2013;94(10):1940–50.
54. BrainLine. Ohio State University TBI Identification Method. 2013. https://www.brainline.org/article/ohio-state-university-tbi-identification-method.
55. Brenner LA, Homaifar BY, Olson-Madden JH, Nagamoto HT, Huggins J, Schneider AL, et al. Prevalence and screening of traumatic brain injury among veterans seeking mental health services. J Head Trauma Rehabil. 2013;28(1):21–30.
56. IOM (Institute of Medicine). Returning home from Iraq and Afghanistan: preliminary assessment of readjustment needs of military personnel, veterans, and their families. Washington, DC: National Academy of Sciences; 2010.
57. Carlson KF, Gilbert TA, Morasco BJ, Wright D, Otterloo JV, Herrndorf A, Cook LJ. Linkage of VA and state prescription drug monitoring program data to examine concurrent opioid and

sedative-hypnotic prescriptions among veterans. Health Serv Res. 2018;53(S3):5285–308. https://doi.org/10.1111/1475-6773.13025.
58. Hudson TJ, Painter JT, Gressler LE, Lu L, Williams JS, Booth BM, et al. Factors associated with opioid initiation in OEF/OIF/OND veterans with traumatic brain injury. Pain Med. 2018;19(4):774–87. https://doi.org/10.1093/pm/pnx208.
59. Adams RS, Corrigan JD, Dams-O'Connor K. Opioid use among individuals with traumatic brain injury: a perfect storm? J Neurotrauma. 2019;37:211–6.
60. Gallagher M, McLeod HJ, McMillan TM. A systematic review of recommended modifications of CBT for people with cognitive impairments following brain injury. Neuropsychol Rehabil. 2019;29(1):1–21.
61. Gros DF, Lancaster CL, Horner MD, Szafranski DD, Back SE. The influence of traumatic brain injury on treatment outcomes of concurrent treatment for PTSD and substance use disorders using prolonged exposure (COPE) in veterans. Compr Psychiatry. 2017;78:48–53.
62. U.S. Department of Veterans Affairs. Polytrauma/TBI system of care. 2016. https://www.polytrauma.va.gov/.
63. Corrigan JD, Bogner JA. Accomodating the symptoms of TBI. n.d.. https://tbi.osu.edu/modules.
64. Silverberg ND, Panenka WJ. Antidepressants for depression after concussion and traumatic brain injury are still best practice. BMC Psychiatry. 2019;19(1):100.
65. Hostetter TA, Hoffmire CA, Forster JE, Adams RS, Stearns-Yoder KA, Brenner LA. Suicide and traumatic brain injury among individuals seeking Veterans Health Administration services between fiscal years 2006 and 2015. J Head Trauma Rehabil. 2019;34:E1–9.
66. Veterans Affairs Mental Illness Research Education and Clinical Centers. Lethal means safety & suicide prevention. n.d. https://www.mirecc.va.gov/lethalmeanssafety/.
67. Greer N, Ackland P, Sayer N, Spoont M, Taylor B, MacDonald R, et al. Relationship of deployment-related mild traumatic brain injury to posttraumatic stress disorder, depressive disorders, substance use disorders, suicidal ideation, and anxiety disorders: a systematic review. Washington, DC; 2019. https://www.hsrd.research.va.gov/publications/esp/tbi-mentalhealth.cfm.
68. Hartlage LC, Durant-Wilson D, Patch PC. Persistent neurobehavioral problems following mild traumatic brain injury. Arch Clin Neuropsychol. 2001;16(6):561–70.
69. U.S. Department of Veterans Affairs. VA suicide prevention resources: what is a safety plan? n.d. https://starttheconversation.veteranscrisisline.net/pdf/what-is-a-safety-plan/.
70. Carroll L, Cassidy JD, Peloso P, Borg J, Von Holst H, Holm L, et al. Prognosis for mild traumatic brain injury: results of the WHO Collaborating Centre Task Force on mild traumatic brain injury. J Rehabil Med. 2004;36:84–105.
71. McCrea M, Iverson GL, McAllister TW, Hammeke TA, Powell MR, Barr WB, Kelly JP. An integrated review of recovery after mild traumatic brain injury (MTBI): implications for clinical management. Clin Neuropsychol. 2009;23(8):1368–90.
72. Orff HJ, Ayalon L, Drummond SPA. Traumatic brain injury and sleep disturbance: a review of current research. J Head Trauma Rehabil. 2009;24(3):155–65.
73. Eapen BC, Jaramillo CA, Tapia RN, Johnson EJ, Cifu DX. Rehabilitation care of combat related TBI: veterans health administration polytrauma system of care. Curr Phys Med Rehabil Rep. 2013;1(3):151–8.
74. Department of Defense. DoD policy guidance for management of mild traumatic brain injury/concussion in the deployed setting. Number 6490.11. Washington, DC; 2012.
75. Agimi Y, Regasa LE, Ivins B, Malik S, Helmick K, Marion D. Role of Department of Defense Policies in identifying traumatic brain injuries among deployed US Service Members, 2001-2016. Am J Public Health. 2018;108(5):683–8. https://doi.org/10.2105/AJPH.2018.304347.
76. Farmer CM, Krull H, Concannon TW, Simmons M, Pillemer F, Ruder T, et al. Understanding treatment of mild traumatic brain injury in the military health system. Rand Health Q. 2017;6(2):11.
77. PsychArmor Institute. Things veterans want you to know. n.d. https://psycharmor.org/courses/15-things-veterans-want-you-to-know/.

Moral Injury in a Military Context

14

Eric Vermetten, Rakesh Jetly, Lorraine Smith-MacDonald, Chelsea Jones, and Suzette Bremault-Phillip

E. Vermetten (✉)
Department of Psychiatry, Leiden University Medical Center, Leiden, The Netherlands

Department Psychiatry, New York University Grossman School of Medicine, New York, NY, USA
e-mail: e.vermetten@lumc.nl

R. Jetly
Canadian Forces Health Services Group HQ, Ottawa, ON, Canada

Institute for Mental Health Research, Ottawa, ON, Canada
e-mail: rakesh@drjetly.com

L. Smith MacDonald
Heroes in Mind, Advocacy and Research Consortium (HiMARC), Faculty of Rehabilitation Medicine, University of Alberta, Edmonton, AB, Canada
e-mail: smithmac@ualberta.ca

C. Jones
Heroes in Mind, Advocacy and Research Consortium (HiMARC), Faculty of Rehabilitation Medicine, University of Alberta, Edmonton, AB, Canada

Department of National Defence, Field Ambulance, Canadian Forces Health Services, Edmonton, AB, Canada
e-mail: cweiman@ualberta.ca

S. Bremault-Phillip
Heroes in Mind, Advocacy and Research Consortium (HiMARC), Faculty of Rehabilitation Medicine, University of Alberta, Edmonton, AB, Canada

Department of Occupational Therapy, Faculty of Rehabilitation Medicine, University of Alberta, Edmonton, AB, Canada
e-mail: Suzette2@ualberta.ca

C. H. Warner, C. A. Castro (eds.), *Veteran and Military Mental Health*,
https://doi.org/10.1007/978-3-031-18009-5_14

Introduction

Growing interest has arisen in recent years regarding Moral Injury (MI). A term used to describe the persistent distress that individuals may develop when they perpetrate, witness, or fail to prevent an act that transgresses their core beliefs [1], MI is increasingly being referred to as a syndrome characterized by guilt, shame, intrusive thoughts, anger and self-condemnation [2]. Individuals may experience moral distress when they are exposed to potentially morally injurious events (pMIES) and/or are unable to act in a manner consistent with their moral requirements due to, for example, external constraints such as "rules of engagement" [3, 4].

While MI is not included in the Diagnostic and Statistical Manual of Mental Disorders: fifth Edition (DSM-5) or officially considered a mental disorder, it shares some similarities with post-traumatic stress disorder (PTSD), most notably within the Criterion D affective domain as defined by DSM-5 [5]. MI may erode a person's self-perception, relationships with self and others, and sense of meaning and place in their family, community and society as a whole. It may also challenge one's faith, beliefs, and value systems. Spirituality and religious beliefs are important factors in MI that have been correlated with post-traumatic growth and are inversely associated with PTSD [6].

Moral injury has potential linkages with other co-occurring conditions. Overlapping symptoms of PTSD and MI include anger, depression, anxiety, insomnia, nightmares, and self-medications [7–10]. Severe violations of beliefs regarding right and wrong, and what is just and fair, can result in intense emotional, cognitive and physical reactions (([1, 11–15], pp. 7–8), including:

> *... self-harming behaviors, such as poor self-care, alcohol and drug abuse, severe recklessness, and parasuicidal behavior, self-handicapping behaviors, such as retreating in the face of success or good feelings, and demoralization, which may entail confusion, bewilderment, futility, hopelessness, and self-loathing. Most damaging is the possibility of enduring changes in self and other beliefs that reflect regressive over-accommodation of moral violation, culpability, or expectations of injustice. This may occur because each re-experiencing and avoidance instance leads to new learning affecting the strength and accessibility of underlying schemas, which, over time, become ingrained and rigid and resistant to countervailing evidence* ([1], p. 701).

Severe suicidal ideation and increased suicide attempts are also reported [7, 8, 16–18]. Shay [11] likens MI, and all psychological injury, to the etiology of physical injury, arguing that it is not the initial event that kills soldiers. "[R]ather it is the complications that arise as they desperately try to manage the aftermath of the initial event, usually with strategies that are maladaptive, dangerous, and even lethal" ([12], p. 292). Physiologically, "[I]t's a kick in the stomach … [It] is coded by the body as a physical attack" ([12], p. 294) "and [the body] reacts with the same massive mobilization" ([11], p. 186).

Populations with which MI has been associated continue to broaden. Initially, MI was described in reference to military members and veterans impacted by war and combat. The phenomenon of MI and moral distress (MD) have more recently been discussed in civilian contexts and among public safety personnel (PSP); i.e., including firefighters, paramedics, police [19, 20], physicians [21], nurses [22], and religious leaders [23]. During the COVID-19 pandemic MI/MD have increasingly been linked to emergency and healthcare services [24].

A better understanding of MI is urgently needed. The clinical community has come to appreciate that combat veterans do not respond well to existing evidence-based PTSD interventions as was once hoped [25–27]. This has led to the recognition that the behaviours and suffering of veterans may not be wholly explained by the traditional "fear-based" paradigm of PTSD [28]. Military combat experiences that result in internal conflict, guilt, ongoing distress [29], disintegration of personhood [30, 31] and moral transgressions [32, 33], often decades after the event [34], are potential drivers for enduring posttraumatic stress and suicide risk [7, 35]. With the number of returning service members who have died by suicide in the US and other NATO nations outnumbering those killed in action on deployment, a greater understanding of military service members' experiences of MI is urgently needed. This may apply equally well to other populations. The concept of MI has emerged as this generation's contribution to addressing psychological injuries [36, 37].

Jonathan Shay was the first to use the term MI [38, 39]. As a psychiatrist at the Boston VA, he worked with Vietnam veterans and listened to their stories. In his 1994 book, *Achilles in Vietnam: Combat Trauma and the Undoing of Character*, Shay compared Vietnam veterans' experience to those immortalized in the epic Greek poems of Homer, such as the Iliad, stating that he aimed to 'put before the public an understanding of catastrophic experiences that not only cause life-long disability but can ruin good character' (p. xiii). Moreover, in his 2002 book, *Odysseus in America: Combat Trauma and the Trials of Homecoming*, Shay emphasized the need to prevent what he heuristically called, "psychological and moral injury in military service" (p. 6). Albert Santoli, a writer who served in Vietnam himself, preserved an oral history by providing narratives of several American soldiers:

> *I have cried my ass off. I don't have any tears left. I first started letting it out in April of 1977. It took two years. I did that because I just couldn't handle being a soldier anymore. Still a fucking soldier. I got out of the Navy in June of '76, but I still acted like one. I guess I still do in a way. I still sleep with one eye open, you know. And I wake up with bad dreams that I have of taking fire and watching people being murdered and being a part of that process. In fact, around this time of year - Christmas time - it gets really heavy for some reason. My wife knows it. Sometimes she feels inadequate because she doesn't know how to deal with that. I get really upset and I have to cry a lot and talk. Once I start it's like for three or four hours. I'm completely exhausted. I cry myself to sleep wherever I am, or I need to go out by myself. People feel inadequate. My wife feels inadequate. I tell her, "There's nothing you can do that can be any more adequate than just to be here." There is no under standing. My mind isn't mature enough. It wasn't then and it isn't now and it's never going to be able to understand murder* ([40], p. 255).

Shay argued that central to the psychological distress and impairment experienced by Vietnam veterans was the undoing of their morality which caused the rupturing of personhood. Despite Shay's observations, the importance of morality and personhood were not included in the DSM-III or in subsequent revisions. The line of scientific inquiry that led to the recognition of MI primarily started to emerge around the experiences of post 9–11 combat veterans receiving care for PTSD [41]. The publication of a landmark paper by Litz et al. [1] regarding MI and moral repair in war veterans preceded a steep increase in the recognition of MI within the academic community that has exponentially increased in the last decade.

Vignette

Tom is a 58 year old veteran who had served in the marines for 4 years. He first presented in 2001 with idiopathic pseudo-epileptic seizures and severe mental health symptoms. He was diagnosed with severe PTSD, yet his underlying trauma was not fully understood. Differential diagnoses included conversion disorder and a possible personality disorder. Up to this point he had been hospitalized and treated with high doses of neuroleptics and sedatives. At this time, the patient was referred to a military treatment unit by a therapist at a regional psychiatric center who suspected the onset of symptoms was related to a military trauma. Trauma-focused therapy resulted in an increase and worsening of symptoms, increased alcohol use and intermittent aggressive outbursts.

Because of the increase in symptoms, the utilization of exposure therapy was reduced. In the course of therapy, it was discovered that while on a host nation training mission in 1980, Tom was engaged in a deadly firefight. He was involved in the killing of other people and witnessed the killing of several unarmed children. The death of the innocent children was particularly troubling. While the incident was never publicly acknowledged, this event had not left his thoughts. When back home with his small unit, he and his peers agreed that the incident was never to be discussed. He committed to avoid thinking about it by working hard and drinking heavily. He was able to function in his daily life until approximately 10 years later when he developed seizures and, as a result, was hospitalized for over a year.

The story unfolded over the course of several years. Tom suffered due to conflict between a need to find a way to reconcile the event, a feeling of disloyalty toward his peers upon the disclosure of the event, and the betrayal to the host nation. He shared his story with his now adult children and found support for his engrained memories. He continues to feel residual guilt and shame regarding the disloyalty to his fellow Marines, but through disclosure and recognition of his suffering is relieved of the dramatic impact that the memories have had on his daily functioning and life.

Vignette

Sam, a Veteran of the conflict in Bosnia, presented with symptoms of PTSD, anhedonia, fatigue, pre-psychotic features, and delusion-like ideas that Bosnians would come to his house and seek revenge for a failed mission. He self-attributed his symptoms to a series of traumatic incidents that transpired in Bosnia. As a corporal, he was exposed to combat involving live fire during which he feared for his life. He felt that his symptoms were driven by these incidents. He was not talkative and Eye movement desensitization and reprocessing (EMDR) did not provide him relief. Referral to various mental health treatment centers did result in some progress in reducing the intensity and functional impairment of his symptoms. After several years of treatment, Sam began to open up to his therapist about his military experiences. In EMDR, he and his therapist appropriately focused on traumatic experiences associated with combat, but did not uncover his guilt and shame until he disclosed a secret that continued to haunt him. He related that, despite being instructed to not make contact with the locals at the gate while protecting a Bosnian enclave, he, like many others, engaged in daily conversations and got to know many from the community. These locals provided him with a large sum of money that he promised to deliver to their relatives after the war due to their certainty that they would not survive. He broke his promise and betrayed their trust, spending the money in Zagreb. Over 8000 people were killed when the enclave was eventually overrun, including those who had entrusted their money to him. He felt guilt and shame associated with his actions and started to become "paranoid," and anticipated that Bosnians would come and take revenge on him. When the doorbell rang, he was afraid and for a long time kept a weapon in his trunk. After disclosure of this pMIE, Sam was able to use his memory of transgression and create positive change in his life. In therapy, he was invited to show pictures of the people of Srebrenica that he had taken during his deployment. He started to reconnect with locals over social media, and set up a campaign aimed at reuniting lost family members.

In both vignettes, the veterans were confronted by difficult decisions. The first vignette involved the betrayal of peers, killing of insurgents, and failing to report knowledge of a failed mission, while the second vignette speaks to breaking a promise and failing to provide aid to civilians. The suffering of these veterans cannot be explained solely by being "overwhelmed" by traumatic events and developing a related fear-based anxiety or phobia. Rather, (in)actions violated both veterans' moral codes. This in turn leads to significant anxiety, hyperarousal, avoidant coping and increased alcohol intake and the silent simmering of shame and guilt within. Memories of the events persisted for years and were suppressed by avoidant cognitions and behavior; there are some things experienced by soldiers that "you just don't talk about." In the first vignette, traumatic memories needed to be released at the price of appearing disloyal to peers. In the second vignette, it was symbolic payback that assuages guilt.

These vignettes highlight that veterans' experiences are complicated and cannot be explained with the single, simple paradigm of fear-based understanding of illnesses such as PTSD [28]. The underlying truth emerges as a veteran comes to trust a therapist, and the therapist attempts to genuinely understand the suffering experienced by the veteran.

Etiology

As we expound on the concept of MI, its assessment, treatment and etiology, agreement on some foundational definitions and concepts is needed. Standardized terminology regarding MI itself, pMIEs, moral emotions and cognitive dissonance, morally challenging interactions, moral dilemmas, moral decisions and trauma will enable MI to be more effectively operationalized and addressed.

Moral Injury

The conceptual understanding of MI continues to evolve. In a systematic study of definitions of MI among military populations, Richardson et al. [42] reviewed 124 articles and found 12 key definitions that were cited across the literature, with themes related to ethics, betrayal, and issues of reconciliation. They found that contradictions between definitions and conceptualizations of MI remain. Some definitions suggest that a specific event or high-stress environment is the foundation of such injuries, whereas others identify one's beliefs or perspective on morality as the origin or cause of these moral wounds. With 9 different themes found in just 12 key definitions, it is apparent that a lack of consistency exists in how MI is being defined and understood across the literature. While this does not suggest that existing definitions of MI are inaccurate or misguided, it does demonstrate that a key next step to strengthening the face validity and reliability of a definition is to test the themes that have emerged through previous definitions in samples of military service members and veteran stakeholders. Doing so would more accurately reflect their experiences and ensure that any other key elements related to MI are not disregarded.

Potentially Morally Injurious Events

While the exact underlying mechanisms of MI are presently unknown, exposure to potentially morally injurious event(s) (pMIE) has been noted to precede MI. In the context of war, pMIEs have been associated with "participating in or witnessing inhumane or cruel actions, failing to prevent the immoral acts of others... engaging in subtle acts or experiencing reactions that, upon reflection, transgress a moral code [or] bearing witness to the aftermath of violence and human carnage" ([1], p. 700). In contrast, PMIEs experienced by healthcare professionals (HCPs) often occur when: (1) a HCP feels responsibility for what happened or cannot act in a patient's best interest; and (2) organizational constraints interfere with best or ethically correct care [43]. The dissonance arising when a perceived transgression is profoundly incongruent with one's moral or ethical beliefs [1], and the way in which the individual appraises and assigns meaning to the event rather than the event itself [44] is believed to lead to the development of MI. In the short term, this may produce severe emotional distress, and in the long term, MI.

Moral Emotions and Cognitive Dissonance

It may be essential to understand moral emotions and cognitive dissonance to comprehend a person's adherence (or lack thereof) to their moral standards when exposed to pMIEs. Defined as emotions "that are linked to the interests or welfare either of society as a whole or at least of persons other than the judge or agent" ([45], p. 276), moral emotions provide the motivation to do good and avoid doing bad [46]. Those experiencing MI may describe feelings of being constrained by an overarching strategy or hierarchical rules that govern their actions, thus being at the mercy of events [47]. Several moral emotions, independent both of a person's perspective (i.e., as witness, betrayer, or victim) or type of pMIE (i.e., act of commission or omission), are thought to be characteristic of MI. These include guilt, regret, grief, sorrow, shame, anger or rage, contempt, disgust or inaction regret [1, 44, 48, 49]. In conjunction with moral emotions, cognitive dissonance may also arise in relation to oneself, others or a higher power (e.g., 'I am a terrible person,' 'my military commanders do not care about me', 'we did bad things,' 'why would my god let this happen?').

Morally Challenging Interactions, Moral Dilemmas and Moral Decisions

PMIEs can include morally challenging interactions, moral decisions and moral dilemmas. Morally challenging interactions are "situations in which an individual is confronted with an intrapersonal "clash" of values caused by an interaction" [50]. Moral decisions are judgments made amidst morally challenging interactions and moral dilemmas that: (a) invoke the fundamental values of the decision-maker; and (b) affect the well-being of others [28]. Moral dilemmas are a special class of moral decisions in which (a) there is a conflict between at least two core values/obligations (i.e., loyalty, obedience, respect for life); (b) acting in a way that is consistent with one underlying value means failing to fulfill the other(s); (c) harm will occur regardless of the option chosen, and; (d) the decision is inescapable and inevitable—some action must be taken [51]. Moral decisions can be difficult, have important moral implications and impact mental health.

PMIEs and PTSD

There is debate as to whether a pMIE "must be" an event that would meet criterion A for PTSD. An argument can be made that it often meets this criteria; however, it may be possible that "moral dilemmas" can exist in the absence of trauma. In the above example, embezzling funds from the victims of Srebrenica is not in and of itself a traumatic event as defined in criteria A for PTSD, yet led to moral distress and indeed "MI" in the veteran. Further discussion and consideration of the difference between an event being perceived as "traumatic" versus "morally injurious" is warranted. It is becoming increasingly important to acknowledge and understand the commonalities and differences associated with exposure to traumatic and potentially morally injurious experiences. While there is a clear overlap between traumatic and pMIEs (i.e., the experience of killing), events such as betrayal by leaders need not be "traumatic" in the traditional sense as defined by the DSM-5. There is accumulating evidence that suggests a link between the perceived transgression of moral values and moral standards (e.g., disproportionate use of force in combat for other reasons than just fulfilling the mission; following orders that were illegal;

failing to provide medical aid; failing to report violent actions; a change in belief about the justification of war) and symptoms of guilt, shame, anger, suicidal ideation and PTSD within military samples and veterans [8, 52, 53]. Future research will assess whether pMIEs may have had an impact on a person's mental state over time and how this could correlate with MI, PTSD, resilience, or other mental health problems. In line with the dissociative subtype of PTSD it may be that if there is a subpopulation within PTSD that has a unique biology driving the symptoms that requires a nuanced treatment there may be a basis for a MI sub-type or dimensional specifier of PTSD.

Epidemiology

MI has been found to be present in a wide range of populations that have been exposed to difficult pMIEs and not limited to military personnel and war veterans. Many civilians, including healthcare professionals, public safety personnel, victims of sexual assault, refugees, and others may experience MI [54]. At least one qualitative study reported that the term MI is useful for exploring medical students' experience in emergency medical settings [55]. Papazoglou and Chopko [56] found that MI was frequently experienced by police officers after suffering repeated trauma. A study of refugees in Switzerland found that MI accounted for 16% of the variance in PTSD symptoms [57]. Some may also experience mental health disorders, such as PTSD, depression, anxiety, or substance use disorders, which may lead to suicidality, cognitive impairment, isolation, and emotional dysregulation causing dysfunction in productivity, relationships, and self-care activities [1, 48, 58]. It is important to note that all of these symptoms, reactions, and responses can be found in clinical diagnoses including PTSD and Major Depressive Disorder. The association between MI and these conditions needs to yet to be better understood.

In the context of more current global conflicts, evidence suggests that pMIEs issues are prevalent. In 2003, 67% of soldiers and Marines reported being unable to help women and children, 52% reported shooting or directing fire at the enemy, 32% reported being directly responsible for the death of an enemy combatant and 20% acknowledged being responsible for the death of a noncombatant [59]. Similar results were reported elsewhere in the same combat theatres [60]. One longitudinal study collected data on behavior, emotional, and biological characteristics at 7 time-points from Dutch International Security Assistance Force (ISAF) military personnel deployed to Afghanistan between 2005 and 2008. The Moral Injury Event Questionnaire—Military Version (MIQ-M) was included as an outcome measure at the 10 year follow up after the combat deployment in Afghanistan to record which pMIEs military personnel had experienced and if some pMIEs were more frequent than others. A total of 458 respondents filled out the MIQ-M. Over 55% of the respondents indicated that they had experienced pMIEs and 5% endorsed having experienced these often. The statement, 'Seeing so much death has changed me' was an example item that was endorsed by more than 40% of the respondents. A third of the respondents indicated that they felt betrayed or let-down by their military/political leaders because of the things they saw/experienced in the war. Nearly 40% indicated that they witnessed or were involved in the death(s) of another person in the war; more than half of these respondents reported having done so more than once.

In the Netherlands, limited research has been conducted into which situations are perceived by soldiers as morally injurious. Rietveld [61] investigated feelings of guilt and shame after deployment among over 1100 young veterans of 14 peacekeeping missions. She reported that a quarter of the veterans surveyed felt guilty and ashamed associated with, (1) being in a "bystander role" after being deployed; (2) possessing a negative attitude towards the population in the deployment area; (3) indirect effects of decisions and actions; (4) attitude and behavior in the context of war and violence; (5) actions and decisions that led to survival or increased the chance of survival, and; (6) normless behavior in the deployment area. Molendijk [62] also researched the morally challenging experiences of Dutch soldiers during missions in Srebrenica and Uruzgan (N = 80). They were especially morally burdened by a conflict of values ("I couldn't do what I knew was right"), a sense of being morally overwhelmed ("We just laughed") and feelings of meaninglessness ("It was one big puppet show") [62]. Similarly, Canadian soldiers often in peacekeeping roles suffered when deployed to places such as the former Yugoslavia and Rwanda. Witnessing atrocities and being unable to act due to rules of engagement created incredible internal conflict that led to suffering in the form of PTSD and MI. Careful examination of General Romeo Dallaire's suffering associated with his experience as a Canadian commander in Rwanda and inability to prevent the horrific genocide more accurately captures the concept of MI versus PTSD [63].

Diagnosis and Assessment

There appears to be agreement that MI is important and contains unique clinical features not fully explained by common mental disorders. As Litz et al. [1] argue, service members and veterans can suffer long-term scars that are not well-captured by the current conceptualizations of PTSD or other adjustment disorders. They did not argue, however, for a new diagnostic category, nor did they want to medicalize or pathologize the moral and ethical distress that service members and veterans may experience. Rather, they believe that the clinical and research dialogue is limited at present because questions about MI are not being adequately addressed. MI in service members and veterans appears to be a distinct phenomenon warranting its own line of inquiry and development of particular intervention strategies. They argue that multi- and interdisciplinary research is needed. There also exists the investigation of MI from the theoretical and empirical bases of moral philosophy, moral psychology, character psychology, and social psychology. This character framework attempts to advance a broader theoretical foundation for MI that has wider applicability to the diversities of human experience [44].

According to Nash [64], MI is a literal wound to the mind, brain, body, and spirit inflicted by a life event that violates deeply held moral expectations of oneself and the world. In keeping with the stress continuum models, MI can be conceived as being on a continuum, with benign or even constructive and exhilarating moral challenges. It is suggested that in a stress injury model, the boundary between normal, reversible moral strains and irreversible (even if repairable) MI is defined by the appearance of distress or alterations in functioning that persist. The persistence of symptoms despite attempts at rest and recovery is a component of diagnostic criteria for other stress-related mental health problems such as depression. Thus, the development of MI may be because of the inability to find resolution or integration of the persistent moral distress rather than merely the PMIE itself. Salient efforts to address MI must include use of accurate measurements of MI and integrated holistic therapeutic approaches, inclusive of spiritual and social components [65].

MI and PTSD, while often co-occurring, may be biologically different [66]. Studies in military personnel and veterans have found that a significant minority of index traumas for PTSD are events that do not primarily evoke fear/threat [14]. Also, MI that are index traumas for PTSD are more strongly associated with emotions that developed after the event than emotions experienced during the event, suggesting that the underlying neurobiology may differ. Recent brain research showed that MI event remembering is associated with enhanced sensory processing and altered top-down control in PTSD samples during autobiographical memory recall [67].

A systematic review summarized the neural correlates of guilt, embarrassment, and shame [68]. Most relevant to understanding the neural correlates of emotional changes associated with development of MI (e.g., guilt, shame) are studies that utilized autobiographical scenarios to induce reexperiencing an emotional state. Guilt was more likely associated with activity in the ventral anterior cingulate cortex, posterior temporal regions and the precuneus; embarrassment more likely with activity in the ventrolateral prefrontal cortex and amygdala; and shame more likely with activity in the dorsolateral prefrontal cortex, posterior cingulate cortex, and sensorimotor cortex. While guilt and shame activated distinct areas of the brain, there were also shared networks that involve emotional processing, self-referential processing, and social cognition. Although methodological approaches to guilt induction varied considerably, a recent meta-analysis of the neural correlates of guilt identified multiple areas, primarily in the left hemisphere [69].

Psychometric Development of MI Assessment: Military

Measures to assess MI as currently understood have only been proposed since 2013. Since then, five measures have emerged to assess the presence of MI among military populations, including two types of assessment tools that measure: (1) both pMIE and MI symptoms, and (2) MI symptoms only. The two scales which measure both pMIE and MI symptoms are the Moral Injury Events Scale (MIES) [70] and the Moral Injury Questionnaire—Military Version (MIQ–M) [71]. The Expressions of Moral Injury Scale—Military Version and the Moral Injury Symptom Scale (MISS) are stand-alone, comprehensive tools for assessing the expressions of MI with good face validity in either a long or short form [72–74]. The Moral Injury Outcome Scale (MIOS) [75] is currently undergoing psychometric testing and validation.

The Moral Injury Events Scale (MIES)

This measure consists of nine pMIE items. An iterative, rational approach was used in scale construction. A team of experts generated a pool of items describing events involving perpetrating, failing to prevent, bearing witness to, learning about, or being the victim of acts that contradict deeply held beliefs and expectations. Instruction to participants is to "indicate how much you agree or disagree with each of the following statements regarding your experiences at any time since [event/deployment….]." Response options are on a Likert scale, ranging from 1 (strongly disagree) to 6 (strongly agree). An even number of response options was chosen to preclude neutral responses. Two items are reverse-keyed; scale scores are generated by reverse coding these two items and then summing across items, with a higher score being indicative of having experienced a greater intensity of events. Of 11 items, 9 address perceived violation of moral beliefs or betrayal by self or others; 2 address perceptions of trust. In later versions 2 items were left out.

Moral Injury Questionnaire-Military Version (MIQ-M)

The MIQ-M was developed as a screening instrument for assessing levels of pMIEs in military populations. The scale lists 20 items that tap into 6 different domains: (1) acts of betrayal (i.e., by peers, leadership, civilians, or self; 3 items); (2) acts of disproportionate violence inflicted on others (5 items); (3) incidents involving death or harm to civilians (4 items); (4) violence within military ranks (2 items); (5) inability to prevent death or suffering (2 items); and (6) ethical dilemmas/moral conflicts (4 items). Respondents are to indicate the frequency of having experienced each of the listed pMIEs in the context of a war-zone deployment(s) on a four-point Likert scale (1 = Never, 2 = Seldom, 3 = Sometimes and 4 = Often). MIQ-M items were developed to provide a unidimensional assessment of exposure to pMIEs. Initial psychometric evidence was reported in a pool of 113 Veterans and showed a 1-factor model providing the best fit to the data for the 6 effect indicators. Higher MIQ-M scores showed convergent validity with exposure to life threatening traumas and was associated with general combat activities/circumstances, worse work/social adjustment, and more PTSD and depressive symptomatology (Currier et al. 2013).

The MIQ-M was recently modified to assess both pMIEs and the defining characteristics of MI (i.e., guilt, shame, difficulty forgiving self and others, and withdrawal) [76]. Exploratory factor analyses suggested a 3-factor model of pMIEs consisting of atrocities of war, psychological consequences of war, and leadership failure or betrayal. The modified MIQ-M factors were correlated with proposed characteristics of MI. Each pMIE factor and associated defining characteristics of MI were positively correlated with symptoms of PTSD, depression, and anxiety, as well as substance use. The modified MIQ-M is a reliable measure of MI that comprises three subscales that are associated with, but is suggestive to be distinct from, mental health outcomes.

The MIES and MIQ-M provide clinicians and researchers with tools to measure exposure to events in a military context with the potential to contravene moral beliefs. These assessment tools can be used to evaluate the prevalence and perceived intensity of potentially injurious war-zone experiences, which is a necessary precursor to evaluating the psychological, social, and spiritual consequences of MI.

Expressions of Moral Injury Scale (EMIS), Military Version (EMIS-M) and Short Form (EMIS-SF)

The Expressions of Moral Injury Scale-Military Version (EMIS-M) was developed as a self-report measure to provide a reliable and valid means of assessing signs of an MI in military populations. This list was drawn from 45 items and reduced to 17. Factor analytic results revealed two distinct factors related to MI expressions directed at both self (nine items) and others (eight items). Self-Directed MI items captured feelings of shame (two items) and guilt (two items) as well as beliefs/attitudes about being unlovable (one item), unforgivable (one item), incapable of moral decision making (one item), self-handicapping behaviours (two items) and acting out (one item) related to committing transgressive acts. In contrast, Other-Directed MI items covered feelings of anger (two items), moral disgust (two items), beliefs/attitudes related to mistrust of others (three items), and revenge fantasies associated with others' acts of perceived wrongdoing (one item). The subscales generated excellent internal consistency and temporal stability over a 6-month period. When compared to measures of PTSD, major depressive disorder, and other relevant constructs (e.g., forgiveness, social support, moral emotions, and combat exposure), EMIS-M scores demonstrated strong convergent, divergent, and incremental validity.

Recently, a brief measure assessing overall MI—the EMIS-M-SF [72] consisting of four items—was developed that represents both self- and other-directed outcomes. Initial results suggest that the EMIS-M-SF holds promise as a short, reliable, and valid assessment of overall outcomes related to a possible MI. In cases when service members or veterans endorse certain items, clinicians may consider giving the full scale to gain a more comprehensive picture of MI-related outcomes and clarify whether the service member's or veteran's painful thoughts and emotions are directed at themselves and/or others. When MI is not a primary treatment target, clinicians might prefer the EMIS-M-SF.

Moral Injury Symptoms Scale-Military Version (MISS-M)

The MISS-M is a reliable and valid measure of MI symptoms that can be used to screen for MI and monitor response to treatment in veterans and active duty military with, or without, diagnosed PTSD [74]. The possible range of scores is from 10 to 100. The total score is an indication of functional impairment caused by MI or distress [74].

These scales have largely followed the definitions by Shay [38] and Litz et al. [1] that focused on MI symptoms acquired during combat, such as feelings of shame, grief, meaninglessness, and remorse for having violated core moral beliefs [77]. Symptoms relate to what one has done (e.g., killed combatants or innocents, dismembered bodies, maltreated others, or deserted comrades during battle), what one has failed to do (e.g., protected innocents or prevented the death of fellow soldiers), and what one has observed others do or fail to do [9]. MI symptoms may also involve intense feelings of betrayal by those in authority, either in or outside of the military, and include religious or spiritual struggles or a complete loss of religious faith resulting from experiences during wartime [77].

The Moral Injury Outcome Scale (MIOS) [75]
Currently undergoing development, psychometric testing and validation by an international research Moral Injury Outcome Scale (MIOS) Consortium, the Moral Injury Outcome Scale (MIOS) is a content-valid measure of moral injury as a multidimensional outcome [78]. The consortium's research suggests that exposure to self- and other-based pMIEs are associated with broad interpersonal/intrapersonal, psychological/behavioral, social, and spiritual/existential impacts and that the difference between moral challenges and MI may be the magnitude and breadth of the symptoms.

Outcome measures that can accurately assess MI are essential to both research efforts and the therapeutic process. Use of such scales heightens clinician awareness of the possible role of exposure to pMIEs and offers insights as to why some service members and veterans have a lack of or poor response to treatment of diagnosed conditions such as PTSD, depressive disorders and substance use disorders.

Psychometric Development of MI Assessment: Other Professions

MI among physicians and other HCPs has received growing attention in the evidence-based literature and media, particularly when discussing issues related to burnout [79] and COVID-19. Clinicians may experience MI when they feel that their ability to deliver care is compromised by the systems being implemented in hospitals, clinics, and medical practices (e.g., insurance, reimbursement, electronic health records, etc.) [80]. During the COVID-19 pandemic, HCPs across the globe have faced difficult ethical/moral decisions given the enormous influx of patients with life-threatening conditions, resource limitations (e.g., ventilators, personal protective equipment, and life-saving medications), as well as having to deal with exposure to the coronavirus themselves and the risk this poses to them and their families [81–83]. HCPs have been stigmatized as vectors of contagion, resulting in their assault, abuse, and isolation during the COVID-19 pandemic, just as they had been during the Severe Acute Respiratory Syndrome (SARS) pandemic [84]. This situation has caused many HCPs to feel a sense of helplessness, shame, and guilt as hundreds of patients every day succumb to the illness [85].

There are multiple psychometrically reliable and validated scales to measure moral distress among HCPs, namely: the Moral Distress Scale [43]; the Moral Distress Scale- Revised [86]; the Moral Distress Risk Scale [87]; Moral Distress Tolerance Scale [88]; Moral Distress Questionnaire [89]; and the Stress of Conscience Questionnaire [90]. Other scales have also been developed and tested within certain health care populations such as the Moral Distress Scale for Psychiatric Nurses [91], the Moral Distress Scale-Pediatric Version [92], or the ICU Nurses Moral Distress Scale [93]. Psychometrically reliable and valid scales, however, to measure MI symptoms in HCPs have only now become available.

A Moral Injury Symptoms Scale-Health Professional (MISS-HP)

The MISS-HP has recently been developed by Zhizhon et al. [24]. This 10-item scale is a measure of MI symptoms that assesses betrayal, guilt, shame, moral concerns, loss of trust, loss of meaning, difficulty forgiving, self-condemnation, religious struggle, and loss of religious/spiritual faith [94]. Response options for each of the 10 items range from 1 to 10 to signify agreement or disagreement with each statement, with a total score ranging from 10 to 100. The higher scores indicate a greater number and severity of MI symptoms [24]. Correlations with common mental conditions (depression and anxiety), well-being, and burnout measures were similar to the EMIS-SF. Factor analysis indicated a three-dimensional structure for the MISS-HP, that explained 59% of the total variance. Using this scale in HCPs in a US hospital revealed a 23.9% prevalence of MI symptoms causing at least moderate functional impairment. Younger age, shorter time in practice, committing medical errors, greater depressive or anxiety symptoms, greater clinician burnout, no religious affiliation, and lower religiosity correlated with MI symptoms [94].

Prevention and Treatment

Although service members may be exposed to traumatic and morally difficult situations throughout their career, military service can also provide a number of benefits and opportunities for growth and resilience that are not possible among civilian populations who will experience unexpected pMIEs in their lifetimes. Training for service members is often specific to battlefield ethics, leadership and resilience.

Battlefield Ethics Training

The profession of arms is fundamentally moral in nature, thus ethical challenges of modern missions need to be addressed by current military ethics educational programs. The Mental Health Advisory Teams (MHAT) ([95]; see also MHAT-V 2008) was the first to systematically investigate battlefield ethical attitudes and behaviors of US soldiers and marines deployed in Iraq and Afghanistan. Investigations by the MHAT showed that standard military ethics training had failed to ensure ethical and moral behaviours in soldiers and Marines. As a result, the MHAT introduced Battlefield Ethics Training Programs based on a chain-teaching instructional model in which senior leaders taught their immediate subordinates using video vignettes from popular movies to highlight lesson objectives. Subordinate leaders in turn taught their subordinates through all levels of military personnel to the lowest echelon. Training occurred in small groups within teams, squads, and platoons to promote discussion. Movie vignettes and leader-led discussions were demonstrated to positively influence the soldiers' understanding of how to interact with and treat noncombatants and reduced reports of ethical misconduct [96].

There is growing evidence that modern missions have added stressors and ethical complexities not seen in previous military operations and that there are links between battlefield stressors and ethical lapses. Asymmetric warfare has been a challenge to traditional military doctrine. Integrating existing research in the area, scenario-based operational ethics training in high-intensity military field training settings has been proposed as an important adjunct to traditional military ethics education and training [97, 98]. Scenario based supported interventions using movie and television clips may also be helpful in a variety of psychoeducational contexts and include evidence-based methods such as group movie therapy, art therapy, and bibliotherapy [96].

Leadership Training

As is often the case in military contexts, poor leadership can aggravate MI and the risk of unethical behaviours. Leaders must demonstrate competence, courage, candor and commitment, while steering the unit in the right direction and maintaining the rules of engagement even during the most difficult times. Commanders must make ethics a top priority throughout the deployment cycle and cannot tolerate violations. Inappropriate soldier actions should be frequently discussed throughout units. Leaders must be personally involved and be aware of their soldiers' perspectives and experiences.

Attention to and an understanding of the bidirectional relationship between moral decision-making and mental health is a crucial component of leaders' responsibility for their soldiers. That is, unethical behaviour increases the risk of mental illness and mental illness increases the risk of ethical transgressions [99, 100]. This is yet another reason leaders need to "know their troops." A culturally-aware and developmentally-focused leadership is seen as a defense against MI [62]. It is also a counter to other harmful effects of what is increasingly described as "toxic leadership" in the military, which has been cited as a common underlying factor of poor unit morale, disillusionment, and failure to respond appropriately to allegations such as sexual assault within the ranks.

This requires leadership initiatives (e.g., education and ethics training, after-action reviews, counseling, postdeployment programs) that mitigate the threat to soldier well-being. Therefore, integrated ethics training must be a part of military education, prior to and during operations. One inherent challenge stems from the fact that service members must make timely, difficult and decisive decisions with competing goals, priorities or values, such as choosing between mission success, civilian safety, force protection, and unit loyalty [101]. Military operations involve decisions requiring ongoing moral justification and can contribute to psychological and moral distress. They are also often associated with an increased likelihood of exposure to life threat and death (loss). Although they have been primarily associated with active combat, these decisions exist throughout the full-spectrum of military operations (e.g., peacekeeping, peacemaking, and humanitarian) (NATO report 2016). For these reasons, leadership training is vital as leaders at all levels are ultimately responsible for the psychological well-being of their soldiers.

Treatment

Given the co-occurrence of MI and PTSD, and widespread dissemination of evidence-based psychotherapies (EBPs) for PTSD, some individuals in the field have hypothesized that EBPs for PTSD are well-positioned to treat MI. Among these treatments, Prolonged Exposure Therapy (PE) and Cognitive Processing Therapy (CPT) are the most established. Yet MI advocates make the case that traditional, empirically validated, fear-based conceptual treatments for PTSD such as Cognitive Behavioral Therapy (CBT), PE, and CPT may not be sufficient to successfully treat or address MI with its strong component of guilt and overwhelming shame ([1], p. 702). At the heart of this, is the concern that the development of post-traumatic syndromes are fear and anxiety based, while MI may be emotionally and relationally based. Mechanisms of change, such as self-forgiveness and self-compassion, which are not integrated into traditional applications of CBT, CPT or PE, may be critical to the treatment of MI. In other words, the shame, guilt, anger, regret and bitterness that accompanies violation of one's own moral code, require a different approach to therapeutic intervention.

Moral Repair is a holistic, biopsychosocial-spiritual process (e.g., body, mind, spirit, community) [102, 103]. Repair may include: (1) *body*: reducing one's stress load, restoring physical health (diet, exercise, play, sleep), and restoring authority of the prefrontal cortex; (2) *mind:* tolerating intense negative moral emotions (e.g., shame, guilt, anger), face personal demons, assess culpability (self and others), and clarify distorted thinking (e.g., overgeneralizations); (3) *spirit:* practicing prayer, meditation, spiritual/religious practices, appreciate beauty, foster relationships self, others, with the Transcendent; and (4) *community*: fostering connection, trust, and love, and seeking true justice rather than revenge. Consideration from a multidimensional perspective is therefore needed to inform both pharmacological and non-pharmacological approaches.

The number and availability of non-PTSD specific approaches are increasing as therapies to address MI are being explored. These include: Adaptive Disclosure Therapy (ADT); Acceptance Commitment Therapy (ACT); Spiritual-Integrated Cognitive Processing Therapy (SICPT); the Impact of Killing in War (IOK); and Trauma-Informed Guilt Reduction Therapy. Approaches focusing on self-forgiveness, spirituality and atonement are also yielding promising findings. Spiritual counseling or retreats for morally injured veterans have also been advocated, such as Soul Repair [77], where a sense of purpose is redeveloped through acts of service and veterans are encouraged to confess their pMIE and receive forgiveness [104]. Nonetheless, the effectiveness of these methods remains poorly understood. As organized religion is in decline in many contexts (e.g., [105]), a means for the non-religious to experience forgiveness may potentially be beneficial to foster well-being in cases of MI. Approaches to treat MI that incorporate ceremonies or rituals may resonate with those within military cultures.

Adaptive Disclosure Therapy

Adaptive Disclosure Therapy [1] is an individualized eight-step pilot program developed for US Marines deployed to Iraq and Afghanistan. Important elements of this therapy include an imaginal dialogue that is held with a forgiving, compassionate moral authority [106]. The approach may be a middle ground between theological and clinical methods. ADT identifies the following phases:

1. Connection, defined as "a strong and genuinely caring and respectful therapeutic relationship" in which, to encourage disclosure, "the therapist must portray unconditional acceptance and the ability to listen to difficult and morally conflicted material without revulsion".
2. Preparation and Education, which helps the soldier understand MI and normalize the path to wellness.
3. Modified Exposure, which includes a "focused reliving of the event."
4. Examination and Integration, which, to provide a baseline, is an exploration of the soldier's moral code and understanding before the war events.
5. Dialogue with a Benevolent Moral Authority, which includes a technique similar to the Gestalt empty chair with a trusted person to whom to tell his/her story.
6. Reparation and Forgiveness, which allows the soldier to make amends and reconnect with personal values.
7. Fostering Reconnection, which includes connecting and reconnecting with others moving toward normalcy in relationships.
8. Planning for the Long Haul, which includes preparing for times when the trauma may be retriggered in the future and skills for managing that.

Acceptance and Commitment Therapy (ACT)

ACT, which was developed during the past decade, comes out of the third wave of cognitive behavioral therapies. While it was not specifically designed for MI, it may be well suited as a treatment for it. ACT stems from a growing body of research [107–110] that supports shifting the focus away from simply treating cognitions to expanding mental skills and flexibility to deal with life's challenges. Patients are supported in mindful awareness of their experience and acceptance techniques ([111], p. 196). The therapeutic work centers on present awareness and managing the ambiguity of cognitions where the trauma and other events of the past are juxtaposed against the "normality" of the present. ACT, with its accent on avoiding rigidity, mindfulness, and skill-building, may have additional contributions by protecting "the construct of MI from developing into an overly medicalized phenomenon" ([111], p. 204). This therapeutic model connects mindful awareness with tolerance or acceptance of unpleasant feelings without a need to do anything in response to them. This combination of thoughts, feelings and behaviors is enhanced by mindful awareness in the present with acceptance of ambiguity. The hope here is to establish a new normal rather than the "fantasy" of turning back the clock to the past. A therapist helps the veteran to understand that the starting point has to be where you are as opposed to where "you wish you were." Evan and Walser [112] have also recently written a self-directed workbook on ACT for MI which may be an asset especially in times or situations where access to trained clinicians is reduced.

The Impact of Killing in War (IOK)

Another relatively new program is the Impact of Killing in War (IOK) [113, 114]. This experimental, six-session course consists of a series of lessons to be used in conjunction with ongoing clinical treatment for PTSD for veterans suffering from MI. The first session takes an educational approach concerning the biological, psychological, and social aspects of killing in war and how these aspects can relate to the development of MI. The later sessions build on this base, looking at meaning, the self-blaming cognitions that develop, the opportunities to experience self-forgiveness, and the development of an action plan to make amends where possible.

> *Look, I don't like to kill people, but I've killed Arabs [note the unconscious dehumanizing of the enemy]. Maybe I'll tell you a story. A car came towards us, in the middle of the [Lebnese] war, with a white flag. Five minutes before another car had come, and there were four Palestinians with RPGs [rocket-propelled grenades] in it - killed three of my friends. So this new Peugeot comes toward us, and we shoot. And there was a family there - three children. And I cried, but I couldn't take the chance. It's a real problem….Children, father, mother. All the family was killed, but we couldn't take the chance (Gaby Bashan, Israeli reservist in Lebanon, 1982* (from [115], quoted in [116], p. 2014).

Trauma-Informed Guilt Reduction Therapy (TrIGR)

Trauma-informed guilt reduction therapy (TrIGR) [117] is a cognitive-behavioral transdiagnostic intervention that offers a potentially useful model and brief protocol (4–6 sessions). TrIGR is built on the model of nonadaptive guilt and shame (NAGS; [118]). Guilt can be adaptive when it helps shape one's actions to be more prosocial and values driven. For example, feeling guilty after violating social distancing norms may lead someone to exercise more caution going forward, which then ameliorates that guilt. In contrast, nonadaptive guilt results when distress is taken as evidence of wrongdoing (e.g., "I feel terrible so I must have done something horribly wrong") and leads to avoidance of thinking about the stressful event. As a result, it may become impossible to evaluate actual evidence and come to an accurate perspective or change one's behavior, thereby maintaining and worsening guilt and distress. The guilt may become shame if someone comes to believe that their role in the stressful event speaks negatively about their value as a person. The NAGS model postulates that this cycle of guilt and shame cognitions and distress is what leads to increased symptom severity and functional problems. Furthermore, the model postulates that guilt and shame play a function for the client in expressing values.

Spiritually-Integrated Cognitive Processing Therapy (SICPT)

Spiritually-Integrated Cognitive Processing Therapy (SICPT) [119] is a novel treatment adapted from CPT to specifically include spiritual resources or targeted spiritual distress, both important components of MI. This 12-week treatment differs from CPT in 5 major ways. First, SICPT specifically targets MI as a major barrier to achieving recovery from PTSD, whereas CPT directly targets PTSD. Second, SICPT targets MI by challenging erroneous interpretations of trauma by focusing on cognitive restructuring using clients' spiritual/religious resources (i.e., spiritual beliefs, practices, sacred writings, values, and motivations) to challenge maladaptive thinking patterns. Third, given the need for moral repair, SICPT employs spiritual tools to help resolve MI and its damaging sequelae, such as shame, guilt, rage, demoralization, and self-handicapping behaviors. Fourth, SICPT also encourages patients to access support from or immersion in a faith community, which can help with recovery and reintegration. Finally, in addition to identifying spiritual resources to aid in recovery, spiritual struggles, which are part of MI, are specifically normalized and addressed in treatment. Spiritual struggles might include: feeling angry at God (or a higher power) for allowing this to happen; feeling punished by God; questioning God's love and one's religious faith; feeling abandoned by God or one's faith community; or a complete loss of faith as a result of severely traumatic experiences. SICPT has also been developed for five religions (Christianity, Judaism, Islam, Buddhism, and Hinduism) for clients who desire a more religion-specific approach.

Spiritually-Oriented Treatments

Currently, there are complimentary spiritually-oriented treatment modalities being explored by clinicians and researchers that are demonstrating early promising results. A review of treatment modalities being used by chaplains in the American Veteran Affairs system noted that pastoral counselling, promoting meaning-making activities, engaging in forgiveness or repair activities, addressing emotional regulation and supporting the use of spiritual practices were helpful to healing MI [120]. Similarly, Canadian Armed Forces mental health chaplains have supported the healing of MI through bridging with other mental health services and supports, facilitating spiritual coping and grounding, reconciling worldviews, resolving anger at a God-figure (not specific to any perspective) and fostering reconciliation [121]. Additional spiritual practices to aid in the recovery of MI may include: prayer; meditation; spiritual/religious practices; spiritual guidance/direction; and the use of narratives, story-telling or spiritual writing [102, 122, 123]. The writing practice of lament, in which a person writes about one's distress to God, has been noted to be a therapeutic means for some service members to express their moral pain and suffering [123, 124]. Moreover, letter writing to facilitate disclosure and augment forgiveness may be less intensive than repeated verbal admissions:

> *To the People of Iraq, please allow me to express my sorrow for all that I have contributed to as an occupier of your country....I became something furthest from what I wanted or set out to be – something vile and disgusting – something I hate....[I] now am sorry and ashamed of the murderer I became....I do have blood on my hands. And it is hard to wash off. (in* [44]*).*

Forgiveness-based experiences have also been found to have a significant impact [125]. Travels to the battleground can ritualize or augment an exposure. While such initiatives have not been reported in literature, several have been undertaken. It is recommended to travel in small groups, preferably not with family, and have a specific itinerary containing places to be visited. Such trips may also allow veterans to connect with locals. Several countries have started initiatives. For the Dutch mission to former Yugoslavia, a recent recommendation was made to promote these 'back with a mission' initiatives. These can be organized with mental health support or chaplains. While more research on this intervention is needed, many nations, such as US veterans returning to Vietnam, have used this "therapeutic" approach for many years [126].

Meaning-Making and Divergent Thinking

Contemporary models of coping suggest that maladjustment after trauma ensues from a mismatch between distressing realities associated with the stressor and one's meaning-making system. Difficulties with meaning making, both global and situational, could serve as a mediating pathway for how pMIEs increase the risk for adjustment problems after warzone service [102, 127]. Challenges in recovery, as observed in cases of MI, may arise to the degree that veterans cannot integrate the appraised reality of their warzone experiences into global meaning and/or cannot accommodate beliefs/values or life goals to "make sense" (situationally) or construct meaning out of these stressors [127]. The process of divergent thinking as it relates to new meaning or 'thinking outside the box' or 'having a corrective experience' may contribute to a new perspective of the situation or self that enables acceptance and personal growth [128]. Such a thought process or method, which typically occurs in a spontaneous, free-flowing, "non-linear" manner such that many ideas are generated in an emergent cognitive fashion, can be used to generate creative ideas by exploring many possible solutions.

Self-Perception and Attachment

One's self-perception and attachments can be fragmented by exposure to pMIEs, fundamentally impacting both the person, and relationships with self and others [102, 129, 130]. When fragmentation occurs, the self tries to restore a sense of coherence, wholeness or vigor. Most symptomatic behaviour that can be seen in MI may be viewed as an emergency attempt to maintain or restore internal cohesion and harmony to a vulnerable unhealthy self [131]. Further, the self and world contain information about relationships, including one's attachment figures, their availability, and the way they are expected to react in times of need and distress [132]. These can also be compromised by MI. Attachment representations are activated in situations of fear and perceived danger and likely affect reactions to fearful and emotionally painful internal and external stimuli.

> *On a fundamental level, "Traumatic events call into question basic human relationships. They breach attachments of family, friendship, love and community, they shatter the construction of the self that is formed and sustained in relations to others. They undermine the belief systems that give meaning to human experiences. They violate the victim's faith in a natural or divine order and cast the victim into a state of existential crisis…Traumatic events destroy the victim's fundamental assumptions about the safety of the world, the positive value of the self, and the meaningful order of creation"* ([133], p. 50, in [134], p. 20).

A realistic appraisal of these stimuli, of one's needs for reassurance and of the potential role of others in alleviating the fear, is guided by secure/autonomous attachment representations. Future research on MI would benefit from further consideration of the role of attachment and connection [135], including within cultural, social, and faith-based communities [102].

Emerging Treatments

Pharmacological and nonpharmacological treatment approaches are currently emerging. While existing FDA approved pharmacotherapy treatments for moral injury are lacking and there is no clear indication for off-label use, a number of noteworthy pharmacotherapy and psychotherapy options are under study.

Psychedelic-assisted therapy In the 1970s in the Netherlands, survivors of concentration camps of WWII were treated with Lysergic acid diethylamide (LSD) psychotherapy to free their mind of the camp. Subsequent psychotherapy was reported to result in lasting positive impacts, but the use of LSD was banned [136]. Recently, new interest has emerged with the use of 3,4-methylenedioxymethamphetamine (MDMA) for combat-related PTSD. Several working models of corrective experiences utilizing psychedelic pharmaceuticals hold promise. Currently, MDMA assisted therapy is finishing phase 3 clinical research trials and the results have been promising for registration for PTSD. Similar results have been found in the use of psilocybin for depression that may be used trans-diagnostically in a similar paradigm for addressing emotions related to the isolation, grief, guilt, and anger of MI. Ayahuasca and other psychedelic compounds are used by some in group settings with indigenous therapists to cleanse themselves and experience healing by what also can be labeled as a corrective experience. These psychedelics may prove to change underlying neural networks and allow for the introduction of ideas that effectively challenge feelings such as guilt and shame.

Intensification of treatment Offering an intensive in-patient program with modalities such as EMDR [137–139] and other psychotherapies can potentially improve outcomes. This therapeutic approach may be effective in allowing patients to open up, break down avoidance patterns, and thus promote therapeutic effectiveness. Such a strategy, while yet to be formally applied to MI, may prove effective with those exposed to pMIEs.

Virtual Reality Exposure Therapies A relatively novel intervention targeting the breakdown of cognitive avoidance is Motion-assisted, Multi-modular Memory Desensitization and Reconsolidation (3MDR). The intervention incorporates exposure therapy, psychotherapy, EMDR, virtual reality, supportive counselling, and treadmill walking. As moving forward opens and encourages divergent thinking, a personalized approach allows disclosure of forgotten memories and the processing of high intensity emotions such as guilt and shame [140]. Three randomized control trials have demonstrated efficacy with low dropout rates among participants who were combat veterans [141–144]. Jones et al. [144] demonstrated a significantly significant reduction in MI symptoms on the MISS-M (n = 11) pre/post 6 sessions of 3MDR.

Soul Repair Drescher et al. [145] work on MI is focused on a treatment called 'Soul Repair'. The authors describe this method as being primarily used by clergy, chaplains, spiritual care providers, and mental health providers. The treatment focuses on "connecting within a supportive community, building friendships, emotional expression through the arts, recovering meaning and purpose through service, and 'deep listening' on the part of the helpers" (p. 53). The central concepts are those of bearing witness and therapeutic presence.

Animal assisted therapies Ferruolo [146] and other clinicians and researchers have observed that veterans with psychological impairments may resist traditional talk therapies and seek alternative treatments. Equine assisted therapy has demonstrated promising outcomes in a myriad of studies around the globe. Ferruolo [146] reported on a pilot study with significant improvement in depression, anxiety, and PTSD in veterans. A recent trial in Dutch veterans in a 12-week program resulted in favorable outcomes. Animal assisted therapies may facilitate a process of self-acceptance that is essential to treatment of MI. Research specific to animal assisted therapies and the effect on MI is emerging and ongoing.

Discussion

In this chapter, the central elements of MI—moral beliefs, pMIEs, and moral suffering—are discussed with reference to the relevant literature. Keeping these elements in mind, an overview was provided of assessments as well as therapeutic approaches. Two case reports served to illustrate that guilt and shame, when left unrecognized and untreated, may contribute to chronic pathology and be a barrier to therapeutic change. The denial or repression of guilt and shame may be the "pressure cooker" that can lead to other presentations including distressing dreams, feelings of anger, self-hatred, distorted cognitions, somatic symptoms, or chronic fatigue. The pMIEs are not necessarily the overwhelming trauma we see in PTSD, although they can be. The patient's wounds and their stories have shaped the life of the individual, much in the same fashion as if they sustained burns or amputations. Although guilt is recognized in DSM-5 as an important feature of PTSD, it has received far less recognition than other symptoms that are associated with fear and intense threat [147].

MI is an emerging construct related to military trauma and stress for which scientific research and potential innovations in clinical practice are sorely needed [1, 33, 148]. Attention is shifting from the amygdalocentric fear-based approach of post-trauma reactions towards a type of disorder in which core drivers are guilt and shame. In the first iteration of the PTSD construct (DSM-III) 'guilt about surviving while others have not or about behavior required for survival' was a symptom of PTSD. This was chiefly the result of the predominance of thinking about the phenomenology of Vietnam veterans and clinical care experience with veterans of war. Consequently, prior to the DSM-III-R, clinicians in VA settings arguably would have frequently seen and attempted to alleviate MI (e.g., [29]). Since then, however, there has been very little attention paid to the lasting impact of moral conflict-colored psychological trauma among war veterans in the clinical science community.

The field of MI interventions are maturing rapidly. The lexicon of MI is predominantly clinical, which can obscure its non-clinical etiology and impact. MI, still a relatively new concept in the psychotrauma field, refers to moral suffering associated with exposure to pMIEs. It is an attractive, but still insufficiently precise, concept that is increasingly used in clinical settings and is broadly interpreted. As a consequence, the concept risks losing clinical utility in the future. It remains unclear if MI warrants a clinical diagnosis, or if it is something that may complicate other conditions such as PTSD. Some have questioned whether it can be a subtype of PTSD such as the dissociative subtype that was recently established in the DSM5. A greater understanding of MI, its assessment and treatment is yet needed to better address the profound human suffering that can result from exposure to pMIEs.

Future research is yet needed in the area of MI. This includes a better conceptual understanding of MI and its relations to PTSD and other conditions (including whether it is a sub-type of or distinct from PTSD), and the underlying neurobiology of MI. Psychometrics and evidence-based interventions also require further consideration. Isolating the neural correlates of MI could be invaluable in guiding development of successful therapies. Of particular interest may be both psychedelic-, virtual-reality and spiritually-integrated psychotherapies. Several gaps exist in current care provision for morally injured veterans, including issues related to spirituality, employment and family functioning, which could ultimately improve veteran well-being [149]. Further, as research has predominantly focused on military populations, an understanding of pMIES and MI experienced by other populations is warranted. Research into community-based, socially-oriented and culturally-specific approaches to MI are also yet required. Finally, direct participation from chaplains, clergy, and religious communities in the treatment of MI may help address the spiritual issues [150]. If we listen empathically to those who struggle following exposure to pMIEs and try to understand their suffering, we will be guided to a better understanding of MI. This generation is well-positioned to expand research and clinical efforts to address psychological injuries such as MI in support of those who continue to support us.

Clinical Pearls

- Moral Injury (MI), a term used to describe the persistent distress that individuals may develop or have when they perpetrate, witness, or fail to prevent an act that transgresses their core beliefs, is increasingly being referred to as a syndrome characterized by guilt, shame, intrusive thoughts, anger and self-condemnation. It is not currently a recognized mental health disorder in the DSM-5.
- While MI may have a trauma component and often coexists with PTSD, it is not exclusively fear-based. Persons can develop MI due to exposure to potentially morally injurious events (pMIES) that result in a fracturing of personal morals, beliefs, values, character and relationships.

- The consequences of MI are found across all health domains including psychological, emotional, relational, social/familial, spiritual and professional.
- Recognizing MI as honorable may reduce stigma and psychological harm, and facilitate help-seeking among uniformed personnel and other trauma-affected populations.
- Assessment and interventions are currently limited.
- Current evidence-based PTSD interventions fail to provide sufficient guidance for topics such as forgiveness, guilt and shame.
- Further research is needed regarding the concept and mechanism of MI, the relationship between MI and PTSD, the experience of MI in various populations, psychometrics, and effective evidence-based interventions.

Acknowledgement The authors also want to express gratitude to the Nyperls-Tans PTSD fund at Leiden University to Dr Vermetten.

References

1. Litz BT, Stein N, Delaney E, Lebowitz L, Nash WP, Silva C, Maguen S. Moral injury and moral repair in war veterans: a preliminary model and intervention strategy. Clin Psychol Rev. 2009;29(8):695–706. https://doi.org/10.1016/j.cpr.2009.07.003.
2. Jinkerson JD. Defining and assessing moral injury: a syndrome perspective. Traumatology. 2016;22(2):122.
3. Berger JT, Hamric AB, Epstein E. Self-inflicted moral distress: opportunity for a fuller exercise of professionalism. J Clin Ethics. 2019;30(4):314–7. https://www.ncbi.nlm.nih.gov/pubmed/31851622. Accessed 11 Apr 2021.
4. Jameton A. What moral distress in nursing history could suggest about the future of health care. AMA J Ethics. 2017;19(6):617–28. https://doi.org/10.1001/journalofethics.2017.19.6.mhst1-1706.
5. American Psychiatric Association. Diagnostic and statistical manual of mental disorders: DSM-5, vol. 10. Washington, DC: American Psychiatric Association; 2013.
6. Koenig HG, Youssef NA, Ames D, Oliver JP, Teng EJ, Haynes K, et al. Moral injury and religiosity in US veterans with posttraumatic stress disorder symptoms. J Nerv Ment Dis. 2018;206(5):325–31. https://doi.org/10.1097/NMD.0000000000000798.
7. Bryan CJ, Bryan AO, Roberge E, Leifker FR, Rozek DC. Moral injury, posttraumatic stress disorder, and suicidal behavior among National Guard personnel. Psychol Trauma. 2018;10(1):36–45. https://doi.org/10.1037/tra0000290.
8. Bryan AO, Bryan CJ, Morrow CE, Etienne N, Ray-Sannerud B. Moral injury, suicidal ideation, and suicide attempts in a military sample. Traumatology. 2014;20(3):154–60.
9. Koenig HG, Youssef NA, Pearce M. Assessment of moral injury in veterans and active duty military personnel with PTSD: a review. Front Psych. 2019;10:443. https://doi.org/10.3389/fpsyt.2019.00443.
10. Wood D. The grunts – damned if they kill, damned if they don't. Huffington Post, March 18, 2014. 2014. http://projects.huffingtonpost.com/moral-injury/the-grunts.
11. Shay J. Casualties. Deadalus. 2011;140(3):179–88.
12. Shay J. The trials of homecoming: Odysseus returns from Iraq/Afghanistan. Smith College Stud Soc Work. 2009;79:286–98.
13. Steenkamp MM, Nash WP, Lebowitz L, Litz BT. How best to treat deployment-related guilt and shame: commentary on Smith, Daux and Rauch (2013). Cogn Behav Pract. 2013;20:471–5.

14. Stein NR, Mills MA, Arditte K, Mendoza C, Borah AM, Resick PA, et al. A scheme for categorizing traumatic military events. Behav Modif. 2012;36(6):787–807. https://doi.org/10.1177/0145445512446945.
15. Thompson M. Moral injury in military operations—a review of the literature and key considerations for the Canadian Armed Forces. Defence Research and Development Canada Scientific Report, DRDC-RDDC-2015-R029, March 2015. 2015. http://cradpdf.drdc-rddc.gc.ca/PDFS/unc203/p801216_A1b.pdf.
16. Bryan CJ, Roberge E, Bryan AO, Ray-Sannerud B, Morrow CE, Etienne N. Guilt as a mediator of the relationship between depression and posttraumatic stress with suicide ideation in two samples of military personnel and veterans. Int J Cogn Ther. 2015;8(2):143–55.
17. Bryan CJ, Ray-Sannerud B, Heron EA. Psychological flexibility as a dimension of resilience for posttraumatic stress, depression, and risk for suicidal ideation among air force personnel. J Contextual Behav Sci. 2015;4(4):263–8.
18. McNair RM. Perpetration-induced traumatic stress in combat veterans. Peace Conflict J Peace Psychol. 2002;8(1):63–72.
19. Canadian Institute for Public Safety Research and Treatment (CIPSRT). Glossary of terms: a shared understanding of the common terms used to describe psychological trauma (version 2.1). Regina, SK: University of Regina; 2019. https://doi.org/10.37119/10294/9055.
20. Papazoglou K, Blumberg DM, Chiongbian VB, Tuttle BM, Kamkar K, Chopko B, et al. The role of moral injury in PTSD among law enforcement officers: a brief report. Front Psychol. 2020;11:310. https://doi.org/10.3389/fpsyg.2020.00310.
21. Lennon RP, Day PG, Marra J. Recognizing moral injury: toward legal intervention for physician burnout. Hast Cent Rep. 2020;50(3):81. https://doi.org/10.1002/hast.1146.
22. Lesley M. Psychoanalytic perspectives on moral injury in nurses on the frontlines of the COVID-19 pandemic. J Am Psychiatr Nurses Assoc. 2020;27:72–6. https://doi.org/10.1177/1078390320960535.
23. Greene T, Bloomfield MAP, Billings J. Psychological trauma and moral injury in religious leaders during COVID-19. Psychol Trauma. 2020;12(S1):S143–5. https://doi.org/10.1037/tra0000641.
24. Zhizhong W, Koenig HG, Yan T, Jing W, Mu S, Hongyu L, Guangtian L. Psychometric properties of the Moral Injury Symptom Scale among Chinese health professionals during the COVID-19 pandemic. BMC Psychiatry. 2020;20(1):556. https://doi.org/10.1186/s12888-020-02954-w.
25. Kitchiner NJ, Lewis C, Roberts NP, Bisson JI. Active duty and ex-serving military personnel with post-traumatic stress disorder treated with psychological therapies: systematic review and meta-analysis. Eur J Psychotraumatol. 2019;10(1):1684226. https://doi.org/10.1080/20008198.2019.1684226.
26. Steenkamp MM, Litz BT, Gray MJ, Lebowitz L, Nash W, Conoscenti L, Amidon A, Lang A. A brief exposure-based intervention for service members with PTSD. Cogn Behav Pract. 2011;18(1):98–107. https://doi.org/10.1016/j.cbpra.2009.08.006.
27. Steenkamp MM, Litz BT, Hoge CW, Marmar CR. Psychotherapy for military-related PTSD: a review of randomized clinical trials. JAMA. 2015;314(5):489–500. https://doi.org/10.1001/jama.2015.8370.
28. Vermetten E, Jetly R. A critical outlook on combat-related PTSD: review and case reports of guilt and shame as drivers for moral injury. Mil Behav Health. 2018;6(2):156–64. https://doi.org/10.1080/21635781.2018.1459973.
29. Friedman MJ. Post-Vietnam syndrome: recognition and management. Psychosomatics. 1981;22(11):931–43. https://doi.org/10.1016/S0033-3182(81)73455-8.
30. Shay J. Achilles in Vietnam: combat trauma and the undoing of character. Scribner; 1994.
31. Shay J. Moral injury. Psychoanal Psychol. 2014;31(2):182–91. https://doi.org/10.1037/a0036090.
32. Drescher KD, Foy DW, Kelly C, Leshner A, Schutz K, Litz B. An exploration of the viability and usefulness of the construct of moral injury in war veterans. Traumatology. 2011;17(1):8–13. https://doi.org/10.1177/1534765610395615.

33. Farnsworth JK, Drescher KD, Evans W, Walser RD. A functional approach to understanding and treating military-related moral injury. J Contextual Behav Sci. 2017;6(4):391–7. https://doi.org/10.1016/j.jcbs.2017.07.003.
34. Kubany ES. A cognitive model of guilt typology in combat-related PTSD. J Trauma Stress. 1994;7(1):3–19. https://doi.org/10.1007/BF02111908.
35. Norman SB, Haller M, Kim HM, Allard CB, Porter KE, Stein MB, et al. Trauma related guilt cognitions partially mediate the relationship between PTSD symptom severity and functioning among returning combat veterans. J Psychiatr Res. 2018;100:56–62. https://doi.org/10.1016/j.jpsychires.2018.02.003.
36. Ames D, Erickson Z, Youssef NA, Arnold I, Adamson CS, Sones AC, et al. Moral injury, religiosity, and suicide risk in U.S. veterans and active duty military with PTSD symptoms. Mil Med. 2019;184(3–4):e271–8. https://doi.org/10.1093/milmed/usy148.
37. Smigelsky MA, Jardin C, Nieuwsma JA, Brancu M, Meador KG, Molloy KG, et al. Religion, spirituality, and suicide risk in Iraq and Afghanistan era veterans. Depress Anxiety. 2020;37(8):728–37. https://doi.org/10.1002/da.23013.
38. Shay J. Moral injury. Psychoanalytic Psychol. 2014;31(2):182–91. https://doi.org/10.1037/a0036090.
39. Shay J. Moral injury. Intertexts. 2012;16(1):57–66. https://doi.org/10.1353/itx.2012.0000.
40. Santoli A. Everything we had: an oral history of the Vietnam war by thirty-three American soldiers who fought it, vol. 2009. Baker and Taylor; 2009.
41. Litz BT, Contractor AA, Rhodes C, Dondanville KA, Jordan AH, Resick PA, et al. Distinct trauma types in military service members seeking treatment for posttraumatic stress disorder. J Trauma Stress. 2018;31(2):286–95.
42. Richardson NM, Lamson AL, Smith M, Eagan SM, Zvonkovic AM, Jensen J. Defining moral injury among military populations: a systematic review. J Trauma Stress. 2020;33(4):575–86. https://doi.org/10.1002/jts.22553.
43. Corley MC, Elswick RK, Gorman M, Clor T. Development and evaluation of a moral distress scale. J Adv Nurs. 2001;33(2):250–6. https://onlinelibrary.wiley.com/doi/pdf/10.1111/j.1365-2648.2001.01658.x?casa_token=upj-EKmwHuMAAAAA%3ASbfs3xuRsMonsWajJw-FOu_rwx95tKwiKzRPG-Pg_Y73GzmCiaW_JbjJ5eshm0IzkgYH_H0N8DX4jA. Accessed 11 Apr 2021.
44. Atuel HR, Barr N, Jones E, Greenberg N, Williamson V, Schumacher MR, et al. Understanding moral injury from a character domain perspective. J Theor Philos Psychol. 2021;41(3):155–73.
45. Haidt J. The moral emotions. 2003.
46. Kroll J, Egan E. Psychiatry, moral worry, and the moral emotions. J Psychiatr Pract. 2004;10(6):352–60.
47. Jones E. Moral injury in a context of trauma. Br J Psychiatry. 2020;216(3):127–8. https://doi.org/10.1192/bjp.2020.46.
48. Frankfurt S, Frazier P. A review of research on moral injury in combat veterans. Mil Psychol. 2016;28(5):318–30.
49. Maguen S, Metzler TJ, Litz BT, Seal KH, Knight SJ, Marmar CR. The impact of killing in war on mental health symptoms and related functioning. J Trauma Stress. 2009;22(5):435–43. https://doi.org/10.1002/jts.20451.
50. de Graaff MC, Schut M, Verweij DE, Vermetten E, Giebels E. Emotional reactions and moral judgment: the effects of morally challenging interactions in military operations. Ethics Behav. 2016;26(1):14–31. https://doi.org/10.1080/10508422.2014.975815.
51. Vermetten E, Jetly R. Moral decisions in military operations and its relevance for mental health practice and outcomes. Moral decisions and military mental health. North Atlantic Treaty Organization STO technical report. AC/323(HFM-179)TP/718. 2016. https://apps.dtic.mil/dtic/tr/fulltext/u2/1048941.pdf. Accessed 11 Apr 2021.
52. Dennis PA, Dennis NM, Van Voorhees EE, Calhoun PS, Dennis MF, Beckham JC. Moral transgression during the Vietnam War: a path analysis of the psychological impact of veterans' involvement in wartime atrocities. Anxiety Stress Coping. 2017;30(2):188–201.

53. Kienzler H. Debating war-trauma and post-traumatic stress disorder (PTSD) in an interdisciplinary arena. Soc Sci Med. 2008;67(2):218–27.
54. Battles AR, Bravo AJ, Kelley ML, White TD, Braitman AL, Hamrick HC. Moral injury and PTSD as mediators of the associations between morally injurious experiences and mental health and substance use. Traumatology. 2018;24(4):246.
55. Murray E, Krahé C, Goodsman D. Are medical students in prehospital care at risk of moral injury? Emerg Med J. 2018;35(10):590–4.
56. Papazoglou K, Chopko B. The role of moral suffering (moral distress and moral injury) in police compassion fatigue and PTSD: an unexplored topic. Front Psychol. 2017;8:1999.
57. Nickerson A, Schnyder U, Bryant RA, Schick M, Mueller J, Morina N. Moral injury in traumatized refugees. Psychother Psychosom. 2015;84(2):122–3.
58. Williamson V, Stevelink SA, Greenberg N. Occupational moral injury and mental health: systematic review and meta-analysis. Br J Psychiatry. 2018;212(6):339–46.
59. Hoge CW, Castro CA, Messer SC, McGurk D, Cotting DI, Koffman RL. Combat duty in Iraq and Afghanistan, mental health problems, and barriers to care. N Engl J Med. 2004;351(1):13–22. https://doi.org/10.1056/NEJMoa040603.
60. Reijnen A, Rademaker AR, Vermetten E, Geuze E. Prevalence of mental health symptoms in Dutch military personnel returning from deployment to Afghanistan: a 2-year longitudinal analysis. Eur Psychiatry. 2015;30(2):341–6. https://doi.org/10.1016/j.eurpsy.2014.05.003.
61. Rietveld N. De gewetensvolle veteraan: schuld-en schaamtebeleving bij veteranen van vredesmissies. 2009.
62. Molendijk T. Moral injury in relation to public debates: the role of societal misrecognition in moral conflict-colored trauma among soldiers. Soc Sci Med. 2018;211:314–20. https://doi.org/10.1016/j.socscimed.2018.06.042.
63. Dallaire R. Waiting for first light: my ongoing battle with PTSD. New York: Vintage Books; 2019.
64. Nash WP. Commentary on the special issue on moral injury: unpacking two models for understanding moral injury. J Trauma Stress. 2019;32(3):465–70. https://doi.org/10.1002/jts.22409.
65. Jin J, Weiman K, Bremault-Phillips S, Vermetten E. Moral injury and recovery in uniformed professionals: lessons from conversations among international students and experts. Front Psychiatry. 2022;1256.
66. Barnes HA, Hurley RA, Taber KH. Moral injury and PTSD: often co-occurring yet mechanistically different. J Neuropsychiatry Clin Neurosci. 2019;31(2):A4–103. https://doi.org/10.1176/appi.neuropsych.19020036.
67. Sun D, Phillips RD, Mulready HL, Zablonski ST, Turner JA, Turner MD, et al. Resting-state brain fluctuation and functional connectivity dissociate moral injury from posttraumatic stress disorder. Depress Anxiety. 2019;36(5):442–52. https://doi.org/10.1002/da.22883.
68. Bastin C, Harrison BJ, Davey CG, Moll J, Whittle S. Feelings of shame, embarrassment and guilt and their neural correlates: a systematic review. Neurosci Biobehav Rev. 2016;71:455–71. https://doi.org/10.1016/j.neubiorev.2016.09.019.
69. Gifuni AJ, Kendal A, Jollant F. Neural mapping of guilt: a quantitative meta-analysis of functional imaging studies. Brain Imaging Behav. 2017;11(4):1164–78. https://doi.org/10.1007/s11682-016-9606-6.
70. Nash WP, Marino Carper TL, Mills MA, Au T, Goldsmith A, Litz BT. Psychometric evaluation of the moral injury events scale. Mil Med. 2013;178(6):646–52.
71. Currier JM, Holland JM, Drescher K, Foy D. Initial psychometric evaluation of the Moral Injury Questionnaire—Military version. Clin Psychol Psychother. 2015;22(1):54–63.
72. Currier JM, Isaak SL, McDermott RC. Validation of the Expressions of Moral Injury Scale-Military version-short form. Clin Psychol Psychother. 2020;27(1):61–8.
73. Currier JM, McDermott RC, Farnsworth JK, Borges LM. Temporal associations between moral injury and posttraumatic stress disorder symptom clusters in military veterans. J Trauma Stress. 2019;32(3):382–92.

74. Koenig H, Ames D, Youssef NA, Oliver JP, Volk F, Teng EJ, Haynes K, Erickson ZD, Arnold I, O'Garo K. Pearce screening for moral injury: the moral injury symptom scale – military version short form. Mil Med. 2018;183(11):e659–65. https://doi.org/10.1093/milmed/usy017.
75. Litz BT, Phelps A, Frankfurt S, Murphy D, Nazarov A, Houle S, Levi-Belz Y, Zerach G, Dell L, Hosseiny F, The Members of the Moral Injury Outcome Scale (MIOS) Consortium. The moral injury outcome scale; 2020.
76. Braitman AL, Battles AR, Kelley ML, Hamrick HC, Cramer RJ, Ehlke S, Bravo AJ. Psychometric properties of a Modified Moral Injury Questionnaire in a military population. Traumatology. 2018;24(4):301.
77. Brock RN, Lettini G. Soul repair: recovering from moral injury after war. Beacon Press; 2012.
78. Yeterian JD, Berke DS, Carney JR, McIntyre-Smith A, St. Cyr K, King L, et al. Defining and measuring moral injury: rationale, design, and preliminary findings from the moral injury outcome scale consortium. J Trauma Stress. 2019;32(3):363–72. https://doi.org/10.1002/jts.22380.
79. Kopacz MS, Ames D, Koenig HG. It's time to talk about physician burnout and moral injury. Lancet Psychiatry. 2019;6(11):e28.
80. Ford EW. Stress, burnout, and moral injury: the state of the healthcare workforce. J Healthc Manag. 2019;64(3):125–7.
81. Lu W, Wang H, Lin Y, Li L. Psychological status of medical workforce during the COVID-19 pandemic: a cross-sectional study. Psychiatry Res. 2020;288:112936.
82. Dean E, Jones A, Yu HPM, Gosselink R, Skinner M. Translating COVID-19 evidence to maximize physical therapists' impact and public health response. Phys Ther. 2020;100(9):1458–64.
83. Favà A, Cucchiari D, Montero N, Toapanta N, Centellas FJ, Vila-Santandreu A, et al. Clinical characteristics and risk factors for severe COVID-19 in hospitalized kidney transplant recipients: a multicentric cohort study. Am J Transplant. 2020;20(11):3030–41.
84. Person B, Sy F, Holton K, Govert B, Liang A, Team SCO, et al. Fear and stigma: the epidemic within the SARS outbreak. Emerg Infect Dis. 2004;10(2):358.
85. Jetly R, Vermetten E, Easterbrook B, Lanius R, McKinnon M. Going to "war": military approach as the antidote to defeating COVID-19. Mil Behav Health. 2020;8(3):243–7.
86. Hamric AB, Borchers CT, Epstein EG. Development and testing of an instrument to measure moral distress in healthcare professionals. AJOB Prim Res. 2012;3(2):1–9. https://doi.org/10.1080/21507716.2011.652337.
87. Schaefer R, Zoboli EL, Vieira MM. Psychometric evaluation of the moral distress risk scale: a methodological study. Nurs Ethics. 2019;26(2):434–42. https://doi.org/10.1177/0969733017707347.
88. Sporrong SK, Höglund AT, Arnetz B. Measuring moral distress in pharmacy and clinical practice. Nurs Ethics. 2006;13(4):416–27.
89. Eizenberg MM, Desivilya HS, Hirschfeld MJ. Moral distress questionnaire for clinical nurses: instrument development. J Adv Nurs. 2009;65(4):885–92. https://doi.org/10.1111/j.1365-2648.2008.04945.x.
90. Glasberg AL, Eriksson S, Dahlqvist V, Lindahl E, Strandberg G, Söderberg A, et al. Development and initial validation of the stress of conscience questionnaire. Nurs Ethics. 2006;13(6):633–48. https://doi.org/10.1177/0969733006069698.
91. Ohnishi K, Ohgushi Y, Nakano M, Fujii H, Tanaka H, Kitaoka K, et al. Moral distress experienced by psychiatric nurses in Japan. Nurs Ethics. 2010;17(6):726–40. https://doi.org/10.1177/0969733010379178.
92. Lazzarin M, Biondi A, Di Mauro S. Moral distress in nurses in oncology and haematology units. Nurs Ethics. 2012;19(2):183–95. https://doi.org/10.1177/0969733011416840.
93. Shoorideh FA, Ashktorab T, Yaghmaei F, Alavi Majd H. Relationship between ICU nurses' moral distress with burnout and anticipated turnover. Nurs Ethics. 2015;22(1):64–76. https://doi.org/10.1177/0969733014534874.

94. Mantri S, Lawson JM, Wang Z, Koenig HG. Prevalence and predictors of moral injury symptoms in health care professionals. J Nerv Ment Dis. 2020;209:174–80. https://doi.org/10.1097/NMD.0000000000001277.
95. Castro CA, McGurk D. The intensity of combat and behavioral health status. Traumatology. 2007;13(4):6–23.
96. Warner CH, Appenzeller GN, Mobbs A, Parker JR, Warner CM, Grieger T, Hoge CW. Effectiveness of battlefield-ethics training during combat deployment: a programme assessment. Lancet. 2011;378(9794):915–24. https://doi.org/10.1016/S0140-6736(11)61039-8.
97. Thompson MM, Jetly R. Battlefield ethics training: integrating ethical scenarios in high-intensity military field exercises. Eur J Psychotraumatol. 2014;5:23668. https://doi.org/10.3402/ejpt.v5.23668.
98. Brémault-Phillips S, Bright KS, Phillips A, Vermetten E. Scenario-based supported interventions for moral injury and posttraumatic stress disorder: data report of film and television references for use with uniformed professionals. Front Psychiatry. 2022;13.
99. Blanc J-RS. Combat exposure and ethical attitudes: preliminary model and mitigation strategy (Doctoral dissertation, Saint Mary's University, Halifax, Nova Scotia, Canada). 2012. http://library2.smu.ca/handle/01/24802. Accessed 11 Apr 2021.
100. Blanc S. Relationship between unethical battlefield conduct and mental health. Moral decisions and military mental health. North Atlantic Treaty Organization STO technical report. AC/323(HFM-179)TP/718. 2018. https://apps.dtic.mil/dtic/tr/fulltext/u2/1048941.pdf. Accessed 11 Apr 2021.
101. Farnsworth JK, Drescher KD, Nieuwsma JA, Walser RB, Currier JM. The role of moral emotions in military trauma: implications for the study and treatment of moral injury. Rev Gen Psychol. 2014;18(4):249–62.
102. Brémault-Phillips S, Pike A, Scarcella F, Cherwick T. Spirituality and moral injury among military personnel: a mini-review. Front Psych. 2019;10:276. https://doi.org/10.3389/fpsyt.2019.00276. PMID: 31110483.
103. Nash WP. Identity and imagination in moral injury and moral repair. Vancouver, BC: Canadian Institute for Military and Veteran Health Research; 2016.
104. Antal CJ, Winings K. Moral injury, soul repair, and creating a place for grace. Relig Educ. 2015;110(4):382–94.
105. Houtman D, Aupers S. The spiritual turn and the decline of tradition: the spread of post-Christian spirituality in 14 Western countries, 1981–2000. J Sci Study Relig. 2007;46(3):305–20.
106. Gray MJ, Schorr Y, Nash W, Lebowitz L, Amidon A, Lansing A, et al. Adaptive disclosure: an open trial of a novel exposure-based intervention for service members with combat-related psychological stress injuries. Behav Ther. 2012;43(2):407–15.
107. Hayes SC, Luoma JB, Bond FW, Masuda A, Lillis J. Acceptance and commitment therapy: model, processes and outcomes. Behav Res Ther. 2006;44(1):1–25.
108. Lappalainen R, Lehtonen T, Skarp E, Taubert E, Ojanen M, Hayes SC. The impact of CBT and ACT models using psychology trainee therapists: a preliminary controlled effectiveness trial. Behav Modif. 2007;31(4):488–511.
109. Powers MB, Vörding MBZVS, Emmelkamp PM. Acceptance and commitment therapy: a metaanalytic review. Psychother Psychosom. 2009;78(2):73–80.
110. Ruiz FJ. A review of acceptance and commitment therapy (ACT) empirical evidence: correlational, experimental psychopathology, component and outcome studies. Int J Psychol Psychol Ther. 2010;10(1):125–62.
111. Nieuwsma JA, Walser RD, Farnsworth JK, Drescher KD, Meador KG, Nash W. Possibilities within acceptance and commitment therapy for approaching moral injury. Curr Psychiatry Rev. 2015;11(3):193–206.
112. Evans WR, Walser RD, Drescher KD, Farnsworth JK. The moral injury workbook: acceptance and commitment therapy skills for moving beyond shame, anger, and trauma to reclaim your values. Oakland: New Harbinger Publications; 2020.

113. Maguen S, Metzler TJ, Bosch J, Marmar CR, Knight SJ, Neylan TC. Killing in combat may be independently associated with suicidal ideation. Depress Anxiety. 2012;29(11):918–23.
114. Maguen S, Burkman K, Madden E, Dinh J, Bosch J, Keyser J, et al. Impact of killing in war: a randomized, controlled pilot trial. J Clin Psychol. 2017;73(9):997–1012.
115. Dyer G. War. New York: Vintage Books; 2005.
116. Grossman D. On killing: the psychological cost of learning to kill in war and society. New York: Open Road Media; 2014.
117. Norman S, Allard C, Browne K, Capone C, Davis B, Kubany E. Trauma informed guilt reduction therapy: treating guilt and shame resulting from trauma and moral injury. Academic Press; 2019.
118. Norman SB, Wilkins KC, Myers US, Allard CB. Trauma informed guilt reduction therapy with combat veterans. Cogn Behav Pract. 2014;21(1):78–88.
119. Pearce M, Haynes K, Rivera NR, Koenig HG. Spiritually integrated cognitive processing therapy: a new treatment for post-traumatic stress disorder that targets moral injury. Global Adv Health Med. 2018;7:2164956118759939. https://doi.org/10.1177/2164956118759939.
120. Drescher KD, Currier JM, Nieuwsma JA, McCormick W, Carroll TD, Sims BM, Cauterucio C. A qualitative examination of VA chaplains' understandings and interventions related to moral injury in military veterans. J Relig Health. 2018;57(6):2444–60. https://doi.org/10.1007/s10943-018-0682-3.
121. Smith-MacDonald LA, Morin JS, Brémault-Phillips S. Spiritual dimensions of moral injury: contributions of mental health chaplains in the Canadian armed forces. Front Psychiatry. 2018;9:592. https://doi.org/10.3389/fpsyt.2018.00592.
122. Doehring C. Military moral injury: an evidence-based intercultural approach to spiritual care. Pastor Psychol. 2018;68:15–30. https://doi.org/10.1007/s11089-018-0813-5.
123. Liebert EA. Accessible spiritual practices to aid in recovery from moral injury. Pastor Psychol. 2019;68(1):41–57. https://doi.org/10.1007/s11089-018-0825-1.
124. Fawson S. Sustaining lamentation for military moral injury: witness poetry that bears the traces of extremity. Pastor Psychol. 2019;68(1):31–40. https://doi.org/10.1007/s11089-018-0855-8.
125. Brémault-Phillips S, Cherwick T, Smith-MacDonald LA, Huh J, Vermetten E. Forgiveness: a key component of healing from moral injury? Front Psychiatry. 2022;13.
126. Tick E. War and the soul: Healing our nation's veterans from post-tramatic stress disorder. Quest Books; 2012.
127. Currier JM, Holland JM, Malott J. Moral injury, meaning making, and mental health in returning veterans. J Clin Psychol. 2015;71(3):229–40.
128. Orkibi H, Ram-Vlasov N. Linking trauma to posttraumatic growth and mental health through emotional and cognitive creativity. Psychol Aesthet Creat Arts. 2019;13(4):416–30. https://doi.org/10.1037/aca0000193.
129. Geuzinge R, Visse M, Duyndam J, Vermetten E. Social embeddedness of firefighters, paramedics, specialized nurses, police officers, and military personnel: systematic review in relation to the risk of traumatization. Front Psych. 2020;11:1450. https://doi.org/10.3389/fpsyt.2020.496663.
130. Nash WP. Moral injury as an identity wound. UCLA/VA Veteran Family Wellness Center. 2021. https://vfwc.ucla.edu/node/451.
131. Kohut H. The restoration of the self. New York: International Universities Press; 1977.
132. Bowlby J. Attachment and loss: volume II: separation, anxiety and anger. London: The Hogarth Press and the Institute of Psycho-analysis; 1973. p. 1–429.
133. Sherman N. The untold war: inside the hearts, minds, and souls of our soldiers. New York: WW Norton & Company; 2010.
134. Stallinga BA. What spills blood wounds spirit: chaplains, spiritual care, and operational stress injury. Reflective practice: formation and supervision in ministry, 1; 2013.
135. Harari D, Bakermans-Kranenburg MJ, De Kloet CS, Geuze E, Vermetten E, Westenberg HGM, Van IJzendoorn MH. Attachment representations in Dutch veterans with and

without deployment-related PTSD. Attach Hum Dev. 2009;11(6):515–36. https://doi.org/10.1080/14616730903282480.
136. Nutt D, Carhart-Harris R. The current status of psychedelics in psychiatry. JAMA Psychiat. 2021;78(2):121–2. https://doi.org/10.1001/jamapsychiatry.2020.2171.
137. Hurley EC. Effective treatment of veterans with PTSD: comparison between intensive daily and weekly EMDR approaches. Front Psychol. 2018;9:1458.
138. Zepeda Méndez M, Nijdam MJ, Ter Heide FJJ, van der Aa N, Olff M. A five-day inpatient EMDR treatment programme for PTSD: pilot study. Eur J Psychotraumatol. 2018;9(1):1425575.
139. Zimmermann P, Biesold KH, Barre K, Lanczik M. Long-term course of post-traumatic stress disorder (PTSD) in German soldiers: effects of inpatient eye movement desensitization and reprocessing therapy and specific trauma characteristics in patients with non-combat-related PTSD. Mil Med. 2007;172(5):456–60.
140. Jones C, Smith-MacDonald L, Miguel-Cruz A, Pike A, van Gelderen M, Lentz L, et al. Virtual reality–based treatment for military members and veterans with combat-related post-traumatic stress disorder: protocol for a multimodular motion-assisted memory desensitization and reconsolidation randomized controlled trial. JMIR Res Protoc. 2020;9(10):e20620.
141. Bisson JI, Van Deursen R, Hannigan B, Kitchiner N, Barawi K, Jones K, et al. Randomized controlled trial of multi-modular motion-assisted memory desensitization and reconsolidation (3MDR) for male military veterans with treatment-resistant post-traumatic stress disorder. Acta Psychiatr Scand. 2020;142(2):141–51.
142. van Gelderen MJ, Nijdam MJ, Haagen JF, Vermetten E. Interactive motion-assisted exposure therapy for veterans with treatment-resistant posttraumatic stress disorder: a randomized controlled trial. Psychother Psychosom. 2020;89(4):215–27.
143. Roy MJ, Bellini P, Kruger SE, Dunbar K, Atallah H, Haight T, Vermetten E. Randomized controlled trial of motion-assisted exposure therapy for posttraumatic stress disorder after mild traumatic brain injury, with and without an eye movement task. Front Virtual Real. 2022;171.
144. Jones C, Smith-MacDonald L, Miguel-Cruz A, Lentz L, Pike A, Brémault-Phillips S. Tackling trauma with technology: treating chronic combat-related PTSD in Canadian Armed Forces personnel and veterans with 3MDR. Annu Rev Cyberther Telemed. 2021;18, In press.
145. Drescher KD, Nieuwsma JA, Swales PJ. Morality and moral injury: insights from theology and health science. Reflective Pract Formation Superv Ministry. 2013;33(1):50–61.
146. Ferruolo DM. Psychosocial equine program for veterans. Soc Work. 2015;61(1):53–60.
147. Pugh LR, Taylor PJ, Berry K. The role of guilt in the development of post-traumatic stress disorder: a systematic review. J Affect Disord. 2015;182:138–50.
148. Griffin BJ, Purcell N, Burkman K, Litz BT, Bryan CJ, Schmitz M, et al. Moral injury: an integrative review. J Trauma Stress. 2019;32(3):350–62.
149. Williamson V, Murphy D, Castro C, Vermetten E, Jetly R, Greenberg N. Moral injury and the need to carry out ethically responsible research. Res Ethics. 2020;17:135–42. https://doi.org/10.1177/1747016120969743.
150. Harris JI, Usset T, Voecks C, Thuras P, Currier J, Erbes C. Spiritually integrated care for PTSD: a randomized controlled trial of "building spiritual strength". Psychiatry Res. 2018;267:420–8. https://doi.org/10.1016/j.psychres.2018.06.045.

Military Sexual Trauma

15

Anne N. Banducci, Colin T. Mahoney, and Amy E. Street

Military sexual trauma (MST) refers to experiences of repeated, threatening sexual harassment or sexual assault during military service. MST substantially and negatively impacts male and female servicemembers, as well as the military itself. MST damages unit cohesion and mission readiness, as it disrupts the trust and bonds formed among servicemembers. The Tailhook sexual assault scandal in 1991 [1] and multiple allegations of sexual assault in the U.S. Air Force Academy that became public in 2003 [2], began to bring the long-standing issue of MST to light. The release of the Oscar nominated film, *The Invisible War*, in 2012, further raised this issue in the public consciousness and helped to motivate lawmakers to propose legislation to protect and support MST survivors [3]. More recently, the experiences of male survivors of MST have been highlighted in the popular press [4, 5]. In this chapter, we provide an overview of the impact, prevalence, prevention, and treatment of MST.

Vignettes

We will use two composite case vignettes throughout this chapter to illustrate the impact of MST on servicemembers. *Maria* is a Black, lesbian, unemployed, female Army veteran in her late 20s who sought treatment for PTSD and depression. She reported a history of a prior suicide attempt and current suicidal ideation. During

A. N. Banducci · A. E. Street (✉)
National Center for PTSD at VA Boston Healthcare System, Boston, MA, USA

Boston University School of Medicine, Boston, MA, USA
e-mail: Anne.banducci@va.gov; Amy.street@va.gov

C. T. Mahoney

National Center for PTSD at VA Boston Healthcare System, Boston, MA, USA

Boston University School of Medicine, Boston, MA, USA

University of Colorado at Colorado Springs and the Lyda Hill Institute for Human Resilience, Colorado Springs, CO, USA
e-mail: cmahoney@uccs.edu

C. H. Warner, C. A. Castro (eds.), *Veteran and Military Mental Health*,
https://doi.org/10.1007/978-3-031-18009-5_15

treatment, Maria disclosed that her father and brothers served in the Army and that she had hoped to build a lifelong career in the military when she joined at 18-years-old. She quickly proved herself during basic training and was particularly admired for her marksmanship. She served in Iraq as a prison guard and frequently did night patrols on her base. Initially, Maria spoke only about PTSD symptoms related to moral injury; she was distressed by witnessing the abuse and neglect of the prisoners she guarded. After developing a trusting relationship with her therapist, Maria disclosed that she had been raped while deployed. The day of her assault, Maria was invited to play cards with members of her unit after work. Although she did not feel like socializing, she wanted to form better working relationships with male servicemembers in her unit, who often excluded her from work-related discussions. When Maria arrived to play cards, she was surprised that only one soldier was present. She attempted to leave after a brief conversation with him, but he tackled her, dragged her to his cot, and raped her. Maria was disgusted, disoriented, and feared for her life. Afterwards, she felt incredibly ashamed and believed she should have defended herself or screamed when the assault occurred. She did not report the assault to anyone, believing that such a report would hurt her military career. She continued to see her assailant throughout her deployment. When their paths crossed, he would often wink or leer at her, causing her to feel angry and frightened about the possibility of future assaults, as well as to worry he told others about what he had done to her. Following her deployment, Maria avoided all relationships because she believed if she got close to or trusted others, that she would get hurt. She also reported significant anger, resulting in difficulties maintaining steady employment and housing, due to frequent conflict with others.

Bill is a middle-aged, heterosexual, White male Marine veteran who presented for treatment for PTSD, alcohol use disorder, and cocaine use disorder. His treatment history included numerous detox and residential substance use treatment programs. Bill waited 30+ years to disclose his MST to a medical provider. He was motivated to disclose his experience after seeing a news story about male victims of MST. He also reported that he did not think he could stop using substances until he dealt with memories of his assault. Bill reports he was assaulted after making a minor mistake in a basic training exercise that caused his unit to finish last in the exercise. That evening, Bill was taking a shower when several Marines attacked him, punched and kicked him, and raped him with a toilet plunger. During the assault they said, *"This is what we do to F*ck-ups."* The next day, Bill went to his sergeant and told him that he was "jumped" in the showers. He did not disclose the details of the sexual assault because he conceptualized the experience as "hazing" and was ashamed that he was not able to prevent it. His sergeant told him to *"do better"* during the next training exercise, so that the other Marines would be less likely to attack him in the future. Following the assault, he became hypervigilant around his fellow Marines, and during target practice he contemplated shooting the Marines who had assaulted him. He saw them daily for a full year after his assault because they were in the same unit and he began drinking heavily to cope with his anxiety, leading to a DUI (driving under the influence) off base. Upon completing his service, he began using cocaine to avoid sleeping (he had nightmares) and continued drinking, a pattern that persisted for decades. He questioned his sexual orientation, despite being attracted to women, and believed the assault made him "less of a man." Bill also reported he had refused his doctor's recommendation for a colonoscopy, despite ongoing gastrointestinal issues, because he was concerned it would trigger memories of his assault.

Epidemiology of MST

Unfortunately, *Maria* and *Bill* are not alone in their experiences. However, given that estimates vary dramatically across studies, the "true" prevalence of MST is difficult to determine. A recent meta-analysis noted that the prevalence of MST ranges across studies from 1 to 70% [6]. Such variation is due to methodological variability across studies, including the population surveyed, the time period assessed, the specific construct being studied (assault vs. harassment vs. both), the specific assessment used, and participants' beliefs about anonymity. Such methodological variability also makes it difficult to clearly compare the prevalence of unwanted sexual assault within and outside of military settings, although many have speculated about aspects of military culture that may contribute to an increased incidence of these experiences (e.g., hypermasculinity, strict hierarchical organizational structure, cultural acceptance of violence, heavy alcohol use, team allegiance) [7, 8].

The Department of Defense (DoD) produces some of the most robust epidemiological work, focusing on past-year prevalence of sexual assault and sexual harassment among military members. Using a widely distributed anonymous survey of active duty servicemembers, the DoD identified that 6.2% of active duty women (around 13,000 women) and 0.7% of active duty men (around 7500 men) were sexually assaulted in the year prior to the survey [9]. Although the estimated prevalence for active duty men remained stable from 2016 to 2018, the estimated prevalence for active duty women significantly increased (4.3% in 2016 to 6.2% in 2018), particularly for younger women (17–24-year-olds). In terms of sexual harassment, 24.2% of active duty women and 6.3% of active duty men indicated at least one experience of sexual harassment in the year prior to the survey [9]. These estimates represent significant increases for both women and men compared to 2016 data (21% and 5%, respectively).

Population-level prevalence data can be obtained from the Veterans Health Administration's (VHA's) universal MST Screening Program, which queries about experiences of sexual harassment or assault experienced throughout military service [10].

VHA Universal MST Screening Program Text

"I'm going to ask you about some things that may have happened to you while you were in the military. We ask all veterans and former Service members these questions because VA offers free care related to these experiences. You can simply say 'yes' or 'no' to these questions or, if you prefer, let me know that you'd rather not answer.

1. When you were in the military, did you ever receive unwanted sexual attention you found threatening (for example touching, cornering, pressure for sexual favors, sexual texts or online messages, or inappropriate verbal remarks, etc.)?
2. When you were in the military, did you ever have sexual contact against your will or when you were unable to say no (for example, after being forced or threatened or to avoid other consequences)?"

Recent data indicates that, among veterans seen at VHA facilities in the past year, 30.4% of women (representing 145,765 veterans) and 1.7% of men (representing 82,067 veterans) endorsed MST (sexual harassment and/or assault) on the two-question screener administered by a healthcare provider [11]. However, these data underestimate the true scope of harassment and assault, as they solely represent veterans who were VA healthcare users and who chose to disclose these experiences to a healthcare provider. In support of the hypothesis that VA screening data underestimate the true prevalence of harassment and assault, Bovin et al. [12] found that male and female veterans were more likely to endorse MST when assessed through structured interviews or anonymous surveys, as compared to VHA's Universal Screening Program. This pattern was particularly striking for male veterans, whose endorsement of harassment and assault experiences was 11 times higher on anonymous surveys than on VHA's Screening Program. For both men and women, this pattern may be explained by concerns about confidentiality or negative social reactions from others, feelings of shame or embarrassment, and stigma associated with sexual assault victimization.

Epidemiological data is a useful tool for characterizing unwanted sexual experiences of servicemembers and can be particularly helpful in understanding how prototypical experiences differ for men and women. Rigorous assessments, via large scale Department of Defense data, indicate that the majority of sexual assaults experienced by service members involve a single perpetrator (58% for men, 64% for women), although about one-third of incidents involved more than one perpetrator (37% for men, 34% for women; [9]). In regard to their "worst" sexual assault experience over the past year, 92% of women reported that their perpetrators were all men. For male victims, perpetrators were most often men (52%), although a sizable minority reported female perpetrators (30%). Women reported that their perpetrators usually included servicemembers (89%), whereas for men this was somewhat less frequent (71%). For both women (62%) and men (57%), most sexual assaults occurred at military installations. Characterizing important differences in men and women's experiences, men (38%) were more likely than women (21%) to describe their sexual assault experiences as hazing and/or bullying, which may help to explain why men were less likely than women to report these experiences to DoD authorities. In 2018, only 30% of women and 17% of men who experienced sexual assault indicated that they had formally reported those experiences.

This same data source also provides important contextual information about men and women's experiences of sexual harassment, using a robust assessment of that construct [9]. In regards to their "worst" sexual harassment experience 79% of women and 68% of men indicated that the experience was ongoing (i.e., happened more than one time). More than half of women (58%) and men (57%) reported that the worst incident involved more than one perpetrator. Among women, perpetrators were mostly men (72%), primarily servicemembers (95%), and all of the same or slightly higher rank. Among men, perpetrators were somewhat less likely to be men (58%), were largely servicemembers (93%), and about 50% were of the same or slightly higher rank.

Etiology of MST Sequelae

Given that MST comprises experiences across a broad range of severity, and that there is variability in environmental and individual resiliency factors, there is not a single prototypical response to MST. Some individuals may recover fully from these experiences, with limited long-term impact on their health and functioning. For those who experience more significant impacts, the severity of these symptoms will vary across and within individuals over time. Like *Maria* and *Bill*, many MST survivors experience chronic mental and physical health symptoms, as well as life disruptions, that are exacerbated by internal or external barriers to seeking care.

Experiences of MST are associated with a range of mental health conditions. MST heightens risk for posttraumatic stress disorder (PTSD), depressive disorders, anxiety disorders, eating disorders, dissociative disorders, and substance use disorders (e.g., [10, 13]). Indeed, MST is as strongly or more strongly associated with PTSD symptoms, as compared to severe combat exposure [14] or civilian sexual assault [15]. Similar to *Maria*, veterans who have experienced MST have elevated rates of suicidal behavior, including suicidal ideation, non-fatal suicide attempts, and non-suicidal self-injury (e.g., [10, 16]), and are significantly more likely to die by suicide than veterans without exposure to MST [17].

The negative impact of MST also extends to physical health. Like *Bill*, men who experienced MST are four times more likely, and women are twice as likely, to report physical health symptoms, as compared to men and women without a history of exposure [18]. Additionally, a history of MST increases the likelihood that both male and female veterans will engage in risky health behaviors, including risky sex behavior [18].

Finally, MST impacts career success. Studies of career impacts of military sexual harassment or assault indicate that these experiences are associated with increased risk of military demotion among servicewomen [19]. Like *Bill* and *Maria*, active duty servicemembers with a history of these experiences are significantly more likely to end their military service and subsequently be unemployed or disabled [13]. Both *Bill* and *Maria* mourned the loss of a career in the military, noting that this was one more thing their perpetrators had taken from them. Not surprisingly, MST experiences are also associated with higher likelihood of difficulties in work due to emotional and physical health problems [19]. Related to evidence of broader struggles in health and functioning, there is evidence of a link between MST and homelessness among women veterans [20]; this issue has been understudied among male veterans.

The significant health impacts associated with MST are not surprising considering the considerable impact of sexual assault that occurs in any context. Rape is one of the traumatic events most strongly associated with PTSD [21] and gender-based violence, including sexual assault, accounts for the largest proportion of PTSD cases worldwide [22]. Sexual assault involves intentional interpersonal victimization (often by a known perpetrator), frequently occurs relatively early in an individual's development, and may represent one of multiple traumatic events across the lifespan—all factors associated with worse mental health outcomes.

In a military context, impacts may be further exacerbated because experiences of MST conflict so strongly with military cultural expectations of loyalty and teamwork. Accordingly, men and women who are victimized by fellow service members may experience a strong sense of betrayal that their "brothers and sisters in arms" intentionally harmed them in this way. Additionally, trust is disrupted in a context where needing to trust those around you is essential; *Maria* pointed out that she never felt safe in Iraq after her rape: "He treated me like I was an animal—how could I trust him or anyone else to protect me from the Iraqis after that?"

Military cultural taboos against reporting fellow servicemembers' inappropriate or illegal behavior may limit disclosure and help-seeking. In addition, realistic concerns about retaliation from perpetrators or others also limits disclosure and help-seeking. As was the case with *Bill*, survivors who do disclose their experience may experience exacerbations in negative mental health sequelae if they perceive responses from leadership to be insufficiently supportive, victim-blaming, or ineffective at stopping the sexual trauma or holding the perpetrator accountable. Sadly, in one sample of female MST survivors, all who disclosed their MST to someone in the military reported experiencing at least one negative reaction their disclosure, with half of the women experiencing some form of retaliation [23, 24].

Another exacerbating factor of the military context is that, as compared to sexual trauma experienced among civilians, for servicemembers escape may be limited. Because of the nature of military service, servicemembers cannot easily quit their jobs and may not be allowed to change their duty stations or work assignments, resulting in ongoing contact with perpetrators. As noted by *Bill*, "I had to see, live, and work with my rapists every day for the next year, and it killed me. Of course I started drinking every chance I got."

Male MST survivors may struggle with an additional unique set of issues, in part explaining why many mental health impacts are worse among male, as compared to female, MST survivors [21, 25]. Because experiencing sexual trauma is not consistent with a traditional masculine identity, many men are not prepared to cope with this experience and feel intense shame in the wake of an assault [26]. Given the preponderance of male perpetrators, many men, like *Bill*, struggle with questions around their sexual orientation following an assault. Further, given that men are less likely than women to disclose these experiences to others, men are less likely to be connected with important informal or formal sources of support that could aid in their recovery.

Prevention

Given the alarmingly high prevalence of sexual harassment and assault in military settings, and the significant negative impact of these experiences on the health and wellbeing of those who have been victimized, primary prevention of sexual trauma is a critical goal. The establishment of the DoD Sexual Assault Prevention and Response Office (SAPRO) in 2005 was a key initial step in establishing DoD-wide policies of effectively preventing and responding to sexual assault. A detailed discussion of DoD prevention strategies is beyond the scope of this chapter, but, in brief, SAPRO has focused on strategies with some evidence base, including bystander intervention training, responsible alcohol consumption promotion, and the creation of violence prevention specialists [27]. Following reports that the incidence of military sexual assault increased from 2016 to 2018, the acting Secretary of Defense, Patrick Shanahan identified additional key actions to prevent and respond to sexual assault in the military, including launching a program to catch serial offenders, improving assessments of the character of military applicants, and enhancing training for junior officers and junior enlisted leaders [28]. It will be important to continue to track the implementation and effectiveness of these initiatives over time to determine their impact on servicemembers.

The DoD has also developed secondary prevention programs aimed at preventing long-term negative health sequalae. A cornerstone of this effort is providing high-quality assistance to sexual assault survivors, through the efforts of Sexual Assault Response Coordinators (SARCs) and Sexual Assault Prevention and Response (SAPR) Victim Advocates, positions that were developed and filled by 2006 and standardized in 2012 [27]. Regarding legal support, the Special Victims' Counsel program ("the Victims' Legal Counsel" in the Navy) provides personalized legal advice and representation to survivors, helping them navigate the military justice system. Survey data demonstrates high levels of satisfaction among survivors using these programs [29].

A cornerstone of DoD's secondary prevention programs is the victim-centered reporting policy, which allows for restricted, or confidential, reporting to specific individuals like victim advocates or healthcare personnel. This policy allows individuals to benefit from victim advocacy, medical and mental healthcare services, and legal advice, without notifying command or law enforcement officials, thereby triggering a criminal investigation [30]. This approach also allows the victim to maintain control over their personal information and provides space and support to carefully consider the decision to participate in a criminal investigation, an approach that is likely to lead to increased unrestricted report rates. In an ongoing debate, many policymakers and survivors have argued that the prosecution of these crimes should occur outside of the chain of command, instead being handled by military prosecutors [31]. Advocates suggest this approach would encourage survivors to engage with the criminal justice system, improve their experiences, and reduce future assaults. Opponents suggest that commanders are critical to enforcing order and discipline in the military and that removing them from the process would result in fewer sexual assault prosecutions. A recently approved pilot program of independent sexual assault prosecutors at military service academies may provide new information on the effectiveness of this approach [32].

Screening and Assessment

Servicemembers and veterans may feel more comfortable disclosing MST when it is discussed within the context of broader assessments of mental health functioning and within a trusting supportive relationship that destigmatizes their experiences [29, 33].

Best Practice Guidelines for Screening and Assessment

- Assess MST within the context of a broader assessment process that gathers background and military history
- Note that you ask ALL clients/patients these questions because these experiences are common
- Provide *clear, concise* descriptors of *specific* behaviors in question (e.g., "were you forced to have sex against your will?"), rather than asking about more technical or emotionally charged terms, like sexual assault or harassment (see VHA Universal MST Screening Program text for example questions)
- If individuals endorse these experiences, thank them for their honesty and validate them:
  - "I really appreciate that you were willing to be honest with me about these experiences."
  - "By telling me about this, you have taken an important step on your path towards recovery."
  - "I am happy to connect you with treatment resources that have been helpful for other veterans who have had similar experiences."
- Know that anyone can be an MST survivor, regardless of demographic characteristics
- Offer respect, information, and support

Given that many survivors have had negative experiences with disclosure in the past, or have waited decades prior to disclosing MST, it is key to respond in a validating, empathic, and nonjudgmental manner when disclosure occurs [34]. When inquiring about and discussing MST, use clear, concise, specific language that fully defines the behaviors in question [23, 24]. For initial screenings, empower survivors to decide whether they want to disclose specific details of their MST. Although it may be necessary to gather additional information about the MST over time (e.g., to assess for Criterion A in PTSD), giving survivors control over what and how much they want to discuss following initial disclosures is key in developing trust. Finally, when survivors disclose these experiences, it can be helpful to normalize their reactions and to provide resources to support them on their path of recovery. Although no survivor should be pushed to report their MST experiences through formal channels, some survivors may wish to talk through the complicated issues involved in a decision to file a formal report with law enforcement officials, thereby triggering a criminal investigation. This issue is best discussed with a victim advocate who is knowledgeable of local civilian and military regulations (either facility-based, from a local rape crisis center, or at DoD's anonymous Self Helpline).

Treatment

Given the range of psychiatric diagnoses associated with experiences of MST, recommended treatment modalities will depend, to a large degree, on the specific symptom patterns reported, underscoring the importance of a comprehensive diagnostic assessment. However, given that PTSD is the diagnosis most closely associated with experiences of MST, a solid knowledge of evidence-based treatments for PTSD is often key to delivering successful care to MST survivors. Clear guidance regarding PTSD treatment can be derived from two recent, rigorous reviews of the PTSD treatment outcome literature, the VA/DoD Clinical Practice Guideline for the Management of PTSD [35] and the International Society for Traumatic Stress Studies PTSD Prevention and Treatment Guidelines [36].

PTSD Treatment Guidelines

VA/DoD Clinical Practice Guidelines for the Management of PTSD

Psychotherapy: Individual, manualized trauma-focused psychotherapies that have a primary component of exposure and/or cognitive restructuring to include prolonged exposure, cognitive processing therapy, eye movement desensitization and reprocessing, specific cognitive behavioral therapies for PTSD, brief eclectic psychotherapy, narrative exposure therapy, and written narrative exposure.

Pharmacotherapy: Sertraline, paroxetine, fluoxetine, or venlafaxine as monotherapy for patients diagnosed with PTSD who choose not to engage in or are unable to access trauma-focused psychotherapy.

ISTSS PTSD prevention and treatment guidelines:

Psychotherapy: Cognitive processing therapy, cognitive therapy, eye movement desensitization and reprocessing, individual CBT with a trauma focus (undifferentiated), and prolonged exposure are strongly recommended for the treatment of adults with PTSD.

Pharmacotherapy: Fluoxetine, paroxetine, sertraline and venlafaxine are identified as interventions with low treatment effects for adults with PTSD.

Of note, both sets of guidelines provide the strongest recommendation for individual, manualized, trauma-focused psychotherapies as first-line treatments for PTSD. Both sets of guidelines also acknowledge that, given more limited evidence for its effectiveness, medication monotherapy is not indicated as a first line treatment for PTSD. VHA/DoD guidelines note that there is moderate evidence for Selective Serotonin Reuptake Inhibitors (SSRIs; Sertraline, Paroxetine, Fluoxetine, Venlafaxine), while also acknowledging that psychopharmacology is only recommended for patients who do not want to engage in psychotherapy. The ISTSS guidelines state that SSRIs can be a recommended treatment when indicated, while acknowledging a low treatment effect for these medications. In terms of other medications, the VHA/DoD guidelines recommend against or strongly against many additional medications including specific antidepressants, antipsychotics and antiepileptics. The ISTSS guidelines indicate that there is insufficient evidence to recommend a similar list of medications, although notes that the antipsychotic medication Quetiapine is a treatment with emerging evidence of efficacy. As new medication-based interventions are developed and tested for their efficacy in PTSD, the recommendations for psychopharmacology-related treatment of PTSD are likely to change. Given the current evidence base, however, for treatment of PTSD, including PTSD due to MST, trauma-focused psychotherapies should be considered first-line treatments. Two of the most strongly supported psychotherapies, Cognitive Processing Therapy [37] and Prolonged Exposure Therapy [38] were originally developed for and tested among sexual assault survivors. CPT includes psychoeducation about PTSD and focuses on challenging maladaptive thoughts and beliefs about safety, trust, power/control, esteem, and intimacy that develop following trauma exposure, in order to impact emotional and behavioral responses [39]. Recent meta-analytic work indicates that 89% of individuals participating in CPT fared better posttreatment than those in inactive control conditions [40], and CPT has shown modest benefits compared to active control treatments among veterans with MST-related PTSD [41]. PE includes psychoeducation about PTSD, breathing retraining to decrease autonomic arousal, repeated recounting of the trauma to teach individuals that their trauma memories are not dangerous and do not need to be avoided, and in vivo exposure to feared real-world situations to decrease fear responses to trauma reminders in the environment. PE intervenes at the level of trauma-related behavior to change thoughts and emotions. A substantial body of research supports the use of PE among survivors of sexual assault [42], with large reductions in symptoms observed following PE among veterans, regardless of trauma type and gender [43], and demonstrated effectiveness among women veterans, most of whom were treated for MST-related PTSD [44].

In our clinical experience, there are several treatment themes that are particularly likely to emerge when treating MST-related PTSD. Given the interpersonal nature of MST, many survivors report difficulties in interpersonal relationships, including struggles with trust and intimacy, problems identifying and setting appropriate boundaries, or unusually strong reactions to hierarchical relationships. Sexual trauma, in general, is strongly associated with self-blame, guilt and shame, and these thoughts and emotions frequently arise among MST survivors. Safety and revictimization may be an area in need of particular focus. Some patients may experience extremes in safety behavior, including global distrust of others, accompanied by hyperattention to personal safety, or a seeming inattention to safety, or vacillation between both extremes. Finally, given the sexual nature of MST, many survivors struggle with questions around their sexuality, extremes in sexual behavior (e.g., only able to engage in sexual behavior while intoxicated or high), or sexual dysfunction.

Of note, the VHA offers *free* care (therapy, medication, outpatient, residential, etc.) for all MST-related mental and physical health conditions, allowing survivors to get much-needed care, regardless of their eligibility for other VHA services. Returning to our case examples, both of whom received care at a VHA facility, *Maria* engaged in a course of CPT. She declined a referral to be evaluated for medications to help with symptom management. Due to employment and economic stressors, she often had difficulties with homework completion in CPT. Nonetheless, as we challenged particular beliefs around trust (e.g., "I cannot trust anyone"), she began to increase her connection with others. PTSD symptoms improved and she began to feel safer in her environment. By emotionally engaging with her trauma memory, she allowed herself to feel the grief she had suppressed and work through her sadness and anger. Cognitive restructuring (i.e., examining the evidence for and against the idea that it was her fault she was raped) allowed her to let go of self-blame and shame. *Bill* engaged in a course of Concurrent Treatment of PTSD and Substance Use Disorders Using Prolonged Exposure (COPE), a treatment modality that integrates PE with cognitive behavior therapy (CBT). Throughout the course of treatment, he worked on CBT skills for sobriety, while repeatedly exposing himself to his trauma memory and to trauma reminders/avoided situations (e.g., gym locker room with men, sitting with his back to the door in a restaurant, building trust in familial relationships by telling his mother he was an MST survivor). Initial imaginal exposures to his trauma memory caused rapid reductions in anxiety. As he repeatedly recalled details of his rape, his perspective on the experience shifted and he stopped blaming himself for his rape, which led to reductions in shame. Later imaginal exposures focused on processing his grief regarding what he described as "a loss of innocence," as well as a loss of a lifelong career in the military. Upon completing COPE, he evidenced clinically significant improvements in PTSD symptoms, was abstinent from substances, and sought a colonoscopy for his gastrointestinal problems.

Additional Resources:
VA MST information and VHA services and services:
https://www.va.gov/find-locations/
www.mentalhealth.va.gov/mst
https://www.mentalhealth.va.gov/msthome/resources.asp
https://www.va.gov/health-care/health-needs-conditions/military-sexual-trauma/
Factsheet for MST survivors:
https://www.mentalhealth.va.gov/docs/mst_general_factsheet.pdf
Self-help mobile app for MST survivors:
Beyond MST—PTSD: National Center for PTSD (va.gov)
Helplines:
Veterans Crisis Line—"Dial 988 and Press 1" www.veteranscrisisline.net
DoD Safe Helpline—(855) 344-5137 www.safehelpline.org
VHA Women Veterans Call Center—1-855-829-6636
National Sexual Assault Hotline (RAINN)—1-800-656-4653
Community resource for male survivors:
www.1in6.org
PTSD treatment overview and free expert consultation for anyone treating veterans with PTSD:
https://www.ptsd.va.gov/understand_tx/tx_basics.asp
PTSDconsult@va.gov or (866) 948-7880

Videos of veterans discussing their experiences recovering from MST:
Military Sexual Trauma | AboutFace (va.gov)
https://maketheconnection.net/conditions/military-sexual-trauma
Finding healthcare and therapists:
https://www.ptsd.va.gov/gethelp/find_therapist.asp
http://www.vetcenter.va.gov
http://www.findcbt.org/FAT/
https://istss.org/public-resources/find-a-clinician.aspx

Conclusions

Military sexual trauma substantially and negatively impacts individual servicemembers and the U.S. military as an institution. It is a costly problem that disrupts the bonds between servicemembers and threatens unit morale. As per DoD reports, *38 men and 33 women are sexually assaulted daily* in the military [45]. MST survivors often suffer in silence for years following these experiences, waiting for decades to seek treatment. As providers, it is our responsibility to create an empathetic and caring environment that can empower those who have experienced MST to face their traumatic memories and move forward on a path of recovery. Further, connecting servicemembers and veterans with evidence-based treatments is essential. They paid a terrible price while serving their country and it is incumbent upon us to provide them with the support and care necessary to heal.

Clinical Pearls

- In 2018, the DoD identified that 6.2% of active duty women (around 13,000 women) and 0.7% of active duty men (around 7500 men) were sexually assaulted, while 24.2% of active duty women and 6.3% of active duty men indicated at least one experience of sexual harassment.
- Most recent data indicates that, among veterans seen at VHA facilities in the past year, 30.4% of women (representing 145,765 veterans) and 1.7% of men (representing 82,067 veterans) endorsed MST (sexual harassment and/or assault) on the two-question screener administered by a healthcare provider. However, these data likely underestimate the true prevalence of harassment and assault, as they solely represent veterans who were VA healthcare users.
- Given that many survivors have had negative experiences with disclosure in the past, or have waited decades prior to disclosing MST, it is key to respond in a validating, empathic, and nonjudgmental manner when disclosure occurs.
- For initial screenings, empower survivors to decide whether they want to disclose specific details of their MST.
- Given the range of psychiatric diagnoses associated with experiences of MST, recommended treatment modalities will depend, to a large degree, on the specific symptom patterns reported, underscoring the importance of a

comprehensive diagnostic assessment. However, given that PTSD is the diagnosis most closely associated with experiences of MST, a solid knowledge of evidence-based treatments for PTSD is often key to delivering successful care to MST survivors.

- Clear guidance regarding PTSD treatment can be derived from two recent, rigorous reviews of the PTSD treatment outcome literature, the VA/DoD Clinical Practice Guideline for the Management of PTSD [35] and the International Society for Traumatic Stress Studies PTSD Prevention and Treatment Guidelines [36].

References

1. Office of the General Inspector: Tailhook report: the official inquiry into the events of Tailhook '91. New York: St. Martin's Press; 2003.
2. Schmitt E, Moss M. Air Force Academy investigated 54 sexual assaults in 10 years. The New York Times. 2003. https://www.nytimes.com/2003/03/07/us/air-force-academy-investigated-54-sexual-assaults-in-10-years.html. Accessed 13 Jul 2021.
3. Dick K The invisible war [film]. Chain Camera Pictures; 2012.
4. Penn N. "Son, men don't get raped". GQ. 2014. https://www.gq.com/story/male-rape-in-the-military. Accessed 13 Jul 2021.
5. Philipps D, Ramic A, Flynn B. Six men tell their stories of sexual assault in the military. The New York Times. 2019. https://www.nytimes.com/interactive/2019/09/10/us/men-military-sexual-assault.html. Accessed 13 Jul 2021.
6. Wilson LC. The prevalence of military sexual trauma: a meta-analysis. Trauma Violence Abuse. 2018;19(5):584–97. https://doi.org/10.1177/1524838016683459.
7. Castro CA, Kintzle S, Schuyler AC, Lucas CL, Warner CH. Sexual assault in the military. Curr Psychiatry Rep. 2015;17(7):54. https://doi.org/10.1007/s11920-015-0596-7.
8. Turchik JA, Wilson SM. Sexual assault in the US military: a review of the literature and recommendations for the future. Aggress Violent Behav. 2010;15(4):267–77. https://doi.org/10.1016/j.avb.2010.01.005.
9. Department of Defense: 2018 workplace and gender relations survey of active duty members. 2019. https://www.sapr.mil/sites/default/files/Annex_1_2018_WGRA_Overview_Report.pdf. Accessed 13 Jul 2021.
10. Kimerling R, Gima K, Smith MW, Street A, Frayne S. The Veterans Health Administration and military sexual trauma. Am J Public Health. 2007;97(12):2160–6. https://doi.org/10.2105/AJPH.2006.092999.
11. Department of Veterans Affairs: veterans ever screened positive for military sexual trauma (MST). 2020. https://reports.vssc.med.va.gov/ReportServer/Pages/ReportViewer.aspx. Accessed 13 Jul 2021.
12. Bovin MJ, Black SK, Kleiman SE, Brown ME, et al. The impact of assessment modality and demographic characteristics on endorsement of military sexual trauma. Womens Health Issues. 2019;29(Suppl 1):S67–73. https://doi.org/10.1016/j.whi.2019.03.005.
13. Millegan J, Wang L, LeardMann CA, Miletich D, Street AE. Sexual trauma and adverse health and occupational outcomes among men serving in the US military. J Trauma Stress. 2016;29(2):132–40. https://doi.org/10.1002/jts.22081.
14. Kang H, Dalager N, Mahan C, Ishii E. The role of sexual assault on the risk of PTSD among gulf war veterans. Ann Epidemiol. 2005;15(3):191–5. https://doi.org/10.1016/j.annepidem.2004.05.009.

15. Himmelfarb N, Yaeger D, Mintz J. Posttraumatic stress disorder in female veterans with military and civilian sexual trauma. J Trauma Stress. 2006;19(6):837–46. https://doi.org/10.1002/jts.20163.
16. Monteith LL, Holiday R, Schneider AL, Forster JE, Bahraini NH. Identifying factors associated with suicidal ideation and suicide attempts following military sexual trauma. J Affect Disord. 2019;252:300–9. https://doi.org/10.1016/j.jad.2019.04.038.
17. Kimerling R, Makin-Byrd K, Louzon S, Ignacio RV, McCarthy JF. Military sexual trauma and suicide mortality. Am J Prev Med. 2016;50(6):684–91. https://doi.org/10.1016/j.amepre.2015.10.019.
18. Schuyler AC, Kintzle S, Lucas CL, Moore H, Castro CA. Military sexual assault (MSA) among veterans in Southern California: associations with physical health, psychological health, and risk behaviors. Traumatology. 2017;23(3):223–34. https://doi.org/10.1037/trm0000098.
19. Millegan J, Milburn EK, LaerdMann CA, Street AE, et al. Recent sexual trauma and adverse health and occupational outcomes among US service women. J Trauma Stress. 2015;28(4):298–306. https://doi.org/10.1002/jts.22028.
20. Washington DL, Yano EM, McGuire J, Hines V, et al. Risk factors for homelessness among women veterans. J Health Care Poor Underserved. 2010;21:82–91. https://doi.org/10.1353/hpu.0.0237.
21. Kessler RC, Sonnega A, Bromet E, Hughes M, Nelson CB. Posttraumatic stress disorder in the National Comorbidity Survey. Arch Gen Psychiatry. 1995;52:1048–60. https://doi.org/10.1001/archpsyc.1995.03950240066012.
22. Kessler RC, Aguilar-Gaxiola S, Alonso J, Benjet C, et al. Trauma and PTSD in the WHO world mental health surveys. Eur J Psychotraumatol. 2017;8(Suppl 5):1353383. https://doi.org/10.1080/20008198.2017.1353383.
23. Dardis CM, Reinhardt KM, Foynes MM, Medoff NE, Street AE. "Who are you going to tell? Who's going to believe you?": women's experiences disclosing military sexual trauma. Psychol Women Q. 2018;42(4):414–29. https://doi.org/10.1177/0361684318796783.
24. Dardis CM, Vento SA, Gradus JL, Street AE. Labeling of deployment sexual harassment experiences among male and female veterans. Psychol Trauma Theory Res Pract Policy. 2018;10(4):452–5. https://doi.org/10.1037/tra0000330.
25. Street AE, Gradus JL, Stafford J, Kelly K. Gender differences in experiences of sexual harassment: data from a male-dominated environment. J Consult Clin Psychol. 2007;75(3):464–74. https://doi.org/10.1037/0022-006X.75.3.464.
26. O'Brien C, Keith J, Shoemaker L. Don't tell: military culture and male rape. Psychol Serv. 2015;12(4):357–65. https://doi.org/10.1037/ser0000049.
27. Department of Defense: 2014-2016 sexual assault prevention strategy. 2014. https://www.sapr.mil/public/docs/prevention/DoD_SAPR_Prevention_Strategy_2014-2016.pdf. Accessed 13 Jul 2021.
28. Shanahan PM. Actions to address and prevent sexual assault in the military [Memorandum]. 2019. https://media.defense.gov/2019/May/02/2002126804/-1/-1/1/ACTIONS-TO-ADDRESS-AND-PREVENT-SEXUAL-ASSAULT-IN-THE-MILITARY.PDF. Accessed 13 Jul 2021.
29. Office of People Analytics: 2016 workplace and gender relations survey of active duty members: overview report (report no. 2017-019). 2017. https://www.sapr.mil/public/docs/reports/FY17_Annual/FY16_Annual_Report_on_Sexual_Assault_in_the_Military_Full_Report_Part2_4.pdf. Accessed 15 Jul 2021.
30. Department of Defense: sexual assault prevention and response (SAPR) program. (DoD Directive 6495.01). 2012. https://www.sapr.mil/public/docs/instructions/DoDI_649501_20130430.pdf. Accessed 12 Jul 2021.
31. House Armed Services Committee: Subcommittee on Military Personnel Hearing: examining the role of the commander in sexual assault prosecutions, 116th Cong. 2019. https://armedservices.house.gov/2019/4/examining-the-role-of-the-commander-in-sexual-assault. Accessed 13 Jul 2021.

32. H.R. 2500: National Defense Authorization Act for Fiscal Year 2020. 116th Congress. 2020. https://www.congress.gov/bill/116th-congress/house-bill/2500. Accessed 13 Jul 2021.
33. Burns B, Grindlay K, Holt K, Manski R, Grossman D. Military sexual trauma among US servicewomen during deployment: a qualitative study. Am J Public Health. 2014;104(2):345–9. https://doi.org/10.2105/AJPH.2013.301576.
34. Street AE, Shin MH, Marchany KE, McCaughey VK, et al. Veterans' perspectives on military sexual trauma-related communication with VHA providers. Psychol Serv. 2019;18(2):249–59. https://doi.org/10.1037/ser0000395.
35. Department of Veterans Affairs, & Department of Defense: VA/DoD clinical practice guideline for the management of posttraumatic stress disorder and acute stress disorder. 2017. https://www.healthquality.va.gov/guidelines/MH/ptsd/VADoDPTSDCPGFinal012418.pdf. Accessed 13 Jul 2021.
36. Berliner L, Bisson JI, Cloitre M, Forbes D, et al. ISTSS PTSD prevention and treatment guidelines methodology and recommendation. 2019. https://istss.org/clinical-resources/treating-trauma/new-istss-prevention-and-treatment-guidelines. Accessed 14 Jul 2021.
37. Resick PA, Monson CM, Chard K. Cognitive processing therapy for PTSD: a comprehensive manual. New York: Guilford Press; 2017.
38. Foa EB, Hembree E, Rothbaum BO. Prolonged exposure therapy for PTSD: emotional processing of traumatic experiences (treatments that work), vol. 1. Oxford: Oxford University Press; 2007.
39. Monson CM, Schnurr PP, Resick PA, Friedman MJ, Young-Xu Y, Stevens SP. Cognitive processing therapy for veterans with military-related posttraumatic stress disorder. J Consult Clin Psychol. 2006;74(5):898–907. https://doi.org/10.1037/0022-006X.74.5.898.
40. Asmundson GJ, Thorisdottir AS, Roden-Foreman JW, Baird SO, et al. A meta-analytic review of cognitive processing therapy for adults with posttraumatic stress disorder. Cogn Behav Ther. 2019;48(1):1–14. https://doi.org/10.1080/16506073.2018.1522371.
41. Surís A, Link-Malcolm J, Chard K, Ahn C, North C. A randomized clinical trial of cognitive processing therapy for veterans with PTSD related to military sexual trauma. J Trauma Stress. 2013;26:28–37. https://doi.org/10.1002/jts.21765.
42. Rothbaum BO, Astin MC, Marsteller F. Prolonged exposure versus eye movement desensitization and reprocessing (EMDR) for PTSD rape victims. J Trauma Stress. 2005;18(6):607–16. https://doi.org/10.1002/jts.20069.
43. Mouilso ER, Tuerk PW, Schnurr PP, Rauch SAM. Addressing the gender gap: prolonged exposure for PTSD in veterans. Psychol Serv. 2016;13(3):308–16. https://doi.org/10.1037/ser0000040.
44. Schnurr PP, Friedman MJ, Engel CC, Foa EB, et al. Cognitive behavioral therapy for posttraumatic stress disorder in women: a randomized controlled trial. JAMA. 2009;297(8):820–30. https://doi.org/10.1001/jama.297.8.820.
45. Department of Defense, & Sexual Assault Prevention and Response Office: Department of Defense annual report on sexual assault in the military: Fiscal year 2019. 2019. https://www.sapr.mil/sites/default/files/DoD_Annual_Report_on_Sexual_Assault_in_the_Military.pdf. Accessed 13 Jul 2021.

16 Understanding Suicide Among Military Service Members and Veterans: Risk and Protective Factors, Theory, and Intervention

Nicholas Barr, Rohul Amin, Sara Kintzle, and Stephanie Watman

Vignette

Corporal (Cpl) Smith is a White, single, 35-year-old male who is a medically retired veteran. He served in the Marines from 2004 to 2009. In 2008, he was deployed to Afghanistan. As an infantryman (military occupational specialty 0311), Cpl Smith and his unit engaged the Taliban insurgents for over a month. He and his unit killed more than 400 insurgents. Cpl Smith personally killed 4 teenaged Taliban insurgents while he was manning a 50 caliber machine gun. He was involved in collecting the remains of the insurgents. After his redeployment to Camp Lejeune, North Carolina, he began to have classic post-traumatic stress (PTSD) symptoms, including nightmares and intrusive thoughts, a heightened startle response, and feelings of irritability and cognitive numbing which led him to drink alcohol most nights. He reported feeling disconnected from his unit, a tight knit group during his deployment. Cpl Smith also began to have chronic low back pain, for which he was

N. Barr (✉)
School of Social Work, University of Nevada Las Vegas, Las Vegas, NV, USA
e-mail: Nicholas.barr@unlv.edu

R. Amin
Uniformed Services University of Health Sciences, Bethesda, MD, USA

National Capital Consortium Psychiatry Residency Program, Bethesda, MD, USA

Walter Reed National Military Medical Center, Bethesda, MD, USA
e-mail: rohul.amin.mil@mail.mil

S. Kintzle
USC Suzanne Dworak-Peck School of Social Work Center for Innovation and Research on Veterans & Military Families, Los Angeles, CA, USA
e-mail: kintzle@usc.edu

S. Watman
UNLV School of Social Work, Las Vegas, NV, USA
e-mail: stephanie.watman@unlv.edu

C. H. Warner, C. A. Castro (eds.), *Veteran and Military Mental Health*,
https://doi.org/10.1007/978-3-031-18009-5_16

prescribed opioid pain medications. Eventually, he received treatment for alcohol use disorder after he was arrested for driving under the influence on base. Despite outpatient interventions, Cpl Smith attempted suicide in early 2009 via overdose using his opioids, an antidepressant, and sleep medications. Soon after, he was referred to the medical evaluation board (MEB) by his military psychiatrist. He was found unfit and failed retention standards for PTSD and chronic low back pain. Cpl Smith did not want to leave the Marine Corps and was angry with his healthcare providers for medical board referral. He was largely unprepared for his transition out of the military and did not have a plan for obtaining civilian employment at the time of his discharge. Since 2009, Cpl Smith has been on chronic opioids for low back pain and continues to be seen in the chronic pain clinic. He is also seen in the behavioral health clinic for PTSD, but has not been able to access evidence-based PTSD interventions, like Prolonged Exposure (PE) or Cognitive Processing Therapy (CPT). When Cpl. Smith first sought treatment, he was wary of therapy and stated that he preferred not to engage in exposure-based treatment when it was initially described to him. Since then, he has not been offered PE or CPT again. He has continued to have suicidal ideations without any attempts since 2009. Cpl Smith has not been able to maintain intimate relationships and reports feeling disconnected from others. His mother lives several hours away and suffers from polysubstance use. She partially relies on Cpl Smith for meeting basic financial needs. Cpl Smith has significant financial difficulties and has come close to becoming homeless on several occasions. He does not have access to firearms and has been sober from alcohol for 5 years.

Introduction

Enormous resources have been devoted to preventing suicides among military service members and veterans, but the problem has persisted despite both research and clinical efforts to understand root causes and develop effective intervention approaches [1]. While the suicide rate among general population U.S. adults has increased in the first decades of the twenty-first century, rates for veterans have increased even more sharply. The 2020 National Veteran's Suicide Report [2] estimates that in 2018 compared to 2005 there was a 47.1% increase in the number of deaths by suicide in the general population of U.S. adults, while the adult population grew from 215 million to 253 million. Among veterans, there was an overall increase of 6.3% in the number of suicides in 2018 compared to 2005, while the veteran population decreased from 24.5 million to 20.1 million. From 2005 to 2018, age and sex-adjusted suicide death rates among veterans rose dramatically. The adjusted rate in 2005 was 18.5 per 100,000; in 2018, it was 27.5 per 100,000, 1.5 times the rate for general population U.S. adults. In 2018, an average of 17.6 veterans died by suicide each day (see Fig. 16.1; [2]).

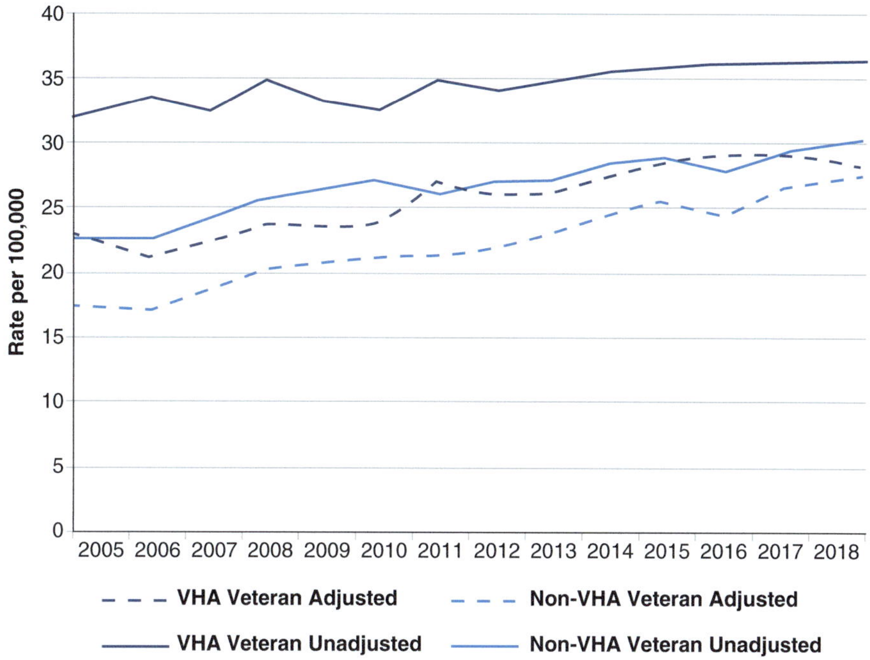

Fig. 16.1 Unadjusted and Age and Sex-Adjusted Suicide Rates for Veterans and Non-Veteran Adults, 2005–2018. 2020 National Veteran Suicide Annual Report

The absolute suicide rates for active duty Service Members also rose over this period. From 2014 to 2019, the suicide rate for active duty Service Members increased from 20.4 to 25.9. The rate for Reserve and National Guard Service Members remained at 20.3, a decrease from 2017 highs of 29.8 for the National Guard as a whole, (35.5 for the Army National Guard) and 25.7 for the Reserve component as a whole (32.1 for the Army Reserve; [2]). However, once controlled for sex and age, current rates are on par with the suicide rates in the general population [2].

From a direct practice perspective, there is an urgent need to synthesize existing empirical knowledge and apply it to clinical practice contexts to identify and intervene with Service Members and veterans at risk for suicide. Bridging the knowledge-practice gap is particularly important for clinicians working with military veterans and Service Members, whether in active duty, Reserve, or National Guard components. The aims of this chapter are to (a) describe the scope of the problem of suicide among military veterans and Service Members; (b) examine risk and protective factors identified in the literature; (c) identify areas that require additional investigation and clarification, and (d) review clinical practice guidelines and offer recommendations for applying empirical knowledge about suicide to inform clinical practice with military populations.

Military service was considered protective against suicidal deaths in the past, though empirical evidence in support of this purported historical effect is mixed. Some previous studies with military populations found evidence of a healthy soldier effect characterized by lower mortality risk and better health outcomes among veterans and military Service Members, particularly younger cohorts, compared to their general population counterparts [3, 4]. However, the negative association between military service and suicide has not been detected in recent studies with modern-era veterans of the conflicts in Afghanistan and Iraq [5]. Across active duty service branches, Reserve, and National Guard components, most suicide decedents were male, enlisted, and under the age of 30.

In 2018, veterans aged 18–34 had the highest suicide rate of any cohort at 45.9 per 100,000, while those over the age of 75 had the lowest rate. However, reflecting veteran population demographics, the highest overall number of suicides in 2018 was among veterans aged 55–74, representing 40% of all veteran deaths by suicide [2]. Veterans who identify as White demonstrated the highest rate of suicide from 2005–2018, while rates were lowest among those who identified as Black. In comparison, among civilians, suicide risk is highest among White men aged 45–64, with the second-highest risk evident among men older than 85 [6]. In addition, suicides among women veterans have increased in both raw numbers and age-adjusted rates from 2005 to 2018. There were 291 suicides among women veterans in 2018 compared to 186 in 2005; in 2018, the age-adjusted suicide rate among women veterans was 2.1 times that of non-veteran women, compared to 1.8 times the rate for non-veteran women in 2005 [2].

While not all military veterans access Veterans Health Administration (VHA) care, VHA records are the most comprehensive source for veterans' behavioral health data. Overall, veterans in VHA care have lower suicide rates than those not in VHA care; from 2005 to 2018, the age and sex-adjusted suicide rate increased by 25.6% for veterans who recently reported using VHA services in comparison to a 57.0% increase among those who did not report VHA service use (see Fig. 16.2). However, it is not clear whether veterans not receiving VHA care received care elsewhere or did not receive care at all; these groups might be expected to have different outcomes. Evidence indicates that suicide rates have consistently been highest among VHA patients with comorbid mental health and substance use disorders receiving mental health treatment; rates are highest for those with bipolar disorder and opioid use disorder [2, 7]. However, there is considerable variability in veterans' mortality and suicide risk by demographic characteristics and service era.

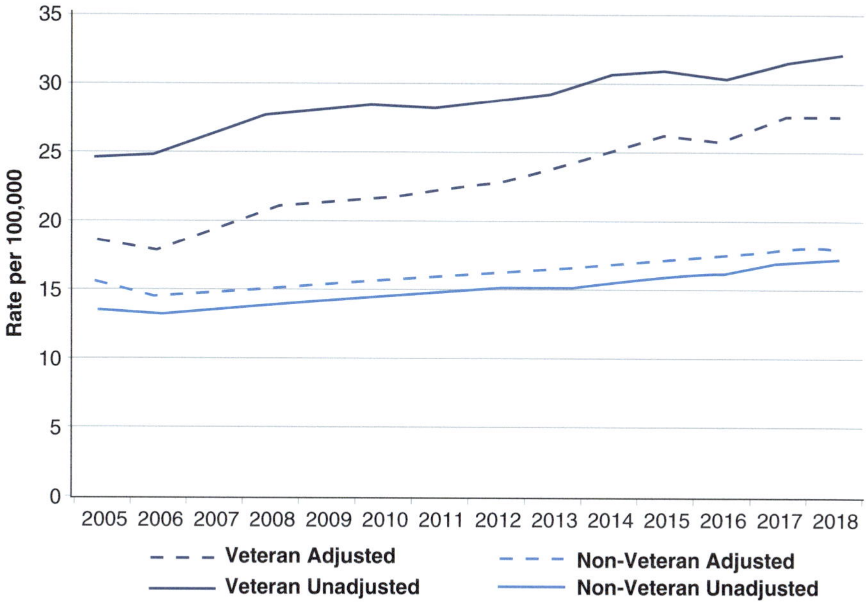

Fig. 16.2 Unadjusted and Age and Sex-Adjusted Suicide Rates, Veterans, by Recent VHA Care, 2005–2018. 2020 National Veteran Suicide Annual Report

Risk Factors by Service Era

Among Vietnam-era veterans, evidence suggests no overall difference in suicide risk compared to the general population [8, 9]. However, certain subgroups of the Vietnam-era cohort display increased risk; those who were deployed, have a post-traumatic stress disorder (PTSD) diagnosis, experienced two or more wounds, or were hospitalized for a combat wound are between 1.76 and 12 times more likely to die by suicide. Similarly, evidence indicates that Gulf War-era veterans as a whole are not at elevated risk of suicide, although they demonstrate increased risk of death from preventable external causes, like automobile accidents, that may reflect a propensity for risk-taking behavior associated with suicidality and the hyperarousal symptom cluster in PTSD [3, 10].

Studies conducted with veterans of Operation Enduring Freedom (OEF) and Operation Iraqi Freedom (OIF) indicate that suicide risk is elevated in this cohort, but findings are complex and nuanced. A 2015 study of 1.3 million active-duty OEF/OIF era Service Members found that suicide risk was 41–61% greater for both those who had ever deployed and those who never deployed compared to civilians, though the risk was highest for veterans who had never deployed [11]. Several interpretations for this finding were offered by the study's authors, including the possibility that those with preexisting risk factors associated with suicide, like mental health problems and substance abuse, were not deployed as a result of these conditions. Another interpretation is that the increased availability of screening, treatment, and counseling programs offered to Service Members who had deployed by DoD and VHA helped mitigate risk. For both veterans who never deployed and those who did, suicide risk was greater among those who recently separated from the military and diminished subsequently. It is also important to note that deployment experiences vary considerably and are likely to impact suicide risk differently for different service branches and components, and over time. A meta-analysis by Bryan et al. [12] found that despite substantial heterogeneity in the relationship between deployment-related predictors (including deployment to a combat zone and combat experience) and suicide risk, a small positive association was evident. Critically, among deployed veterans exposed to killing or atrocities, results showed less heterogeneity and a 43% higher suicide risk for veterans who reported experiences. Thus, while combat experiences appear to be a stronger predictor of suicide risk than deployment, careful assessment is required to clarify the nature of this association. Not surprisingly, the most salient risk factors for suicide among veterans appear to be mental health and substance use problems. One study of veterans receiving VHA care found that, for veterans with a mental health diagnosis, the risk was 77% greater than for those without [8].

A comparison of risk factors among military cohorts suggests an overall risk profile characterized by the presence of a mental health diagnosis such as PTSD or depression; problems with substance use, relationship stress or instability, and medical disability; and access to, knowledge of, and use of firearms. Since 2002, more than 400,000 veterans have received a mental health diagnosis from the VHA [1]. Although there is variability in findings concerning the direct risk of suicide posed by deployment-related stressors in general and combat experiences more specifically, combat experiences are robustly linked to negative mental health outcomes among both active-duty personnel and veterans, and this risk increases with the duration and intensity of combat experience [13, 14]. Mental health disorders like PTSD and depression are well-established risk factors for suicide [15].

Military Service Members and veterans are also more likely to use firearms when attempting suicide than are their general population counterparts. Data show that between 2001 and 2014, 67.8% of male veterans and 40.5% of female veterans who died by suicide used a firearm, in comparison to 52.2% and 31.2% of male and female civilians [7]. These rates have remained stable; in 2018, 68.2% of veteran suicide deaths were by firearm compared to 48.2% of non-veteran adult suicide deaths. Among Service Members, the majority of suicide deaths are also by firearm; 59.6%, 66.2%, and 78.7% of active duty, Reserve, and National Guard Service Members respectively who died by suicide in 2019 used a firearm [2].

Many of the risk factors reviewed here are evident in Cpl Smith's case. Cpl Smith was a Marine infantryman who not only deployed to Afghanistan but also engaged in high-intensity combat, including killing insurgents and clearing their bodies: precisely the type of combat experience most closely linked to suicide risk. Cpl Smith also met the criteria for PTSD, comorbid alcohol use disorder, and experienced chronic low back pain, a perfect storm of physical and psychological distress. Despite being enrolled in medical and psychiatric services, Cpl Smith did not receive PTSD treatments with the strongest basis in evidence, including PE and CPT. Cpl Smith attempted suicide soon after being medically discharged from the Marines—a undesired and destabilizing transition. While he did attempt, he did not die due to the lower lethality associated with overdose as compared to firearms. However, Cpl Smiths ongoing relational and financial problems, in conjunction with this persistent mental and physical health symptoms, place him at great risk for another suicide attempt.

While an elevated risk for suicide is not restricted to veterans or Service Members with combat or deployment experience, it is important to reiterate that suicide risk is not associated with entering the military or simply being a military Service Member or veteran. Rather, evidence suggests that a constellation of stressors, including war-time experience, downstream sequelae like mental health or substance use problems, relationship stress, legal or administrative problems, and financial difficulties, are contextual risk factors. These risk factors can be amplified by disruptive social experiences like unplanned or difficult transitions out of the military and loss of important military social connections. So how can clinicians make sense of these risks in a framework that supports intervention? The following sections review theoretical approaches to organizing and understanding suicide risk in military populations.

Theoretical Considerations

Interpersonal–Psychological Theory of Suicide

Several theoretical approaches have been advanced to account for suicides among military veterans. Although it is beyond the scope of this chapter to explore all relevant theories, we examine two that encompass the broad domains affecting suicide risk among Service Members and veterans with robust support in the research literature. Perhaps the most well-studied is the interpersonal–psychological theory of suicide (IPTS; [16]), which suggests that individuals attempt suicide in the context of three core factors: perceived burdensomeness, thwarted belongingness, and acquired capability for tolerating pain and injury.

Perceived burdensomeness refers to a feeling of being unable to contribute meaningfully in social relationships with important others or society more broadly, whereas thwarted belongingness describes a state of fragmented or absent social connections accompanied by the feeling of profound loneliness. These concepts are consistent with the concept of *anomie*, the experience of social unmooring, isolation, and the breakdown of ties to valued others, originally advanced by Durkheim [17] to describe the psychosocial conditions that lead to suicide. Among Service Members and veterans, burdensomeness can be particularly salient for those who were accustomed to contributing to important mission outcomes as part of a close-knit unit.

The concept of thwarted belonging may hold a special significance in the military context as well; military service is often explicitly linked to identity and a sense of belonging at the institutional, branch, and unit levels. A sense of belonging is protective in active duty personnel [18], and the loss of this special sense of belonging may be particularly distressing to Service Members and veterans. As discussed below, in the vignette of Cpl Smith, the precipitating factor leading to his suicide attempt highlights a threat to his Marine identity. The message he might have received is that the tribe no longer finds him useful or wanted. The threat of thwarted belonging often also may arise from breakups of romantic relationships.

Finally, IPTS predicts that many Service Members and veterans may demonstrate an enhanced capability for suicide by virtue of military training and experiences that habituate them to physical and psychological distress [19]. For military cohorts generally and combat arms occupational specialties in particular, familiarity with firearms is a core component of acquired capability, and this component of IPTS is thus present in the military context to a greater degree than in the civilian context [1].

In the context of IPTS, variables linked to suicide risk can be organized into broader conceptual categories. Functional deficits and disabilities associated with physical and especially mental health diagnoses may contribute to a sense of perceived burdensomeness because they may impede Service Members' and veterans' abilities to find meaningful work or other means of contributing to relationships or society. In addition, stigma associated with mental health problems, like military PTSD, in addition to the direct impact of mental health-related symptoms, may lead to social withdrawal or isolation, compounding the risk posed by perceived burdensomeness and leading to a sense of thwarted belongingness. Finally, Service Members and veterans in general and those with combat experience, in particular, are likely to have an enhanced capability for suicide as a result of habituation to physical stress and access to and familiarity with firearms. This enhanced capability in the context of perceived burdensomeness, thwarted belongingness, and elevated risk of mental health problems represents an important set of risk factors.

Work by Klonsky and May [20] expanded on IPTS by advancing a three-step theory of suicide. In the first step, a combination of psychological pain and hopelessness leads to some degree of suicidal ideation. Next, when pain outweighs social connectedness, ideation increases in severity. Finally, a high degree of pain and a low degree of social connectedness facilitates suicide attempts in the context of dispositional, practical, and acquired capability for completing suicide [20]. Building on with this theoretical framework, research has shown that while some individuals do complete suicide impulsively, suicide models are better characterized by increasingly severe behaviors along a trajectory from ideation to attempts, rather than by a single impulsive behavior resulting in death by suicide [20]. A 2018 review (Klonksy, Saffer, and Bryan) of this ideation-to-action framework emphasized the importance of pain, hopelessness, and acquired capability for bridging the gap between suicide ideation and suicide attempt. This is consistent with the risk and resilience framework advanced by IPTS, wherein social connectedness and the ability to contribute meaningfully buffer against the risk conferred by psychological pain, social isolation, perceived burdensomeness, and capability for suicide.

Military Transition Theory

Military transition theory [1] describes the social processes and conditions that define key transition points in military Service Members' career trajectories and how they can lead to the development of thwarted belongingness, perceived burdensomeness, and the acquired ability to complete suicide. Perhaps the most salient military transition experience is the move from active or reserve duty status to veteran status. This entails shifting from military culture to civilian culture, producing changes in relationships, social norms and values, work context, and personal and social identity. Military transition theory identifies three interacting and overlapping phases to describe the progression of Service Members' transition out of the military. The first phase, approaching the military transition, outlines the personal identity, social, cultural, and economic factors that lay the foundation of the transition trajectory. This phase can be understood to represent the groundwork the Service Member has done to prepare for the transition to civilian status. It may include behaviors like planning for civilian employment or enrolling in higher education, obtaining civilian housing, managing healthcare and benefits paperwork, connecting with civilian family members and friends, and reflecting on how the transition may impact identity. The second phase, managing the transition, refers to an individual, community and organizational factors that affect the individual progression from Service Member to civilian. This phase includes behaviors that new veterans engage in to adapt to and maintain their new lives as veterans, including managing civilian employment, adjusting to civilian norms and values, and connecting with veterans' services and opportunities that contribute to the development of post-military life. The final phase, assessing the transition, describes outcomes associated with the transition. The key outcomes domains include work, family, health, general well-being, and community [21].

Military transition theory illustrates how changes in determinants of social, economic, and personal identity that accompany the transition to civilian status may create susceptibility to negative mental and behavioral health outcomes, including suicidal behavior. Castro and Kintzle [1] apply the theory to demonstrate vulnerability to acts of self-harm among both older and younger veterans, describing how the development of perceived burdensomeness and thwarted belongingness may be influenced by distinct temporal factors unique to each group. The authors described the impact of the transition from middle to later life, a period often filled with increased feelings of burdensomeness and lack of belongingness, as the Hemingway effect. Physical and psychological health tends to deteriorate later in life, especially if injuries were incurred while serving in the military [22]. Family members and close friends, especially friends with combat and military experience, begin dying, significantly disrupting the veterans' social support network and thus their sense of belongingness [23]. Identifying older veterans who are entering this transition phase of their lives can help provide critical support and address unmet physical and psychological health needs to ensure a sense of social connection and belonging is retained in older adulthood.

Military transition theory can also be applied to make sense of observed vulnerability to suicidality among younger Service Members and veterans. OEF/OIF era veterans often rejoin civilian communities characterized by a lack of familiarity with military culture [24]. Military transition theory suggests that this lack of shared military cultural identity can impede the development of an effective social support network as well as a sense of community belongingness. In addition, OEF/OIF era veterans may have encountered difficulties translating their military experience into civilian employment opportunities with the same level of responsibility, team cohesion, and social prestige, particularly in the context of the global economic crisis of the late 2000s. These challenges are even greater for veterans with nonroutine or punitive military discharge status, whose transitions are more likely to be unplanned and to reflect existing behavioral health problems [25]. Veterans' with nonroutine discharge status demonstrate more physical and mental health challenges than routinely discharged veterans, as well as social stigma, an increased risk for suicide, and more barriers to accessing physical and mental health services [25, 26]. Along with challenges to personal identity and unmet psychological and physical health needs, these impediments can complicate the transitions of younger veterans; if they are not addressed promptly, thwarted belongingness may ensue. Military transition theory explicates how thwarted belongingness and burdensomeness are particularly salient risks at specific junctions in veterans' transition trajectories; understanding where along the transition trajectory risks are greatest allows for development and targeting of interventions to support the development of a healthy veteran identity.

In light of these theoretical considerations, a picture of suicide risk framed by an enhanced capability for suicide in the context of mental and behavioral health challenges, physical health problems, and the downstream sequelae of perceived burdensomeness and thwarted belongingness in the context of poor military transitions, begins to emerge.

For Cpl Smith, the loss of his identity as Marine following his discharge, as well as his deteriorating psychological and physical health, lead to feelings of burdensomeness and thwarted belonging. Cpl Smith had been close to members of his unit, but his psychiatric symptoms made socializing in public uncomfortable, and he lost touch with many of his battle buddies. When they did connect, Cpl Smith didn't want to disclose his diagnoses or symptoms and found himself avoiding their company. Cpl Smith also faced serious financial challenges and had difficulty securing civilian employment. He felt ashamed of not being able to provide more support to his mother, which lead to more isolation.

Protective Factors and Suicide Prevention Interventions

While recent VHA and DoD reporting showed an increase in age and sex-adjusted suicide rates for military Service Members and veterans from 2005 to 2018, both institutions have made substantial efforts to decrease suicides in these groups. VHA clinics have attempted to increase mental health treatment access, including hiring additional professional mental health counselors, expanding telehealth programs, and establishing a 24/7 crisis hotline [7, 12]. Additional VHA efforts to address veterans' suicide risk include bolstering mental health services for women, providing mobile apps designed to assist with self-management of mental health problems, and expanding partnerships with community-based counseling centers [7].

DoD initially recognized an increase in rates during the early years of deployments to Iraq prompting the initial Mental Health Assessment Team reviews and subsequently made efforts throughout their organizations to increase awareness, enhance first line leader recognition, educate about and normalize deployment transitions, and improve access to mental health care. Beginning in 2009, the Army and the National Institute of Mental Health (NIMH) formed a partnership to fund a large research team to develop and implement the Army Study to Assess Risk and Resilience in Servicemembers (Army STARRS). While the initial study terminated in 2015 with over 100,000 participants, ongoing longitudinal data collection efforts continue under the STARRS paradigm with the goal of building on existing STARRS data to further produce actionable findings in support of improving Service Members resilience and reducing military suicides (see https://starrs-ls.org/). Informed by these data, DoD has invested in prevention strategies including strengthening economic supports and access to and delivery of suicide care; creating protective environments by attempting to change norms and behaviors around firearm storage and access; expanding the availability of peer to peer supports; teaching coping skills; and identifying those at highest risk [2]. However, that latter initiatives began as pilot interventions in 2019 and 2020, and outcome data is not yet available. Despite these and additional efforts to reduce suicides and improve access to mental health services for active-duty personnel and veterans, suicide rates have proven resistant to change, particularly among those, like Cpl Smith, with several overlapping risk factors. Overall, there remains a dearth of empirical evidence from a systematic investigation of interventions designed specifically to reduce suicides among Service Members and veterans.

In civilian studies, variables associated with social support, like feelings of family responsibility and purpose in life, are consistently linked with reduced risk of suicide. Social support and sense of purpose have also been found to exert protective effects against suicidal ideation in military populations [27, 28]. In addition, mixed evidence suggests that unit cohesion, a term used to describe social support afforded by interpersonal connections and task orientation within military units, may offer some protective effect against suicide among service members [29, 30]. A recent study of approximately 500 Army Soldiers also found that leadership qualities like providing meaning and purpose in addition to unit cohesion were associated with lower baseline rates of suicidal ideation and suicide death during deployment, though only leadership purpose demonstrated a significant association with suicide outcomes 3 months following return from deployment [31]. Despite these findings, there has been relatively little empirical investigation of factors that might protect against suicide among Service Members and veterans, further hindering prevention efforts. One promising approach has been the collaborative assessment and management of suicidality [32]. This approach to suicide prevention among veterans has demonstrated feasibility, acceptability, and effectiveness in reducing suicides among veterans compared to usual treatment [33, 34]. Both its individual treatment framework and group iteration focus explicitly on reducing veteran suicide by targeting primary drivers of suicidal behaviors assessed on an individual and ongoing basis. In addition to assisting suicidal veterans with developing adaptive strategies for coping with suicide risk factors and ideation, the framework focuses on building social connectedness as a means of combating thwarted belongingness [34]. This intervention strategy exemplifies the movement of suicide prevention efforts toward a focus on resilience, which is broadly concerned with psychosocial factors that protect against negative mental and behavioral health outcomes following exposure to stressors.

Debate continues concerning the definition and operationalization of the resilience construct, but evidence suggests that certain psychological skills may protect against the development of PTSD and other mental health problems following exposure to high-stress situations, such as combat. As a result, these skills might serve as useful targets for upstream preventive interventions, even if they do not target specific drivers of suicidality. For example, mindfulness, or the ability to focus nonjudgmental attention on present-moment thoughts, emotions, and behavioral urges without attempts to change them [35], has been linked to improvements in adaptive coping behavior and stress management [36]. In addition, because both Service Members and veterans consistently demonstrate a preference for self-management of mild to moderate mental health symptoms [2, 37, 38], self-guided mindfulness practices may represent a low barrier path to acquiring emotion regulation and attention control skills that facilitate adaptive coping.

Studies investigating domain-focused mindfulness-based interventions with veterans are have demonstrated promising preliminary results. A study of veterans in a residential PTSD treatment program [39] found that increased mindfulness operationalized as cognitive and emotional awareness skills was associated with reduced clinician-rated measures of PTSD and depressive symptoms. A separate study of 34 Marine reservists [40] showed that more time spent in attention control practice was associated with lower perceived stress. Despite these empirical links between attention control and nonjudgmental awareness domains and psychological resilience, there has been little investigation of the potential for mindfulness training to buffer against downstream behaviors, like suicidality, associated with military-specific risk factors. While evidence based PTSD interventions like prolonged exposure therapy and cognitive processing therapy ought to be the first-line treatments, research shows that only 6.3% of veterans with PTSD seeking VHA care actually receive at least one session of PTSD-specific treatment, and most treatments received are non-trauma focused these treatments [41].

In addition to intervening to improve psychological skills associated with resilience, veteran suicide prevention efforts could benefit from holistic interventions that address critical determinants of Service Members' multiple postservice transitions. Because suicide is a complex phenomenon, multiple, overlapping intervention strategies applied at the individual, group, and institutional levels are likely to have the best chance of lowering suicide rates. Military transition theory suggests that Service Members and veterans with mental health problems are most vulnerable to suicidal urges and behaviors during periods of upheaval in social support networks and employment (or other activities that provide a sense of contributing to valued others or society) because these disruptions may trigger feelings of thwarted belongingness and perceived burdensomeness [1]. In addition to screening for mental health problems and efforts to improve psychological coping skills before deployment or exposure to other military stressors, interventions designed to prevent veteran suicides must take broader social and contextual factors into account and emphasize the importance of developing robust social support systems and improving veterans' transitional outcomes.

The theoretical emphasis on the importance of a sense of belonging and meaning in the prevention of veterans' suicide is bolstered by empirical evidence. In a study of Vietnam veterans [42], those who were more resilient, operationalized by evincing a high number of lifetime traumas but low psychological distress, scored higher on measures of perceived purpose in life, social support, and community integration. Similarly, several studies investigating resilience among OIF/OEF veterans show that lower perceived unit support and postdeployment social support were associated with higher rates of PTSD and depression, mental health problems with well-established links to suicidal behaviors [28, 43]. Cpl Smith joined the Marines in his early 20s and deployed to Afghanistan soon after. Other than his mother and a few high school buddies, he did not have close civilian relationships before joining and did not have a social network to return to after his discharge. In addition, Cpl Smith did not have access to a broad range of adaptive coping skills. His family of origin was also characterized by maladaptive emotion regulation behaviors; his mother used substances for most of his childhood, and he grew up without his father in the home. Before his discharge, Cpl Smith would typically manage his stress by drinking. While Cpl Smith's strengths include his commitment to his sobriety and his consistency regarding medical and behavioral health appointments, his PTSD symptoms and associated psychological pain have not remitted. This highlights that while the VHA access to care appears to be appropriate, Cpl Smith may not be receiving evidence-based PTSD therapies given their poor penetration real-world clinical practice with veterans. While everything may be done well, this veteran will still have non-modifiable social and biological risks that will remain a threat for chronic suicide risks.

Clinical Management

Clinicians serving military Service Members or veterans in any practice context may encounter those at risk for suicide. While epidemiological studies have identified risk factors at the aggregate level, suicide remains difficult to predict reliably because of low base rates and the fact that many individuals who share risk factors do not go on to attempt or complete suicide. For example, while mental health diagnoses are common risk factors for suicide, DoD data suggests that only about 44%

of 2019 military suicide decedents had mental health conditions [2]. In light of the challenges inherent in identifying Service Members and veterans at risk for suicide and improving suicide prevention, the VA and DoD Cinical Practice Guideline for the Assessment and Management of Patients at Risk for Suicide [44] has advanced several clinical practice guidelines to help prevent suicide in military populations.

Themes derived from patient-driven focus groups involved in the VA/DoD report emphasize the importance of building trust between clinicians and patients, defined by consistent, open, and respectful communication around care. Additional themes include the importance of providing patients with comprehensive information related to risk factors and prevention interventions, including complementary and alternative therapies; a coordinated treatment team approach to facilitate information sharing and support integrated care plans oriented to patient needs; the involvement of patient's families and support networks in care when consistent with patient preferences; and the need to destigmatize the culture around suicide prevention and treatment-seeking in DoD and VA systems [44]. In addition to these guiding themes, the report details a comprehensive algorithmic approach to assessing suicide risk in individual patients—consistent with the report's recommendations, we urge clinicians to examine and adapt these decision tree algorithms to their specific patient contexts. Finally, the report offers a list of specific intervention recommendations accompanied by quality of evidence ratings across the following phases:

Screening and Evaluation

Providers can conduct this by using the Patient Health Questionnaire-9 item 9 to identify suicide risk and conducting a thorough assessment of risk factors including current and past suicidal ideation and attempts, psychiatric conditions and symptoms, prior hospitalizations, recent stressors, and access to lethal means and firearms in particular [44]. Screening is recommended in both primary and specialty care settings and is a low-risk intervention; evidence shows that screening for suicide ideation or behaviors does not increase risk for suicide [45, 46].

Non-pharmacologic Risk Management and Treatments

These include the use of cognitive behavior therapy, dialectical behavior therapy, or problem-solving therapy depending on patient diagnostic characteristics, and development of a crisis response plan for those with ideation or a history of suicide attempts. For clinicians working with military Service Members, the crisis response plan will also require informing command, assessing barriers to care with special attention to stigma, enrolling the Service Member in risk management tracking, and ensuring follow-up during transitions. Case management may offer another way to support treatment engagement and follow through, though there is mixed evidence for its effectiveness in preventing suicide. A retrospective analysis examining changes in suicide rates among VHA enrolled veterans from 2005–2009 found that while increased mental health staffing at VHA clinics was associated with reduced suicide rates, case management did not demonstrate a significant correlation [47]. However, [48] study of case management to facilitate tracking across the deployment cycle did show benefits for reducing suicide risk in Service Members [48]. This study of a U.S. Army division over a 15 month deployment cycle to Iraq found that, when coupled with a case management program to ensure service members remained engaged in treatment, those who deployed with active mental health conditions under treatment had significantly lower incidence of suicide behaviors than those who did not have screening or case management [48]. Thus, in an active duty context where Service Members may be moving frequently, case management can help to facilitate treatment engagement. Given the requirements to inform the commander, clinicians should especially focus on limits of confidentiality around this area when initiating care for active duty Service Members [44].

The specific instances when healthcare providers should notify commanders concerning a Service Member are outlined in the Department of Defense Instructions 6490.08 [49]. These include harm to self or others, admission or discharge from inpatient mental health or substance abuse treatment facility, or enrollment or discharge from any substance abuse treatment programs. Additionally, a commander needs to be notified if the clinician judges the patient to have impulsivity, reliability or judgment concerns that may pose a threat to the military mission. For example, a patient with mania whose military job is working on highly classified cyberwarfare programs may cause damage to national security unless the commander is tracking and is able to mitigate this risk by temporarily removing the patient's access. Therefore, any conditions that may interfere with duty or impair the Service Member requires commander notification. Civilian clinicians may be hesitant and protective of the patient's privacy. However, commanders are important stakeholders who can help deploy a significant amount of care and support to assist the individual Service Member in crises. Additional information about limits to confidentiality and commander exemptions to the Health Insurance Portability and Accountability Act (HIPAA) and be found in the Limits of Confidentiality section of this book.

An important component of psychosocial risk mitigation is removing access to firearms. For active-duty Service Members, a commander can lawfully remove service-issued firearms. Additionally, if the patient resides on a military base, the commander may also order the placement of personal firearms in the unit's armory. However, personal-owned firearms stored off-base cannot be removed involuntarily by a commander despite personal firearms being the most commonly used method of suicide by Service Members [50]. The commander does have the authority to restrict the individual Service Member to the military base as a step towards mitigating risk. This highlights the importance of engagement and initiation of a productive relationship with the commander.

For veterans, usual clinical interventions based on local jurisdictions and laws need to be implemented to reduce access to firearms. For the majority of encounters, the most important factor is the therapeutic alliance and voluntary removal of firearms as the most prudent strategy.

Pharmacologic Treatments

VA/DoD [44] guidelines further describe several pharmacologic interventions with empirical support. These may include a short term ketamine infusion as an adjunctive treatment for reducing acute risk; according to the guidelines, 0.5 mg/kg has moderate evidence for improvement of acute suicide ideation within 24 h of treatment with a moderate effect size persisting for 1 week [44, 51]. In select cases, lithium may be considered although this need to be balanced with the low LD-50 and risk of overdose. Clozapine should be considered in schizophrenia or schizoaffective disorders [44]. Additionally, there may be a role for the treatment of insomnia in suicidal patients where reduced suicidal ideations have been shown with the use of zolpidem [52]. However, the type of hypnotic to use is unclear and there are also concerns of an increase in suicidality with zolpidem [53] and benzodiazepines [54].

Post-acute Care

The posttreatment initiation and posthospitalization periods are critical for intervention. A 2015 Army STARRS study of Soldier's psychiatric hospitalizations from 2004–2009 found that 12% of all Army suicides during the study period occurred in the 12 months following hospitalization, a rate of 239 per 100,000 person years compared to 18.5 per 100,000 person years in the Army as a whole [55]. Another Army STARRS study found that, of the Army suicides from 2004–2009, 41.5% occurred among the 12% of Soldiers who were seen outpatient by mental health specialists, with the highest risk period within 26 weeks of mental health visits [55]. As these findings make clear, engaging Service Members and veterans in evidence-based post-acute care is essential. This includes sending postcards or other caring communications for 1–2 years in addition to treatment as usual following psychiatric hospitalization, offering a home visit to support participation in outpatient care, offering the World Health Organization Brief Intervention and Contract modality, and maintaining reduced access to lethal means following suicide ideation or attempt [44].

We encourage clinicians to review the full 2019 VA and DoD report for additional details and resources related to the recommendations described here.

Clinical Approach

Understand, Identify, and Assess Risk and Protective Factors

As with all clinical practice, careful, ongoing assessment of risk and protective factors identified in the literature is critical. In the context of military suicide, risk factors include ready access to firearms; symptoms of PTSD and depression associated with perceived burdensomeness, thwarted belongingness, and social disruption;

substance use behavior; and difficult transitions, among others. On the other hand, social and contextual factors associated with resilience, like social support, sense of purpose, and adaptive coping and emotion regulation skills, are protective. Identifying these factors, understanding their relationship with suicide risk, and intervening to reduce risks and buttress protective factors are critical components of suicide prevention. Because transitions represent particularly risky periods for veterans due to effects on social connectedness, additional care should be taken during these periods.

Focus on Preventing Risk Factors and Strengthening Protective Factors

For the majority of individuals, thoughts of suicide develop over time as risk factors emerge, protective factors erode, and components of IPTS converge. For practitioners who work with military populations, upstream prevention through intervention at the first signs of difficulty can prevent the accumulation of risk factors. For example, in the veteran context, identifying difficulty finding or maintaining employment may not typically represent a point of suicide prevention, but lack of meaningful employment can interfere with identity development, building new social networks, and financially stability postservice, while also creating anger, frustration, regret, and disappointment. For Service Members coming home from deployments or overseas rotations, readjusting to life with partners and children who have developed a new routine may prove particularly challenging. Although the path may be long, there is a connection between these factors and eventually perceived burdensomeness and thwarted belongingness. Clinicians should recognize the development of even one risk factor as an essential point of intervention in suicide prevention. In addition to the guidelines reviewed above, this might include helping individuals find meaning in their life postservice, encouraging the development of a robust social network by focusing on strengthening relationships with family and friends, providing support related to securing postservice employment, and most critically, addressing unmet physical and psychological health issues as soon as possible. A brief summary of potential interventions is outlined in Table 16.1.

Consider the Complexity of Interventions

Intervention must take into account the complex interplay of psychosocial factors that drive suicide risk among Service Members and veterans. A patient-centered focus on assessing and intervening from a person-in-environment perspective provides an approach well suited to addressing the dynamic constellation of risk factors that contribute to suicide. Although no single intervention can address all mental health risks and social stressors, careful assessment and collaboration with clients or patients can yield a roadmap for treatment wherein immediate risks are addressed and adaptive psychological coping skills and prosocial behaviors are developed

Table 16.1 Risk domains and intervention approaches

Risk domains	Biological	Psychological	Social	Additional notes
Behavioral health	Sleep, diet, exercise, medications	Cognitive therapy for suicidal patients; evidence-based psychotherapy for primary diagnosis	Reduce isolation and develop a plan for strengthening social connections Command notification if indicated for active duty	Consider chaplain referral who can provide absolute confidentiality
Substance use	Medication-assisted treatments; naloxone; treatment of BH conditions	Motivational interviewing; individual psychotherapies	AA, smart recovery, group therapies Command notification if indicated for active duty	
Financial	N/A	Stress management and coping techniques	VA financial support programs	
Occupational	Physical therapy; occupational therapy to improve physical functioning if needed	Job coaching; interviewing skills practice	Community rehabilitative programs Military and veteran educational programs such as GI bill Command notification if indicated for active duty Medical evaluation board referral if active duty	
Legal	N/A	Legal education	Linkage to providers Refer to commander and/or JAG (legal) for active duty	

Table 16.1 (continued)

Risk domains	Biological	Psychological	Social	Additional notes
Relational	Mood, anger, concentration treatment with medications if indicated; treatment of sexual dysfunction with phosphodiesterase-5 inhibitors or specialty referrals for dyspareunia or other sexual disorders	Individual psychotherapies	Partner/couples counseling; occupational and financial stability	Military chaplains offer couples retreats
Access to firearms	N/A	Develop a coping plan for storage when in distress	Remove access; engage family and friends Command notification and command authority	

over time. At a minimum, for clinicians serving military populations, adequate training in evidence-based screening and treatments for PTSD, depression, and suicide risk approaches is critical [56].

Future Direction

There remains much to learn about how to prevent suicide in veterans and which interventions are most effective with this population. Staying vigilant about research with new and emerging findings on the topic is essential to preventing military suicide. Clinicians must stay informed regarding current best practices and supporting evidence.

These recommendations largely reflect guidelines for good practice regarding suicide risk for any individual, and are by no means meant to replace current best practices for suicide assessment and prevention. In the veteran context, however, additional attention is required to address military-specific stressors. Consistent with military transition theory, these include a special focus on identified transition periods such as separation from the military, marriage or family disruption, beginning college or a civilian job, following inpatient hospitalization, or aging.

This chapter is not a comprehensive review of all Service Member and veteran suicide data; rather, we endeavored to synthesize the most well-researched risk and protective factors and intervention recommendations for Service Member and veteran suicide prevention and examine them in a theoretical context that facilitates their application to this unique population. Clinicians serving Service Members and veterans are a critical resource for reducing suicides, and we hope the recommendations we outlined will support their work with this population.

Cpl Smith has experienced trauma including direct killing, alcohol use disorder, opioid use disorder, and chronic pain. The vignette also highlights significant dysfunction consistent with perceived burdensomeness and thwarted belonging; the veteran has been unable to secure meaningful employment and lacks intimate social connections. In addition, his mother suffers from polysubstance abuse, which may convey a predisposition to substance use problems for the veteran through social learning and biological pathways. The convergence of these factors threatens financial instability and presents an imminent risk for homelessness. This veteran is hanging by a thread. His disability money is his lifeline for now, and he relies completely on VHA for his medical care. Cpl Smith requires collaborative, ongoing, evidence-based care in order to reduce modify risk factors for suicide and support development of adaptive coping across psychosocial domains.

Clinical Pearls

- Remember: suicide risk is not associated with entering the military or simply being a military Service Member or veteran. Overlapping stressors like war-time experience, mental health and substance use problems, relationship stress, legal or administrative problems, and financial difficulties, are contextual risk factors amplified by disruptive social experiences and loss of important social connections
- Work to build and maintain a trusting, validating, open, and honest clinical relationship with military-connected individuals. Service Members and veterans have often had unique experiences that require extra effort from clinicians to understand
- Assess for risk factors like psychiatric conditions and symptoms including substance use and sleep quality, previous hospitalizations, recent psychosocial stressors including important transitions, and availability of firearms
- Use presented theories to organize thinking around risk and protective factors and to highlight critical periods of greater risk for suicide
- Employ a collaborative, patient-centered approach and apprise patients of treatment and prevention methods, including complementary and alternative therapies
- Involve trusted members of the patient's social network in prevention and care strategies when consistent with patient preferences
- Develop a plan for restricting lethal means, particularly firearms, when patients endorse high risk behaviors like suicidal ideation or intent

References

1. Castro CA, Kintzle S. Suicides in the military: the post-modern combat veteran and the Hemingway effect. Curr Psychiatry Rep. 2014;16(8):460.
2. U.S. Department of Veterans Affairs Office of Mental Health and Suicide Prevention. National veteran suicide prevention annual report 2020. 2020. https://www.mentalhealth.va.gov/docs/datasheets/2020/2020_National_Veteran_Suicide_Prevention_Annual_Report_508.pdf. Accessed 22 Feb 2021.

3. Kang HK, Bullman TA. Mortality among U.S. veterans of the Persian Gulf War. N Engl J Med. 1996;335(20):1498–504.
4. Seltzer CC, Jablon S. Effects of selection on mortality. Am J Epidemiol. 1974;100(5):367–72.
5. Bollinger MJ, Schmidt S, Pugh JA, Parson HM, et al. Erosion of the healthy soldier effect in veterans of US military service in Iraq and Afghanistan. Popul Health Metrics. 2015;13(1):1–12.
6. Murphy SL, Xu JQ, Kochanek KD, Arias E, Tejada-Vera B. Deaths: final data for 2018. National Vital Statistics Reports, vol. 69 no 13. Hyattsville, MD: National Center for Health Statistics; 2020.
7. Veterans' Health Administration. Suicide among veterans and other Americans 2001–2014. August 3, 2016. https://www.mentalhealth.va.gov/docs/2016suicidedatareport.pdf. Accessed 19 July 2021.
8. Bruce ML. Suicide risk and prevention in veteran populations. Ann N Y Acad Sci. 2010;1208(1):98–103.
9. Kang HK, Bullman TA. Is there an epidemic of suicides among current and former U.S. military personnel? Ann Epidemiol. 2009;19(10):757–60.
10. Barr NU, Sullivan K, Kintzle S, Castro CA. PTSD symptoms, suicidality and non-suicidal risk to life behavior in a mixed sample of pre- and post-9/11 veterans. Soc Work Mental Health. 2016;14:465–73.
11. Kang HK, Bullman TA, Smolenski DJ, Skopp NA, et al. Suicide risk among 1.3 million veterans who were on active duty during the Iraq and Afghanistan wars. Ann Epidemiol. 2015;25(2):96–100.
12. Bryan CJ, Jennings KW, Jobes DA, Bradley JC. Understanding and preventing military suicide. Arch Suicide Res. 2012;16(2):95–110.
13. Castro CA, McGurk D. The intensity of combat and behavioral health status. Traumatology. 2007;13(4):6–23.
14. LeardMann CA, Powell TM, Smith TC, Bell MR, et al. Risk factors associated with suicide in current and former US military personnel. JAMA. 2013;310(5):496.
15. Bachynski KE, Canham-Chervak M, Black SA, Dada EO, et al. Mental health risk factors for suicides in the US Army, 2007–8. Inj Prev. 2012;18(6):405–12.
16. Joiner TE. Why people die by suicide. Cambridge, MA: Harvard University Press; 2005.
17. Pope W. Durkheim's suicide: a classic analyzed. Chicago: University of Chicago Press; 1976.
18. Bryan CJ, Heron EA. Belonging protects against postdeployment depression in military personnel. Depress Anxiety. 2015;32(5):349–55.
19. Bryan CJ, Bryan AO, May AM, Harris JA, Baker JC. Depression, suicide risk, and declining to answer firearm-related survey items among military personnel and veterans. Suicide and Life-Threatening Behavior. 2021;51(2):197–202.
20. Klonsky ED, May A. Rethinking impulsivity in suicide. Suicide Life Threat Behav. 2010;40(6):612–9.
21. Kintzle S, Castro CA. Examining veteran transition to the workplace through military transition theory. In: Harms PD, Perrewe PL, editors. Occupational stress and well-being in military contexts. Bingley: Emerald Publishing Limited; 2018. p. 117–27.
22. Crum-Cianflone NF. The millennium cohort study: answering long-term health concerns of US Military Service members by integrating longitudinal survey data with Military Health System Records. Part 2. Pre-deployment. 2013. https://apps.dtic.mil/sti/pdfs/ADA620647.pdf. Accessed 19 July 2021.
23. Nicholson NR Jr. Social isolation in older adults: an evolutionary concept analysis. J Adv Nurs. 2009;65(6):1342–52.
24. Pease JL, Billera M, Gerard G. Military culture and the transition to civilian life: suicide risk and other considerations. Soc Work. 2015;61(1):83–6.
25. Barr N, Kintzle S, Alday E, Castro C. How does discharge status impact suicide risk in military veterans?. Social Work in Mental Health. 2019;17(1), 48–58.
26. Gundlapalli AV, Fargo JD, Metraux S, Carter ME, et al. Military misconduct and homelessness among US veterans separated from active duty, 2001-2012. JAMA. 2015;314(8):832–4.

27. Lemaire CM, Graham DP. Factors associated with suicidal ideation in OEF/OIF veterans. J Affect Disord. 2011;130(1–2):231–8.
28. Pietrzak RH, Johnson DC, Goldstein MB, Malley JC, Southwick SM. Psychological resilience and postdeployment social support protect against traumatic stress and depressive symptoms in soldiers returning from operations enduring freedom and Iraqi freedom. Depress Anxiety. 2009;26(8):745–51.
29. Mitchell MM, Gallaway MS, Millikan AM, Bell M. Interaction of combat exposure and unit cohesion in predicting suicide-related ideation among post-deployment soldiers. Suicide Life Threat Behav. 2012;42(5):486–94.
30. Wilk JE, Bliese PD, Kim PY, Thomas JL, et al. Relationship of combat experiences to alcohol misuse among U.S. soldiers returning from the Iraq war. Drug Alcohol Depend. 2010;108:115–21.
31. Trachik B, Oakey-Frost N, Ganulin ML, Adler AB, et al. Military suicide prevention: the importance of leadership behaviors as an upstream suicide prevention target. Suicide Life Threat Behav. 2021;51(2):316–24.
32. Jobes DA. The collaborative assessment and management of suicidality (CAMS): An evolving evidence-based clinical approach to suicidal risk. Suicide and life-threatening behavior. 2012;42(6):640–53.
33. Ellis TE, Green KL, Allen JG, Jobes DA, Nadorff MR. Collaborative assessment and management of suicidality in an inpatient setting: results of a pilot study. Psychotherapy. 2012;49(1):72.
34. Johnson LL, O'Connor SS, Kaminer B, Jobes DA, Gutierrez PM. Suicide-focused group therapy for veterans. Military Behavioral Health. 2014;2:327–36. http://doi.org/10.1080/21635781.2014.963762.
35. Kabat-Zinn J. An outpatient program in behavioral medicine for chronic pain patients based on the practice of mindfulness meditation: theoretical considerations and preliminary results. Gen Hosp Psychiatry. 1982;4(1):33–47.
36. Farb NAS, Anderson AK, Segal ZV. The mindful brain and emotion regulation in mood disorders. Can J Psychiatry. 2012;57(2):70–7.
37. Barr N, Kintzle S. Can mindfulness help to predict veterans' mental health service utilization? Soc Work. 2019;64(4):329–38.
38. Barr N, Kintzle S, Alday E, Castro C. How does discharge status impact suicide risk in military veterans? Soc Work Ment Health. 2019;17(1):48–58.
39. Owens GP, Walter KH, Chard KM, Davis PA. Changes in mindfulness skills and treatment response among veterans in residential PTSD treatment. Psychol Trauma Theory Res Pract Policy. 2012;4(2):221–8.
40. Stanley EA, Schaldach JM, Kiyonaga A, Jha AP. Mindfulness-based mind fitness training: a case study of a high-stress predeployment military cohort. Cogn Behav Pract. 2011;18(4):566–76.
41. Shiner B, D'Avolio LW, Nguyen TM, et al. Measuring use of evidence based psychotherapy for posttraumatic stress disorder. Admin Pol Ment Health. 2013;40(4):311–8.
42. Pietrzak RH, Cook JM. Psychological resilience in older U.S. veterans: results from the national health and resilience in veterans study. Depress Anxiety. 2013;30(5):432–43.
43. Pietrzak RH, Johnson DC, Goldstein MB, Malley JC, Southwick SM. Psychological resilience and postdeployment social support protect against traumatic stress and depressive symptoms in soldiers returning from Operations Enduring Freedom and Iraqi Freedom. Depression and Anxiety. 2009;26:745–51. http://doi.org/10.1002/da.20558.
44. U.S. Department of Veterans Affairs & U.S. Department of Defense. Clinical practice guidelines for the assessment and management of patients at risk for suicide. 2019. https://www.healthquality.va.gov/guidelines/MH/srb/VADoDSuicideRiskFullCPGFinal5088212019.pdf. Accessed 1 May 2021.
45. Harris KM, Goh MT. Is suicide assessment harmful to participants? Findings from a randomized controlled trial. Int J Ment Health Nurs. 2017;26(2):181–90.
46. Law MK, Furr RM, Arnold EM, Mneimne M, et al. Does assessing suicidality frequently and repeatedly cause harm? A randomized control study. Psychol Assess. 2015;27(4):1171–81.

47. Katz IR, Kemp JE, Blow FC, McCarthy JF, Bossarte RM. Changes in suicide rates and in mental health staffing in the veterans health administration, 2005–2009. Psychiatr Serv. 2013;64(7):620–5.
48. Warner CH, Appenzeller GN, Parker JR, Warner CM, Hoge CW. Effectiveness of mental health screening and coordination of in-theater care prior to deployment to Iraq: a cohort study. Am J Psychiatr. 2011;168(4):378–85.
49. U.S. Department of Defense. Department of Defense Instruction 6490.08. August 17, 2011. https://www.esd.whs.mil/Portals/54/Documents/DD/issuances/dodi/649008p.pdf. Accessed 10 May 2021.
50. Hoyt T, Repke DM. Development and implementation of US Army guidelines for managing soldiers at risk of suicide. Mil Med. 2019;184(Supplement_1):426–31.
51. Wilkinson ST, Ballard ED, Bloch MH, Mathew SJ, et al. The effect of a single dose of intravenous ketamine on suicidal ideation: a systematic review and individual participant data meta-analysis. Am J Psychiatr. 2018;175(2):150–8.
52. McCall WV, Benca RM, Rosenquist PB, Youssef NA, et al. Reducing suicidal ideation through insomnia treatment (REST-IT): a randomized clinical trial. Am J Psychiatr. 2019;176(11):957–65.
53. Cho CH, Jee HJ, Nam YJ, An H, et al. Temporal association between zolpidem medication and the risk of suicide: a 12-year population-based, retrospective cohort study. Sci Rep. 2020;10(1):1–8.
54. Cato V, Holländare F, Nordenskjöld A, Sellin T. Association between benzodiazepines and suicide risk: a matched case-control study. BMC Psychiatry. 2019;19(1):1–7.
55. Kessler RC, Stein MB, Petukhova MV, Bliese P, et al. Predicting suicides after outpatient mental health visits in the Army Study to Assess Risk and Resilience in Servicemembers (Army STARRS). Mol Psychiatry. 2017;22(4):544–51.
56. Rudd MD, Goulding J, Bryan CJ. Student veterans: a national survey exploring psychological symptoms and suicide risk. Prof Psychol Res Pract. 2011;42(5):354–60.

17 Substance and Prescription Misuse in Military and Veteran Populations

James Rachal, Christian C. Schrader, April Schindler, and Veronica Ridpath

Vignette

John was a 20 year old young man in the early 1970s from an industrial area in the Midwest United States who was drafted to go to serve in Vietnam as an infantryman. Prior to his drafting, he had smoked cigarettes a handful of times and consumed alcohol during several parties with his friends but did not routinely use either. While in Vietnam, John had significant combat exposure, witnessed several of his platoon mates killed in action, and on at least one occasion was himself injured with shrapnel. Shortly after his arrival to Vietnam, John began smoking regularly, initially to help stay awake during guard duty and then just "out of routine." After his injury, he was prescribed narcotic pain medication. He began increasing the amount he was taking and after his prescription ran out began obtaining opiates through non-medical sources. Upon his return from Vietnam, John began working as a steel worker at a local mill. Over the subsequent years, he continued to smoke, his alcohol consumption increased, and his drug use expanded. Over the years he had multiple events at work in which he failed to show up due to his intoxication/hangover or presenting to the work place under the influence. Over the next decade he was fired from numerous jobs and eventually became unable to obtain a job. After repeatedly stealing from or mistreating his friends and family they quit supporting him and he became homeless panhandling and engaging in other illicit behaviors to continue to obtain drugs and alcohol. On one morning, John's body was found by the local policy under a bridge underpass having died from a drug overdose.

J. Rachal (✉)
Atrium Health, Charlotte, NC, USA
e-mail: james.rachal@atriumhealth.org

C. C. Schrader
US Army Psychiatry Residency Program, Carl R. Darnall Army Medical Center, Fort Hood, TX, USA

A. Schindler · V. Ridpath
Atrium Health, Sandra and Leon Levine Psychiatry Residency Program, Charlotte, NC, USA

C. H. Warner, C. A. Castro (eds.), *Veteran and Military Mental Health*,
https://doi.org/10.1007/978-3-031-18009-5_17

Introduction

The case of Joseph above highlights the potential impacts of untreated substance and prescription misuse. These impacts are by no means unique to our military and veteran population as the United States is currently mired in an opioid epidemic across the nation. However, there are several military and veteran unique aspects to these conditions that are important for mental health clinicians to consider and a recent study found that more than one in ten veterans who present to the VA for the first time meet criteria for a substance use disorder [1]. One of the most significant impacts of military service is the exposure and cultural environment to substance use, as well as the potential combat and operational stress exposures. History of combat exposure, hospitalization during deployment, or combat related injuries placed veterans at increased risk for substance use disorders [1].

Additionally, studies of veterans of Iraq and Afghanistan have suggested that 58% suffer from a mental health conditions such as PTSD (55%), depressive disorders (45%), and alcohol dependence (13%) [2]. These conditions all have strong co-morbidities with the development of substance use disorders. Untreated, these substance use disorders can lead to other significant complications including homelessness and suicide. Since 2003, nearly one-third of all suicides and almost half of suicide attempts in the United States Army have involved alcohol or drug use [1] and a recent study of veterans found that those receiving high doses of opiates prescriptions were more than twice as likely to die of suicide [3]. US veterans are estimated to account for over 10% of the national homeless population [4] and a 2014 study found that nearly 70% of homeless veterans also had a substance use disorder [5]. Further, there is a strong link between veteran homelessness. The topics of homelessness and suicide are covered in greater detail in other chapters of this book, but it is important that clinicians keep these areas in mind when considering substance use in this population.

Specific to the military, substance use disorders have a significant negative impact on the mission readiness of our armed forces and upon the daily lives of US service members and veterans. Treatment for service members and for the veteran population can be more difficult than for civilians. Not only for the active treatment but also difficulties in navigating administrative regulations, policies and guidelines for each population. Many service members work in fields that require they be able to safely access or be reliable enough to use or train with explosives, heavy weapons, heavy military vehicles, or complex tasks involving interests of national security. Many veterans continue to work as contractors in the same field as their active duty position so their risk is often similar. Substance use disorders may impair functionality and put the mission at risk. This is why treatment is often overseen by clinicians working for the Department of Defense (DoD). For military service members, their commanding officers are often knowledgeable about, and involved in, referral to services for substance use disorder (SUD) treatment and are aware of how the service member is performing in treatment. This may be due to various reasons, including military regulation, oversight and monitoring of personnel who may have access to high risk or high-value equipment, information and monitoring to ensure that personnel are available to deploy around the world for military missions [6].

Epidemiology Specific to Military and Veteran Personnel

As identified by SAMHSA, the highest risk population for substance use disorders are youth transitioning into adulthood, approximately 18 to 25 years of age [7]. The cohort generally represents young servicemembers in the active, reserve and National Guard populations. 43% of the armed forces personnel are under the age of 25. This population accounts for 2/3 of the positive drug tests within the armed forces. The DoD has identified substance related disorders as an issue impacting sustainment, readiness for deployment, and the ability of soldiers or their counterparts to adequately perform their duties. As such the military has a wide variety of resources available to their populations to assist with overcoming substance abuse or addictions related issues that may not be available or easily accessible within the civilian population. Other major risks include chronic pain, the presence of mental illness, or a history of past diagnosis of SUD. In the veteran and military population, combat exposure and history of deployments correlates with increased prevalence of alcohol and nicotine use disorders.

Illicit substance use within the military achieved significant attention during the Vietnam War era. According to historical documents approximately 42% of US military personnel in Vietnam had used opioids at least once, and half of those individuals had reported physical dependence or symptoms of physical dependence at some time [8]. Although historic numbers were elevated, military drug use trends have continued to decline over the last few decades and are now lower than comparable civilian workforce. In 2009, 1.2% of all DoD uniformed personnel tested positive for illicit substances and the decline continued to 2016 with 0.85% positive for illicit substance use or prescription misuse. In 2016, the United States Army had a 0.95% positive urine drug screen rate, the Navy a 0.38%positive rate, the Air Force a 0.34% positive rate, and the United States Marine Corp a 0.53% positive rate. Civilian data from that same year demonstrated an equivalent positive rate of 4.2% for the same tested substances [9, 10].

Civilian vs DoD Military, Illicit Positives	2010	2012	2014	2016
General Civilian Workforce (% positive)	4.2	4.1	4.7	4.2
DoD Military Personnel (% positive)	1.1	0.9	0.9	0.9

Table references [1, 11]

Although illicit substance use is significantly lower than rates amongst the civilian population, even when age and demographically matched, alcohol and nicotine use disorders remain common and commonly diagnosed amongst military service members [12].

Alcohol use disorder diagnoses (DSM-IV) are more common amongst males than females at a rate of 10.5% vs. 4.8%. Illicit substance use in male veterans had self-reported at 4.8% vs 2.4% for female veterans [13]. The veteran population is more likely to be seen in non-military health care settings, however, and would represent the majority of what is seen off military installations for direct and ancillary care. For this population specifically, reported rate of substance use is increased as compared to the active-duty military, with 3.5% reporting illicit substance use (inclusive of cannabis use), and 1.7% use of illicit other than cannabis [14].

Alcohol

Mr. James is a 45-year-old service member with 21 years of service time who presented to a psychiatrist with a request to be seen outside of normal substance use disorder treatment channels due to his personal concerns for becoming overly reliant on alcohol. He disclosed 10+ years of daily drinking, with his intake reported to have increased to approximately 12 to 14 drinks daily. He cited one year of personal attempts to cut down, only to have drinking increase after those periods of attempted reduction. At present he feels he needs 2 to 3 drinks throughout the day just to get through the day without his hands shaking and to reduce cravings for more. He had no past medication assisted treatment or rehabilitation efforts and had never attended 12 step program meetings. He reported no previous service related or veterans care related substance treatment due to fears that it would negatively impact his career, which to date had been very successful.

Combating alcohol use within the military and veteran populations is a difficult task since it is part of the cultural norm within the populations. Studies have shown increased alcohol use disorder (AUD) diagnoses compared to civilian counterparts [12, 15]. Alcohol use degrades performance and function in both social and occupational settings. Military commands and veterans outreach organizations have identified prevention and treatment remains key to maintenance of a stable and healthy organization, as well as health maintenance for the individual [16]. Early intervention, screening and treatment is required in both populations. Within the active duty military population, proactive treatment is warranted to ensure intoxication or withdrawal does not pose a personal or environmental risk. Military personnel are often required to work with and maintain explosives, weaponry, heavy vehicles, helicopters and aircraft. Additionally, veterans use their expertise in military grade equipment in a high-risk civilian job or have co-morbid conditions which will likely improve with treatment of an underlying AUD. Providing preventive or early treatment to maintain functional status, requires screening in the clinical setting using targeted questioning and motivational interviewing techniques [17].

Unfortunately, AUD remains undertreated pharmacologically, despite the numerous FDA-approved low-cost and minimal side effect medications. Current clinical practice guidelines recommend naltrexone and acamprosate as first-line treatment strategies for moderate or severe AUD. Topiramate and gabapentin remain second line treatment strategies and are also clinically effective in individuals who suffer chronic migraines and or chronic pain, respectively. The medications are available within the military healthcare system for prescription, and while naltrexone is a medication that can only be prescribed to a military member by a psychiatrist at a military treatment facility, gabapentin can be prescribed by any licensed independent practitioner. In treating acute withdrawals, the practitioner needs to determine the potential viability of outpatient versus inpatient treatment. In cases where there is a history of complicated withdrawal, inpatient management should be considered. Outpatient withdrawal management should not be attempted unless the individual can be evaluated daily for 3–5 days for symptom monitoring and for dose adjustment of the benzodiazepines.

Pharmacologic intervention is most effective when combined with patient-tailored behavioral interventions. The VA/DOD recommends offering patients at least one of the following evidence-based interventions: Alcoholics Anonymous (or other 12-step peer support groups), motivational enhancement therapy (aka motivational interviewing), community reinforcement approach, behavioral couples therapy, and/or cognitive behavioral therapy for AUD. For those requiring more comprehensive oversight, intensive outpatient and inpatient rehabilitation centers remain viable options. While the evidence widely supports reduction in alcohol use and increase in abstinence at follow up, outcomes have not shown to differ significantly between inpatient and intensive outpatient service settings [18]. Prior studies have supported better outcomes as measured in reduced daily intake for those severely impaired, but definitive evidence remains elusive [19].

Recommended Treatment Strategies for AUD, in Military and Veteran Populations

- Screen for alcohol use at every visit.
- Offer referral to treatment or 12 Step information to all who screen positive.
- Offer medication management (naltrexone, acamprosate as first line) to assist with recovery and relapse prevention.
- Make the appropriate diagnosis on the medical record, and ensure the record is sent to the nurse case manager who oversees care coordination for the military (Tricare) or VA beneficiaries.

Nicotine

Service member, Sam, used tobacco rarely prior to joining the Marines after high school. He had a history of childhood abuse which he never disclosed to anyone and always had been dysphoric with passive suicidal thoughts. He found boot camp to be very challenging emotionally. A friend recommended e-cigarettes to help manage his anxiety, and he began using them. He liked the fact he could take a quick "puff" almost anywhere and anytime when he needed a "pick me up." Later, he was deployed to Baghdad. He found the days long and boring mixed with the stress of rocket attacks at night. He was not able to take e-cigarettes to his deployment but still needed "help" managing his "anxiety." He began smoking combustible cigarettes. His use further increased to two packs a day after he was in a fire fight and his closest friend died. Upon his return from deployment, he continued to smoke 2 packs a day and had escalating suicidal thoughts. Eventually he presented to behavioral health for depression.

Nicotine use disorder remains a concern in the United States military and veteran population. A 2011 study showed 24% of the military population smoked compared to 19% of the American population. The Marine Corp reported the highest use and the Air Force the lowest [20]. The use of smokeless tobacco among military members remains high as well. One survey showing 19.5% of military personnel using smokeless tobacco [21].

Recent antismoking initiatives including limiting tobacco advertising in military publications, limiting discounted tobacco prices, and increased focus by primary care and dental clinics to ask about interest in quitting have shown promise. A recent study showed a decrease in tobacco use in the Army by 7% from 2013–2017 [22]. Despite this, 22% of veterans enrolled at the VA still smoke [23] with a quit rate of 12% annually [24]. Both are higher than the general population. The higher quit rate is likely due to age and poorer health status of the veterans. Like service member Sam, a 2006 study shows that 38% of smokers started after joining the military [25]. Factors include the young age of recruit, lack of other activities, and a need for socialization. Combat also plays a role in smoking initiation. The deployed environment is a mix of extreme stress and boredom. Further, deployed environments limit the use of other mind- and mood-altering substances leaving tobacco as the only one permitted. Nonsmokers have 60% higher odds of starting smoking after deployment and past smokers have a 30% higher odds of reinitiating smoking [26]. Additionally, nearly a quarter of Iraq and Afghanistan war veterans are diagnosed with PTSD, and individuals with a PTSD diagnosis have an even higher risk of tobacco use disorder [27]. The service member from the vignette had a history of childhood trauma that was exacerbated by his deployment experience. Increase in tobacco use followed.

Electronic cigarettes are the newest tobacco delivery devices used by both civilians and military members. 35.7% of military members have used e-cigarettes and 12.4% are current users according to a recent survey in 2014. This is compared to 12.6% and 3.7% respectively for the United States population [28]. Military members who were younger, tobacco user and had a low perception of harm from e-cigarettes were at increased risk of use [29]. A study by Little of USAF members who used e-cigarettes showed the service members perceived e-cigarettes as unharmful, cool gadgets that are easy to use. Like service member Sam, military members who used e-cigarettes perceived them as a way for "emotional management" and a way to fit in. E-cigarettes also make it easier to circumvent tobacco restrictions during technical training [30]. Air Force members' tobacco use is restricted during training; however, e-cigarettes are much more difficult to detect and, thus, are often used in the dorms. There is also the measure of convenience that the smoker would not have to go to the tobacco use area to smoke and could even conceal it and use it in the workplace. There is also the misperception that bystanders would not be at risk for secondhand smoke despite growing evidence of toxicity [30]. Our member from the vignette showed how easily the transition from e-cigarettes to combustible cigarettes is made.

Along with the economic impacts of smoking there are also serious health consequences and readiness concerns. Military personnel that smoke have more difficulty with physical fitness tests than non-smokers [31, 32]. Studies have shown that smokers are less fit for duty and have difficulty passing the physical fitness test when compared to being overweight [33]. Another study found that Navy females that were smokers were likely to be hospitalized ½ day more than nonsmokers [34]. Smokers are also slower to adapt to the dark and lower awareness of dim lighting. This could have adverse consequences in combat theatre.

Further smoking has shown to hasten hearing loss which is especially concerning since many military personnel are in situations that may already accelerate hearing loss (combat, flight line etc.) [35]. There was a study in 2019 that showed an association between nicotine dependence and onset of suicidal ideation with progression to unplanned suicide attempts. Tobacco users that achieved long term abstinence have improved mental health outcomes relative to those where dependence persist [36]. It should be noted that in military aviators, tobacco use has a unique set of hazards. Use before bedtime can disrupt pilot's ability to obtain restorative sleep and increase risk of inflight error. Withdrawal from nicotine can trigger anger, anxiety and difficulty concentrating all of which can pose significant risk to inflight safety. Lastly carbon monoxide poisoning decreases resistance to hypoxia at altitude and significantly degrades visual performance [22].

Whether smokeless tobacco, combustible tobacco, or e-cigarettes there is strong evidentiary support for asking about the members willingness to quit during health care appointments. Starting out using motivational interviewing techniques to help the patient find their motivation for change is a useful first step [37]. A recent study showed proactive outreach (identifying smokers and contacting them by phone with someone trained in motivational interviewing) can be effective especially with members who suffer with PTSD [27].

Nicotine gum was introduced in 1984 as a prescription for smoking cessation. Since then, other forms of replacement have been introduced both prescription and nonprescription [38]. Nicotine replacement with behavioral therapy has had variable efficacy with smoking cessation but has been shown to be more efficacious than placebo [37]. Both bupropion and varenicline with behavioral therapy have been shown to have greater efficacy than nicotine replacement [23, 39]. Varenicline has shown the greatest success overall [22]. Another consideration when treating military personnel is their specific job type. Members who are on flight status or who are involved with nuclear weapons are often not allowed to take certain medication to maintain their readiness. Any medication used by members on flight status or involved with nuclear weapons should only be prescribed by providers at a military treatment facility [22].

VA/DoD Guidelines and Recommended Strategies for NUD in Military and Veterans

- Ask about tobacco use at every visit
- Advise to quit
- Assess willingness to quit
- Promote motivation to quit
- Educate about treatment options
- Assist in setting a quit date, initiate counseling, initiate pharmacotherapy, offer self-help materials
- Contact 1–2 weeks after quit date to reassess

Cannabinoids

"I just can't get the nightmares to stop any other way, doc." David had come to the office with the complaint of slowly worsening anxiety. His drug screen was positive for THC. He admits that he smokes marijuana nightly as he believes it is the only thing that has helped with pain and sleep. "I've tried to give it up, but I won't sleep for days."

The use, abuse, and perceived medicinal value of marijuana is a very polarizing subject among service members and civilians. Legislative actions at the state level have created a murky landscape with some states legalizing the recreational or medical use of cannabis while it remains a Schedule I drug at the federal level. Active service members are held to federal standards and subject to disciplinary action for cannabis use whereas veterans like David may be using cannabis with the intent to treat medical and psychiatric concerns. In states that have legalized recreational use, cannabis-related ER visits have increased dramatically [40]. Marketing has truly outpaced research and at the time of publication the legality and decriminalization of cannabis and cannabis products remains in flux.

Cannabis

When screening for cannabis use, traditional cannabis flower and derivatives remain the most used forms. Service members describe smoking "bowls," "blunts," "joints," or "bongs" and quantify use in terms of numbers of each or grams of product consumed. Quantifying use becomes more difficult when patients are using waxes and resinous products as these products are significantly more potent. Psychoactive effects of cannabis are derived primarily from delta-9-tetrahydrocannabinol (THC) which is attenuated by a coexisting compound, cannabidiol (CBD). Potency of cannabis flower has itself changed, with average cannabis THC percentage in 1995 at just 4% and increasing to 12% in 2014 while CBD percentage declined [41].

The initial desired effects of euphoria, relaxation, sleep, and altered perception of time are often followed by heightened anxiety, paranoia, and amotivation. A particularly insidious effect of cannabis use is that users have poor appraisal of their capabilities during use, reporting improvement in cognition and skills such as attention and coordination when studies show statistically significant decline in performance [42].

Veterans and others who suffer from PTSD may report improvement in nightmares and sleep duration, and there is evidence in the literature to support this. Use of THC and CBD has been shown to have some REM sleep suppression, which reduces or eliminates the stage of sleep when nightmares occur [43]. The effect is abruptly reversed with discontinuation and can cause "REM rebound" during cannabis withdrawal syndrome with associated vivid dreams and nightmares. Those experiencing this may relapse or escalate use in response. THC use has been found to worsen symptoms of psychosis, increase the development of bipolar disorder and psychotic disorders, such as schizophrenia, particularly when used by adolescents, and while some studies have found a mild reduction in anxiety, the evidence quality is low [44].

Cannabidiol

Cannabidiol (CBD) is considered the non-psychoactive component of cannabis and is marketed for many psychiatric and medical indications without FDA approval. Epidiolex is the only FDA-approved cannabidiol and not accessible by most patients due to the narrow application. Approved for two rare childhood seizure disorders as a second line treatment, it is a CBD isolate available by prescription only [45]. Presently CBD is being studied for applications in anxiety, psychotic disorders and addictions, however the research is not conclusive [46].

The most concerning aspect of supplementation with cannabis products is the lack of regulation by the FDA. Patients who utilize CBD are generally using products of questionable purity derived from industrial hemp. The US FDA sends warning letters frequently to companies based on inaccurate labeling [47]. Products have been removed for higher than allowable levels of THC and other impurities. CBD is an inhibitor of enzymes CYP-3A4 and CYP-2D6, and can increase serum concentrations of SSRIs, opioids, TCAs, benzodiazepines, antipsychotics, antiretrovirals, macrolides, some statins, and warfarin [48]. This can lower the therapeutic dose for prescribed medications and increase the risk for medication adverse effects.

Delta-8 THC and Synthetic Cannabinoids

In states where traditional cannabis products are not legally available, there is a robust market for synthetic cannabinoids. Delta-8 THC is popular and is a nearly identical molecule to the delta-9-THC that makes cannabis psychoactive. There is limited peer reviewed research on the substance, however it is less potent pharmacologically [49]. It is however cross-reactive on urine drug screens and will test positive for THC.

Synthetic cannabinoids known by street names such as K2 and spice may be purchased legally or added as adulterants to other cannabis products [50]. The substances may not be detected on a drug screen and effects can vary drastically from paranoia and profound anxiety, to psychosis or delirium. Patients who try to cut back on their own can find a prolonged withdrawal period characterized by restlessness, anger, irritability, cravings, anxiety, vivid dreams and loss of appetite [51]. There are no FDA-approved treatments for the cannabis withdrawal syndrome, but supportive medications can be used to address symptoms.

Management of Marijuana Withdrawal

- Withdrawal symptoms peak between days 3–5 and generally resolve by three weeks and is dependent on potency of product and chronicity of use.
- In recent studies, women generally have more severe symptoms than men.
- No FDA approved medications for treatment. Mirtazapine and zolpidem are helpful for sleep disturbance acutely, but have no overall benefit for preventing relapse.
- Quetiapine and venlafaxine exacerbate withdrawal symptoms and increase risk of relapse [51].

Veterans Administration Stance on Marijuana

- VA clinicians may not recommend medical marijuana, fill out paperwork supporting the use of medical marijuana, prescribe or recommend the use of CBD, THC productions, or derivatives for non-FDA approved indications.
- VA pharmacies will not fill medical marijuana prescriptions nor will VA pharmacies pay for medical marijuana from other sources.
- Veterans will not be denied VA benefits because of marijuana use and are encouraged to discuss use with their provider for treatment purposes.
- Use of marijuana is prohibited on VA grounds as it is under federal law [52]

Department of Defense Stance on Marijuana

The DoD has stringent regulations regarding the use of cannabinoids and derivatives. Army Regulation 600–85: The Army Substance Use Program details regulations that clarify prohibition of all cannabinoid and hemp products, including CBD, and clarify that service members will be subject to referral to disciplinary action should they engage in the use of these products. Prescription medication Epidiolex is excluded from this prohibition but included is the use of any synthetic cannabinoid such as "K2" or "spice" or substances mimicking the effects of cannabis. These are routinely tested in urine drug screens and positive drug screens may be referred for treatment or disciplinary action.

Benzodiazepines

Ms. Rose is a 39-year-old Army veteran who presents to a community health clinic complaining of insomnia. Last month, she began individual psychotherapy to address military sexual trauma and now has difficulty falling and staying asleep. She reveals increasing alcohol intake of at least ½ bottle of wine per night after work to "calm the nerves" and help her fall asleep. She says clonazepam has been helpful in the past. Review of the EMR and PDMP reveals a recently filled script for hydrocodone-acetaminophen 5 mg–325 mg which was prescribed for chronic back pain from injuries sustained in the service as well as monthly refills of clonazepam 1 mg TID for the past 3 years. She reports her former prescriber at the VA will no longer refill clonazepam due to the new addition of opioids.

Benzodiazepine use, misuse and addiction has been rapidly growing in the US. It is the third most commonly misused substance in the US [53]. Benzodiazepine misuse has been described as an "overlooked" epidemic [54]. As of 2016, 12.6% adults reported benzodiazepine use in the past year. Adults aged 50–64 have the highest prescribed use (12.9%) while young adults (18–25 years) having the highest rates of misuse (5.2%) [55]. A recent Harvard Review found very limited evidence to support the use of benzodiazepines in older adults for any approved indication [56]. Among veterans, prescribing rates in older adults are dropping (3% as of 2017) due to considerable education efforts on the part of VA DoD [57]. Ambulatory prescribing of benzodiazepines continues to climb, and veterans like Ms. Rose may present to civilian clinics in this context. A recent study revealed ambulatory care visits for benzodiazepines have doubled between 2003 and 2015, and primary care visits accounted for 52.3% of all such visits [58]. Perhaps, most concerning is co-prescribing of benzodiazepines with opioids has quadrupled during this same period [58].

Alongside rising use of prescribed benzodiazepines, there is growing use of illicit novel benzodiazepines that can be more potent and less detectable by conventional UDS screening. These new psychoactive substances, or "designer benzodiazepines," have similar structures to FDA-approved benzodiazepines although they have no proven medical use. Some have never even been formally studied prior to human consumption. There is limited information about specific pharmacodynamic actions, metabolic profiles, risks, and addiction or overdose potential. The "designer benzodiazepines" have not specifically been studied in veteran populations. Designer agents are typically manufactured outside the US and sold online for a nominal fee [59]. There is growing concern for lethal contaminants, such as fen tanyl, and they are often used in combination with other substances. Novel substances can typically be detected with confirmatory urine mass spectrometry [60, 61].

Inappropriate use of benzodiazepines remains a considerable problem carrying significant risk, comorbidity, and mortality, especially for veterans. The general risks of benzodiazepine use include tolerance, dependence, and withdrawal. Worsening anxiety, cognitive decline, persistent and rebound insomnia, falls, accidental injuries, increased healthcare utilization, and death are risks of use [54]. For patients like Ms. Rose who combine CNS depressants, there is a specific danger of respiratory depression, hypoxemic brain injury and death [62]. For US veterans overall, the odds of adverse outcomes with concomitant opioid use (opioid and benzodiazepine prescriptions that overlap for at least 7 days) is 1.36 times more likely than for opioid-only prescriptions alone [63]. In fact, half of deaths from drug overdose in US veterans occur when veterans simultaneously take benzodiazepines and opioids, independent of benzodiazepine dose [64]. In response, the FDA issued a black box warning against co-prescribed benzos and opioids. However, a veteran with moderate to severe opioid use disorder (OUD) and long-term benzodiazepine use should still be considered for opioid agonist medications to treat OUD. In this case, the prescriber would work closely with the veteran to taper them off the benzodiazepine while treating the OUD.

VA/DoD Guidelines and Recommended Strategies for Benzodiazepines in Military and Veterans

For veterans with PTSD, the VA/DoD 2017 Practice Guideline for the Management of PTSD discourages against benzodiazepine use given their lack of efficacy and risk of dependency [65, 66]. Veterans with PTSD who take benzodiazepines have increased risk of hospitalization, emergency room visits, mental health visits, and all-cause mortality [67, 68]. Sadly, these same veterans have significantly increased risk of suicidal ideation, suicide attempts and death by suicide [67]. Even still, the VA found that up to 30% of veterans are prescribed benzodiazepines [65, 66].

Veterans with concurrent use of CNS depressants (opioids, alcohol, skeletal muscle relaxants, gabapentinoids, etc.), comorbid conditions (in particular, with a history of substance use disorders, chronic pain, COPD, and PTSD), and adults under age 65 are considered highest risk for benzodiazepine use disorder [69]. Such veterans are at increased risk of adverse events, overdose, and death, necessitating continuous screening, close monitoring, clinical documentation of medical necessity, and treatment optimization [70].

Risk Mitigation

To mitigate the risk when prescribing benzodiazepines, consider implementing the following practices:

- Routine urine drug screening
- Screen for illicit medication use (± confirmatory testing)
- Pill counts
- PDMP review when prescribing narcotics
- Deprescribe (slowly taper) patients on long-term benzodiazepines
- If medically necessary, prescribe for short term in low doses. Clearly document the necessity and discussion of risks.

The VA has implemented targeted interventions to change prescribing practices for veterans. These resources are available for all prescribers to access and disseminate. The VA DoD has published resources to assist prescribers in educating themselves, their patients, and assist providers in discussions about risks of use and tapering strategies for benzodiazepines (https://www.pbm.va.gov/PBM/academicdetailingservice/Benzodiazepines.asp).

Stimulants

Mr. S is a 28-year-old partnered, Caucasian Army veteran with no documented medical history who presents to the clinic complaining of poor concentration and memory. He says he cannot keep up with nursing school studies. He has been drinking 3–4 cups of strong, home brewed coffee throughout the day to "help focus and stay on task." He reports having a similar problem while serving in Special Forces for which he "chewed Adderall like candy" between ages 22–24. He denies any behavioral or academic issues in childhood. He denies depression and anxiety. He smokes cannabis nightly to fall asleep and is ambivalent about how cannabis use may be affecting his attention, memory, and performance in college. He asks to be restarted on Adderall for self-reported ADHD.

The use of stimulants has steadily increased worldwide over the last decade, to include the use of prescribed stimulants (amphetamine and methylphenidate), non-medical use of pharmaceutical stimulants, methamphetamine and cocaine. Recently, the US has seen a slight decrease in misuse of pharmaceutical stimulants and an increase in methamphetamine use [71]. Cocaine remains one of the more commonly abused substances worldwide. Each of these substances will be addressed in the following paragraphs. Nicotine-based stimulants are discussed independently elsewhere in the chapter.

Methamphetamine/Amphetamine

The annual prevalence of stimulant use, both prescribed and illicit use, is estimated at 3.3% [71]. There is a growing concern over the non-medical use of stimulants other than methamphetamine. Nearly 2% of people over age 12 report misuse of pharmaceutical stimulants in the past year and 0.7% report using methamphetamine [71]. As compared to non-veterans, veterans meet criteria for lifetime history of stimulant use disorder at a slightly higher rate (2.2% vs 1.7) [72]. Stimulants are the second most abused drug in the world, and veterans are no exception.

In veteran populations, initial prescriptions for stimulants rose three-fold between 2001 and 2012, with an even greater increase (eightfold!) in adults aged 18–44 [73]. Other subgroups with increased rates of stimulant prescriptions include females, adults aged 45–64, and veterans in the US South region. Shockingly, 3 out of 5 stimulant prescriptions (64.7% overall) were written for off-label use. Studies indicate that the off-label, non-medical use of stimulants places veterans at high risk for subsequent amphetamine use disorder [73].

For veterans receiving prescribed stimulants, there are mixed findings concerning potential risks. It is well documented that appropriate treatment of ADHD with stimulants reduces the risks of developing subsequent substance use disorders [74]. However, those with ADHD are at elevated risk of comorbid SUD at baseline. In fact, 1 of 10 veterans with an incident stimulant prescription have at least one documented SUD at baseline. There is a subset of veterans for whom one should exercise increased caution when initiating stimulant medications due to the risk of developing a subsequent amphetamine use disorder [73]:

- Those with increased baseline SUD
- Younger age
- White non-Hispanic
- Male gender
- Unmarried
- No service connection, no insurance

For Mr. S, he has a questionable history of ADHD and self-reports a history of misusing stimulants and cannabis. This in addition to his age, gender, and ethnicity all increase his risk of developing a subsequent amphetamine use disorder. The prudent clinician should proceed cautiously with a thorough medical and psychiatric evaluation before considering prescribed stimulants.

The health consequences for amphetamine/methamphetamine abuse in the veteran population include cardiovascular complications, heart failure, more frequent healthcare utilization, and unintentional overdose [75]. While rare, there are reports of methamphetamine containing fentanyl and other high potency synthetic opioid analogues making recreational use of illicit amphetamines even more dangerous and potentially lethal.

Treatment of stimulant/amphetamine use disorder is challenging and there is low quality evidence for pharmacologic interventions. There have been studies to suggest benefits with high-dose methylphenidate. However, VA DoD clinical practice guidelines discourage pharmacologic treatments and recommend cognitive behavioral therapy (CBT) and/or recovery focused behavioral therapy in combination with contingency management [65, 66].

Cocaine

The estimated annual prevalence of cocaine use in the US is approximately 2% [71]. Compared to non-veterans, veterans met criteria for a lifetime history of cocaine use disorder at a similar rate of 2.4% [72]. Cocaine is a stimulant with high addictive potential and is associated with similar health complications as with other stimulants, including cardiovascular, neurologic, psychiatric, and behavioral effects [76]. As one of the most common drugs of abuse worldwide, it remains one of the more difficult substance use disorders to treat. In 2013, cocaine was the third most common reason for veterans who sought inpatient substance abuse treatment, after alcohol and heroin [7]. Unfortunately, there are no FDA-approved treatments for cocaine use disorder.

In addition to the health complications of stimulant abuse, cocaine use has been shown to result in structural and functional brain changes in veterans, including alterations in the striatal reward circuitry, impaired inhibitory control of the dorsolateral prefrontal cortex, as well as other insular, orbitofrontal and prefrontal changes that affect decision-making and response to cravings [77]. Many of these changes persist despite prolonged abstinence. Furthermore, cocaine carries a high risk of suicide and overdose among veterans [78]. As with other illicit substances, the growing concern for contaminants, such as fentanyl, further increase the risk of unintentional overdose and death. Cocaine use disorder is a complicated disease with significant morbidity and mortality warranting further research to identify successful treatment strategies.

Treatment

The general treatment strategy for stimulant use disorders favor psychosocial interventions involving [79]:

- Cognitive behavioral therapy
- Motivational enhancement therapy
- Contingency management

Pharmacotherapies have thus far yielded unimpressive results and are not encouraged by the current VA DoD cocaine use disorder treatment guidelines [76, 80].

Opiates

Mr. Salyer is a 23-year-old male service member and was seen in the emergency room due to altered mental status and multiple positives on the urine drug test. He presented in a mud-stained military uniform, disheveled and unwashed, with tired, bloodshot eyes. His accompanying escort (equally dirty, though presenting much better combed hair and a shave) relates that he was a brought for an acute evaluation due to periods of not being able to be aroused, irritability, poor work performance, and finding a canteen filled with vodka and a small tin with white pills and white powder residue. He was mildly sedated in the interview and generally non-cooperative. A review of his medical record showed a history of prescription opiates over the last year and half due to intermittent knee pain.

The misuse of prescription drugs, particularly opioids, and prescription-initiated substance use disorders is on the rise within the United States. The most recent data from the 2016 National Survey on Drug Use and Health (NSDUH) reports data on misuse of prescription drugs in the four categories which include pain relievers, tranquilizers, stimulants, and sedatives [81]. Over six million Americans aged 12 years or older reported misuse of prescription drugs at least once in the past month. More than half of these individuals reported misuse of prescription pain relievers in the past the month followed by tranquilizers, prescription stimulants, and prescription sedatives. An even greater number of Americans, almost 12 million, reported misuse of opioids in 2016, with over 95% of these individuals reporting misuse of prescription pain relievers. Of the seven million people identified to have an illicit drug use disorder in 2016, prescription pain relievers were the second most common disorder reported [82, 83].

The most common formulation of prescription pain relievers misused in the survey was hydrocodone products, followed by oxycodone products, and a much smaller percentage of misuse with fentanyl, buprenorphine, and methadone. Pain was the most common reason for misuse of prescription pain relievers; however, other reasons reported included to get high, relax, help with sleep, calm troubled emotions, or to simply experiment with the drug [81]. Military personnel and veterans remain at increased risk in the above factors due to high levels of musculoskeletal injury during training or deployment, the sleep disruption caused by high operational tempo or mission requirements, or to alleviate the emotional distress from an underlying depression, anxiety or trauma-based disorder post combat. Re-developing early intervention and treatment strategies for pain and other causal factors that may lead to prescription substance abuse has been a high priority in keeping service members healthy and mission capable.

For many years, opioids have been the most common prescription treatment for pain; however, clinical practices are transforming the approach to management of pain within the civilian and military populations [84]. There are several risks associated with long-term opioid therapy which include drug tolerance, addiction, and risk of overdose. In order to reduce initial opiate contact, a large re-focus has taken place in early treatment and physical therapy for musculoskeletal injuries in this highly athletic population (active duty military) and amongst the veteran population who often push through their day with remnants of injuries sustained while on active duty status [85].

Several interventions across the civilian and military cultures have been created in response the opioid epidemic with the goal of reducing prescription opiate misuse and prevention of prescription initiation substance use disorder [86]. Several states have created prescription drug monitoring programs (PDMPs) that are electronic databases used to track the prescribing and dispensing of controlled prescription drugs to patients. Some research has shown a decrease in rates of opioid prescribing and overdose in some states that use PDMPs [87, 88]. While many are state dependent, the military healthcare system utilizes a prescription database accessible within the current electronic medical record, allowing providers to track and monitor all medications dosed at any site for their patients. This functionality allows for ease of tracking past pain treatments and prescription over-use within the military system, and when coupled to PDMP monitoring provides a comprehensive assessment of controlled substance use over time. Newly released results from a study that looked at data for opioid prescription patterns between 2006 and 2014 within military treatment facilities or through TRICARE reveal a decrease in opioid use patterns in both civilian and military populations, more pronounced in military populations [89].

Management of low back pain and opioid therapy for chronic pain is addressed in two clinical practice guidelines by the DOD & the VA, where an emphasis is placed on non-pharmacologic and non-opioid pharmacologic therapies for chronic pain such as occupational therapy, physical therapy, and non-opioid pain medications as first line treatments [65, 66]. In the 2015 updates, the VA and DoD released guidelines for management of substance use disorders including opioid use disorder. There is strong recommendation to treat opioid use disorders with medication-assisted treatment using opioid agonists such as methadone or buprenorphine over taper or psychosocial treatment alone. There is moderate evidence for recommendation to use naltrexone, an opioid antagonist for treatment of opioid use disorder. Both of those treatments have been integrated into the ongoing roll out of intensive outpatient and residential treatment programs within the DoD and VA systems of care, and widely supported by the addictions medicine specialists in the services.

Buprenorphine represents a medication and treatment strategy for both pain (as buprenorphine formulation) and opiate use disorder (as the buprenorphine/naloxone combination medication) [90] which in the recent decade has received renewed interest and research in the United States. It has been used successfully in many European countries over that same time in the harm reduction model of addictions treatment and approved for use in the US by the FDA in the 1980s. Unlike full agonists, buprenorphine has been shown to have no immunosuppressive effects, its breakdown and elimination are not altered in the geriatric population or in cases of renal dysfunction, and risk of respiratory depression is much lower [91].

In cases where opioid therapy is warranted, it is recommended that the clinician do a complete opioid risk assessment which include complete biopsychosocial assessment including assessment for behavioral health issues, prior substance use history, and family history. Risk mitigation strategies for long-term opioid therapy include written informed consent and opioid treatment agreements, routine urine drug testing, quarterly checks of the state database system for prescription drugs, monitoring for overdose potential and suicidality, prescribing of naloxone as rescue medication, and frequent follow up at a minimum every three months [92].

Recommended Treatment Strategies for Opiate Related Disorders in Military and Veterans

- Avoid opiate prescriptions if clinically appropriate.
- Switch to buprenorphine as an alternate to chronic opiate prescriptions.
- Obtain and check the prescription monitoring database for your state, prior to prescribing opiates.
- Refer to an addiction specialist for medication assisted therapy in cases where opiate use impairs social and occupational function.

Other Medication Abuse and Misuse

Mr. Seymour is a 25 year old US Air Force member. He presents to you for a command directed evaluation after being apprehended by an air marshal on a civilian flight. While in mid-air, he began telling everyone on the aircraft to take cover, there were terrorists on board. His urine drug screen is negative and no one in his command has noted any unusual behavior other than this incident. You do an exhaustive evaluation of the gentleman, and he denies any other psychiatric concerns. On your review of substance use, he denies any illicit substances and only minimal alcohol. When asking about non-prescription medication, he admits to taking several tablets containing dextromethorphan to help him "dance better with his daughter."

Controlled substances are often in the spotlight for medication overuse and diversion; however, there are several other medications that can be misused or abused. Prescription drug abuse can be difficult to detect. Practitioners who work with patients with a history of substance use often take care to avoid the use of medications with known abuse potential. However, substance use disorders are often more behavioral than related to a specific substance. Distress tolerance and the ability to endure unpleasant or uncomfortable internal states can improve with treatment for substance use disorders. A lack of improvement can be predictive for relapse [93].

Gabapentin

Gabapentin has indications for neuropathic pain and anxiety, as well as evidence that it may reduce alcohol cravings. Gabapentin is widely prescribed and readily accessible. In one study, between 40% and 65% of those with a prescription for gabapentin reported taking more than prescribed at least once, and between 15% and 22% of patients with opioid use disorder reported mixing with gabapentin [94]. The potentiating effect of gabapentin to increase sedation and anxiolytic effect of other depressants is part of the abuse potential, and it has been found to increase the risk of opioid related death [95].

Muscle Relaxants

Skeletal muscle relaxants are often used in patients with chronic pain. Those that are considered less reinforcing and non-scheduled are preferred. There is however a continued risk of abuse, again with supratherapeutic doses and when combined with other depressant substances. All centrally acting muscle relaxants, including methocarbamol, which has historically been thought to be less sedating, carry the risk of respiratory depression when mixed with other depressants [96]. Baclofen is a GABA mediated agent and is used long term in patients with traumatic spinal cord for spasticity and even for management of alcohol use disorder [97]. However, abrupt discontinuation, particularly if patients have been taking higher than prescribed doses, can lead to a GABA rebound and delirium.

Antihistamines and Over the Counter Medications

Diphenhydramine abuse is not uncommon as it is readily accessible, undetectable by standard drug screen, and provides rapid anxiolytic and sedative effect. Abuse may go unnoticed until patients present to emergency services with tachycardia, diaphoresis, tremor, seizure, and altered mental status [98]. Other antihistamines produce a similar effect. Another cough and cold medicine, dextromethorphan, can be abused for its euphoric and hallucinogenic potential, as it can be a potent dissociative [58]. Special care needs to be taken if dextromethorphan abuse is suspected as many of these products are compounded with acetaminophen and liver injury can occur due to unintentional acetaminophen overdose.

Treatment Recommendations

- Screen for high-risk behavior including taking more medication than prescribed, mixing medications with alcohol or other depressants, using sedating medications in high-risk situations such as driving or operating machinery.
- Include screening for depression and anxiety disorders as well as psychosocial stressors

Access to Substance Use Disorder Care

Access to care for service members for assessment or treatment for substance related disorders occurs by one of 3 main routes. The first is self-referral for treatment, though often a senior officer has unofficially advised the individual to go seek help before a formal recommendation is made. This is most common with legal substances, especially when impairment is severe. The second route is that of the command directed evaluation through behavioral health services. This occurs when the commanding officer or supervisor has ordered the individual to appear for a formal psychiatric assessment and often due to observed occupational or social impairment, or due to a serious alcohol or drug related event such as a DUI [99].

The results of that evaluation are returned to the service member's commander so that they may determine how best to use the individual in a work environment, as well as knowledge about limitations to work. The third category of service members seen for treatment are those who have been found to be positive on a routine urine drug test performed regularly through the DoD drug monitoring protocols [100]. These last cases carry potential legal consequences because the urine drug tests have approved chain of custody as well as being confirmed by centralized laboratory through gas or liquid chromatography. All three however, receive the same assessment and treatment as any other. Following ASAM criteria almost every military installation will have access to military behavioral health outpatient services at level 1. Larger installations with more robust behavioral healthcare resources onsite will have access to level II.5 intensive outpatient programs which typically run in 4-to-6-week cycles. Services for residential treatment at level 2.5 to 3.5 at the largest medical facilities is also offered, with patients at sites not offering residential treatment being transferred for care when needed. If access to care issues present themselves treatment may be referred to civilian rehabilitation programs.

Treatment for those within the service may involve 28-day rehabilitation programs in conjunction with the Veterans Affairs (VA), attendance in a military oriented intensive outpatient program for substance use treatment, or routine outpatient care with a licensed counselor and monitoring with routine drug or alcohol testing. Increased monitoring or treatment requirements may be needed for pilots, those with national security clearances, and or high risk jobs in dealing with explosives or heaven weaponry with risk of catastrophic failure. Failure of the service member of treatment or rehabilitation, or with any positive urine drug screen for illicit substances, may result in a misconduct separation from service as well as disciplinary action which could impact the service members pay and rank.

For veteran care, a referral is requested by the veteran themself or by a clinician hired by the VA or the DoD for in VA substance use treatment, which can include inpatient admission, rehabilitation, intensive outpatient therapy, or routine outpatient therapy. The VA system has very robust substance use treatment options and often represent an integrated care model with the other comorbid diagnoses also in treatment. Within this system of care, options range from level I outpatient treatment offered at most city level veterans care centers, intensive outpatient level II programs of which there are usually multiple in every state, level III residential treatments of which there are usually at least one in every state or a nearby state, and approximately half the states with dedicated opioid maintenance treatment clinics. The goal of both systems in treating substance use disorders is to restore to full physical and mental function so the service member or veteran is reliable, healthy, and without social or occupational dysfunction.

Conclusion

Substance use disorders continue to exact a heavy toll on our veterans and service members. The military has a unique culture and presents stressors that can be much different than the civilian environment. Members can spend months isolated from the family and friends whether at home or abroad can endure traumas that they may not have expected. Likewise, the many unique settings in the military and rules and regulations can be stressful. The risk for substance use in many members and veterans is higher than the general population due to factors before joining the military and compounded by events during their time in service. John from the opening vignette demonstrates the risk factors for substance abuse and the downward economic and social drift that some members who abuse substances endure. While all current or former military members who abuse substances do not end up being eventual victims of overdose, there is no doubt substance use disorders have an adverse effect on those it touches and great societal cost associated.

While there are many similarities between the military and civilian sector in substance use and treatment of substance use disorders, there remain important differences. Many of the differences are due to the culture of the military and the effect the treatment may have on the overall mission. The military and Veteran's Administration are focused on decreasing substance use and abuse.

Recommendations and clinical practice guidelines are included in this chapter and help the clinician navigate the differences from the civilian community. Your local Veteran's Administration Hospital and local military treatment facilities offer a variety of unique treatment option for military members and veterans.

Clinical Pearls

- Active "full time" service members need additional monitoring of SUD treatment by DoD clinicians.
- Generally, service members and veterans have robust SUD treatment options through the military or the VA
- Current clinical practice guidelines recommend naltrexone and acamprosate as first-line treatment strategies for moderate or severe alcohol use disorder.
- Screen for tobacco and alcohol use disorders at every visit.
- Varenicline is the most efficacious medication for smoking cessation.
- Withdrawal symptoms from Marijuana peak between days 3–5 and generally resolve by three weeks and is dependent on potency of product and chronicity of use
- Quetiapine and venlafaxine exacerbate marijuana withdrawal symptoms and increase risk or relapse
- To mitigate risks when prescribing benzodiazepines, consider routine urine drug screen and discontinuation of any opiates
- Stimulant treatment has shown unimpressive results with pharmacologic management and the most effective therapies have been primarily psychotherapy
- Avoid opiate prescriptions if clinically appropriate.
- Switch to buprenorphine as an alternate to chronic opiate prescriptions.
- Obtain and check the prescription monitoring database for your state, prior to prescribing opiates.
- Any medication or substance can be abused or diverted, making the clinical interview crucial.
- DSM criteria for substance use disorders include domains such as persisting use despite consequences, legal, social or interpersonal problems with use and physical consequences that include withdrawal and tolerance or harmful physical effects [101].

References

1. Teeters JB, Lancaster CL, Brown DG, Back SE. Substance use disorders in military veterans: prevalence and treatment challenges. Subst Abus Rehabil. 2017;8:69–77.
2. Brancu M, Wagner H, Morey R, et al. The Post-Deployment Mental Health (PDMH) study and repository: a multi-site study of US Afghanistan and Iraq era veterans. Int J Methods Psychiatr Res. 2017;26(3):e1570.
3. Ilgen M, Bohnert A, Ganoczy D, et al. Opioid dose and risk of suicide. Pain. 2016;157(5):1079–84.
4. Perl L. Veterans and homelessness. Washington, DC: Congressional Research Service Report for Congress; 2013.

5. Substance Abuse and Mental Health Services Administration (SAMHSA). Veteran's primary substance of abuse is alcohol in treatment admissions. The CBHSQ Report. 2015. Available at: https://www.samhsa.gov/data/sites/default/files/report_2111/Spotlight-2111.html. Accessed 27 Apr 2021.
6. Defense Health Agency. Procedural instruction 6025.15, management of problematic substance use by DoD personnel. 2019.
7. Substance Abuse and Mental Health Services Administration (SAMHSA). 2019 National Survey of Drug Use and Health (NSDUH). 2019. Available at: https://www.samhsa.gov/data/release/2019-national-survey-drug-use-and-health-nsduh-releases. Accessed 29 Mar 2021.
8. Department of Defense (DoD). Status of drug use in the department of defense. 2015.
9. Center for Behavioral Health Statistics and Quality (BHSQ). Key substance use and mental health indicators in the United States: Results from the 2015 National Survey on Drug Use and Health (HHS Publication No. SMA 16-4984, NSDUH Series H-51). 2016.
10. Quest diagnostics, drug testing tables, Available at: https://www.questdiagnostics.com/home/physicians/health-trends/drug-testing/. Accessed 20 May 2020.
11. Meadows SO, Engel CC, Collins RL, et al. Health related behaviors survey: substance use among U.S. active-duty service members. Santa Monica, CA: RAND Corporation; 2018.
12. Institute of Medicine (IOM). Substance use disorders in the US armed forces. Washington, DC: National Academies Press; 2013.
13. Seal KH, Cohen G, Waldrop A, et al. Substance use disorders in Iraq and Afghanistan veterans in VA healthcare, 2001–2010: Implications for screening, diagnosis and treatment. Drug Alcohol Depend. 2011;116(1–3):93–101.
14. National Institute on Drug Abuse (NIDA). Substance use and military life drug facts. 2019. Available at https://www.drugabuse.gov/publications/drugfacts/substance-use-military-life Accessed 17 April 2021.
15. Edelman EJ, Fiellin DA. Alcohol use. Ann Intern Med. 2016;165(5):379–80.
16. Watkins KE, Ober AJ, Lamp K, et al. Collaborative care for opioid and alcohol use disorders in primary care: The SUMMIT randomized clinical trial. JAMA Intern Med. 2017;177(10):1480–8.
17. McCarty D, Braude L, Lyman DR, et al. Substance abuse intensive outpatient programs: assessing the evidence. Psychiatr Serv. 2014;65(6):718–26.
18. Friedrichs A, Spies M, Härter M, Buchholz A. Patient preferences and shared decision making in the treatment of substance use disorders: a systematic review of the literature. PLoS One. 2016;11(1):e0145817.
19. Mooney SR, Horton PA, Trakowski JH Jr, et al. Military inpatient residential treatment of substance abuse disorders: the Eisenhower Army Medical Center experience. Mil Med. 2014;179(6):674–8.
20. Barles FM, Higgins WB, Pflieger JC, et al. Health related behaviors survey of active duty military personnel. Fairfax VA: ICF International INC; 2013.
21. Severson HH, Peterson AL, Andrews JA, et al. Smokeless tobacco cessation in military personnel: a randomized control trial. Nicotine Tob Res. 2009;11:730–8.
22. Dailey JI, Wilson KC. Impact of smoking and smoking cessation medication in aviators. Curr Psychiatry Rep. 2019;21:1–5.
23. Schrader C, Lenton A, Gertonson P, et al. Redeveloping substance abuse treatment for military personnel. Curr Psychiatry Rep. 2018;20:1–8.
24. Barnett PG, Chow A, Flores NE, et al. Changes in Veteran tobacco use identified in electronic medical records. Am J Prev Med. 2017;53:e9–e18.
25. Grier T, Knapik JJ, Canada S, Canham-Chervak M, et al. Tobacco use prevalence and factors associated with tobacco use in new U.S. Army personnel. J Addict Dis. 2010;29:284–93.
26. Smith B, Ryan MA, Wingard DL, et al. Cigarette smoking and military deployment: a prospective evaluation. Am J Prev Med. 2008;35:539–46.
27. Hammett PJ, Japuntich SJ, Sherman SE, et al. Proactive tobacco treatment for veterans with posttraumatic stress disorder. Psychol Trauma Theory Res Pract Policy. 2021;13:114–22.

28. Lin J, Kangmin Z, Hoang PK, et al. Electronic cigarette use and related factors among active duty service members in the U.S. military. Mil Med. 2020;185:418–27.
29. Dixit D, Herbst E, Das S. E-cigarette use and perceptions among veterans receiving outpatient treatment in Veterans Affairs substance use and mental health clinics. Mil Med. 2021;186:24–9.
30. Little MA, Pebley K, Porter K, et al. 'I think smoking's the same, but the toys have changed.' Understanding facilitators of e-cigarette use among air force personnel. J Addict Prevent. 2020;8:1–16.
31. Bahrke MS, Baur TS, Poland DF, et al. Tobacco use and performance on the US Army Physical Fitness Test. Mil Med. 1988;153(5):229–35.
32. Conway TL, Cronan TA. Smoking and physical fitness among Navy shipboard men. Mil Med. 1988;153:589–94.
33. Haddock CK, Pyle SA, Poston WS, et al. Smoking and body weight as markers of fitness for duty among US military personnel. Mil Med. 2007;172:527–32.
34. Woodruff SI, Conway TL, Shilington AM, et al. Cigarette smoking and subsequent hospitalization in a cohort of young U.S. Navy female recruits. Nicotine Tob Res. 2010;12:365–73.
35. Truth initiative. Military: the tobacco industry has targeted the military for decades. Truth initiative: inspiring tobacco free lives. Washington DC; 2018.
36. Campbell-Sills L, Kessler RC, Ursano RJ, et al. Nicotine dependence and pre-enlistment suicidal behavior among U.S. Army soldiers. Am J Prev Med. 2019;56:420–8.
37. Wynn WP, Stroman RT, Almgren MM, et al. The pharmacist "toolbox" for smoking cessation: a review of methods, medicines, and novel means to help patients along the path of smoking reduction to smoking cessation. J Pharm Pract. 2012;25:591–9.
38. Carpenter MJ, Jardin BF, Burris JL, et al. Clinical strategies to enhance the efficacy of nicotine replacement therapy for smoking cessation: a review of the literature. Drugs. 2013;73:407–26.
39. Taylor GM, Taylor AE, Thomas KH, Jones T, et al. The effectiveness of varenicline versus nicotine replacement therapy on long-term smoking cessation in primary care: a prospective cohort study of electronic medical records. Int J Epidemiol. 2017;46(6):1948–57.
40. Marijuana's impact on California: 2020: cannabis-related ER visits and admissions skyrocket after medical and recreational marijuana laws. Mo Med. 2021;118(1):22–23.
41. ElSohly MA, Mehmedic Z, Foster S, Gon C, et al. Changes in cannabis potency over the last 2 decades (1995-2014): analysis of current data in the United States. Biol Psychiatry. 2016;79(7):613–9.
42. Volkow ND, Swanson JM, Evins AE, et al. Effects of cannabis use on human behavior, including cognition, motivation, and psychosis: a review. JAMA Psychiat. 2016;73(3):292–7.
43. Schierenbeck T, Riemann D, Berger M, Hornyak M. Effect of illicit recreational drugs upon sleep: cocaine, ecstasy and marijuana. Sleep Med Rev. 2008;12(5):381–9.
44. Black N, Stockings E, Campbell G, Tran LT, Zagic D, Hall WD, Farrell M, Degenhardt L. Cannabinoids for the treatment of mental disorders and symptoms of mental disorders: a systematic review and meta-analysis. Lancet Psychiatry. 2019;6(12):995–1010.
45. Greenwich Biosciences, Inc. EPIDIOLEX® (cannabidiol). 2020. Available at https://www.epidiolex.com/. Accessed 20 Feb 2021.
46. Blessing EM, Steenkamp MM, Manzanares J, Marmar CR. Cannabidiol as a potential treatment for anxiety disorders. Neurotherapeutics. 2015;12(4):825–36.
47. VanDolah HJ, Bauer BA, Mauck KF. Clinicians' guide to cannabidiol and hemp oils. Mayo Clin Proc. 2019;94(9):1840–51.
48. Zendulka O, Dovrtělová G, Nosková K, et al. Cannabinoids and cytochrome P450 interactions. Curr Drug Metab. 2016;17(3):206–26.
49. Thomas BF, Crompton DR, Martin BR. Characterization of the lipophilicity of natural and synthetic analogs of delta 9-tetrahydrocannabinol and its relationship to pharmacological potency. J Pharmacol Exp Ther. 1990;255(2):624–30.
50. Synthetic cannabinoids: What are they? What are their effects? 2018. Available at https://www.cdc.gov/nceh/hsb/chemicals/sc/default.html Accessed 20 Feb 2021.

51. Bonnet U, Preuss UW. The cannabis withdrawal syndrome: current insights. Subst Abus Rehabil. 2017;8:9–3.
52. US Department of Veterans Affairs. VA and Marijuana – what veterans need to know. US Department of Veterans Affairs. 2017. VA.gov: Veterans Affairs. Available at https://www.publichealth.va.gov/marijuana.asp. Accessed 21 Mar 2021.
53. Votaw VR, Geyer R, Rieselbach MM, McHugh RK. The epidemiology of benzodiazepine misuse: A systematic review. Drug Alcohol Depend. 2019;200:95–114.
54. Lembke A, Papac J, Humphreys K. Our other prescription drug problem. N Engl J Med. 2018;378(8):693–5.
55. Maust DT, Lin LA, Blow FC. Benzodiazepine use and misuse among adults in the United States. Psychiatr Serv. 2019;70(2):97–106.
56. Gerlach LB, Wiechers IR, Maust DT. Prescription benzodiazepine use among older adults: a critical review. Harv Rev Psychiatry. 2018;26(5):264–73.
57. Maust DT, Kim HM, Wiechers IR, Ignacio RV, Bohnert ASB, Blow FC. Benzodiazepine use among Medicare, commercially insured, and veteran older adults, 2013-2017. J Am Geriatr Soc. 2021;69(1):98–105.
58. Agarwal SD, Landon BE. Patterns in outpatient benzodiazepine prescribing in the United States. JAMA Netw Open. 2019;2(1):e187399.
59. Moosman B, Auwärter V. Designer benzodiazepines: Another class of new psychoactive substances. Handb Exp Pharmacol. 2018;252:383–410.
60. Greenblatt HK, Greenblatt DJ. Designer benzodiazepines: A review of published data and public health significance. Clin Pharmacol Drug Dev. 2019;8(3):266–9.
61. Zawilska JB, Wojcieszak J. An expanding world of new psychoactive substances - designer benzodiazepines. Neurotoxicology. 2019;73:8–16.
62. White JM, Irvine RJ. Mechanisms of fatal opioid overdose. Addiction. 1999;94(7):961–72.
63. Gressler LE, Martin BC, Hudson TJ, Painter JT. Relationship between concomitant benzodiazepine-opioid use and adverse outcomes among US veterans. Pain. 2018;159(3):451–9.
64. Park TW, Saitz R, Ganoczy D, Ilgen MA, Bohnert AS. Benzodiazepine prescribing patterns and deaths from drug overdose amonth US veterans receiving opioid analgesics: case-cohort study. BMJ. 2015;350:h2698.
65. Veterans Affairs and Department of Defense (VA DoD). Clinical practice guideline for opioid therapy for chronic pain. Version 3.0. Washington, DC: Department of Veterans Affairs and Department of Defense; 2017.
66. Veterans Affairs and Department of Defense (VA DoD). The Management of posttraumatic stress disorder workgroup: clinical practice guideline for the management of posttraumatic stress disorder and acute stress disorder. Version 3.0. Department of Veterans Affairs, Department of Defense. 2017. Available at: https://www.healthquality.va.gov/guidelines/MH/ptsd/VADoDPTSDCPGFinal012418.pdf. Accessed 27 Feb 2021.
67. Deka R, Bryan CJ, LaFleur J, Oderda G, Atherton A, Stevens V. Benzodiazepines, health care utilization, and suicidal behavior in veterans with posttraumatic stress disorder. J Clin Psychiatry. 2018;79(6):17m12038.
68. Hawkins EJ, Goldberg SB, Malte CA, Saxon AJ. New coprescription of opioids and benzodiazepines and mortality among Veterans Affairs patients with posttraumatic stress disorder. J Clin Psychiatry. 2019;80(4):18m12689.
69. Donovan LM, Malte CA, Spece LJ, et al. Risks of benzodiazepines in Chronic Obstructive Pulmonary Disease with comorbid posttraumatic stress disorder. Ann Am Thorac Soc. 2019;16(1):82–90.
70. Gudin JA, Mogali S, Jones JD, Comer SD. Risks, managment, and monitoring of combination opioid, benzodiazepines, and/or alcohol use. Postgrad Med. 2013;125(4):115–30.
71. United Nations Office on Drugs and Crime (UNODC). World drug report 2020. Austria, United Nations publication, Sales No. E.20.XI.6. 2020.
72. Boden MT, Hoggatt KJ. Substance use disorders among veterans in a nationally representative sample: prevalence and associated functioning and treatment utilization. J Stud Alcohol Drugs. 2018;79(6):853–61.

73. Westover AN, Nakonezny PA, Halm EA, Adinoff B. Risk of amphetamine use disorder and mortality among incident users of prescribed stimulant medications in the veterans administration. Addiction. 2018;113(5):857–67.
74. Posner J, Polanczyk GV, Sonuga-Barke E. Attention-deficit hyperactivity disorder. Lancet. 2020;395(10222):450–62.
75. Nishimura M, Ma J, Fox S, Toomu A, et al. Characteristics and outcomes of methamphetamine abuse among veterans with heart failure. Am J Cardiol. 2019;124(6):907–11.
76. Chan B, Kondo K, Freeman M, Ayers C, Montgomery J, Kansagara D. Pharmacotherapy for cocaine use disorder - a systematic review and meta-analysis. J Gen Intern Med. 2019;34(12):2858–73.
77. He Q, Huang X, Turel O, Schulte M, Huang D, Thames A, Bechara A, Hser YI. Presumed structural and functional neural recovery after long-term abstinence from cocaine in male military veterans. Prog Neuro-Psychopharmacol Biol Psychiatry. 2018;84(Pt A):18–29.
78. Bohnert KM, Ilgen MA, Louzon S, McCarthy JF, Katz IR. Substance use disorders and the risk of suicide mortality among men and women in the US Veterans Health Administration. Addiction. 2017;112(7):1193–201.
79. Kampman KM. The treatment of cocaine use disorder. Sci Adv. 2019;5(10):eaax1532.
80. Veterans Affairs and Department of Defense (VA DoD). Clinical practice guideline for the management of substance use disorders, Version 3.0. 2015. Available at: https://www.healthquality.va.gov/guidelines/MH/sud/VADODSUDCPGRevised22216.pdf. Accessed 12 Mar 2021.
81. Losby J, Hyatt J, Kanter M, et al. Safer and more appropriate opioid prescribing: a large healthcare system's comprehensive approach. J Eval Clin Pract. 2017;23(6):1173–9.
82. Guy G, Pasalic E, Zhang K. Emergency department visits involving opioid overdoses, U.S., 2010-2014. Am J Prev Med. 2018;54:37–9.
83. Kazanis W, Pugh MJ, Tami C, et al. Opioid use patterns among active duty service members and civilians: 2006-2014. Mil Med. 2018;183:3–4.
84. Schuchat A, Houry D, Guy G. New data on opioid use and prescribing in the United States. JAMA. 2017;318(5):425–6.
85. Simon K, Worthy S, Barnes M, et al. Abuse-deterrent formulations: transitioning the pharmaceutical market to improve public health and safety. Ther Adv Drug Saf. 2015;6(2):67–79.
86. Johnson H, Paulozzi L, Porucznik C, et al. Decline in drug overdose deaths after state policy changes - Florida, 2010-2012. MMWR Morb Mortal Wkly Rep. 2014;63(26):569–74.
87. Franklin G, Sabel J, Jones CM, et al. A comprehensive approach to address the prescription opioid epidemic in Washington state: milestones and lessons learned. Am J Public Health. 2015;105(3):463–9.
88. Rutkow L, Chang HY, Daubresse M, et al. Effect of Florida's prescription drug monitoring program and pill mill laws on opioid prescribing and use. JAMA Intern Med. 2015;175(10):1642–9.
89. Dowell D, Haegerich TM, Chou R. CDC guideline for prescribing opioids for chronic pain – United States, 2016. MMWR Recomm Rep. 2016;65(RR-1):1–49.
90. Roux P, Sullivan MA, Cohen J, et al. Buprenorphine/naloxone as a promising therapeutic option for opioid abusing patients with chronic pain: reduction of pain, opioid withdrawal symptoms, and abuse liability of oral oxycodone. Pain. 2013;154(8):1442–8.
91. Kress H. Clinical update on the pharmacology, efficacy and safety of transdermal buprenorphine. Eur J Pain. 2009;13(3):219–30.
92. American Society of Addiction Medicine. The ASAM Criteria: treatment criteria for addictive, substance-related, and co-occurring conditions. 3rd ed. Carson City, NV: The Change Companies; 2013.
93. Reese ED, Conway CC, Anand D, Bauer DJ, Daughters SB. Distress tolerance trajectories following substance use treatment. J Consult Clin Psychol. 2019;87(7):645–56.
94. Smith RV, Havens JR, Walsh SL. Gabapentin misuse, abuse and diversion: a systematic review. Addiction. 2016;111(7):1160–74.

95. Gomes T, Juurlink DN, Antoniou T, Mamdani MM, et al. Gabapentin, opioids, and the risk of opioid-related death: a population-based nested case-control study. PLoS Med. 2017;14(10):e1002396.
96. See S, Ginzburg R. Choosing a skeletal muscle relaxant. Am Fam Physician. 2008;78(3):365–70.
97. Liu J, Wang LN. Baclofen for alcohol withdrawal. Cochrane Database Syst Rev. 2019;2019(11):CD008502.
98. Saran JS, Barbano RL, Schult R, Wiegand TJ, Selioutski O. Chronic diphenhydramine abuse and withdrawal: a diagnostic challenge. Neurol Clinical Pract. 2017;7(5):439–41.
99. Department of Defense (DoD). Department of Defense Instruction (DODI) 6490.04, mental health evaluations of members of the military services. 2013.
100. Department of Defense (DoD). Department of Defense Instruction (DODI) 1010.16, technical procedures for the military personnel drug abuse testing program. 2020.
101. Hasin DS, O'Brien CP, Auriacombe M, et al. DSM-5 criteria for substance use disorders: recommendations and rationale. Am J Psychiatry. 2013;170(8):834–51.

Sleep Disorders

18

Vincent F. Capaldi II and Guido Simonelli

Vignette

A 48 year old, male, active duty, US Air Force, Lieutenant Colonel, physician with 21 years time in military service presents for a retirement physical. The patient reports that he has been struggling with insomnia for the past 10 years. He reports that he has difficulty getting to sleep and staying asleep most night, waking 3–4 times per night to urinate. The patient's wife reports loud snoring and that the patient appears to gasp for air 3–4 times per week. The patient endorses excessive daytime somnolence, often falling asleep at work, stoplights, and watching television on the weekend. He reports that he takes medication for hypertension and drinks 5–6 cups of coffee during the daytime to, "get me through the day."

Introduction

Sleep is an essential component of well-being [1], yet short sleep and poor sleep quality are ubiquitous in the military. The scope of this issue was highlighted in a recent study that found approximately 49% of a large active duty military cohort

V. F. Capaldi II (✉)
Department of Psychiatry, Uniformed Services University of the Health Sciences, Bethesda, MD, USA
e-mail: Vincent.f.capaldi.mil@health.mil

G. Simonelli
Department of Psychiatry, Uniformed Services University of the Health Sciences, Bethesda, MD, USA

Department of Medicine, Universite de Montreal, Montreal, QC, Canada

Center for Advanced Studies in Sleep Medicine, Hospital du Sacre-Coeur de, Montreal, QC, Canada
e-mail: Guido.simonelli@umontreal.ca

C. H. Warner, C. A. Castro (eds.), *Veteran and Military Mental Health*,
https://doi.org/10.1007/978-3-031-18009-5_18

reported sleeping less than the 7 h per night [2]. Both the National Sleep Foundation and the American Academy of Sleep Medicine recommend at least 7 h per night for individuals aged 18–25, the average age of vulnerable military recruits [3]. Even though in the general population the prevalence of insomnia is estimated to be 6–10% [4], in uniformed service members the prevalence is estimated to be almost 50%[2]. There are several factors that may explain the large difference in prevalence estimates between civilian and those in uniform (or veterans). One often cited factor is military culture, comprised of shift work and vigorous conditioning, which may necessitate sleep restriction and erratic sleep patterns over the course of training or deployment (lasting up to 12–18 months) [5, 6]. For example, the prevalence of insomnia was estimated 24–54% of veterans who served in Operation Enduring Freedom, Operation Iraqi Freedom, and Operation New Dawn in 2013 [7, 8]. The volume of hypnotic medications prescribed to 15–20% of all deployed service members underscores the extent of sleep deficiency among service members [9, 10].

Independently of age and sex, active duty members have a higher prevalence of sedative hypnotic prescription compared to non-active duty service members [10]. Further, to illustrate the magnitude of the problem, a recent study of active duty service members showed that 50% of pilots reported falling asleep in the cockpit at least once, and over 50% of all soldiers attribute mistakes made in the field to sleepiness [11, 12]. Insomnia and/or insomnia-like symptoms are also a major public health issue for veterans, who have a two to three times higher prevalence of insomnia than in the general U.S. adult population [9]. In veterans, insomnia, sleep-related disordered breathing, and nightmares have been associated with suicide attempts, and treatment for sleep disorders is correlated to a reduced risk for suicide attempts in veterans [13]. After accounting for demographics, health behaviors and posttraumatic stress disorder diagnosis, veterans who reported lower household assets, lower food security, greater discrimination, and lower subjective social status are at a higher risk of being short sleepers [14].

Patients that feel they "cannot fall asleep or stay asleep", "cannot stay awake" or "have problems when sleeping" often approach mental health providers for help. In this chapter we discuss in a practical way these three chief complains often brought up by patients.

Assessing Sleep

The most essential tool that mental health practitioners should always use is a sleep diary, there are many sleep diaries available. The American Academy of Sleep Medicine provides a standardized form in their website [15, 16] and the Veterans Affairs (VA) Department offers an android/iOS application that also provides sleep diary functionality. Ideally, an objective sleep measure should be coupled with a sleep diary. The most commonly used objective measure is actigraphy recordings, and if not possible, the potential use of sleep tracking apps may be advised although with the caveat that these may not be validated measures. These sleep measures will provide the patient's sleep onset latency, wake after sleep onset, sleep efficiency, total sleep time, as well as informing on influencing factors such as caffeine use, exercise and use of prescribed medication. The sleep assessment is also dependent on the patient's compliance, as to wear the prescribed device and filling the sleep diary daily and accurately.

Besides the sleep diary and sleep tracking devices. There are a number of validated sleep questionnaires that may help in both the initial assessment and throughout the course of the treatment. Among those, the most used are the Insomnia Severity Index (ISI—past week symptoms) [17], the Pittsburgh Sleep Quality Index (PSQI—past insomnia symptoms) [18] and the Epworth Sleepiness Scale (ESS—past month sleepiness) [19]. Although these measures are not essential to diagnose a sleep disorder, these questionnaires have normed values and should help assess the patient's initial symptoms, as well as potential treatment efficacy.

If there are suspicions of the presence of a sleep breathing disorder, narcolepsy, or restless leg syndrome, patients should be referred to a sleep center for in lab or at home polysomnographic assessment. In the sections below we provide some further guidance.

Insomnia ("I Cannot Fall Asleep or Stay Asleep")

A 22 year old female active duty, junior enlisted, US Army medic with two years time in military service presents with difficulty initiating sleep. She states that it has been difficult for her to get to sleep and wake up for morning physical training. She states that she has received two negative counseling statements due to missing physical training. She states that she has always been a night owl and has always found it difficult to wake up for early morning classes in high school. She relates that she gets into bed around 2300 but does not fall asleep until 0030. She has tried taking melatonin but it has not helped her get to sleep. She has a normal BMI and does not snore. Mallampati class I.

Etiology

Poor sleep quality, increased sleep latency, shortened sleep duration, difficulty with sleep maintenance and daytime impairments are typical symptoms of insomnia [4]. The American Academy of Sleep Medicine defines insomnia as the subjective perception of difficulty with sleep initiation, duration, consolidation, or quality that occurs despite adequate opportunity for sleep, and that results in some form of daytime impairment [20]. It has been hypothesized that there are two distinctive phenotypes of insomniacs, one that is objectively a short sleeper and the one that is not [21, 22]. The first one is argued to be the most harmful for health and well-being, in particular given the extensive link between sleep duration and health [23]. Symptoms of insomnia independent, of objective sleep duration, are nevertheless associated with increased both psychological and physical morbidity and increased mortality [24]. There are symptoms that may be somewhat specific to service members, and those may involve sleep onset during briefings, irritability with people at work and at home, and difficulty maintaining work schedules (e.g. morning formation), which can persist even after retirement from military life [5].

The Spielman Model for Chronic Insomnia posits 3 components: predisposing factors, precipitating factors, and perpetuating factors [25]. Using this model as a framework there are several distinctive factors that put service members at risk for chronic insomnia.

Predisposing factors include classic risk factors for insomnia such as sex, age, ethnicity and family history. For example it's been shown that women have higher rates of insomnia [26]. Similarly, young people by virtue of their natural propensity for delayed sleep phase disorder may be at a higher risk for insomnia [27].

Precipitating factors often include stress related episodes that trigger insomnia symptoms [25]. For example, an acute event that triggers insomnia may become the nidus of persistent maladaptive sleep patterns. In military populations, precipitating factors could be auditory disturbances and anxiety during the sleep opportunity during deployment.

Perpetuating factors include factors that might be seen to maintain or even exacerbate the problem, and thus contribute to the insidious nature of chronic insomnia. Exposure to combat, shiftwork and deployment in general can all lead to long lasting change in sleep habits of service members. For example, in a 14-month longitudinal study in Air Force, deployment status and having experienced trauma were associated with higher physical and emotional fatigue, and increased risk for burnout, all common symptoms of insomnia. In sum, it is important for the providers to understand that the impact of military life on sleep habits can start soon with pre-deployment activities and last long after returning home [7].

Diagnosis and Assessment

It can be challenging to parse out an organic sleep disorder such as insomnia from effect of environmental disruptors of sleep of service members and veterans [28]. For this reason, classically, some sleep disorders such as insomnia used to be categorized in primary and secondary [29]. Because these subtypes of insomnia categories did not aid clinician in choosing effective treatments modalities or prognosticating the success of treatment, the International Classification of Sleep Disorders, Third Edition (ICSD-3) and the Diagnostic and Statistical Manual of Mental Disorders, Fifth Edition: DSM-5 streamlined the diagnosis of insomnia disorder [30]. Accordingly, the diagnosis has been reduced to categorizing insomnia by duration, rather than etiology. Therefore, the only difference in the diagnostic criteria for short-term and chronic insomnia is the duration of symptoms over time. Table 18.1 shows the main differences and similarities between the ICSD-3 and the DSM-5 classification of insomnia.

As per the AASM guidelines, the initial diagnosis of insomnia should include a comprehensive sleep assessment as well as medical, substance use and detailed

Table 18.1 Comparison and Similarities of the ICSD-3 and DSM-5 classifications of insomnia

ICSD-3 insomnia classifications	**DSM-5 insomnia classifications**
Chronic insomnia **Short-term insomnia**—No DSM-5 equivalence **Other insomnia disorder**	**Insomnia disorder**—similar to ICSD-3 diagnosis of chronic insomnia **Other specified insomnia disorder**
1. A self-reported complaint of poor sleep quality including one of the following: – Difficulties initiating sleep – Difficulties maintaining sleep – Waking up earlier than desired.	
2. Sleep difficulties occur despite adequate sleep opportunity.	
3. Impaired sleep produces deficits in daytime function[a]	
4. Sleep difficulty occurs three nights per week and is present for three months ICSD-3—Symptoms lasting <3 months can be coded 'Short-term insomnia' DSM-5—Symptoms lasting <3 months, but meeting all other criteria, can be coded Other specified insomnia disorder'	
Terms that have been removed: Acute insomnia Stress-related insomnia Transient insomnia Primary insomnia Secondary insomnia Comorbid insomnia	

[a] The DSM-5 emphasizes sleep disturbance must cause clinically significant distress or impairment across personal, vocational, behavioral, social, educational or other areas of functioning

psychiatric history [31]. It is recommended that providers use standardized questionnaires, two-week sleep log and actigraphy to rule out secondary causes of insomnia symptoms and to help inform treatment [32]. The use of actigraphy is recommended as it provides objective data on sleep onset latency and may help identify circadian phase pathology such as advances or delayed sleep phase disorder. In some cases polysomnography is also recommended to rule out sleep disordered breathing, and a multiple sleep latency test to rule out other causes of excessive daytime somnolence, such as narcolepsy [15, 31].

There are a number of psychiatric conditions, which present with significant insomnia symptoms. For this reason, the health provider should always first rule out other medical and psychiatric comorbidity. Among the most common conditions that should be ruled out are: thyroid disease, chronic obstructive pulmonary disease, congestive heart failure, major depressive disorder, bipolar disorder, generalized anxiety disorder, and post-traumatic stress disorder [4]. There are also a number of sleep disorder that are associated with insomnia symptoms. For example, obstructive sleep apnea and both restless leg syndrome and period limb movement disorder have been associated with insomnia [27]. Both these disorders should be ruled out with a sleep study, and if present, should be treated in addition to the insomnia treatment.

Once other causes of insomnia have been ruled out in the differential, environmental disruptors of sleep should be carefully assessed in service members. For example, when deployed members are exposed to light at night, noise and air pollution from aircrafts as well as indirect fire, which all are linked to deficient sleep [28]. Additionally, changes in their duty station or deployment may abruptly change their sleeping environment and thus can precipitate insomnia. Preventive measures in the field may consist of sleep protective gear such as eye masks and ear plugs, as well as strict sleep habits including limiting caffeine in the late hours and maintaining consistent bedtimes and wake up times. Treatment of insomnia in the field is particular difficult, and veterans who have insomnia may be resistant to seeking medical treatment due to stigma related to seeking behavioral health support [33]. Further, it has been shown that beliefs about mental health conditions as a weakness are associated with decreased access to mental health services [7, 34].

Prevention and Treatment

The main goal of insomnia treatment is to improve both sleep quality and quantity, and to reduce daytime impairment associated with insomnia [29]. The main treatments of insomnia are psychological and behavioral modifications via CBTi and a military adapted Brief Behavioral Treatment for insomnia (BBTi), pharmacotherapy, and alternative therapy options for which there is limited evidence [35, 36]. Current guidelines recommend behavioral treatments as the first line approach [35]. These main treatments when used in combination are associated with an increase in total sleep time and decreased sleep onset latency. These treatments may be applied in military populations, both in active duty service members and veterans.

Cognitive Behavioral Therapy for Insomnia

The term CBTi encompasses a variety of techniques that includes cognitive alteration, relaxation, sleep hygiene, stimulus control therapy, and sleep restriction. It is common for patients to get caught in a vicious cycle of worry over lack of sleep, excessive time in bed, fatigue and work impairment. The goal of CBTi is to reduce both anxiety and unrealistic expectations about patients' sleep. Through this techniques the patients learn through Socratic questioning how to identify and mitigate cognitive distortions before, during, and after sleep. During this treatment, the patient completes a sleep diary that is designed to provide the health provider with self-reported data on bed timing, medication administration, caffeine intake, exercise, nocturnal awakenings as well as self-reported sleep quality. The use of a sleep diary is a key component of CBTi as it reduces retrospective assessment, and thus potentially reducing recall bias and exaggeration of symptoms. For military providers it is very important to emphasize the importance of the sleep diary, as it has been reported that veterans and Service Members often forget to complete the diary on a daily basis and solely rely on memory to record data points over several nights. One strategy to improve compliance is to send daily reminders to the patients, and to add time stamps to record the timing of each entry.

There are a number of factors that make insomnia treatment challenging for the deployed community. The main challenges are multiple time zone changes that alter circadian rhythm, chronic sleep restriction, night operations and shiftwork, physical and emotional stress, and excessive caffeine intake [5, 28]. Further, it has also been shown that traumatic combat experiences can have an impact on the development of insomnia. For veterans exposed to trauma, CBTi is particularly useful, as it has been shown that it is an effective treatment, especially when insomnia is comorbid with anxiety, depression and post-traumatic stress disorder. For example, in a study of veterans who had never had psychotherapy, CBTi was first used to treat symptoms of insomnia, and then exposure therapy was used to treat PTSD symptoms [6]. Both insomnia and PTSD symptoms significantly improved, suggesting that CBTi should be used in combination with other therapies.

The main CBTi techniques are: CBTi with behavioral analysis (CBTi-BA), sleep restriction therapy, stimulus control, sleep hygiene and mental relaxation. CBTi-BA consist in discusses the influence and consequence of Service Member's behavior on their insomnia. This technique is often used in the presence of psychological comorbidities such as depression which can be resistant to pharmacologic treatments [37]. Studies comparing the CBTi-BA versus treatment as usual show that CBTi-BA group had a higher reduction both insomnia and depressive symptoms as well as reduction in hypnotic medication use [37]. This technique has been primarily shown to be successful in civilian communities but it may be particular challenging in a deployed setting as Service Members lack some control over their schedules are not necessarily able to choose behavioral modifications that may influence their sleep pattern. CBT-i-BA should however be highly considered in life after deployment and in veterans.

Sleep restriction therapy is based on the solely principle that the patient should not stay in bed when awake [35]. The provider should calculate the patients sleep efficiency as total sleep time divided by time in bed to understand whether sleep restriction therapy is needed. If needed, the provider should recommend to the patient to restrict their time in bed for activities other than sleep or sex. It is hypothesizes that reducing time in bed reduces exposure to potential anxiety at bedtime, reducing mental pressure to sleep. This therapy can be very effective by targeting both homeostatic and circadian control systems and resetting the patients' sleep pattern. In the context of deployment, alternating schedules and rotating shift make sleep restriction therapy difficult. From a practical stand point, it could be recommended that Service Members who are significantly impaired by insomnia due to rotating schedules should be moved to larger base camps, where higher manpower could allow fixed schedules, making sleep therapy feasible.

A third CBTi technique is stimulus control therapy. In this classical condition technique the goal is to re-associate bedtime with sleep [18]. The main tactics used in this therapy is to encourage patients to go to bed only when they are sleepy, to maintain consistent rise time and to avoid naps. The concept underlying this therapy is simple yet effective: the conditioned stimulus of lying in bed is paired with the unconditioned stimulus of being tired. Further, wake promoting activities such as watching TV, talking on the phone, exercising vigorously, and eating large meals are discouraged immediately before bedtime [28]. Stimulus control therapy can be difficult to utilize in the context of deployment, where bedtimes are dependent on mission requirements, and naps are a commonly used counter-fatigue measure to enhance combat efficacy.

Sleep hygiene is a helpful technique when used in combination with other parts of CBTi for patients and consist on the adjustment and improvement of habitual sleep patterns [35]. The idea behind this technique is also simple, and revolves around replacing wake-promoting behaviors with sleep-promoting behaviors. Typical adjustments that the health provider should encourage can include light exercise in the late afternoon, a light snack before bed, at least 1 h wind-down time before bed, a comfortable dark room for sleep, regular sleep schedule, and limiting alcohol intake [28]. Some of these sleep-promoting habits are able to be applied in deployed settings, such as exercising for example. Habits related to sleep timing consistency and rooming quality may not be feasible in the operational context.

The final component that we will discuss in this chapter is mental relaxation, a key component of CBTi. Strategies for winding-down should be particularly encouraged in deployed populations. These activities could include muscle relaxation, meditation and yoga, which have all been associated with improved sleep. The main goal of these activities is to alleviate anxiety and mental pressure, which can be particularly high during deployment. The VA/DoD have developed several android/iOS applications to assist with breathing and relaxation techniques.

Due to the shortage of clinicians, the Brief Behavioral Treatment for insomnia (BBTi) was developed based on CBTi. The BBTi consist of two in-person sessions, and two follow up telephone sessions over a four-week period. The BBTi has standardized sessions based on three CBTi techniques: sleep restriction, sleep hygiene, and stimulus control. This intervention has been successfully tested in combat-exposed veterans compared to control conditions. BBTi treatment shows a significant reduction in insomnia severity and improvement in sleep quality at six months post treatment. The brevity, effectiveness, and the existence of a military adapted language version (BBTi-MV) make this a cost-effective promising intervention for military and veteran communities. Large-scale training in and implementation of CBT-I in veterans have been demonstrated to be effective and feasible, and greater focus on patient adherence may lead to enhanced outcomes [34].

Pharmacotherapy

The primary goal of pharmacotherapy is to promote sleep onset and sleep maintenance without next-day side effects such as grogginess, fatigue or headaches [38]. There are three classes of medications that the FDA has approved for insomnia treatment: benzodiazepine gamma-aminobutyric acid receptor agonists (BZPs), nonbenzodiazepine GABAA receptor agonists (non-BZPs), orexin receptor antagonists, and melatonin receptor agonists. Because BZPs and non-BZPs side effect includes impaired performance through daytime sedation, cognitive impairment, motor incoordination and transient amnesia, these medications should be used with caution in the operational environment and patients should be closed monitored. An advantage of pharmacotherapy compared to behavioral treatment is that pharmacotherapy can be fast acting. In the same way that pharmacotherapy can act fast, it is common for patients to develop tolerance and dependence on these medications. This can be a problem as patients may require a higher dose for a similar effect resulting in greater side effects, coupled with the fact that there limited evidence of long-term safety of the use of these drugs [38].

An important factor when considering BZPs and non-BZPs medications is their half-life, which can range 1.5 h for zaleplon to more than 24 h for some benzodiazepines [38]. The longer the half-life of the medications, the greater the likelihood for the individuals to sleep through the night. An important disadvantage of longer half-life medications is the likelihood of next-day sedation, a critical component of readiness. Even though these individuals may be able to sleep through the night, they may experience difficulty waking up in the morning and feel groggy for several hours, resulting in increased safety risks. On the other hand, short-acting medications are less likely to cause next day sedation, and they may help individuals fall asleep. The caveat of these medications however is that once the medication wear off, the individuals may experience middle-of-the-night awakenings and difficulty sleeping the rest of the night. An important consideration for the psychiatrist is to assess whether the insomnia is onset insomnia, sleep maintenance insomnia (middle insomnia), late insomnia (terminal) [39]. Although this is an old classification, this information may sometimes be helpful in determining the most appropriate treatment modality for a patient. As an example, a patient with sleep onset insomnia may respond better to a short acting benzodiazepine, whereas a patient with maintenance insomnia might respond better to a longer acting non-benzodiazepine hypnotic. Suvorexant is the newest FDA approved insomnia medication on the market [38]. Suvorexant, given that it works on the orexin, wake promoting system, may have less sleep inertia [40]. While using this medication, Service Member may be able to respond to alarms/awake from sleep faster. Work being done at Walter Reed Army Institute of Research is investigating the ability for Service Members to perform while on sleep inducing medications such as suvorexant and zolpidem. Another drug group include selective melatonin receptor agonist, which primarily includes FDA approved Ramelteon. Ramelteon is a highly selective melatonin receptor type 1 and type 2 agonist, unlike non-prescription melatonin, which is nonselective for all three melatonin receptors. Ramelteon reduces time to fall asleep without next-day associated psychomotor nor memory impairment. Ramelteon has less of an immediate effect, but less likelihood of dependence [38].

Alternative Therapies

There a number of alternative medical treatments for which there are limited evidence for. These treatments are likely to appeal to populations that may actively avoid medication use and favor a holistic approach to health. To name a few, these alternative medical treatments include: mindfulness-based therapies (MBTs) mindfulness, tai chi, acupuncture, hypnosis and biofeedback for example [41]. Mindfulness-based therapies have shown significant improvement in insomnia symptoms and fatigue compare to sleep hygiene controls. It has been hypothesizes that meditation may lead to reduced rumination, and thus decreasing bedtime anxiety. Some advantages of mindfulness-based therapies is that they are low cost, can be done in groups or individually, there are ample options available online and can take as short as few minutes [41]. MBTs should be recommended pre, during and post-deployment, as well as during transition to civilian life.

Hypersomnia ("I Cannot Stay Awake")

52 y/o AD USA O7 with 30 years TIS presents with excessive daytime somnolence. The patient reports that he falls asleep in the early afternoon despite taking modafinil 300 mg PO daily. He drinks 6 cups of coffee daily and 2 five hour energy drinks. He notes that despite his best efforts he cannot stay awake and senior leaders are noticing. The patient has a BMI of 30, snores, and his wife endorses significant snoring at nighttime.

Etiology

Complains about not being able to stay awake during the day are fairly common in both military and civilian populations. As it was described earlier in this chapter, the first step is to have the patients complete a sleep diary as well as validated questionnaires. The sleep diary should provide information on whether sleepiness is present despite sleeping normal amounts. Even though normal amounts for adults are between 7–9 h per night, it is possible for some individuals to need more for optimal health and performance [3]. If sleepiness is likely due to insufficient sleep opportunity, some of the strategies described in the CBTi section should be implemented. Further, the use of questionnaires should inform on the severity of the daytime somnolence.

Diagnosis and Assessment

Obstructive Sleep Apnea (OSA)

A reasonable amount of sleepiness in the context of sufficient sleep is likely due obstructive sleep apnea [42]. OSA is characterized by multiple apneic events throughout the night due to airway obstruction. The breathing pauses result in microarousals, preventing the patients from having a restful and restorative sleep [43]. In adults, one of the main causes of daytime somnolence is OSA. The main phenotype of OSA include a number of predictors that have been outlined in the acronym STOP-BANG [44]:

- S: Do you snore loudly?
- T: Do you feel tired or fatigued during the daytime?
- O: Has anyone observed you stop breathing while asleep?
- P: Do you have high blood pressure?

- B: Is your B MI greater than 35?
- A: Is your age greater than 50?
- N: Is your neck circumference greater than 40 cm?
- G: Is your gender male?

The scoring of the STOP-BANG is simple. The health practitioner should add one point for each positive symptom, a score greater than 3 is highly suggestive of OSA [44]. These patients should be referred to a sleep disorder specialist for an overnight in-lab polysomnography or a home sleep test. These tests measure a number of different variables to quantify how many times per hour a person stops breathing, has periods of low oxygen (hypopneic events) or has high carbon dioxide (hypercapnic events). The apnea-hypopnea index (AHI) on polysomnography reports represents the number of apneic or hypoapneic events per hour. A score greater than 5–15 indicates mild OSA, moderate is 15–30 and severe is generally >30 [43]. OSA is increasingly common in military populations, and it may be attributable to a number of factors that include the persistence of maladaptive sleep practices from combat deployments, sleep deprivation, and fragmentation, which is known to exacerbate sleep disordered breathing and comorbid service-related disorders (anxiety, depression, PTSD, and mild TBI) [45, 46].

Narcolepsy

Narcolepsy is a rare sleep disorder that also causes excessive daytime somnolence. A large majority of narcoleptic patients experience sleep attacks [47]. A sleep attack can be described at the sudden urge to fall asleep in inappropriate situation. These attacks although are short, usually last between 5–30 min. Narcoleptic patients may also experience loss of muscle tone during these episodes, which is known as cataplexy. Cataplexy is more likely to happen if the person is either excited or frightened [47]. Patients with narcolepsy will also complain of disrupted sleep.

Mental health practitioners should always consider common differential diagnosis such as OSA, sleep deprivation, shift work, medications, drugs, alcohol dependence, and neurological conditions (i.e., seizure disorder). The most common cause of narcolepsy symptoms is insufficient sleep syndrome. If narcolepsy is suspected, the patient should be referred to a sleep specialist. The main studies that the sleep specialist will require are an overnight polysomnography as well as a multiple sleep latency test (MSLT) [47].

Prevention and Treatment

All patients complaining of an inability to stay awake during the daytime should have a documented driving precaution. Patients who cannot maintain wakefulness should be recommended not to drive until they have been adequately treated. If a provider suspects narcolepsy, some states require mandated reporting. Consult your local DMV regulations for reporting requirements. Narcolepsynetwork.org provides a state by state list of current reporting requirements. Additionally, active duty military personnel should receive a medical profile which informs their units of these restrictions to limit the service members' accessibility to weapons and equipment.

Obstructive Sleep Apnea

The gold standard for the treatment of OSA is continuous positive airway pressure (CPAP) device. Using a mask over the nose and/or mouth (or a cannula), the device keeps the airways open and thus reduces the number of apneic events during the course of the night. CPAP adherence have been long been studied and there are different strategies that should be used to improve adherence. For example, there is evidence that tailored approaches such as support from a psychologist using exposure therapy and systematic desensitization, or the use of hypnotic in some cases may help the participants in acclimating to the use of CPAP, in particular to the mask. OSA treatment in the operational setting may be challenging due to austere environment, including the lack of electricity to feed the CPAP device. In these cases, an oral appliance may be recommended in conjunction with sleep hygiene tips in lieu of the CPAP device. In rare cases, patients may elect surgery as a treatment technique instead of CPAP or oral appliance devices.

Narcolepsy

Untreated narcoleptic patients should be informed about safety risk associated with their daytime sleepiness. A sleep specialist will likely chose pharmacotherapy as first line of treatment [47].

Other Sleep Disturbances ("I Am Having Problems When Sleeping")

A 19 year old, female, active duty, female, US Navy sailor presents with difficulty staying asleep most nights of the week. She was recently diagnosed with PTSD due to military sexual assault. The patient notes that she is fearful about going to sleep because of the vivid recurrent nightmares that she experiences related to her sexual assault while deployed on the ship. She has recently started using Benadryl to get to sleep nightly.

Etiology

During the sleep assessment the patient may report presence of nightmares, complaint about restless leg syndrome (and periodic limb movements) or somnambulism. The first two are far more common that the later ones. For example, a retrospective study on 500 active duty United States military personnel who underwent a sleep medicine evaluation and polysomnography at our sleep center found that almost a third of individuals reported having weekly nightmares [48]. This study also highlighted that even though there is a high prevalence of nightmares in active duty, nightmares were not the main reason for which they came to the sleep center. It is important for mental health practitioners to inquire about the presence of nightmares [48].

Diagnosis and Assessment

Nightmares

Nightmares are common symptoms of an underlying psychiatric condition. Post-traumatic stress disorder if the most common psychiatric condition associated with nightmares [49]. Nightmares secondary to some medications (or medication withdrawal) should also be considered during the comprehensive sleep assessment.

Periodic Limb Movements and Restless Leg Syndrome

Periodic limb movements (PLMS) are limb movements that are stereotypic and that mainly occur during nonREM sleep. Restless leg syndrome's main difference with PLMS is that it occurs as the patient is falling asleep. During this condition is common for the patient to experience a sensation of creeping, crawling, tingling, or burning sensations in the calf area that is relieved with movement. Under both of these conditions the patients should be referred to a sleep specialist for evaluation. While PSG is not necessary for diagnosis, many patients undergo PSG to rule out other causes of sleep symptoms such as OSA. For restless leg syndrome there are two common underlying conditions that should be investigated. The first one is iron-deficiency and the second is peripheral neuropathy, often causes by diabetes.

Prevention and Treatment

Nightmares

There are several approaches that should be considered for the treatment of nightmares in the context of PTSD. Some PTSD treatment techniques, while overall decreasing PTSD symptoms may initially precipitate in increased nightmare symptoms. These techniques include prolonged exposure therapy, cognitive processing therapy, or eye movement desensitization and reprocessing (EMDR). A psychiatrist may prescribe alpha blockers (such as prazosin) to decrease sympathetic response to nightmares during the night. Like with most medications it is important to weigh in the risk and benefits of the specific pharmacotherapeutic approach, and for them to be used on a time-limited basis. Non-pharmacologic techniques have been shown to be effective and include imagery rehearsal therapy and guided imagery.

Periodic Limb Movements and Restless Leg Syndrome

If the sleep disorder is caused by an underlying condition, the focus of the treatment should be underlying cause [50]. Some patients although complain about muscle jerks during sleep onset, often described a sensation of tripping or "falling off a cliff", should be informed that these are normal myoclonic jerks or twitches that are considered normal and require no follow-up. Restless leg syndrome may be otherwise treated with dopaminergic medications or iron supplementation [50]. It is important to recognize that dopaminergic medications may carry significant psychiatric side effects including hallucinations and increased propensity for pleasure seeking because of increased dopaminergic activation [50].

Future Directions

Sleep complaints are among the most common concerns raised by patients presenting to a military behavioral health provider. Military behavioral health providers should master the initial assessment and treatment of insomnia. Military behavioral health providers should also recognize when to refer a patient for further evaluations when they are presenting with symptoms concerning for OSA, RLS, PLMS, narcolepsy or other symptoms of hypersomnia. Behavioral health providers should only use hypnotic medications on a time limited basis and should refer to a sleep specialist if the patient requires a sleep aid for more than 6 months. Likewise, behavioral health providers should refrain from prescribing simulants for daytime somnolence. These patients should be referred to a sleep specialist for evaluation and treatment.

Clinical Pearls

- Even though in the general population the prevalence of insomnia is estimated to be 6–10% [4], in uniformed service members the prevalence is estimated to be almost 50%[2]. There are several factors that may explain the large difference in prevalence estimates between civilian and those in uniform (or veterans) including military culture, comprised of shift work and vigorous conditioning, which may necessitate sleep restriction and erratic sleep patterns over the course of training or deployment (lasting up to 12–18 months) [5, 6].
- The most essential tool that mental health practitioners should always use is a sleep diary while the most commonly used objective tool is sleep actigraphy.
- In accordance with the Spielman Model for Chronic Insomnia, military service members and veterans have several distinctive factors that place them at increased risk for insomnia.
- The initial diagnosis of insomnia should include a comprehensive sleep assessment as well as medical, substance use and detailed psychiatric history [43]. It is recommended that providers use standardized questionnaires, two-week sleep log and actigraphy to rule out secondary causes of insomnia symptoms and to help inform treatment [32].
- The main treatments of insomnia are psychological and behavioral modifications via CBTi and a military adapted Brief Behavioral Treatment for insomnia (BBTi), pharmacotherapy, and alternative therapy options for which there is limited evidence [35, 36]. Current guidelines recommend behavioral treatments as the first line approach [35].

- All patients complaining of an inability to stay awake during the daytime should have a documented driving precaution. Patients who cannot maintain wakefulness should be recommended not to drive until they have been adequately treated. Specifically for active duty military personnel, this would include a medical profile communication to their unit commander.
- Behavioral health providers should only use hypnotic medications on a time limited basis and should refer to a sleep specialist if the patient requires a sleep aid for more than 6 months.

References

1. Luyster FS, Strollo PJ, Zee PC, Walsh JK. Sleep: a health imperative. Sleep. 2012;35(6):727–34. https://doi.org/10.5665/sleep.1846.
2. Seelig AD, Jacobson IG, Donoho CJ, Trone DW, et al. Sleep and health resilience metrics in a large military cohort. Sleep. 2016;39(5):1111–20.
3. Watson NF, Badr MS, Belenky G, Bliwise DL, et al. Joint consensus statement of the american academy of sleep medicine and sleep research society on the recommended amount of sleep for a healthy adult: methodology and discussion. Sleep. 2015;38(8):1161–83. https://doi.org/10.5665/sleep.4886.
4. Roth T. Insomnia: definition, prevalence, etiology, and consequences. J Clin Sleep Med. 2007;3(5 Suppl):S7–10.
5. Good CH, Brager AJ, Capaldi VF. Mysliwiec: sleep in the United States military. Neuropsychopharmacology. 2020;45(1):176–91. https://doi.org/10.1038/s41386-019-0431-7.
6. Wright KM, Britt TW, Bliese PD, Adler AB, et al. Insomnia as predictor versus outcome of PTSD and depression among Iraq combat veterans. J Clin Psychol. 2011;67(12):1240–58. https://doi.org/10.1002/jclp.20845.
7. Bramoweth AD, Germain A. Deployment-related insomnia in military personnel and veterans. Curr Psychiatry Rep. 2013;15(10):401. https://doi.org/10.1007/s11920-013-0401-4.
8. McLay RN, Klam WP, Volkert SL. Insomnia is the most commonly reported symptom and predicts other symptoms of post-traumatic stress disorder in U.S. service members returning from military deployments. Mil Med. 2010;175(10):759–62. https://doi.org/10.7205/milmed-d-10-00193.
9. Ford ES, Wheaton AG, Cunningham TJ, Giles WH, et al. Trends in outpatient visits for insomnia, sleep apnea, and prescriptions for sleep medications among US adults: findings from the National Ambulatory Medical Care survey 1999-2010. Sleep. 2014;37(8):1283–93. https://doi.org/10.5665/sleep.3914.
10. Thelus Jean R, Hou Y, Masterson J, Kress A, Mysliwiec V. Prescription patterns of sedative hypnotic medications in the military health system. J Clin Sleep Med. 2019;15(6):873–9. https://doi.org/10.5664/jcsm.7840.
11. Vinokur AD, Pierce PF, Lewandowski-Romps L, Hobfoll SE, Galea S. Effects of war exposure on air force personnel's mental health, job burnout and other organizational related outcomes. J Occup Health Psychol. 2011;16(1):3–17. https://doi.org/10.1037/a0021617.
12. Williams SG, Collen J, Wickwire E, Lettieri CJ, Mysliwiec V. The impact of sleep on soldier performance. Curr Psychiatry Rep. 2014;16(8):459. https://doi.org/10.1007/s11920-014-0459-7.
13. Pigeon WR, Britton PC, Ilgen MA, Chapman B, Conner KR. Sleep disturbance preceding suicide among veterans. Am J Public Health. 2012;102(Suppl 1):S93–7. https://doi.org/10.2105/AJPH.2011.300470.

14. Widome R, Jensen A, Fu SS. Socioeconomic disparities in sleep duration among veterans of the US wars in Iraq and Afghanistan. Am J Public Health. 2015;105(2):e70–4. https://doi.org/10.2105/ajph.2014.302375.
15. Morgenthaler T, Alessi C, Friedman L, Owens J, et al. Practice parameters for the use of actigraphy in the assessment of sleep and sleep disorders: an update for 2007. Sleep. 2007;30(4):519–29.
16. Morgenthaler TI, Lee-Chiong T, Alessi C, Friedman L, et al. Practice parameters for the clinical evaluation and treatment of circadian rhythm sleep disorders. An American Academy of Sleep Medicine report. Sleep. 2007;30(11):1445–59.
17. Bastien CH, Vallieres A, Morin CM. Validation of the Insomnia Severity Index as an outcome measure for insomnia research. Sleep Med. 2001;2(4):297–307.
18. Buysse DJ, Reynolds CF, Monk TH, Berman SR, Kupfer DJ. The Pittsburgh Sleep Quality Index: a new instrument for psychiatric practice and research. Psychiatry Res. 1989;28(2):193–213.
19. Lapin BR, Bena JF, Walia HK, Moul DE. The Epworth sleepiness scale: validation of one-dimensional factor structure in a large clinical sample. J Clin Sleep Med. 2018;14(8):1293–301. https://doi.org/10.5664/jcsm.7258.
20. Buysse DJ. Chapter 75 - Insomnia: recent developments and future directions. In: Kryger MH, Roth TR, Dement WC, editors. Principles and practice of sleep medicine. 5th ed. Philadelphia: W.B. Saunders; 2011. p. 822–6.
21. Vgontzas AN, Liao D, Bixler EO, Chrousos GP, Vela-Bueno A. Insomnia with objective short sleep duration is associated with a high risk for hypertension. Sleep. 2009;32(4):491–7.
22. Vgontzas AN, Lin HM, Papaliaga M, Calhoun S, et al. Short sleep duration and obesity: the role of emotional stress and sleep disturbances. Int J Obes. 2008;32(5):801–9. https://doi.org/10.1038/ijo.2008.4.
23. Cappuccio FP, D'Elia L, Strazzullo P, Miller MA. Sleep duration and all-cause mortality: a systematic review and meta-analysis of prospective studies. Sleep. 2010;33(5):585–92.
24. Sofi F, Cesari F, Casini A, Macchi C, et al. Insomnia and risk of cardiovascular disease: a meta-analysis. Eur J Prev Cardiol. 2014;21(1):57–64. https://doi.org/10.1177/2047487312460020.
25. Spielman AJ, Caruso LS, Glovinsky PB. A behavioral perspective on insomnia treatment. Psychiatr Clin North Am. 1987;10(4):541–53.
26. Zhang B, Wing YK. Sex differences in insomnia: a meta-analysis. Sleep. 2006;29(1):85–93. https://doi.org/10.1093/sleep/29.1.85.
27. Mysliwiec V, Gill J, Lee H, Baxter T, et al. Sleep disorders in US military personnel: a high rate of comorbid insomnia and obstructive sleep apnea. Chest. 2013;144(2):549–57. https://doi.org/10.1378/chest.13-0088.
28. Mantua J, Bessey A, Sowden WJ, Chabuz R, et al. A Review of Environmental Barriers to Obtaining Adequate Sleep in the Military Operational Context. Mil Med. 2019;184(7–8):e259–66. https://doi.org/10.1093/milmed/usz029.
29. Morin CM, Benca RM. Insomnia nature, diagnosis, and treatment. Handb Clin Neurol. 2011;99:723–46. https://doi.org/10.1016/B978-0-444-52007-4.00004-7.
30. Diagnostic and statistical manual of mental disorders: DSM-5™, 5th ed. Arlington, VA: American Psychiatric Publishing, Inc; 2013.
31. Schutte-Rodin S, Broch L, Buysse D, Dorsey C, et al. Clinical guideline for the evaluation and management of chronic insomnia in adults. J Clin Sleep Med. 2008;4(5):487–504.
32. Carney CE, Buysse DJ, Ancoli-Israel S, Edinger JD, et al. The consensus sleep diary: standardizing prospective sleep self-monitoring. Sleep. 2012;35(2):287–302. https://doi.org/10.5665/sleep.1642.
33. Campbell DG, Bonner LM, Bolkan C, Lanto AB, et al. Stigma predicts treatment preferences and care engagement among veterans affairs primary care patients with depression. Ann Behav Med. 2016;50(4):533–44. https://doi.org/10.1007/s12160-016-9780-1.
34. Trockel M, Karlin BE, Taylor CB, Manber R. Cognitive Behavioral Therapy for insomnia with Veterans: evaluation of effectiveness and correlates of treatment outcomes. Behav Res Ther. 2014;53:41–6. https://doi.org/10.1016/j.brat.2013.11.006.

35. Sateia MJ, Buysse DJ. Chapter 83 - Treatment guidelines for insomnia. In: Kryger MH, Roth T, Dement WC, editors. Principles and practice of sleep medicine. 5th ed. Philadelphia: W.B. Saunders; 2011. p. 931–7.
36. Weil JV. Principals and practice of sleep medicine. In: Kryger MH, Roth T, Dement WC, editors. Principles and practice of sleep medicine. 5th ed. Philadelphia: W.B. Saunders; 2011. p. 242–53.
37. Ayabe N, Okajima I, Nakajima S, Inoue Y, et al. Effectiveness of cognitive behavioral therapy for pharmacotherapy-resistant chronic insomnia: a multi-center randomized controlled trial in Japan. Sleep Med. 2018;50:105–12. https://doi.org/10.1016/j.sleep.2018.05.038.
38. Sateia MJ, Buysse DJ, Krystal AD, Neubauer DN, et al. Clinical practice guideline for the pharmacologic treatment of chronic insomnia in adults: an American Academy of Sleep Medicine clinical practice guideline. J Clin Sleep Med. 2017;13(2):307–49. https://doi.org/10.5664/jcsm.6470.
39. Harvey AG, Spielman AJ. Chapter 77 - Insomnia: diagnosis, assessment, and outcomes. In: Kryger MH, Roth T, Dement WC, editors. Principles and practice of sleep medicine. 5th ed. Philadelphia: W.B. Saunders; 2011. p. 838–49.
40. Kishi T, Matsunaga S, Iwata N. Suvorexant for primary insomnia: a systematic review and meta-analysis of randomized placebo-controlled trials. PLoS One. 2015;10(8):e0136910. https://doi.org/10.1371/journal.pone.0136910.
41. Gong H, Ni CX, Liu YZ, Zhang Y, et al. Mindfulness meditation for insomnia: a meta-analysis of randomized controlled trials. J Psychosom Res. 2016;89:1–6. https://doi.org/10.1016/j.jpsychores.2016.07.016.
42. Chervin RD. Sleepiness, fatigue, tiredness, and lack of energy in obstructive sleep apnea. Chest. 2000;118(2):372–9.
43. Schwartz AR, Patil SP, Laffan AM, Polotsky V, et al. Obesity and obstructive sleep apnea: pathogenic mechanisms and therapeutic approaches. Proc Am Thorac Soc. 2008;5(2):185–92. https://doi.org/10.1513/pats.200708-137MG.
44. Chung F, Abdullah HR, Liao P. STOP-bang questionnaire: a practical approach to screen for obstructive sleep apnea. Chest. 2016;149(3):631–8. https://doi.org/10.1378/chest.15-0903.
45. Hoge CW, McGurk D, Thomas JL, Cox AL, et al. Mild traumatic brain injury in U.S. Soldiers returning from Iraq. N Engl J Med. 2008;358(5):453–63. https://doi.org/10.1056/NEJMoa072972.
46. Mysliwiec V, McGraw L, Pierce R, Smith P, et al. Sleep disorders and associated medical comorbidities in active duty military personnel. Sleep. 2013;36(2):167–74. https://doi.org/10.5665/sleep.2364.
47. Koziorynska EI, Rodriguez AJ. Narcolepsy: clinical approach to etiology, diagnosis, and treatment. Rev Neurol Dis. 2011;8(3–4):e97–106.
48. Creamer JL, Brock MS, Matsangas P, Motamedi VA, Mysliwiec V. Nightmares in United States military personnel with sleep disturbances. J Clin Sleep Med. 2018;14(3):419–26. https://doi.org/10.5664/jcsm.6990.
49. Germain A. Sleep disturbances as the hallmark of PTSD: where are we now? Am J Psychiatry. 2013;170(4):372–82. https://doi.org/10.1176/appi.ajp.2012.12040432.
50. Aurora RN, Kristo DA, Bista SR, Rowley JA, et al. The treatment of restless legs syndrome and periodic limb movement disorder in adults--an update for 2012: practice parameters with an evidence-based systematic review and meta-analyses: an American Academy of Sleep Medicine Clinical Practice Guideline. Sleep. 2012;35(8):1039–62. https://doi.org/10.5665/sleep.1988.

Addressing Veteran Homelessness

19

Benjamin F. Henwood and Sonya Gabrielian

Introduction

During the past decade, homelessness among U.S. veterans has been reduced by nearly half [1]. Most of this decline has been attributed to the success of the U.S. Department of Housing and Urban Development-U.S. Department of Veterans Affairs (VA) Supported Housing program (HUD-VASH, the VA's permanent supportive housing program) and its adoption of a Housing First approach [1]. Housing First is guided by several key principles that include: (1) immediate access to permanent housing; (2) no treatment or sobriety requirements (either before or after being housed); (3) availability of a flexible array of health and social services; and (4) choice in the type and frequency of housing and supportive services [2, 3]. For most homeless veterans—regardless of mental illness, substance use disorders, or co-occurring disorders—HUD-VASH has been associated with improved housing and clinical outcomes [4, 5]. Still, HUD-VASH is not appropriate for all homeless veterans, and it may work better for some than others [4, 6]. There can be significant challenges to engaging and enrolling some veterans in HUD-VASH [7]. The VA and its community partners use several other services to address veteran homelessness, including transitional housing, residential rehabilitation, assertive community treatment, homeless outreach, and patient-centered medical homes tailored for homeless veterans (also known as homeless patient-aligned care teams). In this chapter, we discuss contextual factors relevant to working with homeless veterans who have mental illness, substance use disorders, or co-occurring disorders and share best practices that meet the needs of homeless veterans. Throughout the chapter, we use case examples to help bridge the gap between the research literature and frontline practice.

B. F. Henwood (✉) · S. Gabrielian
Suzanne Dworak-Peck School of Social Work, University of Southern California, Los Angeles, CA, USA
e-mail: bhenwood@usc.edu; Sonya.gabrielian@va.gov

C. H. Warner, C. A. Castro (eds.), *Veteran and Military Mental Health*, https://doi.org/10.1007/978-3-031-18009-5_19

Vignette

Jeff, who was married with two children, served in the U.S. Air Force toward the end of the Vietnam War. After his successful return and reentry, a divorce was the catalyst for increased daily alcohol use, loss of employment, and becoming homeless for the first time. After spending almost 2 years without a stable place to live that included stays at an emergency shelter, his sons' homes, and on the streets, Jeff went to his local VA and enrolled in a substance use disorder treatment program. After a year of sobriety and living temporarily with his oldest son, Jeff relapsed and became homeless again. When he eventually enrolled in a treatment program for a second time almost a year later, he was diagnosed with bipolar disorder and prescribed Zyprexa. After 6 weeks, Jeff left his treatment program and returned to living on the streets, in part because he did not like the way Zyprexa made him feel. A local outreach team attempted to engage Jeff, who was not interested in exploring other treatment options but was willing to apply for housing. After supporting Jeff for several months through the application process, a social worker who worked with the outreach team informed Jeff that he had been approved for HUD-VASH. Jeff moved into an apartment 6 weeks later but continued to drink every day. After nearly 6 months in his apartment with twice-a-month home visits from a social worker, Jeff informed his social worker that he wanted to return to residential treatment to help repair his relationship with his son. Jeff and his treating psychiatrist discussed how Zyprexa made him feel and found a new medication that he could tolerate. Jeff now regularly sees his son, who comes to his apartment where he has been living for the past 18 months.

There are several key points to highlight from Jeff's case. The first is why a veteran becomes homeless in the first place. Often, mental illness and substance use are part of the story but should be thought of as an important risk factor rather than an explanation [8]. As in Jeff's case, a precipitating event such as a divorce, death in the family, losing a job, or another loss or transition (e.g., re-entry from military to civilian life) is often a major contributing factor. Trauma is also an important consideration that may have occurred as part of childhood adversity or interpersonal violence rather than from combat experience while on active duty, which was not part of Jeff's experience in the service.

Equally important to individual risk factors is how systems are designed to respond to at-risk veterans. For Jeff, it's not clear what preventive services, if any, were available. Could interpersonal therapy have saved his marriage? Why wasn't he diagnosed earlier with bipolar disorder? What if unemployment benefits or affordable housing were more readily available? We also see that although Jeff at times proactively engaged in on-site treatment at the VA after he became homeless, assertive outreach was needed while Jeff was living on the streets and in his apartment to help him engage in treatment and services that he felt he needed and was ready for. The use of a harm reduction approach was also important so that Jeff was not disqualified from housing and did not feel judged for continuing to drink after moving into his own apartment, which opened the door later for more effective treatment and longer-term housing stability [9, 10]. This is generally consistent with taking a veteran-centered approach to facilitate shared decision-making when prescribing psychiatric medication [11], which appears to have happened the second time Jeff engaged in psychiatric services but not the first time, when he stopped treatment. Finally, it is not uncommon for veterans to maintain housing stability for a year or more in HUD-VASH, but improved social outcomes are less robust [5]. In Jeff's case, reconnecting with his son was an important part of his recovery from mental illness, alcohol abuse, and homelessness, but for many veterans, establishing meaningful connections remains a challenge [12].

Before tackling some of these key points, we will first examine the epidemiology of mental illness and substance use disorders among homeless veterans and consider differences in pathways to homelessness, including those between veterans who served in Vietnam versus those who served in Operation Enduring Freedom, Operation Iraqi Freedom, or Operation New Dawn.

Epidemiology of Behavioral Health Conditions Among Homeless Veterans

Like Jeff, many veterans who experience homelessness also have mental illness, substance use disorders, or co-occurring disorders. In fact, the presence of these conditions regardless of veteran status is one of the strongest risk factors for homelessness [13–15]. Veterans with certain behavioral health conditions such as illicit substance use or psychotic disorders including schizophrenia may be more at risk of homelessness [15]. For example, one large-scale study found that a diagnosis of schizophrenia increased a veteran's odds of homelessness by approximately three times; the presence of any illicit drug use disorder increased a veteran's odds of experiencing homelessness by nearly eight times; and veterans with an alcohol use disorder such as Jeff are nearly five times more likely to experienced recent homelessness than veterans without this disorder [16]. Having a co-occurring mental illness also decreases the likelihood of effective engagement and retention in care and social services [7].

In general, there is limited research examining specific military experiences, such as the psychological impact of combat exposure or military sexual trauma, and homelessness [17]. There is also limited research showing a strong connection between posttraumatic stress disorder, which is more prevalent among veterans than the general population, and veteran homelessness [15, 18]. Some research has found that screening positive for posttraumatic stress disorder increases the likelihood of experiencing homelessness among female but not male veterans [19, 20]. Nevertheless, we know that military-related trauma (physical, emotional, or sexual) can increase the risk of developing mental illness, substance use disorders, or both [21], which are strong risk factors for homelessness [13–15]. Rates of military sexual trauma are particularly high among women, with close to 40% of female homeless veterans who received VA services screening positive; although slightly more than 3% male homeless veterans [22] report military sexual trauma, the total number of men and women who have these experiences is approximately equal [23].

In terms of prevalence, recent data from the largest survey of homeless veterans to date showed that mental illness was highly prevalent in this population, with 33% reporting severe psychological distress during the past 2 weeks and 35% reporting receipt of psychiatric medication in the last 30 days [24]. Rates of active substance use disorders were also notable, with 29% reporting an alcohol problem and 14% reporting a drug problem. Interestingly, a study that used cluster analysis to classify homeless veterans into groups with shared clinical characteristics found three distinct clusters: (a) those with "addiction" issues (92%), a heterogeneous group with substance use disorders, depression, bipolar disorders, and adjustment disorders; (b) those with "psychosis" (6.5%), encompassing people with schizophrenia and other psychotic disorders, and sometimes with comorbid affective disorders or substance use disorders; and (c) those with "personality disorders" (1.6%), including people with personality disorders, sometimes with accompanying adjustment disorders, but without comorbid substance use disorders [25]. This underscores the need to integrate psychiatric and substance abuse treatment to effectively serve homeless veterans.

It's important to note that although most homeless veterans served during the Vietnam era [26], those who served in more recent conflicts who were diagnosed with a mental health condition when discharged from active duty also have high risk and are growing in number. In fact, research from the National Center on Homelessness among veterans has shown that the 18% of veterans of Operation Enduring Freedom, Operation Iraqi Freedom, or Operation New Dawn who were diagnosed with a mental health condition make up close to half of this era's homeless veterans [27]. Some have attributed differences in risk and pathways to homelessness between younger and older veterans to the fact that many Vietnam-era veterans were recruited via the draft, whereas veterans of recent conflicts come from an all-volunteer military [19, 28]. For Vietnam-era veterans, psychiatric and substance use disorders experienced after military discharge, along with postmilitary social isolation, were strong predictors of homelessness, whereas younger veterans were found to have higher rates of symptoms consistent with childhood conduct disorder and instability in their family of origin; they were also disproportionately African American and never married [28]. Differences in age cohorts are also seen among the nonveteran homeless population [29].

Specialty Primary Care Settings for Homeless Veterans

Although the VA is known for providing comprehensive services and health care access that are more robust than many community resources for nonveterans, adjustment challenges subsequent to military discharge may outweigh the protective benefits of available VA services to prevent and treat homelessness for a portion of vulnerable veterans [17]. Accordingly, many VA facilities and some community providers have developed innovative models of primary care that are tailored to the needs of homeless persons who struggle to access mainstream primary care services [30, 31]. The VA-based homeless patient-aligned care team program was developed in 2010 to provide interdisciplinary, team-based care tailored to homeless veterans at more than 65 VA medical centers. Though specific adaptations for homeless veterans vary by site—including practices to increase access (e.g., walk-in care) and service delivery in nontraditional locations (e.g., streets and shelters)–studies have shown that these programs are associated with lower rates of emergency department use and hospitalization, increased engagement in ambulatory care services, identification of undiagnosed health conditions, and improved housing outcomes [32]. This model was based on more than 20 years of learning how best to provide primary care to people experiencing homelessness through programs that were part of a national demonstration project that started in 1985 [32].

Team-Based Care

The importance of team-based care that is at the core of the homeless patient-aligned care team model can be seen in other homelessness service models used in and outside of the VA. Assertive community treatment is a long-standing evidence-based practice [33] that has been used to help people with serious mental illness live independently in the community since the 1960s; it has been adapted for use in Housing First [34] and medical home models [35]. A team approach is associated with multiple advantages for homeless veterans, including the ability of different team members to work with a veteran in multiple settings and domains. This results in having more information in the treatment team than any single service provider could access individually. For example, an employment specialist may be the first to learn about the reemergence of a veteran's psychiatric symptoms in the context of helping them finding a job. Sharing information and coordinating services in the context of an interdisciplinary team can ensure that services and treatment are complementary. One challenge of the team approach, however, is the risk of blurring boundaries between professional roles. Even a role as clearly medical as prescribing medication can become partly a case management issue if a veteran is living on the streets and cannot easily keep or store daily medication. Daily medication delivery may be possible but must be coordinated with a case manager. Similar issues arise in terms of whether money management is a clinical or housing issue if a person decides to stop paying rent. Although psychiatrists are ultimately responsible for the medications they prescribe, they also have a responsibility to ensure that other team members understand medication decisions. Social service staff members also have a responsibility to consult with the psychiatrist if they have knowledge about a veteran's medication regimens, jointly developing a comprehensive medication support plan. Although changes in prescribed medication and support occur based on a medication's effectiveness and corresponding side-effects, they also need to be responsive to a homeless veteran's daily routines that at times can vary from week to week. Daily team meetings are often necessary to reduce potential blurring of roles and boundaries among team members and ensure optimal operation. Of course, it is important to note merely colocating a psychiatrist with other disciplines such as social work and nursing does not constitute an effective team approach.

Psychiatrists, whether as a team leader or other member of the team, can support teamwork that involves a coherent approach among team members, a shared practice ideology, clear and open communication, mutual respect and understanding of roles, and separate and defined domains of responsibility.

A team-based approach can also support the use of harm reduction that is considered a best practice in homelessness services [10]. For some, harm reduction, which requires a practical and creative approach to both clinical work and housing management, can be difficult to navigate with homeless veterans who have substance use or co-occurring disorders. Harm reduction is a consumer-directed intervention in which the effectiveness in treatment is often measured in untraditional or smaller increments using highly individualized metrics, such as working with veterans to help them limit beer intake to a "40-ouncer" a day as opposed to a six-pack; spend fewer days in the hospital or jail during the next 6 months; or spend $20 less on drugs this month. The following vignette is provided to illustrate the often difficult and uneasy resolutions that emerge when working with a harm reduction approach. The vignette shows some of the compromises that must be made and that outcomes may be less than ideal for both the veteran and treatment team.

Vignette

Bobby is a 52-year-old African American veteran with schizophrenia and alcohol use disorder who has had multiple hospitalizations due to nonadherence to medication. He had spent many years homeless and drinking, including a period when he lived under a bridge with other individuals who were homeless. After 6 months of outreach and engagement, Bobby finally agreed to an initial evaluation with the psychiatrist. During the evaluation, Bobby told the psychiatrist that he did not need psychiatric care or medication in part because he had self-healing powers. He refused to meet with the psychiatrist again but easily accepted the offer of an apartment and was engaged with the team during the selection of an apartment and move-in period. After spending some time isolated in his apartment, he decided to resume contact with some of the other people from the under the bridge with whom he drank heavily, and eventually three of those contacts moved into his apartment. When the team informed Bobby that he was in violation of his lease agreement and was under scrutiny by his building's superintendent, he confessed that he felt powerless to have them leave. On several occasions after disturbances were reported by the superintendent, the team and the psychiatrist attempted to encourage and empower Bobby to continue to engage with his social networks but to do so away from his apartment. The psychiatrist made several home visits and used motivational interviewing techniques to understand Bobby's perspective on drinking and suggest several strategies for lessening or changing the context of his drinking. Though Bobby said drinking made him feel calmer, his speech and behavior while sober was not always coherent, and intermittently he became very agitated. A few days later, during a routine home visit, the team observed that Bobby had been putting out cigarettes on paper towels and that he had left a burner on the stove lit when not in use. This behavior was of grave concern to the team, which had him involuntarily hospitalized because he presented a danger to himself and others in the building. After Bobby was discharged from the hospital, the team psychiatrist met with him again, and he continued to refuse formal treatment and medication. The team offered to relocate Bobby to another apartment to make it more difficult for his previous acquaintances to reengage, to which he readily agreed. The psychiatrist encouraged Bobby to attend at least some group therapy sessions or drop by the VA regularly to avoid being in the apartment and feeling lonely.

Over the next year, Bobby remained very symptomatic but at the same time became more engaged with the team, including meeting with the team psychiatrist. Notably, during this time, Bobby's dangerous self-destructive behaviors did not recur. However, Bobby was eventually rehospitalized due to an episode of severe agitation and threatening behavior at the office when he did not receive the amount of money from his VA benefits that he was expecting. After this hospitalization, Bobby said he would be amenable to working with his psychiatrist to find a medication that would work better for him.

Bobby's case illustrates the creativity, long-term commitment, assertive outreach, and compromise that is often required to effectively maintain housing and treatment for veterans who have experienced homelessness. It reflects the numerous situations that can lead to conflicting or problematic interactions between housing and clinical services, including problematic behaviors resulting from nonadherence to medications, substance abuse, hoarding, nonpayment of rent, people squatting in an apartment, inability to maintain an apartment, medical disability, loneliness and vulnerability, and involuntary hospitalizations.

The vignette illustrated several of these challenges, highlighting how an interdisciplinary team can work with veterans in crisis to help them access and maintain an apartment while navigating relationships to avoid eviction. Although team-based services may not always be available to homeless veterans, it is important to recognize their advantages, especially with veterans with more significant mental illness, substance use disorders, or co-occurring disorders.

Housing Services Along the Continuum of Care

Although the central role of the HUD-VASH program was previously described, it is important to note that other programs are available to homeless veterans. Other housing services are offered along a continuum, including street outreach, emergency shelters, transitional housing, residential treatment, and independent housing. The Domiciliary Care for Homeless Veterans program and the Grant and Per Diem programs are two large VA efforts that operate on this continuum; these programs offer residential rehabilitation for homeless veterans and are operated by the VA and its community partners, respectively. Prevention services and rapid rehousing services are also available through the Supportive Services for Veteran Families program [36]. Rapid rehousing programs offer short-term subsidies and support to quickly house homeless veterans and prevent homelessness for those at imminent risk of homelessness. Supportive Services for Veteran Families serves veterans with and without families; its rapid rehousing services are delivered via VA's community partners.

Vignette

Carmen is a 28-year-old Navy veteran with a 2-year-old daughter. She completed one combat tour and experienced sexual trauma while on active duty. Following to these traumatic experiences, she has posttraumatic stress disorder and amphetamine use disorder. In addition, she has struggled to maintain steady employment and stable housing. After becoming involved with the criminal justice system due to her substance use and temporarily losing custody of her child, her case was diverted to a collaborative justice court. She learned that completion of a residential rehabilitation program, followed by an intensive outpatient program, could clear her criminal charges and help her reunify with her daughter. Prior to applying for HUD-VASH, she opted to enter the women's track at the Domiciliary Care for Homeless Veterans program for 6 months of residential rehabilitation for her co-occurring disorders. She received cognitive processing therapy for her posttraumatic stress disorder, psychosocial rehabilitation for her substance use disorder, and medication management. She found the comradery of the women's track at the Domiciliary and its intensive services helped with her long-term recovery from homelessness.

The continuum-of-care paradigm is rooted in the belief that treatment facilitates skills needed to sustain independent, permanent housing. Though HUD-VASH has been shown to be more effective [2] than the continuum of care in population-based studies, this vignette illustrates that available services along this continuum enable shared decision making, allowing veterans and their clinicians to develop treatment plans to facilitate exits from homelessness. Commonly, as in Carmen's case, veterans elect to address their psychiatric symptoms, substance use disorders, or co-occurring disorders in residential treatment before transitioning to independent housing.

Regardless of veterans' paths to HUD-VASH or other permanent housing, a fundamental problem of overall recovery beyond the acquisition of permanent housing remains. Based on the larger mental health literature, recovery for homeless veterans must involve a deeper process of building a meaningful and fulfilling life that includes autonomy and social relationships [37]. The extent to which this occurs with formerly homeless veterans with mental illness or substance use disorders who are engaged in HUD-VASH is unclear [12] and requires further research on how this can be achieved. In addition, some homeless veterans who enroll in supported housing programs disengage prematurely, before receiving permanent housing [38], whereas others who attain housing subsequently lose it and return to homelessness [39, 40]. Further research is needed to understand how best to support those who are not successful in Housing First programs and to facilitate recovery and social integration for homeless veterans who are successfully housed via HUD-VASH.

Addressing Suicidal Behavior Among Homeless Veterans

Suicidal ideation and attempts are highly prevalent among homeless adults, regardless of veteran status [13, 41]. Suicide attempts among homeless veterans are much higher than the rate of suicide attempts among all veterans, but suicidal behaviors likely predate homelessness episodes [42]. Given the VA's mission to end veteran suicide and the significant vulnerability to suicidal behaviors seen among homeless veterans, embedding suicide prevention strategies in homelessness services is critical. Currently, the VA's suicide prevention initiative employs multiple modalities, including a crisis line (available via telephone, text message, or instant message), services from designated suicide prevention coordinators, outreach efforts, and training on safety assessments and safety planning. Clinicians working with homeless veterans need to be cognizant of this population's elevated suicide risk and the potential value of linking this group to suicide prevention efforts. Even in HUD-VASH, teams need to continually evaluate for suicide risk, because although moving into an apartment can be experienced as a positive experience, it also represents a transition period when veterans are at heightened risk and unfortunately can result in them feeling more isolated than when homeless.

Future Directions

Mental illness, substance use disorders, and co-occurring disorders are highly prevalent among veterans experiencing homelessness. Yet even among veterans with these behavioral health problems, only a minority experience homelessness [8]. The VA and its community partners offer diverse services tailored to the psychiatric, medical, and social vulnerabilities of this population, including specialized primary care clinics, other team-based services, HUD-VASH, and housing programs along the continuum of care. Though many of these programs employ evidence-based practices that improve housing and health for persons experiencing homelessness, a subset of veterans with mental health problems struggle in these programs and experience recurrent homelessness. Even the veterans who successfully use services to attain and retain housing often see limited gains in their community functioning, such as connections with family and friends or vocational activities. Implementation approaches (e.g., adapting psychosocial treatment used for people with serious mental illness for those experiencing homelessness) may hold potential to substantively improve the health, housing, and functional outcomes of highly vulnerable veterans with homelessness experiences.

The novel coronavirus (COVID-19) pandemic has been particularly disruptive for homeless veterans with mental illness, substance use disorders, and co-occurring disorders. This group is disproportionally burdened by the pandemic, which has posed profound health risks and diminished access to medical, mental health, addiction treatment, and social services [43, 44]. Though the VA and community-based health systems rapidly adopted virtual care modalities [45], little is known about changes to this population's access to mental health care and housing resources during the pandemic. There are ongoing efforts to use digital navigators for veterans with low technology literacy; developing standardized practices to increase digital competence among veterans with homelessness experiences may prove valuable [46]. Even beyond the pandemic—particularly for homeless veterans in rural or underresourced communities—virtual care approaches may serve as critical adjuncts to existing services. The pandemic is an impetus to optimize these technologies for homeless veterans.

Last, novel programs—for example, low-barrier, protected outdoor environments ("safe camping") where veterans experiencing homelessness can live, access hygiene resources and food, and receive services—hold potential to improve services for the most vulnerable homeless veterans who fall through the cracks of existing services offered by the VA and its community partners. These low-barrier, recovery-oriented programs provide an entry point into care, helping homeless veterans achieve their immediate goals while providing nonmandated linkages to services. These directions hold promise for achieving the overarching goal of eliminating veteran homelessness and improving the overall functioning of homeless veterans who use the VA and community-based housing and health care services.

Clinical Pearls

- Mental illness, especially schizophrenia and substance use disorders, should be thought of as an important risk factor rather than an explanation for veteran homelessness [8].
- There is limited research examining connections between veteran homelessness and specific military experiences, such as the psychological impact of combat exposure or military sexual trauma, or military PTSD.
- The VA Healthcare system offers a homeless patient-aligned care team program to provide interdisciplinary, team-based care tailored to homeless veterans at more than 65 VA medical centers around the country.
- A team-based approach in caring for homeless veterans provides greater information sharing to better coordinate support resources and support harm reduction.
- The VA and other support organizations offer a continuum, of support services for homeless veterans including street outreach, emergency shelters, transitional housing, residential treatment, and independent housing.
- Suicide attempts among homeless veterans are much higher than the rate of suicide attempts among all veterans, but suicidal behaviors likely predate homelessness episodes [42].

References

1. Henry M, Watt R, Mahathey A, Ouellette J, Sitler A. The 2019 annual homelessness assessment report (AHAR) to congress. 2020. Available at https://www.hudexchange.info/resource/5948/2019-ahar-part-1-pit-estimates-of-homelessness-in-the-us/. Accessed 20 July 2021.
2. O'Connell MJ, Rosenheck RA. Supported housing: twenty-five years of the Housing and Urban Development-Veterans Affairs Supported Housing (HUD-VASH) program. In: Tsai J, editor. Homelessness among U.S. veterans: critical perspectives. Oxford: Oxford University Press; 2019. p. 77–108.
3. Padgett D, Henwood BF, Tsemberis SJ. Housing First: ending homelessness, transforming systems, and changing lives. Oxford University Press; 2016.

4. Gabrielian S, Gores AM, Gelberg L, Tsai J. Mental illness and substance use disorder among homeless veterans. In: Tsai J, editor. Homelessness among U.S. veterans: critical perspectives. Oxford: Oxford University Press; 2019. p. 77–108.
5. Montgomery AE, Hill LL, Kane V, Culhane DP. Housing chronically homeless veterans: evaluating the efficacy of a Housing First approach to HUD-VASH. J Community Psychol. 2013;41(4):505–14.
6. Tsai J, Rosenheck RA, Kane V. Homeless female US veterans in a national supported housing program: comparison of individual characteristics and outcomes with male veterans. Psychol Serv. 2014;11(3):309–16.
7. Montgomery AE, Cusack M, Blonigen DM, Gabrielian S, et al. Factors associated with veterans' access to permanent supportive housing. Psychiatr Serv. 2016;67(8):870–7.
8. Montgomery AE, Metraux S, Culhane D. Rethinking homelessness prevention among persons with serious mental illness. Soc Issues Policy Rev. 2013;7(1):58–82.
9. Collins SE, Clifasefi SL, Dana EA, Adrasik MP, et al. Where harm reduction meets Housing First: exploring alcohol's role in a project-based housing first setting. Int J Drug Policy. 2012;23(2):111–9.
10. Tsemberis S, Gulcur L, Nakae M. Housing First, consumer choice, and harm reduction for homeless individuals with a dual diagnosis. Am J Public Health. 2004;94(4):651–6.
11. Deegan PE, Drake RE. Shared decision making and medication management in the recovery process. Psychiatr Serv. 2006;57(11):1636–9.
12. Tsai J, Mares AS, Rosenheck RA. Does housing chronically homeless adults lead to social integration? Psychiatr Serv. 2012;63(5):427–34.
13. Folsom DP, Hawthorne W, Lindamer L, Gilmer T, et al. Prevalence and risk factors for homelessness and utilization of mental health services among 10,340 patients with serious mental illness in a large public mental health system. Am J Psychiatr. 2005;162(2):370–6.
14. Susser E, Moore R, Link B. Risk factors for homelessness. Epidemiol Rev. 1993;15(2):546–56.
15. Tsai J, Rosenheck RA. Risk factors for homelessness among US veterans. Epidemiol Rev. 2015;37(1):177–95.
16. Edens EL, Kasprow W, Tsai J, Rosencheck RA. Association of substance use and VA service-connected disability benefits with risk of homelessness among veterans. Am J Addict. 2011;20(5):412–9.
17. Balshem H, Christensen V, Tuepker A, Kansagara D. A critical review of the literature regarding homelessness among veterans. 2011. Available at https://www.hsrd.research.va.gov/publications/esp/homelessness.cfm. Accessed 20 July 2021.
18. O'Connell MJ, Kasprow W, Rosenheck RA. Rates and risk factors for homelessness after successful housing in a sample of formerly homeless veterans. Psychiatr Serv. 2008;59(3):268–75.
19. Rosenheck R, Fontana A. A model of homelessness among male veterans of the Vietnam War generation. Am J Psychiatry. 1994;151(3):421–7.
20. Washington DL, Yano EM, McGuire J, Hines V, et al. Risk factors for homelessness among women veterans. J Health Care Poor Underserved. 2010;21(1):82–91.
21. Murdoch M, Nichol MD. Women veterans' experience with domestic violence and with sexual harassment while in the military. Arch Fam Med. 1995;4(5):411–8.
22. Pavao J, Turchik JA, Hyun JK, Karpenko J, et al. Military sexual trauma among homeless veterans. J Gen Intern Med. 2013;28(Suppl. 2):S536–41.
23. Bell ME, Turchik JA, Karpenko JA. Impact of gender on reactions to military sexual assault and harassment. Health Soc Work. 2014;39(1):25–33.
24. Kertesz SG, DeRussy AJ, Kim YI, Polio DE, et al. Comparison of patient experience between primary care settings tailored for homeless clientele and mainstream settings: a large, multisite survey. Med Care. 2021;59(6):495–503.
25. Goldstein G, Luther JF, Jacoby AM, Haas GL, Gordon AJ. A preliminary classification system for homeless veterans with mental illness. Psychol Serv. 2008;5(1):36–48.
26. National Coalition for Homeless Veterans. FAQ about homeless veterans. n.d.. Available at http://nchv.org/index.php/news/media/background_and_statistics/. Accessed 20 July 2021.

27. Metraux S, Clegg LX, Daigh JD, Culhane DP, Kane V. Risk factors for becoming homeless among a cohort of veterans who served in the era of the Iraq and Afghanistan conflicts. Am J Public Health. 2013;103(S2):S255–61.
28. Tessler R, Rosenheck R, Gamache G. Comparison of homeless veterans with other homeless men in a large clinical outreach program. Psychiatry Q. 2002;73(2):109–19.
29. Culhane DP, Metraux S, Byrne T, Stino M, Bainbridge J. The age structure of contemporary homelessness: evidence and implications for public policy. Anal Soc Issues Public Policy. 2013;13(1):228–44.
30. O'Toole TP, Johnson EE, Aiello R, Kane V, Pape L. Tailoring care to vulnerable populations by incorporating social determinants of health: the Veterans Health Administration's "Homeless Patient Aligned Care Team" program. Prev Chronic Dis. 2016;13:150567.
31. Zlotnick C, Zerger S, Wolfe PB. Health care for the homeless: wshat we have learned in the past 30 years and what's next. Am J Public Health. 2013;103(S2):S199–205.
32. O'Toole TP. Primary care for homeless veterans. In: Tsai J, editor. Homelessness among U.S. veterans: critical perspectives. Oxford: Oxford University Press; 2019. p. 61–75.
33. Padgett DK, Henwood BF. Moving into the fourth decade of ACT. Psychiatr Serv. 2011;62(6):605.
34. Matejkowski J, Draine J. Investigating the impact of Housing First on ACT fidelity. Community Ment Health J. 2009;45(1):6–11.
35. Vanderlip ER, Henwood BF, Hrouda D, Meyer PS, et al. Systematic literature review of general health care interventions within programs of assertive community treatment. Psychiatr Serv. 2017;68(3):218–24.
36. Byrne T, Treglia D, Culhane DP, Kuhn J, Kane V. Predictors of homelessness among families and single adults after exit from homelessness prevention and rapid re-housing programs: evidence from the Department of Veterans Affairs Supportive Services for Veteran Families program. Hous Policy Debate. 2016;26(1):252–75.
37. Davidson L, Roe D. Recovery from versus recovery in serious mental illness: one strategy for lessening confusion plaguing recovery. J Ment Health. 2007;16(4):459–70.
38. Gabrielian S, Burns AV, Nanda N, Hellemann G, et al. Factors associated with premature exits from supported housing. Psychiatr Serv. 2016;67(1):86–93.
39. Cusack M, Montgomery AE, Blonigen D, Gabrielian S, Marsh L. Veteran returns to homelessness following exits from permanent supportive housing: health and supportive services use proximal to exit. Fam Soc. 2016;97(3):221–9.
40. Gabrielian S, Hamilton AB, Alexandrino A, Hellemann G, Young AS. "They're homeless in a home": retaining homeless-experienced consumers in supported housing. Psychol Serv. 2017;14(2):154–66.
41. Goldstein G, Luther JF, Haas GL. Medical, psychiatric and demographic factors associated with suicidal behavior in homeless veterans. Psychiatry Res. 2012;199(1):37–43.
42. Bommersbach TJ, Stefanovics EA, Rhee TG, Tsai J, Rosenheck RA. Suicide attempts and homelessness: timing of attempts among recently homeless, past homeless, and never homeless adults. Psychiatr Serv. 2020;71(12):1225–31.
43. Jordan RE, Adab P, Cheng KK. Covid-19: risk factors for severe disease and death. BMJ. 2020;368:m1198.
44. Kirby T. Efforts escalate to protect homeless people from COVID-19 in UK. Lancet Respir Med. 2020;8(5):447–9.
45. Heyworth L, Kirsh S, Zulman D, Kizer KW. Expanding access through virtual care: the VA's early experience with Covid-19. NEJM Catalyst. 2020. https://catalyst.nejm.org/doi/full/10.1056/CAT.20.0327.
46. Raja PV, Gabrielian S, Doran N. Access to care for veterans with serious mental illness during the COVID-19 pandemic. Psychiatr Serv. 2021;72(11):1324–7.

Mental Health of LGBT Service Members and Veterans

20

Kathleen A. McNamara, Jillian C. Shipherd, and Terry Adirim

Lesbian, Gay, Bisexual and Transgender U.S. Military Personnel: Prevalence and History

In military and veteran communities, about 5% of individuals are lesbian, gay, bisexual, or transgender (LGBT; [1]), with an estimated one million veterans and 75,000 actively serving personnel identifying as LGBT [2, 3]. Women appear to be over-represented in this population with servicewomen and female veterans being twice as likely to identify as lesbian or bisexual than their civilian counterparts. Younger Service members (under age 35) are more likely to identify as LGB than older members (aged 35 and older) [4]. Cultural, religious, and political messaging, as well as resulting local, state, and federal policies regarding this population have been found to impact LGBT individuals' self-conceptualization, mental wellbeing, physical health, and a number of other aspects of life satisfaction [5–8]). As a result

Disclaimer: The view(s) expressed herein are those of the authors and do not reflect the official policy or position of the Department of the Air Force, the Department of Defense, the Department of Veterans Affairs, or the U.S. Government.

K. A. McNamara (✉)
Nellis Air Force Base, Las Vegas, NV, USA

J. C. Shipherd
Lesbian, Gay, Bisexual, and Transgender (LGBT) Health Program, Veterans Health Administration, Washington, DC, USA

National Center for PTSD, VA Boston Healthcare System, Boston, MA, USA

Boston University School of Medicine, Boston, MA, USA
e-mail: Jillian.Shipherd@va.gov

T. Adirim
Department of Preventive Medicine and Biostatistics, F. Edward Hebert School of Medicine, Uniformed Services University of the Health Sciences, Bethesda, MD, USA

C. H. Warner, C. A. Castro (eds.), *Veteran and Military Mental Health*,
https://doi.org/10.1007/978-3-031-18009-5_20

of policy changes over the years, more and more Service members and veterans will seek care for issues related to LGBT health, requiring clinicians practicing within the military and veteran health systems to recognize the issues and to acquire the knowledge of the treatments required to care for these individuals. This care can include better awareness of health disparities and preventive screens, more inclusive sexual health assessments, mental health care to address sequelae of stress stigma and discrimination, as well as gender affirmation therapy for transgender Service members and veterans. This awareness should also include sensitivity to the need of older LGBT veterans who may have served under restrictive policies and who are fearful of disclosure. Healthcare professionals should be aware of the historical factors at play in an LGBT patients' clinical presentation, as well as the uniquely influential role they play in providing LGBT-affirming healthcare, especially among military personnel and veterans.

Throughout this chapter we will use the term "LGBT." We acknowledge that this community often uses other terminology such as queer, pansexual, and gender expansive; however, the majority of research on this population has not yet incorporated such terms in their data collection nor publications. Therefore, we use "LGBT" to reflect existing literature. Healthcare providers should mirror their patient's self-defining language and check for clarity if needed.

LGBT Terminology

Jessica is a 35-year-old African American gender nonbinary lesbian veteran who separated from the U.S. Air Force as a Major 5 years ago after 12 years of service. She/they present for mental health care to address work-related anxiety as she/they was recently promoted at the educational institution in which she/they works. Jessica presents with a gender nonbinary appearance: a masculine haircut and clothing, polished nails, and feminine makeup. Jessica reports being "gender nonbinary" on her intake paperwork and requests use of either pronouns "she" or "they." Jessica selects "lesbian" on her intake paperwork and states that she/they is exclusively attracted to and dates cisgender women and transgender women and has been in a monogamous relationship with her girlfriend for many years.

The terms "lesbian" and "gay" can indicate a romantic interest, sexual attraction, and/or intimate behavior with others of the same gender. Like those who identify as "heterosexual" or "straight," individuals who identify themselves as lesbian or gay are "monosexual," or are more often attracted to only one gender. In contrast, "bisexual" or "pansexual" individuals are attracted to people of their gender as well as those of other genders. Sexual orientation, behavior, and/or identity are distinct and can change over the lifespan. Thus, knowing someone's sexual orientation doesn't tell you about their sexual behavior and vice versa. It is important to note that gender identity is distinct from sexual attraction or orientation. Individuals whose current gender identity corresponds with their sex assigned at birth (typically female or male) are considered "cisgender," while those whose current gender identity is dissimilar from sex assigned at birth are commonly called "transgender" or "gender diverse." Some people identify as "nonbinary," "gender fluid," or "genderqueer" in which individuals present in a manner outside of society's binary gender norms. Use of the singular "they," as portrayed in the vignette above, is a personal pronoun option, commonly employed by individuals who do not identify as male or female. As in the example above, a patient may indicate use of both "she/they" or "he/they" pronouns.

In this example, Jessica has clearly identified her gender, pronoun(s), and sexual orientation. These demographic factors may or may not be related to her/their work-related anxiety for which she/they presents to the clinic for care. The provider should reflect the patient's self-identifying language in their communication with and about the patient verbally and in their notes. In the clinical interview, it is apparent that Jessica is pleased with her/their gender presentation and does not meet criteria for any gender-related diagnosis. She/they is evaluated to meet criteria for an adjustment disorder related to her/their work stress. Her/their provider documents Jessica's gender presentation and pronouns in her/their medical record, the provider openly discusses Jessica's partnership with a woman in the context of the partner providing significant social support, and the provider uses respectful, non-judgmental language and tone while discussing Jessica's case at weekly group supervision with other providers. Thus, Jessica is treated for work anxiety with LGBT-inclusive care by her medical provider, but the focus of the treatment is on work anxiety unrelated to her gender identity or sexual orientation.

Disclosure Considerations in a Military Environment

Rafael is a 28 year old Hispanic cisgender gay male Sergeant in the U.S. Army. He presents for an annual physical health exam and the medical technician asks him the typical intake questions, including his sexual history. Rafael has exclusively been in romantic partnerships with cisgender men. Since joining the military, Rafael consistently responds that he is sexually abstinent, as he is unsure whether his medical technicians and providers are compassionate and competent in LGBT matters. In the civilian medical clinic he frequented prior to joining the military, there were rainbow flag stickers, representing an LGBT-friendly climate, on the entrance door, in the lobby, and in the exam room. There had also been a document labeled "LGBT Healthcare Bills of Rights" prominently displayed on the lobby wall, and the intake form had an exhaustive list of sexual orientations, gender identities, and pronouns to choose from. In that clinic, he was forthcoming in all questions related to his sexual health. Rafael had looked for similar indications of an LGBT-friendly climate at the military medical treatment facilities where he had been served over the past few years, but had found none of these inclusivity indicators. Although he had questions related to pain during sex and assistive reproductive technology, he opted not to ask any of these questions, as he feared homophobic responses and misinformation, which some of his gay and bisexual friends had experienced in other military medical clinics.

Research indicates that Rafael's hesitance to disclose his same-sex sexual behavior and minoritized sexual orientation is a common concern among LGB Service members. Despite "Don't Ask, Don't Tell" (DADT) repeal, sexual minoritized

Service members and veterans are cautious about disclosing their sexual orientation and behavior, fearing homophobic or biphobic responses from healthcare providers, therapists, religious personnel, rejection from members of their unit, and even violence [9, 10]. Indeed, the language of the DADT repeal stated "Sexual orientation is a personal and private matter. DoD components, including the Services are not authorized to request, collect, or maintain information about the sexual orientation of Service members except when it is an essential part of an otherwise appropriate investigation or other official action" [11]. Thus, the culture of DADT remained even after the revocation, including asking about a Service member's sexual orientation as part of health care.

Outness to fellow Service members varies by disclosure recipient, with one study finding relatively low outness to chaplains (33%), moderately high outness to military medical providers (76%) and the highest outness to other LGBT friends in their unit (93% of respondents; [12]). Certain demographic characteristics have been found to be associated with different levels of outness, with Officers, unpartnered personnel, and bisexuals reporting lower odds of being out to fellow Service members compared to those who are enlisted, partnered personnel, lesbian women and gay men [12].

Transgender Service members report high levels of outness to both LGBT and non-LGBT military friends, commanders, and helping professionals (at least 80% reported being out to these entities) in an effort to access needed medical and logistical resources [12]. In one qualitative study on LGBT outness in the military since DADT repeal, LGBT respondents noted a continued hesitance to disclose, noting a fear that anti-LGBT sentiment remains amongst fellow personnel and concern that there may be negative career repercussions to disclosure [9]. One study found that gay and bisexual male Service members were only comfortable disclosing their sexual orientation to their military health care provider if the provider initiated the conversation about the members' sexual orientation, however unsurprisingly, only 5% of medical providers inquired about same-sex sexual activity among their patients [13, 14]. Similar findings are noted in the veteran literature, with both providers and veterans expecting that the other will raise the issue if it is relevant to their care [15]. In the military setting, junior providers were significantly more comfortable assessing the sexual health needs of LGB individuals compared to senior providers [14]. The overall picture that emerges from these studies is that barriers for disclosure of LGB identity, even to healthcare providers, persist following DADT repeal.

Providers should take measures to proactively communicate an LGBT-inclusive environment in their clinics. In the case vignette above, Rafael sought visual clues that his military medical providers were LGBT-inclusive, yet found none. The American Medical Association recommends the following tips for creating an LGBT-inclusive practice: Provide visual clues that your practice is a safe place for LGBT-disclosure by displaying a LGBT Health Care Bill of Rights [16], brochures and materials about LGBT-health concerns, customize intake forms to be LGBT-inclusive (included in Diagnostic and Treatment Consideration with the LGBT Patient Population below), ensure providers and staff are educated on inclusive, bias-free language, and educate providers on health concerns and treatments specific to this population [17, 18].

Military Policies Impacting LGBT Service

When treating members of a historically discriminated-against group, it is imperative that providers consider the legacy such institutionalized discrimination may leave in its wake. Since its inception, the U.S. military has situated minoritized sexual and gender identities as critical considerations in determining fitness for military duty. Suspected or confirmed same-sex intimate behavior was cause for rejection from military accession, or separation from service until 2011. While LGB-intolerance in the military took various forms over several decades, the Department of Defense (DoD) sentiment was, in sum: "Homosexuality is incompatible with military service… The presence of such members adversely affects the ability of the armed forces to maintain discipline, good order, and morale" [19]. In a purported effort to improve the wellbeing of lesbian, gay, and bisexual military members and stem the sense of fear and exclusion they experienced at work, the Don't Ask, Don't Tell, Don't Pursue (DADT) policy was signed into law in 1993 [20]. Under this policy, LGB Service members were permitted to serve, however under the condition that they refrain from disclosing their identity to others [2, 3]. Between 1993 and 2011 at least 14,000 Service members were discharged under DADT [2, 3]. Years of advocacy on behalf of Service members desiring open LGB service, highlighting DADT's cost on military readiness and on LGB Service members and their families, resulted in DADT being revoked in 2011 [11]. Yet as discussed above the culture of DADT remained as military personnel were discouraged from asking about sexual orientation, even in health care.

It is important to note that the DADT policy addressed same-sex behavior and interest only (i.e. sexual orientation). Gender identity and expression were not overtly spoken to by DADT, and official policies on transgender service have been non-linear. A repeal of the ban on transgender individuals serving in the military went into effect in 2016, however, was contested by the subsequent presidential administration beginning in 2017 [21]. Legal cases contesting reinstatement of the ban ensued, with one reaching the U.S. Supreme Court; ultimately, the so-called "transgender ban" was officially reinstated in April 2019 [22–24]. In January 2021, upon inauguration of a new U.S. president, the transgender ban on military service was again repealed, allowing individuals who meet certain physical and psychological fitness criteria to serve [25]. According to Schvey et al., transgender individuals are overrepresented 2:1 in the military as compared with the general population [26]. Estimates of the number of Service members who are transgender are as high as 12,800; however, there is some evidence that many if not most are hiding their gender identity due at least in part to the reversal in policy and concerns for impacts on their military career. As of this writing, same-sex intimate behavior, openly identifying as a member of a minoritized sexual orientation, and incongruence between one's sex assigned at birth and current gender identity are officially no longer cause for rejection from military service.

Mental and Physical Health Disparities by LGBT and Non-LGBT Military Populations

Nathan is a 22-year-old bisexual White cisgender male veteran who was medically discharged from the U.S. Navy after 3 years of service due to persistent low mood and posttraumatic stress that was negatively impacting his functioning and was not responsive to treatment. After a medical evaluation board, he was deemed unfit for continued military service. Nathan presents to a VA Community Outpatient Clinic to establish mental health care and address posttrauma symptoms, chronic suicidal ideation, and increased alcohol use which is negatively impacting his relationships. In his first PTSD support group at the VA clinic, a fellow group member makes homophobic comments including a desire to kill any gay or bisexual males he encounters. Others in the group laugh at his comment. Nathan thinks about leaving the group as the homophobia and biphobia in the group is upsetting. Per VA policy, the therapist leading the group comments: "As you know, VA Serves all Who Served and making any Veteran feel unsafe or uncomfortable is unacceptable in this group. We talked about that at the first session as one of our ground rules." The therapist then addresses the group member who made the offending comment: "You never know someone's identity. You can either apologize to the group or we can discuss finding you another treatment, the choice is yours." The group member apologized to the group saying "I'm sorry if I made someone uncomfortable. This is just how we talked to each other when we were active duty." The therapist then commented: "If anyone in the group was bothered by what was said, I am happy to follow-up with you individually. Please just let me know how I can support you. And as always, it's also OK to leave me a voicemail asking for additional support." Nathan felt supported by the therapist but is still wary of the other members of the group, and unsure if this is the best treatment for him.

A narrative review of the health and well-being of LGBT personnel and veterans found that Nathan's clinical presentation is not uncommon. Likely due to minority stress [7, 27] LGBT veterans experience consistently poorer mental and physical health compared to their non-LGBT military counterparts [5, 28–32]). As a whole, LGBT personnel and veterans have been found to be at heightened risk for suicidal ideation, suicide attempts, substance misuse, anxiety, trauma exposure and post-traumatic stress, mood disorders, homelessness, and some physical health concerns such as hypertension, tobacco-related diseases, and HIV [30, 33–35]. Almost one in three LGB Service members reported psychological distress levels consistent with serious distress, which was found to be nearly twice the percentage of non-LGB Service members [4]. Health disparities by subgroups of minoritized sexual orientation and gender identities have also been found in actively serving personnel, with cisgender lesbian and bisexual servicewomen at heightened risk for problematic alcohol and tobacco use than heterosexual servicewomen [36]. Cisgender gay and bisexual servicemen were found to be at seven times the odds of suicidality than cisgender heterosexual servicemen, and transgender personnel were at significantly heightened risk for anxiety, PTSD, depression, and suicidality than cisgender personnel [36]. A prevailing finding in the years since DADT repeal is that LGB-inclusive policy has not translated into a universally LGB-accepting climate [9, 12, 37]. Moreover, every service member and veteran has a sexual orientation and a gender identity, but the lack of routine data collection on these identity characteristics in routine healthcare has been problematic for the culture of inclusivity and has hampered research efforts [38].

As seen in the examples above, continued anti-LGBT sentiment pervades some military and veteran communities. The dominant group (White, heterosexual, cisgender servicemen) perceive minoritized groups to be more accepted than people in those groups perceive themselves [39]. The therapist from the above example can consider specifically emphasizing the importance of safety for marginalized populations when they facilitate future PTSD support groups. Setting ground rules at the start of a new group leads with an expectation of inclusive, unbiased, non-violent language among participants, and makes it easier to intervene when problems arise (e.g., referencing those "ground rules"). The therapist should always intervene when biased, violent language is used, inviting the members to reflect on the purpose of the group, and recommit to a cohesive environment [40]. For example, another approach could be for the therapist to step in immediately following a member's homophobic and violent comment with the following: "We need to take a pause. Comments about harming other people based on their sexual orientation, for example, won't be tolerated in this group. This is a therapeutic environment, and a purpose of this group is to form a supportive, cohesive bond with one another. Does anyone have any concerns with that?" This boundary may need to be set several times in different ways. Medical providers working with military personnel or veterans can have a significant impact on hastening the movement of social norms to match inclusive policy.

Rachel is a 25-year-old White transgender Active Duty servicewoman diagnosed with gender dysphoria by a military psychiatrist in 2017. With her primary care provider, the support of her therapist, and unit Commander, she developed a plan for transition that included initiating hormone treatment and upon completion of her transition, a change in her gender marker in the Defense Enrollment Eligibility Reporting System (DEERS), the official database of Service members. As she was approaching 9 months of hormone therapy, she completed a request for gender affirming surgery, specifically vaginoplasty, through the Department of Defense's Supplemental Health Care Program in order to undergo the vaginoplasty surgery at a medical center with the appropriate expertise in the civilian sector. It is required that Service members work with their unit Commanders on timing of any surgeries to mitigate any impacts to the unit and to the Service member's career.

Over the year of gender transition, Rachel has been subjected to teasing and comments as she appears more feminine while at work. She expresses concerns to her therapist about escalation of these encounters and fears of reporting these harassing incidents due to concern that retaliation may occur.

Serving in the Military adds a layer of complexity to the process of transitioning, which can contribute to a Service member's stress if they are not properly supported. Service members currently must have a medical plan and the time required for surgical procedures and recovery must be approved by the Service Member's Commander. Additionally, if a Service member requires a type of surgery not performed within one of the Military Health System (MHS) hospitals, they must undergo an approval process to undergo the procedure at a non-MHS facility. The process of transitioning is highly individualized and some Service members do not undergo surgeries. Many will require hormone therapy, which does not interfere with military service. Rachel has chosen to undergo a surgical procedure and that is supported by her medical team. Commanders can support Service members planning surgical procedures by guiding them in their decision-making regarding timing of procedures. Comprehensive information on Commanders' duties and responsibilities are available in the 2016 "Transgender Service in the U.S. Military: An Implementation Handbook" available at https://dod.defense.gov/Portals/1/features/2016/0616_policy/DoDTGHandbook_093016.pdf

The process of transitioning can elicit reactions from others that can contribute to distress such as the harassment experienced by Rachel in the vignette above. Providing support during transition is critical to a transitioning Service member's mental health and well-being. With Rachel's permission, her medical personnel can educate Rachel's Commander and unit about gender transition as a means of preventing misinformation about people who are transgender and to avoid incidents of harassment. Per DoD guidance, transgender Service members must be protected from anti-transgender discrimination in the workplace [25]. It is incumbent upon the Commander to ensure that Rachel is treated with dignity and respect, that Rachel's privacy is respected and that her colleagues' personal beliefs regarding transgender issues will not lead to a lack of respect and mistreatment. As the leader, the Commander needs to clearly communicate that treating each other with respect is the upmost priority and that Service members who disrespect others will be held accountable. The transgender member, Commander, and medical provider can work together to determine the best course of action to ensure an inclusive climate. This may consist of monthly check ins between the three individuals to ensure the transgender member is accessing needed care, to navigate any logistical challenges, and to get a pulse on the unit climate. If interested in additional resources, Commanders are encouraged to contact the Equal Opportunity office of their respective branch.

Considering transgender military service, a study conducted from 2017 to 2018 found the highest rates of support for open transgender service were among LGBT Service members [41]. Cisgender heterosexual women and Black and Hispanic Service members were found to be significantly more likely to support open transgender service when compared to cisgender heterosexual men, and White Service members, respectively [41]. Overall, 82% of cisgender LGB, and 57% of cisgender heterosexual personnel supported open transgender service [41].

Diagnostic and Treatment Considerations with the LGBT Patient Population

LGBT military personnel and veterans have reported that they expect discrimination when seeking care [13, 31, 37, 42–44]. Thus, the long history of LGBT people being discriminated against, even in health care settings, is important to consider. This includes psychological diagnoses associated with marginalized sexual and gender identities. For example, the American Psychiatric Association (APA) removed the diagnosis of Homosexuality from the Diagnostic and Statistical Manual of Mental Disorders in 1973, but Gender Dysphoria remains in the most recent edition [45] and 'high-risk homosexual behavior' is coded in the ICD system [46]. Currently, the consensus among major medical bodies such as the American Medical Association, American Psychiatric Association, American Psychological Association, and American Academy of Pediatrics is one that rejects historical positions pathologizing minoritized sexual and gender identities, and now advocates for LGBT-affirming policies and healthcare, respecting one's right to self-knowledge and self-identification [47–50]. This affirming stance is based on data that anti-LGBT societal messaging, targeted violence against minoritized people, internalization of anti-LGBT sentiment, and lack of protective factors lead to poorer health among LGBT people [7, 51].

Assessment

Assessment of a patient's sexual orientation and gender identity should be routine. Unfortunately, VHA and DoD electronic health records do not currently gather sexual orientation and gender identity as routine demographic variables. To provide LGBT-inclusive intake forms, consider the following approach.

What is your current gender identity? (Check all that apply)

- ❐ Man
- ❐ Woman
- ❐ Transgender man
- ❐ Transgender woman
- ❐ Genderqueer/gender diverse/nonbinary
- ❐ Different identity e.g., transsexual, two-spirit, bigender, etc., (please state): _______
- ❐ Prefer to not say

What is your current sexual orientation? (Check all that apply)

- ❐ Straight/Heterosexual
- ❐ Gay or Lesbian
- ❐ Bisexual
- ❐ Queer/Pansexual

❐ Other sexual orientation (please state): _____________
❐ Prefer to not say

As a healthcare provider, also be aware that knowing a person's sexual orientation, doesn't give you information about their sexual behavior. If that is relevant in your setting, then asking questions about identity and sexual activity can include a question such as:

Routine assessment of sexual functioning is important in healthcare. To better take care of you, can you tell me who you have sex with? (Check all that apply)

❐ Men
❐ Women
❐ Transgender and gender diverse people
❐ Other (please state): _____________________
❐ Prefer to not say

Treatment

All high-quality care is person centric. It is important to use language that the person feels comfortable with and that they feel understood in care. All people have various aspects of themselves that are key to how they understand themselves and their role in the world. Consider how the intersecting identities of having a LGBT identity and also being a Service member or veteran might be important (or not) to the person you are treating. Are there also other important aspects of their identity that require cultural humility by you as a provider, including being from a different race, ethnicity, or religious belief? Understanding the complexities of these various intersecting identities will help you provide culturally competent care.

VA-Specific Policies and Care Options

Once Service members leave the Armed Forces and become a veteran, they have options about where they receive their ongoing healthcare. The majority (about 70%) of military veterans get their healthcare coverage outside VHA, typically through employer-based health care plans. However, for about nine million veterans, VHA is the source for their healthcare, and it is estimated that at least 250,000 VHA patients are LGBT veterans [52, 53]. While VHA does not routinely gather data on sexual orientation and gender identity, this figure is based on a predicted one million veterans with LGBT identities in the US and current rates of VHA utilization. Thus, VHA is likely the largest provider of LGBT care in the U.S.

For veterans, it is important to understand the policies and ways in which VHA addresses the needs of veterans with LGBT and related identities, especially since VHA policies differ from DoD. First, it is important to recognize that VHA never had a "Don't Ask, Don't Tell" policy. Despite being welcome to seek care, many veterans were not aware that policies were different at VHA from DoD. At the time of this writing, VHA has Directives for the provision of care to veterans with lesbian, gay and bisexual identities and for veterans with transgender and intersex identities [54, 55]. These policies guarantee access to a healthcare environment that is affirming of the veteran's identity and prohibits attempts at changing or converting identities.

Sam is a 73-year-old African American gay identified cisgender veteran who served in the Marines under 'Don't Ask, Don't Tell' and receives a service-connected disability check every month from the VA for a back injury he sustained during his military service. Sam watched friends be discharged from the military for their LGBT identities and hears stories in the news and from other people about discrimination against LGBT people in healthcare settings. He has never talked about his sexual orientation with a medical provider for fear that he will lose his disability check and/or access to medical treatment.

Sam's life-partner of 30 years Bill died last year from colon cancer. Sam has been grieving and is increasingly depressed, so he asks if he can see a therapist for depression. The therapist begins by asking Sam questions, including about his current symptoms, recent stressors, and about several aspects of his identity including racial identification and sexual orientation. Sam is uncomfortable and says "maybe therapy isn't for me, you are asking too many personal questions that I am just not comfortable answering." The therapist validates that Sam's reaction is common and says "It's important that you know that anything you say is confidential. I am only allowed to break that rule if you are thinking of killing yourself or someone else, or if you tell me about child or elder abuse. I am required to report those things. But everything else says between us." Sam asks if VBA will learn of what he shares in therapy because he is dependent on his disability payments. After some discussion, the therapist learns of Sam's fears of being "outed" as a gay man and that his benefits will be taken away. The therapist assures Sam that coming out about his sexual orientation is entirely up to him beyond the walls of the therapy room and that VA benefits cannot be taken away due to his identity. They agree that the therapist will not document his sexual orientation in the chart notes and will reference Bill's death only as "death of a spouse". Sam is relieved and is able to open up in therapy and process his loss. Months later, when Sam's depression has lifted and rapport established, Sam asks to shift the focus of treatment to talking about a coming out to other VA healthcare providers.

It is VHA policy that all veterans should feel welcome and valued at VHA facilities, and Directives 1340 and 1341 assist in setting these expectations [54, 55]. Moreover, the VHA's non-discrimination policy includes sexual orientation, gender identity and gender expression as protected and allows veterans to self-define who "counts" as family (VHA(b)). At every VHA hospital, a LGBT Veteran Care Coordinator is available to provide education to staff and to address any issues veterans encounter [56, 57]. A virtual course in transgender health in VHA has graduated nearly 900 providers who learned about all aspects of transgender care [58, 59]. Several online education programs help providers know about culturally competent care, including 12 brief topic-focused trainings about topics relevant to transgender and gender diverse care (now publicly available) and 8 new trainings that are in development about care for veterans with LGB and related identities [60]. In addition, any VHA provider can ask a question about a transgender veteran's treatment plan (with the veteran's consent) through their electronic medical record. An expert interdisciplinary team reviews the chart and responds with advice about next steps in the care [58, 59, 61]. Recently, it was identified that rural transgender veterans had trouble accessing voice and communication interventions because neither local community nor VHA providers had the expertise. Therefore, a program to set up virtual care with trained speech language pathologists was launched so that all transgender veterans using VHA had access to the same high-quality services. VHA is also training a new generation of providers with expertise in LGBT Health at ten VHA hospitals through LGBT Health Fellowships [62]. Through these strategies, VHA hopes to assist the healthcare system in addressing the needs of veterans with LGBT and related identities. For more information about any of these programs, policies or additional information, please visit the LGBT Health Program website [63].

Clinical Pearls

- Assessment of a patient's sexual orientation and gender identity, ideally on intake paperwork and in the clinical interview, should be routine and done with appreciation of historical discrimination.
- Clinic leaders should ensure policies, procedures, and clinical environment proactively communicate an LGBT-inclusive environment.
- Avoid over-emphasis on LGBT identity among patients for whom the presenting concern is unrelated to their sexual or gender identity. While everyone's sexuality and gender are important aspects in their life history, which we acknowledge in the overall narrative of their lives, these demographic factors may be irrelevant to the problems at hand.
- It is incumbent upon behavioral health providers to treat LGBT patients with affirming, inclusive care, especially considering the history of harm done to this population in the military environment.
- Due to minoritization of identities, LGBT service members and veterans are at heightened risk for a variety of mental health conditions. Routine assessments for trauma exposure, including intimate partner violence, depression, substance abuse and suicidal thoughts should be conducted regularly.

References

1. Davis L, Grifka A, Williams K, et al. 2016. Workplace and gender relations survey of active duty members. https://sapr.mil/public/docs/reports/FY17_Annual/FY16_Annual_Report_on_Sexual_Assault_in_the_Military_Full_Report_Part2_4.pdf. Accessed 1 Apr 2021.
2. Gates GJ. Discharges under the Don't Ask, Don't Tell policy: women and racial/ethnic minorities. The Williams Institute, UCLA School of Law; 2010a.

3. Gates GJ. Lesbian, gay, and bisexual men and women in the US military: updated estimates. The Williams Institute, UCLA School of Law; 2010b. http://williamsinstitute.law.ucla.edu/wp-content/uploads/Gates-GLBmilitaryUpdate-May-20101.pdf. Accessed 7 May 2021.
4. Meadows SO, Engel CC, Collins RL, et al. 2018. Department of Defense Health Related Behaviors Survey (HRBS) Results for the Active Component. https://www.rand.org/pubs/research_reports/RR4222.html. Accessed 7 May 2021.
5. Blosnich JR, Farmer GW, Lee JGL, et al. Health inequalities among sexual minority adults: evidence from ten US states. Am J Prev Med. 2014;46:337–49.
6. Hatzenbuehler ML. How does sexual minority stigma 'get under the skin'? A psychological mediation framework. Psychol Bull. 2009;135:707–30.
7. Meyer IH. Prejudice, social stress, and mental health in lesbian, gay, and bisexual populations: conceptual issues and research evidence. Psychol Bull. 2003;129(5):674–97.
8. Pachankis JE, Cochran SD, Mays VM. The mental health of sexual minority adults in and out of the closet: a population-based study. J Consult Clin Psychol. 2015;83(5):890–901.
9. McNamara KA, Lucas CL, Goldbach JT, et al. "You don't want to be a candidate for punishment": a qualitative analysis of LGBT service member "outness". Sexuality Res Soc Policy. 2020a;18:144–59.
10. Schuyler A, Klemmer C, Mamey M, et al. Experiences of sexual harassment, stalking, and sexual assault during military service among LGBT and non-LGBT service members. J Trauma Stress. 2020;33(3):257–66.
11. Personnel and Readiness. Repeal of 'Don't, Ask, Don't Tell.' 20 Sept 2011. http://archive.defense.gov/home/features/2010/0610_dadt/USD-PR-DADT_Repeal_Day_Memo_20Sep.pdf. Accessed 26 Apr 2021.
12. McNamara KA, Lucas CL, Goldbach JT, et al. "Even if the policy changes, the culture remains the same:" a mixed methods analysis of LGBT service members' "outness" patterns. Armed Forces Soc. 2020b.
13. Biddix JM, Fogel CI, Perry Black B. Comfort levels of active duty gay/bisexual male service members in the military healthcare system. Mil Med. 2013;178:1335–40.
14. Rerucha CM, Runser LA, Ee JS, Hersey EG. Military healthcare providers' knowledge and comfort regarding the medical care of active duty lesbian, gay, and bisexual patients. LGBT Health. 2018;5(1):86–90. https://doi.org/10.1089/lgbt.2016.0210.
15. Sherman M, Kauth M, Shipherd JC, Street R. Communication between VA providers and sexual and gender minority veterans: a pilot study. Psychol Serv. 2014a;11(2):235–42.
16. LGBT Health Link. Healthcare Bill of Rights. n.d. https://healthcarebillofrights.org/. Accessed 26 Apr 2021.
17. American Medical Association (AMA). Creating an LGBTQ-friendly practice. n.d.-a. https://www.ama-assn.org/delivering-care/population-care/creating-lgbtq-friendly-practice. Accessed 26 Apr 2021.
18. Stanford Medicine. LGBTQ Medical Education Research Group: resources. n.d. https://med.stanford.edu/lgbt/resources.html. Accessed 26 Apr 2021.
19. DoD Instruction Number 1332.14. Subject: enlisted administrative separations. 1981. https://archive.defense.gov/news/DoDI%201332%2014%20-%20REVISIONS%20032510.pdf. Accessed 26 Apr 2021.
20. Don't Ask Don't Tell, 10 U.S.C. § 654. 1993 (Repealed 2010). https://www.gpo.gov/fdsys/pkg/USCODE-2010-title10/pdf/USCODE-2010-title10-subtitleA-partII-chap37-sec654.pdf.
21. Trump DJ. [@realDonaldTrump]: "After consultation with my Generals…" 26 July 2017. https://twitter.com/realDonaldTrump/status/890193981585444864. Accessed 26 Apr 2021.
22. DTM-19-004-Directive-type Memorandum (DTM)-19-004 - Military Service by Transgender Persons and Persons with Gender Dysphoria. Office of the Deputy Secretary of Defense. 2019. https://health.mil/Reference-Center/Policies/2020/03/17/Military-Service-by-Transgender-Persons-and-Persons-with-Gender-Dysphoria. Published 2019. Accessed 06 January 2013.
23. Trump v. Karnoski. 22 Jan 2019. https://www.scotusblog.com/case-files/cases/trump-v-karnoski/. Accessed 26 Apr 2021.

24. U.S. DoD. Secretary of defense Ash Carter announces policy for transgender service members. 2016a. https://www.defense.gov/News/News-Releases/News-Release-View/Article/821675/secretary-of-defense-ash-carter-announcespolicy-for-transgender-service-members/. Accessed 26 Apr 2021.
25. White House Memo. DoD announces policy updates for transgender military service. 31 Mar 2021. https://www.defense.gov/Newsroom/Releases/Release/Article/2557220/dod-announces-policy-updates-for-transgender-military-service/. Accessed 21 Apr 2021.
26. Schvey N, Blubaugh I, Morettini A, et al. Military family physicians readiness for treating patients with gender dyphoria. JAMA Intern Med. 2017;177(5):727–9.
27. Hendricks ML, Testa RJ. A conceptual framework for clinical work with transgender and gender nonconforming clients: an adaptation of the minority stress model. Prof Psychol Res Pract. 2012;43(5):460–7.
28. Lehavot K, Simpson TL, Shipherd JC, et al. Factors associated with suicidality among a national sample of transgender veterans. Suicide Life Threat Behav. 2016a;46(5):507–24.
29. Lehavot K, Rillamas-Sun E, Weitlauf J, et al. Mortality in postmenopausal women by sexual orientation and veteran status. Gerontologist. 2016b;56 Suppl 1(1):S150–62.
30. Mark K, McNamara K, Gribble R, et al. The health and well-being of LGBTQ serving and ex-serving personnel: a narrative review. Int Rev Psychiatry. 2019;31:75–94.
31. Shipherd JC, Ruben MA, Livingston NA, et al. Treatment experiences among LGBT veterans with discrimination-based trauma exposure: a pilot study. J Trauma Dissociation. 2018a;19:461–75.
32. Shipherd JC, Darling JE, Klap RS, et al. Experiences in VHA and impact on healthcare utilization: comparisons between LGBT and non-LGBT women veteran. LGBT Health. 2018b;5(5):303–11.
33. Blosnich JR, Boyer TL, Brown GR, et al. Differences in methods of suicide death among transgender and non-transgender patients in the Veterans Health Administration, 1999-2016. Med Care. 2021;59:S31–5.
34. Boyer TL, Youk AO, Haas AP, et al. Suicide, homicide, and all-cause mortality among transgender and non-transgender patients in the Veterans Health Administration. LGBT Health. 2021;8(3):173–80.
35. Montgomery AE, Shipherd JC, Kauth MR, et al. Use of Veterans Health Administration homeless programs among transgender and non-transgender veterans experiencing self-reported housing instability. J Health Care Poor Underserved. 2020;31:909–19.
36. Holloway I, Green D, Pickering C, et al. Mental health and health risk behaviors of active duty sexual minority and transgender service members in the United States military. LGBT Health. 2021;8:152–61.
37. Ruben MA, Livingston NA, Berke DS, et al. LGBT veterans' experiences of discrimination in healthcare and their relation to health outcomes: a pilot study examining the moderating role of provider communication. Health Equity. 2019;3:480–8.
38. Government Accountability Office. VA Health Care: better data needed to assess the health outcomes of lesbian, gay, bisexual, and transgender veterans. Oct 2020. https://www.gao.gov/assets/gao-21-69.pdf. Accessed 26 Apr 2021.
39. Green D, Holloway IW, Pickering CE, et al. Group perceptions of acceptance of racial/ethnic, sexual and gender minorities in the United States military, military behavioral health, 2020.
40. Yalom I. The theory and practice of group psychotherapy. 2d ed. New York: Basic Books; 1975.
41. Dunlap S, Holloway I, Pickering C, et al. Support for transgender military service from active duty United States military personnel. Sex Res Soc Policy. 2021;18:137–43.
42. Lutwak N, Byne W, Erickson-Schroth L, et al. Transgender veterans are inadequately understood by healthcare providers. Mil Med. 2014;179:483–5.
43. Mount SD, Steelman SM, Hertlein KM. "I'm not sure I trust the system yet": lesbian service member experiences with mental health care. Military Psychol (American Psychological Association). 2015;27:115–27.
44. Sherman M, Kauth M, Ridener L, et al. An empirical investigation of challenges and recommendations for welcoming sexual and gender minority veterans into VA care. Prof Psychol Res Pract. 2014b;45:433–42.

45. American Psychiatric Association. Diagnostic and statistical manual of mental disorders. 5th ed. Washington, DC: American Psychiatric Association; 2013.
46. ICD-10-CM. Diagnosis Code: Z72.52: high risk homosexual behavior. 2021. https://icdlist.com/icd-10/Z72.52. Accessed 11 May 2021.
47. American Academy of Pediatrics (AAP). Office-based care for lesbian, gay, bisexual, transgender, and questioning youth. n.d. https://pediatrics.aappublications.org/content/132/1/198. Accessed 10 May 2021.
48. American Medical Association (AMA). Policies on lesbian, gay, bisexual, transgender & queer (LGBTQ) issues. n.d.-b. https://www.ama-assn.org/delivering-care/population-care/policies-lesbian-gay-bisexual-transgender-queer-lgbtq-issues. Accessed 10 May 2021.
49. American Psychiatric Association (APA). Position statement on issues related to sexual orientation and gender minority status. July 2020. https://www.psychiatry.org/File%20Library/About-APA/Organization-Documents-Policies/Policies/Position-Sexual-Orientation-Gender-Minority-Status.pdf. Accessed 10 May 2021.
50. American Psychological Association (APA). APA policy statements on LGBT concerns. n.d. https://www.apa.org/pi/lgbt/resources/policy. Accessed 10 May 2021.
51. Castro CA, Goldbach J. The perpetrator hypothesis: victimization involving LGBT service members. In: Roberts L, Warner C, editors. Military and veteran mental health. New York, NY: Springer; 2018.
52. Kauth MR, Shipherd JC. Transforming a system: improving patient-centered care for sexual and gender minority veterans. LGBT Health. 2016;3(3):1–3.
53. Veterans Health Administration: VHA. About VHA. n.d.-a. https://www.va.gov/health/about-vha.asp. Accessed on 10 May 2021.
54. VHA Directive 1340(2). Provision of health care for veterans who identify as lesbian, gay or bisexual. Amended 26 June 2020. https://www.va.gov/vhapublications/ViewPublication.asp?pub_ID=5438. Accessed 10 May 2021.
55. VHA Directive 1341(2). Providing Health Care for Transgender and Intersex Veterans. Amended 26 June 2020. https://www.va.gov/vhapublications/ViewPublication.asp?pub_ID=6431. Accessed 10 May 2021.
56. VA Facilities with LGBT Program Websites. n.d. https://www.patientcare.va.gov/LGBT/VAFacilities.asp. Accessed 10 May 2021.
57. Valentine SE, Shipherd JC, Smith AM, et al. Improving affirming care for sexual and gender minority veterans. Psychol Serv. 2019;18(2):205–15.
58. Shipherd JC, Kauth MR, Firek AF, et al. Interdisciplinary transgender veteran care: development of a core curriculum for VHA providers. Transgender Health. 2016a;1:54–62.
59. Shipherd JC, Kauth MR, Matza A. Nationwide interdisciplinary e-consultation on transgender care in the Veterans Health Administration. Telemed J E Health. 2016b;22(12):1008–12.
60. VHA Train. n.d. https://www.train.org/vha/welcome. Accessed 10 May 2021.
61. Kauth MR, Shipherd JC, Lindsay JA, et al. Teleconsultation and training of VHA providers on transgender care: implementation of a multisite hub system. Telemed J EHealth. 2015;21:1012–8.
62. LGBT Veteran Services. U.S. Department of Veteran Affairs. n.d. https://www.patientcare.va.gov/LGBT/LGBT_Veteran_Training.asp. Accessed 10 May 2021.
63. Patient Care Services. n.d. Veterans with lesbian, gay, bisexual and transgender (LGBT) and related identities. https://www.patientcare.va.gov/LGBT/index.asp. Accessed 10 May 2021.

Combating Military and Veteran Mental Health Provider Burnout and Enhancing Resiliency

21

Rachel M. Sullivan, Christopher H. Warner, Matthew S. Heller, and Elspeth Cameron Ritchie

Vignette

Captain S is a 31 year old U.S. Army psychiatrist who recently graduated from a military psychiatry residency training program and arrived at his first duty location with a military unit in Texas that had just deployed to Iraq. Shortly after his arrival, Captain S joined the team in Iraq for 12 months. He had not met any of the medical providers or other service members that he was deploying with and his duties would include both serving as a mental health provider to more than 20,000 service members and an advisor to the senior leaders in this area of the country.

While deployed, Captain S was routinely exposed to indirect fire and had several near-miss events where incoming mortar fire landed in close proximity to his location. Additionally, he was asked to attend all of the memorial services for the service members who were killed in action in his region.

R. M. Sullivan
Department of Psychiatry, Uniformed Services University of Health Sciences, Bethesda, MD, USA

Department of Behavioral Health, Tripler Army Medical Center, Honolulu, HI, USA
e-mail: Rachel.m.sullivan18.mil@health.mil

C. H. Warner (✉)
Department of Psychiatry, Uniformed Services University of Health Sciences, Bethesda, MD, USA

E. C. Ritchie
Department of Psychiatry, Uniformed Services University of Health Sciences, Bethesda, MD, USA

Med-Star Washington Hospital Center, Georgetown University School of Medicine, George Washington University School of Medicine, Washington, DC, USA

M. S. Heller
Walter Reed National Military Medical Center, Bethesda, MD, USA
e-mail: Matthew.s.heller4.mil@mail.mil

C. H. Warner, C. A. Castro (eds.), *Veteran and Military Mental Health*,
https://doi.org/10.1007/978-3-031-18009-5_21

One group of deaths weighed heavily upon him. One of the individuals killed was a service member who was an active patient of Captain S and who he considered removing temporarily from a mission due to worsening depressive symptoms and reports by the service member of decreased focus. Captain S had discussed this recommendation with the service member's unit leader but was swayed to not remove the service member after the leader cited how critical he was to the mission.

At the memorial service, Captain S learned that his patient was responsible for identifying possible improvised explosive devices along the road they were traveling and had not seen the device that killed all five service members. Captain S continued to wonder if the service member missed identifying the device due to his symptoms and felt responsible for the deaths of that team.

Upon return from deployment, Captain S was rapidly asked to resume full duties. The mental health department at his hospital had only three psychiatrists on the installation, including him, and he would be responsible for all of the outpatient psychiatric care for the more than 25,000 active duty service members on the installation. Due to the increasing demand, he was asked to waive his post-deployment leave.

Over the course of the next 6–12 months, he continued to see high levels of demand, worked extended hours, and suicide rates at the installation were climbing. This led to additional questions about what else the mental health team could do to support the installation. As this progressed, Captain S felt himself becoming increasingly tired, more sarcastic and frustrated about work and military service, and began questioning why he even went into medicine in the first place.

Introduction

Captain S is suffering from burnout and may also be suffering from compassion fatigue. Burnout is marked by the triad of emotional exhaustion, depersonalization, and a low sense of personal accomplishment from work; it can have significant overlap with compassion fatigue [1]. Compassion fatigue is defined as reduced empathic capacity or client interest manifested through mental and emotional reactions from exposure to the traumatizing experiences of others, and is sometimes associated with secondary traumatic stress [2]. Of note, one United States Army model suggested that burnout, secondary stress, and the provider's own primary and operational stress exposures combine to result in provider fatigue [3].

Over the past several years, national research on health care resiliency has focused on the concept of burnout, as it is a growing national public health concern due to its impact on patient safety, quality of care, and retention of health care employees. Even prior to the COVID-19 pandemic, health care clinician burnout was noted to be high, with a recent National Academy of Medicine report citing national levels of burnout in physicians and nurses ranging from 35% to 54% [1].

The pandemic and its unique demands on the medical community have only increased those levels with the most recent annual MEDSCAPE National Physician Burnout and Suicide report citing that 42% of all physicians responding indicated they had burnout (41% for psychiatrists). Even more concerning was that 13% of respondents reported considering suicide with 1% of the more than 12,000 respondents citing that they had attempted suicide [4].

The drivers for this growing public health problem are numerous and health care provider burnout is a complex problem; however, the general themes being investigated are the influences of workload demand, administrative tasks and responsibilities, the impacts of technology, effects of health care policies, decisions, and external factors on front line health care delivery [1]. These issues are at a crisis level because they influence two key aspects of health care, both the retention/continuation of personnel within the practice of medicine, and also on the quality and safety of care that is delivered.

Military and veteran mental health providers face some additional challenges in addition to the current burnout crisis, many of which are highlighted in the case of Captain S. As of this writing, the United States has been continuously at war for nearly two decades. One study noted that there were over 5000 mental health professionals within the Department of Defense, many of whom have deployed, some multiple times to employ combat and operational stress control [5].

A separate chapter in this book outlines the principles and practices involved, but of key concern for this topic is that the military's employment of deployed mental health professionals involves placing them in close proximity to front lines and increasing their personal risk of trauma exposure, as well as exposing them to high volumes of patients with recent traumatic experiences. Furthermore, many military and veteran mental health professionals have seen the increased workload, impacts of trauma, and readiness supporting requirements at their facilities which support both service members and family members. This has led to concerns that this population of mental health providers are at an increased risk for provider fatigue, secondary stress, and burnout [3].

Many early studies looking at military medical and mental health personnel focused on rates of depression and posttraumatic stress disorder. One of the initial studies, focused specifically on burnout in military mental health providers, noting that levels were comparable to those seen in civilian mental health providers [6]. However, subsequent research, which examined timeframes further along into the Global War on Terror, noted elevated levels of depression, distress, impaired functioning and work/family related stress in military medical personnel compared to other military personnel [7]. Additionally, nearly 1 in every 5 military mental health providers met all four criteria for a diagnosis of secondary traumatic stress [8].

Understanding Burnout

A 12-stage model for burnout was initially proposed by Freudenberger in the 1970s and was subsequently reduced to a 5-phase model (honeymoon, onset of stress, chronic stress, burnout, and habitual burnout) [9]. The initial honeymoon phase is marked by enthusiasm, high energy levels, a sense of a need to prove oneself, and a high level of job satisfaction. To help illustrate and understand this model, let's return to our case of CPT S. He arrived at his first duty station after completing his residency, motivated to take on new challenges and seeking to establish a strong reputation as a military psychiatrist. He was excited to participate in his first deployment and to have an oppportunity to treat patients in a unique environment.

However, CPT S did not employ any positive coping strategies: in his deployed environment he failed to obtain adequate sleep and was working at various hours day and night, with few to no days off, leading to an increase in physical, mental, and emotional exhaustion. He began to not only experience these environmental stressors but also concerns about his physical safety and some frustration with the increasing workload, unsure whether his efforts are making a difference. This increasing sense of stagnation leads to the onset of stress phase. The most common symptoms that begin to appear during this phase are the same as anyone under stress and include increasing irritability, decreasing sleep quality, headaches, decreased social activities, difficulty focusing, anxiety, and challenges in decision making.

Unfortunately for CPT S, he still has a long time to continue in his deployment when these symptoms began and had a limited number of peers in his field who were able to help reduce the workload. With increasing clinical demands coupled with increased physical exhaustion, CPT S found himself being less efficient at work and as such, his days felt longer and longer. In his initial exuberance upon arrival he established a high bar for service delivery, then struggled to maintain those levels, leading to reduced personal time and limited to no time for physical exercise. Increasing frustration coupled with the moral injury that he experienced over his decision to not remove his patient from the mission, pushed CPT S into the chronic stress phase. At this stage, he started experiencing chronic fatigue, apathy, increased procrastination, social withdrawal, and a growing sense of resentment.

CPT S completed his deployment, returning to his family feeling bitter and questioning the purpose of his work and whether he made a difference. Subsequently, he watched the majority of service members be allowed to have time off and focus on a reset of military activities, he was immediately pushed to continue to work hard due to the post-deployment mental health needs of the unit that he supported. On top of this, his hospital regularly added administrative requirements and mandatory trainings on tasks such as managing blood products that did not pertain to his work, without giving him additional time to accomplish these tasks.

By this point, CPT S focused on negative events and problems, had lost confidence in his clinical skills and abilities, was neglecting personal responsibilities with his family, and was experiencing a growing number of physical ailments from his mental and physical fatigue, including recurrent headaches and GI symptoms. His work production continued to fall and his colleagues noticed some questionable medical decision making in some of his case management. His supervisor started receiving complaints from patients and unit leaders about his behavior and attitude in various engagements. As mentioned previously, by this time, CPT S was displaying the hallmarks of burnout.

Unfortunately, CPT S did not see a way out of his situation and was becoming increasingly indifferent not only about his role as a military psychiatrist but about medicine in general. Without an effective intervention, CPT S will move into the habitual burnout phase marked by chronic sadness, fatigue, and depression. As highlighted in the CPT S case, this not only becomes problematic at work, but impacts his personal relationships, health, and overall quality of life.

While the case of CPT S highlights how burnout can develop in a military psychiatrist and emphasizes some of the unique stressors that our military mental health personnel of all disciplines face, it is by no means a condition unique to our uniformed mental health providers. The reality is that the long-term mental health demands of our military and veteran population place significant stress on all mental health personnel caring for this population, to include civilians and contract staff.

Military and veteran mental health providers are facing many of the same stressors as CPT S. They are working in settings where despite continuous efforts to increase staff and expand capabilities, there remain challenges for service members and veterans trying to access mental health services. Providers are forced to choose between rapidly accessible initial evaluation or maintaining panel sizes that allow them the opportunity to deliver evidence-based treatments in a timely manner. Additionally, patient panels with complex illness and challenging personality traits are an inherent part of work within the military and VA systems.

Individuals who serve in the military deploy, leaving their families. They then must face the challenge of reintegrating with them while still being asked to manage ever increasing workload demands. Military and veteran mental health providers are frequently subjected to military and organizational leadership and community concerns, expectations, feedback, and criticisms about issues such as suicide, substance abuse, domestic violence, homelessness, and posttraumatic stress disorder. Additionally, they must manage their military careers, including professional military education, additional military duties, non-deployment missions, fitness and training requirements, and all of the other tasks associated with wearing the uniform for which providers are rarely given protected time to accomplish.

Lastly, our providers are increasingly subjected to the same pressures of cost-effective managed care that has led to an epidemic of burnout in the civilian sector over past decades. Prior authorizations, frustrating electronic health records, increasing administrative burdens, and decreasing resources with the same or increased work demands are all factors that civilian, VA, and military medical institutions share.

Factors Impacting Provider Resiliency and Burnout

There is evidence that interventions focused on the organizational level can mitigate burnout, placing both power and responsibility in the hands of healthcare leaders [1]. However, there is no one set prescription to implement; just as each system is unique, the mitigating techniques available to healthcare leaders differ as well. This section will begin by introducing a cognitive framework for conceptualizing burnout within a complex system. Next we will review burnout factors that are supported by the emerging literature, broken down into key categories. Lastly we will review best practices for combating these factors both at the organizational and individual level.

Work System Model

A simple way to approach this complex issue is to consider the interplay between the individual, the work environment, and job expectations termed the *work system* [10]. The work system captures everything that impacts the worker's ability to approach their work in either an effective or impeded way. Examples include the work culture, the individual's own personal needs and traits, land decisions made at all levels above and below the worker.

While personal traits of employees are not modifiable by their supervisors, culture, processes, acceptable workplace behaviors, expectations, and standards are. CPT S may have traits at baseline that contribute to low personal resilience, but his work environment did not promote his well-being by denying him time off. While there were short-term benefits to having additional coverage, his supervisor's decision to keep him at work decreased his long-term efficiency and his willingness to remain in uniform once his initial commitment to the military was complete. If CPT S continues to practice in a system that prioritizes short-term benefits with minimal consideration for the long-term, then his decision to leave the service when he's finished with his obligation will be the obvious choice.

Combine this with inefficient workflows, demands from higher management that do not match the resources of the clinic, challenging patient panels, poor behavior from CPT S's co-workers that goes unchecked by supervisors, as well as a heavy administrative burden, and the path to burnout becomes clear.

Job Demands/Job Resources Model

A useful way to categorize environmental factors in the work system is using the Job Demands and Job Resources dichotomy, as outlined by the National Academy of Medicine report on clinician burnout, illustrated by the figure below [1].

Job demands	Job resources
• Workload	• Organizational culture
• Time pressure, encroachment on personal time	• Meaning in work
• Workflow, interruptions, distractions	• Values aligned with expectations and incentives
• Patient complexity and acuity	• Autonomy
• Administrative burden	• Rewards
• Moral distress	• Professional relationships
• Inadequate technology	• Work-life integration

Job Demands

Workload—Traditionally, clinicians work intense, long hours, always putting patients first. Yet burnout has not always been at the epidemic levels we see today, implying that hard work and long hours do not tell the whole story. There is ample evidence that excessive workload is associated with increased worker stress, decreased job performance, and an increase in errors and accidents. However, there is conflicting evidence regarding an excessive workload's impact on burnout [11, 12].

It's a much clearer picture when it comes to scheduling and hours worked. Data surveying 7288 U.S. physicians showed that for every extra hour worked above 51.8 h per week, the odds of burnout symptoms increase by about 2% [13]. Additionally, night call increased the risk of burnout by 3–9% for every additional night per week, and another study showed an additional 2% increase for each hour spent charting at home per week [13–17].

Time Pressure and Encroachment on Personal Time—A shifting culture from that of private practice to one of employed clinicians and managed care has reduced clinician autonomy on how to spend time in favor of an emphasis on cost savings and increasing provider demands. Budget cuts drive worsening staffing ratios on inpatient units and increase productivity expectations in outpatient clinics, leading to shorter office visits and minimal protected time for charting, returning patient calls, or administrative tasks [18]. This leads to professional tasks bleeding into personal and off-duty time. Administrators erroneously conclude that they have increased productivity without cost, when in fact the cost is absorbed by the providers themselves, who are at increased risk of staff burnout. The parent organization inherits long-term costs such as lower retention, decreased care quality, and decreased provider productivity [1].

Other unprotected and increasingly uncompensated but necessary time obligations include continuing education requirements from licensing and board certification bodies, as well as the time investment needed to keep up with an increasingly complex body of medical knowledge via reading and literature review. In addition, academic centers have not decreased their expectations of scholarly work to achieve academic advancement, yet the time allotted for these pursuits has steadily diminished. Collectively, these factors have all led to the encroachment of professional tasks into personal time for health care professionals to a much greater degree than for most other fields [19–22].

Workflow, Interruptions, and Distractions—Poorly designed workflow leads to chaotic environments and increased time pressure, making it difficult to complete simple tasks efficiently and effectively, with emotional exhaustion as the result [23]. Interruptions add to cognitive burden, delay task completion, and increase the risk of forgetting tasks [24]. Distractions, such as poorly designed electronic health records, are likely associated with burnout [25].

Patient Complexity and Acuity—The more complex and acute a provider's patient panel is, the higher the theoretical risk for burnout and secondary trauma. One study looked at patient factors in providers who treated Operation Enduring Freedom/Operation Iraqi Freedom veterans, and theorized that patient age, likelihood of patient redeployment, comorbid conditions, patient attendance issues, and elevated risk for suicide and aggression were associated with higher risk of burnout [26]. There are no available studies that evaluate whether or not treating patients with secondary gain, personality disorders, or malingering increases burnout, but anecdotal evidence suggests that these challenges may also take a toll on clinician well-being.

Administrative Burden—As captured by the [4] Burnout Report, administrative burden is one of the top concerns for clinicians. 58% of respondents chose "bureaucratic tasks" as a key factor leading to burnout [4]. These administrative tasks can be subdivided into patient-related tasks such as looking up labs, navigating a complicated electronic health record in order to search for patient data and non-patient-related tasks such as ancillary duties, required workplace trainings not related to day to day job, billing-related tasks, complex employment-related tasks such as payroll systems, etc.

Moral Distress—Moral distress or moral injury is the persistent distress that individuals may develop when they perpetrate, witness, or fail to prevent an act that transgresses their core beliefs. This topic is discuss in greater detail in another chapter in this book. For health care professionals, pressure to violate one's ethical principles can come from patients, one's clinical team, the healthcare organization, or the external environment/political climate [27, 28]. In the long term, moral distress may lead to an unstable workforce, as several studies of clinicians showed that nearly 20% of them considered leaving their jobs due to a morally distressing work environment [28, 29].

Inadequate Technology—One observational study showed that physicians spent 47.2% of their time interacting with the electronic health record, twice the time they spent with patients, while another showed that physicians spent 61% of their 11 h workday charting [18, 30]. A third study showed that users were almost 4 times more likely to report burnout with increased hours charting, and that these users attributed the increased burnout specifically to the electronic health record [31]. One of the most common criticisms of modern electronic health records is their lack of focus on facilitating high-quality patient care. Most electronic health records are designed for billing, compliance, and documentation requirements, not the clinical aspects of patient care [32].

Job Resources

Organizational Culture—An organization's culture is manifested by its decisions, to include resource allocation, devotion to staff development, and leadership behaviors. For example, having inadequate time set aside for professional development was an independent predictor for burnout in a study of 783 physicians [33]. Healthcare providers who perceive poor work climate and environment are more likely to experience burnout [34–37]. These findings were also reproduced within the Military Health System [38].

One additional factor for mental health staff not faced by other specialties is the stigma associated with the work, with increased risk of burnout for staff who report feeling stigmatized due to their chosen field [39]. To add insult to injury, the perception of stigma faced by providers who personally seek mental healthcare was also associated with increasing burnout rates [40]. While this stigma begins in society at large, organizations can perpetuate this problem through the institutional culture as well.

Conversely, a positive organizational culture is protective and leads to improved patient outcomes, staff retention, and job satisfaction, while at the same time decreasing burnout and compassion fatigue [34, 37, 41, 42]. One study of 88,605 U.S. Department of Veterans Affairs staff showed that alignment between employee values and the organization's behaviors and decisions was associated with more favorable perceptions of organizational culture, which in turn was related to employee satisfaction and improved worker engagement [43].

Meaning in Work—The meaning and purpose of clinician's work is crucial in professional satisfaction and identity, while finding meaning in one's work prevents burnout among clinicians [44, 45]. In contrast, when clinicians find dissonance between what they find meaningful and their work tasks, burnout and work stress increase significantly [46]. Physicians who report spending less than 20% of their time on meaningful work have higher rates of burnout [46].

Values Aligned with Expectations and Incentives—If an individual's values are at odds with what is expected and incentivized, burnout will result. One longitudinal survey of primary care physicians working in a large hospital system found that values dissonance, along with too high workload and decreased job control, were the largest drivers of burnout [47].

Autonomy—Autonomy is defined as the amount of freedom an individual has to control and plan work activities, along with the input he or she has in making decisions that affect work. Several studies show that physicians with perceived low levels of autonomy have significantly increased levels of burnout, independent of many possible confounding factors such as work–life integration, partner support, and current work-related stressors [23, 47, 48]. This is an increasingly challenging problem as high-level workplace standardization increases, removing decision making from local supervisors and clinicians alike.

Rewards—Clinicians experience intrinsic rewards when they perceive work as meaningful, have job control, feel mastery over challenging work, feel respected, and are able to connect with their team [49]. The extrinsic reward that seems to matter most is feeling appreciated; one study of pharmacists found that salary was not a predictor of burnout, but feeling that one's contributions were underappreciated by others doubled the odds of burnout [50]. Many studies have found no correlation between salary and burnout for medical staff, though one found that concerns about future earnings was an independent predictor of burnout among neurosurgeons [33, 51].

Professional Relationships—Good interpersonal relationships between staff and patients, colleagues, and in cross-discipline interactions are protective; while the converse is true for negative, high-conflict relationships [52, 53]. Several studies show that having positive support from colleagues decreases the risk of burnout among clinicians [54, 55]. A work system attempting to improve this might prioritize collegiality and empower front-line managers to correct any unacceptable behavior.

Work-life Integration—This is the combination of personal and professional responsibilities and activities. It is in contrast to the previously preferred term work–life balance, which inherently segregates the two and has been shown to be more cognitively draining. Lower satisfaction with work–life integration is associated with a higher risk of burnout [33, 56, 57]. When healthy work–life integration does not occur, work–home conflicts may increase and in turn increase the risk of burnout [57]. Therefore a work environment aiming to improve this factor might prioritize making time for employee's family and personal needs along with work demands.

Individual Factors

Continuing with the theoretical model of the work system, we will now consider the factors that each individual brings to the equation. Each individual has a unique makeup of traits (personality, baseline health and physical capacity), states (sleep deficit, short-term illness, acute stressors, mood), and roles (parent, spouse, caregiver, other personal demands and roles). Individuals also have varying capacity for resilience.

Traits

Personality is commonly sorted into the "Big 5" traits: openness, conscientiousness, extraversion, agreeableness, and neuroticism. Studies have found that neuroticism, perfectionism, and introversion place the individual at increased risk for burnout [58, 59]. Others have shown that other aspects of personality such as having an easygoing or receptive personality, high self-efficacy, confident decision-making, and an internal locus of control are protective against burnout [60–62].

Personality and locus of control have been theorized to influence the selection and use of coping behaviors, which then impacts overall well-being [63]. Emotion-focused coping styles, such as wishful thinking, can moderate stress to some degree but ultimately increase the risk of burnout while avoidance increases the risk of burnout as well [64]. Coping via problem-solving is correlated with a decreased risk of burnout [65]. All told, it is hypothesized that about 10% of an individual's burnout risk can be attributed to coping strategies [64, 65].

States

Stress and burnout go hand in hand, as is manifest throughout this chapter, with both acute and chronic stressors contributing to burnout. Sleep deprivation is common among medical staff, and many studies show direct correlation between fatigue and burnout [66]. Sleep deprivation also causes cognitive impairment, which is associated with increased burnout, decreased professional fulfillment, and increased self-reported clinically significant medical errors [67]. Other theoretical contributors might include short-term and chronic illnesses, as well as fluctuations in mood.

Roles

Work-related stressors can impact home life and relationships with partners and children [68, 69]). Several studies have shown that low spousal support is associated with high emotional exhaustion and therefore increased burnout risk [57, 70–72]. Many studies conclude that women are at increased risk for burnout relative to their male colleagues after adjusting for other personal and professional factors, which may also be related to traditional female roles and societal expectations [16, 19, 20, 69, 73]. According to the most recent Medscape article this disparity is large, with 51% of women endorsing burnout symptoms, compared to 36% of men [4].

For military providers, the dual agency role may also impact burnout. It has been well documented that military psychiatrists commonly confront the dilemma of "dual allegiance", in which they are bound to both meet the needs of the patient they are treating while attempting to do what is in the best interest of the mission [74]. This potential conflict might introduce moral injury when the best interests of the patient and the military do not align, are perceived by the provider.

Resilience

Resilience has no agreed upon definition in the medical literature. In general it is the ability to persevere and perhaps even grow when faced by challenges, to remain well despite stressors, and to maintain performance despite adversity. It includes the ability to self-monitor, self-regulate, and maintain an attitude that allows engagement with difficult work-related challenges. Resilience is considered a continuous, dynamic state that can be strengthened and modified to a certain degree [75]. No studies have shown that medical professionals have lower resiliency than the general population, and one might argue that they are perhaps more resilient, having self-selected for such demanding work [1].

One study found that mindfulness and improved sleep increased resilience and decreased burnout [76]. Regular sleep, exercise, protecting time with family and friends, talking about feelings and engaging in recreation or hobbies have all been associated with a lower risk of burnout and increased resilience [16, 77–79]. In general, these studies conclude that caring for one's physical well-being, improving one's social connectedness, and protecting time away from work for other areas of interest are crucial to maintaining resilience in staff.

Combating Burnout and Enhancing Resiliency

As described above, the ability to decrease burnout lies within the power of healthcare organizations and leaders. However, each organization is different, so the first challenge is to identify the factors and opportunities within each work system. The groundbreaking 2019 report on burnout from the National Academy of Medicine proposes a framework for designing a healthcare system focused on decreasing burnout amongst providers, as outlined below [1].

National Academy of Medicine Guidelines for Designing Well-Being Systems

Values, Systems Approach, and Leadership

- Align organizational structures and processes with organizational and workforce values (respect, justice, compassion, diversity of views).
- Use a systems approach to proactively improve professional well-being while supporting patient care.
- Engage and commit leadership at all organizational levels to address clinician burnout and improve professional well-being.

Work System Redesign

- Enhance the meaning and purpose of work and deliver value to patients.
- Provide adequate resources and environment (e.g., staffing, scheduling, workload, opportunities to learn, greater job control, usable technologies, adequate physical environment) to support clinicians' work.
- Design work systems that encourage and facilitate relational care (team work), collaboration, communication, and professionalism.

Implementation

- Build infrastructure for a well-being system that has adequate organizational resources, processes, and structures, continually learns and improves, and is accountable.
- Design reward systems that align with organizational and professional values to support professional well-being.
- Nurture (establish and sustain) organizational culture that supports change management, psychological safety, vulnerability, and peer support.
- Use human-centered design processes to co-design, implement, and continually improve solutions and interventions that address clinician burnout.

In addition to proposing the above guidelines, the National Academy of Medicine also set the following goals to combat burnout and enhance professional well-being:

National Academy of Medicine Goals to Enhance Well-being

1. *Create Positive Work Environments:* Transform health care work systems by creating positive work environments that prevent and reduce burnout, foster professional well-being, and support quality care.
2. *Create Positive Learning Environments:* Transform health professions education and training to optimize learning environments that prevent and reduce burnout and foster professional well-being.
3. *Reduce Administrative Burden*: Prevent and reduce the negative consequences on clinicians' professional well-being that result from laws, regulations, policies, and standards promulgated by health care policy, regulatory, and standards-setting entities, including government agencies (federal, state, and local), professional organizations, and accreditors.
4. *Enable Technology Solutions:* Optimize the use of health information technologies to support clinicians in providing high-quality patient care.
5. *Provide Support to Clinicians and Learners:* Reduce the stigma and eliminate the barriers associated with obtaining the support and services needed to prevent and alleviate burnout symptoms, facilitate recovery from burnout, and foster professional well-being among learners and practicing clinicians.
6. *Invest in Research:* Provide dedicated funding for research on clinician professional well-being.

Considering the recommendations above, imagine CPT S in a healthcare system designed with the well-being of staff in mind. Upon return from deployment, his leaders would recognize the need for him to spend time away from work to rest, recharge, and reconnect with friends and loved ones. Upon return, his clinic would be optimally staffed to allow him to work no more than 51 h per week on average, and overnight call would be minimized or eliminated. He would be encouraged to take time away from work to speak with someone about the troubling events of his deployment instead of feeling scrutinized or stigmatized for seeking help.

Workflow would be optimized to allow him to spend the majority of his time on what he finds most meaningful, while ancillary duties and administrative burdens would be minimized or assigned to support staff. The clinic's EHR would be designed for ease of data access and optimal patient care, so it would complement clinical work, not be a source of burnout and stress. A well-designed work system would allow CPT S to provide the highest quality patient care, which in turn would help his patients, help him derive meaning from his work, help him continue to gain mastery, and help him build a positive, resilient professional identity. Whenever possible, he would be given the autonomy to determine his workflow and work processes and schedule, and his leaders would ensure a positive environment where incentives and rewards were aligned with patient-centered and provider-centered values.

Role of the Psychiatrist in Addressing Burnout in a Patient

There are over 5000 mental health professionals within the Department of Defense [5] and over 50,000 medical personnel in the United States Army alone [3], as well as, countless more throughout the Military Health System and the VA. Like CPT S, they are at risk for burnout and may seek counseling and care. There are multiple psychometric scales that can be used to assess and quantify levels of burnout. One such tool is available for Military Health System and VA providers to either self-assess or complete and share with their provider through the VA's National Center for PTSD website (www.ptsd.va.gov/professional/treat/care/toolkits/provider/SelfAssessmentProQOL.asp). This particular site includes interpretation of the results and recommended actions.

Psychiatrists who are caring for providers who are experiencing burnout should consider which factors they can influence in the work system model. If they are a provider who also works within the system or has access to organizational leadership, then they may be able to impact job demands and job resources which arguably would have the broadest impact. Unfortunately, in most cases, psychiatrists will not be able to influence organizational factors and as such, must focus on the individual factors. Individually, the symptoms of depression, anxiety, grief, and stress should be addressed based on case presentation. Just as importantly, the treatment plan should look at the underlying drivers for the burnout and consider what can be done in terms of education, sleep, activity, nutrition, and mindfulness to address burnout and if necessary, occupational changes.

Role of Military/VA Graduate Medical/Health Programs

As previously noted, organizational culture and climate play an important role in the levels of burnout. Many discussions about these factors begin with a discussion of onboarding and how an individual is welcomed into the hospital or organization. Many providers in the military and VA health systems are trained internally. Nearly all of the military's uniformed medical force is trained through the military's own graduate medical education programs. The majority of civilian providers working in these federal systems completed their graduate medical education within either a VA or Military Health System facility. Graduate medical education programs are vital to maintaining the capabilities and readiness of Department of Defense and VA so that they can meet their mission requirements now and in the future.

These educational programs are charged with helping the learner create a life-long professional identity, build healthy habits to sustain a lifetime of challenging work, and learn optimal professional communication and team building skills in order to become future healthcare leaders. The importance of valuing and protecting these graduate medical education programs cannot be overstated, as they are the foundation for everything that will come later in the learner's career. A culture of inquiry and life-long learning begins during training, and can be sustained only through intrinsic motivation and ongoing systemic support.

While in theory trainees in all mental health training programs are at risk, the large majority of studies focus on physician trainees. For physicians, burnout often begins in medical school. One study of 2682 medical students showed that burnout was independently associated with self-reported unprofessional conduct to include increased cheating, plagiarism, and poor patient care, as evidenced by lying about aspects of the physical exam, and lying about tests ordered, etc. [80]. These habits, if formed early, have dire consequences for the future of any medical system graduating such learners. Residents also suffer significant levels of burnout, with evidence that this impairs knowledge acquisition. One study of 16,000 residents showed a step-wise reduction in the residents' performance on their in-service exam, correlating directly with worsening burnout symptoms [81]. Since acquiring knowledge and developing professionalism are the most important, fundamental tasks of graduate medical and health education, institutions should make every effort to avoid burnout in learners.

Students are just as sensitive to the job demands/resources model as their supervisors, and they are no less sensitive to the faults of the work system in which they train. They find spending more time on EHRs than with patients challenging, are not strangers to work-life conflicts, and do better when they are able to delegate administrative tasks [82]. Recent research reveals some additional ways to improve the learning environment and decrease burnout in physician learners. One study showed that student perception of high-quality learning environments and receiving timely feedback from supervisors decreased depressive symptoms, even in the context of long hours [83]. Students will work hard, as long as it's in the service of their education and with faculty engagement, involvement and support.

Future Directions

Burnout within the health care community is a growing public health concern and is not unique to military or veteran care. However, the unique challenges of working as a provider within the military and veteran health systems creates additional burden and may negatively impact the ability of these departments to meet their mission. There is increased emphasis within both systems to address the resiliency of their health care teams and prevent burnout, but challenges will likely remain including stigma faced by health care personnel seeking assistance. The recent COVID-19 pandemic has brought this topic to the forefront and has led to increasing novel uses of phone applications that promote self-assessment, self-care, and peer to peer support, as well as, increased organizational awareness and commitment to prevention. Future research efforts must be focused on identifying strategies and mechanisms that stabilize our medical force while maintaining high quality care and patient safety, with a significant emphasis on what changes and advances will be required within the military and veterans affairs' organizational culture.

Clinical Pearls

- Burnout can be understood using the work systems model
- Each work system is unique, with differing challenges and opportunities to combat burnout
- Leaders have the ability to change the organization to decrease burnout for all staff
- Individual Factors that contribute to burnout include traits, states, and resilience. About 10% of burnout risk can be attributed to one's coping strategies. - In most cases, psychiatrists will not be able to influence the organizational factors and as such, must focus on the individual factors.
- Treatment plans should not only address symptoms of depression, anxiety, grief, and stress but should also look at the underlying drivers for the burnout and consider what can be done in terms of education, sleep, activity, nutrition, and mindfulness to address burnout and if necessary, occupational changes.
- Compassion fatigue and stigma (both the stigma of working in the field and the stigma of seeking care) are significant risks for mental health staff, especially for those who work with patients exposed to wartime trauma.
- Graduate Medical/Health Education program effectiveness is compromised when learners suffer from burnout

References

1. National Academies of Sciences. Engineering, and medicine: taking action against clinician burnout: a systems approach to professional Well-being. Washington, DC: The National Academies Press; 2019.
2. Cieslak R, Anderson V, Bock J, Moore BA, et. al. Secondary traumatic stress among mental health providers working with the military: prevalence and its work- and exposure related correlates. J Nerv Ment Dis. 2013;201:917–25.
3. Penachek MA, Bicknell GC, Landry L. Provider fatigue and provider resiliency training. In: Ritchie EC, editor. Combat and operational behavioral health. Washington, DC: Department of the Army, Office of The Surgeon General, Borden Institute; 2011. p. 375–89.
4. Medscape. Death by 1000 Cuts: Medscape National Physician Burnout and Suicide Report 2021. 2021. https://www.medscape.com/slideshow/2021-lifestyle-burnout-6013456. Accessed on 14 June 2021.
5. Lester PB, Taylor LC, Hawkins SA, Landry L. Current directions in military health-care provider resilience. Curr Psychiatry Rep. 2015;17:6.
6. Ballenger-Browning KK, Schmitz KJ, Rothacker JA, Hammer PS, et al. Predictors of burnout among military mental health providers. Mil Med. 2011;176:253–60.
7. Hickling EJ, Gibbons S, Barnett SD, Watts D. The psychological impact of deployment on OEF/OIF healthcare providers. J Trauma Stress. 2011;24:726–34.
8. Kintzle S, Yarvis JS, Bride BE. Secondary traumatic stress in military primary and mental health care providers. Mil Med. 2013;178:1310–5.
9. De Hert S. Burnout in healthcare workers: prevalence, impact, and preventative strategies. Local Reg Anesth. 2020;13:171–83.
10. Carayon P. The balance theory and the work system model. Twenty years later. Int J Hum Comput Interact. 2009;25(5):313–27.
11. Xu J, Reale C, Slagle JM, Anders S, et al. Facilitated nurse medication-related event reporting to improve medication management quality and safety in intensive care units. Nurs Res. 2017;66(5):337–49.

12. Young MS, Brookhuis KA, Wickens CD, Hancock PA. State of science: mental workload in ergonomics. Ergonomics. 2015;58(1):1–17.
13. Dyrbye LN, Varkey P, Boone SL, Satele DV, Sloan JA, Shanafelt TD. Physician satisfaction and burnout at different career stages. Mayo Clin Proc. 2013;88(12):1358–67.
14. Dyrbye LN, Shanafelt TD, Balch CM, Satele D, et al. Relationship between work–home conflicts and burnout among American surgeons: a comparison by sex. Arch Surg. 2011;146(2):211–7.
15. Shanafelt TD, Balch CM, Bechamps GJ, Russel T, et al. Burnout and career satisfaction among American surgeons. Ann Surg. 2009;250(3):463–70.
16. Shanafelt TD, Oreskovich MR, Dyrbye LN, Satele DV, et al. Avoiding burnout: the personal health habits and wellness practices of U.S. surgeons. Ann Surg. 2012b;255(4):625–33.
17. Shanafelt TD, Gradishar WJ, Kosty M, Satele D, Chew H, Horn L, Clark B, Hanley AE, Chu Q, Pippen J, Sloan J, Raymond M. Burnout and career satisfaction among U.S. oncologists. J Clin Oncology. 2014;32(7):678–86.
18. Arndt BG, Beasley JW, Watkinson MD, Temte JL, et al. Tethered to the EHR: primary care physician workload assessment using EHR event log data and time–motion observations. Ann Fam Med. 2017;15(5):419–26.
19. Shanafelt TD, Boone S, Tan L, Dyrbye LN, et al. Burnout and satisfaction with work–life balance among U.S. physicians relative to the general U.S. population. Arch Intern Med. 2012a;172(18):1377–85.
20. Shanafelt TD, Hasan O, Dyrbye LN, Sinsky C, et al. Changes in burnout and satisfaction with work–life balance in physicians and the general U.S. working population between 2011 and 2014. Mayo Clin Proc. 2015;90(12):1600–13.
21. Shanafelt TD, Sinsky DC, Dyrbye LN, Trockel M, West CP. Burnout among physicians compared with individuals with a professional or doctoral degree in a field outside of medicine. Mayo Clin Proc. 2019a;94(3):549–51.
22. Shanafelt TD, West CP, Sinsky C, Trockel M, et al. Changes in burnout and satisfaction with work–life integration in physicians and the general U.S. working population between 2011 and 2017. Mayo Clin Proc. 2019b;94(9):1681–94.
23. Linzer M, Manwell LB, Williams ES, Bobula JA, et al. Working conditions in primary care: physician reactions and care quality. Ann Intern Med. 2009;151(1):28–36.
24. Grundgeiger T, Sanderson P, MacDougall HG, Venkatesh B. Interruption management in the intensive care unit: predicting resumption times and assessing distributed support. J Exp Psychol Appl. 2010;16(4):317–34.
25. Gregory ME, Russo E, Singh H. Electronic health record alert-related workload as a predictor of burnout in primary care providers. Appl Clin Inform. 2017;8(3):686–97.
26. Horrell SC, Holohan DR, Didion LM, Vance GT. Treating traumatized OEF/OIF veterans: how does trauma treatment affect the clinician? Prof Psychol Res Pract. 2011;42(1):79–86.
27. Burston AS, Tuckett AG. Moral distress in nursing: contributing factors, outcomes and interventions. Nurs Ethics. 2013;20(3):312–24.
28. Dodek PM, Wong H, Norena M, Ayas N, et al. Moral distress in intensive care unit professionals is associated with profession, age, and years of experience. J Crit Care. 2016;31(1):178–82.
29. Whitehead PB, Herbertson RK, Hamric AB, Epstein EG, Fisher JM. Moral distress among healthcare professionals: report of an institution-wide survey. J Nurs Scholarsh. 2015;47(2):117–25.
30. Sinsky C, Colligan L, Li L, Prgomet M, et al. Allocation of physician time in ambulatory practice: a time and motion study in 4 specialties. Ann Intern Med. 2016;165(11):753–60.
31. Robertson SL, Robinson MD, Reid A. Electronic health record effects on work–life balance and burnout within the I3 population collaborative. J Grad Med Educ. 2017;9(4):479–84.
32. Downing NL, Bates DW, Longhurst CA. Physician burnout in the electronic health record era: are we ignoring the real cause? Ann Intern Med. 2018;169(1):50–1.
33. McAbee JH, Ragel BT, McCartney S, Jones GM, et al. Factors associated with career satisfaction and burnout among U.S. neurosurgeons: results of a nationwide survey. J Neurosurg. 2015;123(1):161–73.

34. Aiken LH, Sermeus W, Van Den Heede K, Sloane DM, et al. Patient safety, satisfaction, and quality of hospital care: cross sectional surveys of nurses and patients in 12 countries in Europe and the United States. BMJ. 2012;344(7851):e1717.
35. Green AE, Albanese BJ, Shapiro NM, Aarons GA. The roles of individual and organizational factors in burnout among community-based mental health service providers. Psychol Serv. 2014;11(1):41–9.
36. Hanrahan NP, Aiken LH, McClaine L, Hanlon AL. Relationship between psychiatric nurse work environments and nurse burnout in acute care general hospitals. Issues Ment Health Nurs. 2010;31(3):198–207.
37. McHugh MD, Ma C. Wage, work environment, and staffing: effects on nurse outcomes. Policy Polit Nurs Pract. 2014;15:72–80.
38. Patrician PA, Shang J, Lake ET. Organizational determinants of work outcomes and quality care ratings among Army medical department registered nurses. Res Nurs Health. 2010;33(2):99–110.
39. Rössler W. Stress, burnout, and job dissatisfaction in mental health workers. Eur Arch Psychiatry Clin Neurosci. 2012;262(Suppl 2):S65–9.
40. Mitake T, Iwasaki S, Deguchi Y, Nitta T, et al. Relationship between burnout and mental-illness-related stigma among nonprofessional occupational mental health staff. Biomed Res Int. 2019;2019:5921703.
41. Lake ET, Sanders J, Duan R, Riman KA, et al. A metaanalysis of the associations between the nurse work environment in hospitals and 4 sets of outcomes. Med Care. 2019;57(5):353–61.
42. Wei H, Sewell K, Wood G, Rose M. The state of the science of nurse work environments in the United States: a systematic review. Int J Nurs Sci. 2018;5:287–300.
43. Foglia MB, Cohen JH, Pearlman RA, Bottrell MM, Fox E. Perceptions of ethical leadership and the ethical environment and culture: integrated ethics TM staff survey data from the VA health care system. AJOB Prim Res. 2013;4(1):44–58.
44. Ben-Itzhak SJ, Dvash MM, Rosenberg N, Halpern P. Sense of meaning as a predictor of burnout in emergency physicians in Israel: a national survey. Clin Exp Emerg Med. 2015;2(4):217–25.
45. Tak HJ, Curlin FA, Yoon JD. Association of intrinsic motivating factors and markers of physician well-being: a national physician survey. J Gen Intern Med. 2017;32(7):739–46.
46. Shanafelt TD. Enhancing meaning in work: a prescription for preventing physician burnout and promoting patient-centered care. JAMA. 2009;302(12):1338–40.
47. Gregory ST, Menser T. Burnout among primary care physicians: a test of the areas of worklife model. J Healthc Manag. 2015;60(2):133–48.
48. Campbell DA, Sonnad S, Eckhauser FE, Campbell K, Greenfield LJ. Burnout among American surgeons. Surgery. 2001;130:696–705.
49. Deci EL, Ryan RM. Intrinsic motivation and self-determination in human behavior. New York: Plenum Press; 1985.
50. Jones G, Roe N, Louden L, Tubbs C. Factors associated with burnout among US Hospital clinical pharmacy practitioners: results of a Nationwide pilot survey. Hosp Pharm. 2017;52(11):742–51.
51. Keeton K, Fenner DE, Johnson TR, Hayward RA. Predictors of physician career satisfaction, work–life balance, and burnout. Obstet Gynecol. 2007;109(4):949–55.
52. Embriaco N, Azoulay E, Barrau K, Kentish N, et al. High level of burnout in intensivists: prevalence and associated factors. Am J Respir Crit Care Med. 2007a;175(7):686–92.
53. Embriaco N, Papazian L, Kentish-Barnes N, Pchard F, Azoulay E. Burnout syndrome among critical care healthcare workers. Curr Opin Crit Care. 2007b;13(5):482–8.
54. Adriaenssens JV, De Gucht V, Maes S. Determinants and prevalence of burnout in emergency nurses: a systematic review of 25 years of research. Int J Nurs Stud. 2015;52(2):649–61.
55. Hyman SA, Shotwell MS, Michaels DR, Han X, et al. A survey evaluating burnout, health status, depression, reported alcohol and substance use, and social support of anesthesiologists. Anesth Analg. 2017;125(6):2009–18.
56. Anandarajah AP, Quill TE, Privitera MR. Adopting the quadruple aim: the University of Rochester Medical Center experience: moving from physician burnout to physician resilience. Am J Med. 2018;131(8):979–86.

57. Oskrochi YM, Maruthappu M, Henriksson M, Davis AH, Shalhoub J. Beyond the body: a systematic review of the nonphysical effects of a surgical career. Surgery. 2016;159(2):650–64.
58. McManus IC, Keeling CA, Paice E. Stress, burnout and doctors' attitudes to work are determined by personality and learning style: a twelve-year longitudinal study of UK medical graduates. BMC Med. 2004;2:29.
59. Shimizutani M, Odagiri Y, Ohya Y, Shimomitsu T, et al. Relationship of nurse burnout with personality characteristics and coping behaviors. Ind Health. 2008;46(4):326–35.
60. Fida R, Lasching HKS, Leiter MP. The protective role of self-efficacy against workplace incivility and burnout in nursing: a time-lagged study. Health Care Manag Rev. 2018;43(1):21–9.
61. Moreno-Jiménez B, Rodríguez-Carvajal R, Hernández EG, Benadero MEM. Terminal versus non-terminal care in physician burnout: the role of decision-making processes and attitudes to death. Salud Mental. 2008;31(2):93–101.
62. Partlak Günüşen N, Ustün B, Erdem S. Work stress and emotional exhaustion in nurses: the mediating role of internal locus of control. Res Theory Nurs Pract. 2014;28(3):260–8.
63. Haybatollahi M, Gyekye SA. The moderating effects of locus of control and job level on the relationship between workload and coping behaviour among Finnish nurses. J Nurs Manag. 2014;22(6):811–21.
64. Pejuskovic B, Lecic-Tosevski D, Priebe S, Toskovic O. Burnout syndrome among physicians—the role of personality dimensions and coping strategies. Psychiatr Danub. 2011;23(4):389–95.
65. Payne N. Occupational stressors and coping as determinants of burnout in female hospice nurses. J Adv Nurs. 2001;33(3):396–405.
66. Stewart NH, Arora VM. The impact of sleep and circadian disorders on physician burnout. Chest. 2019;156(5):1022–30.
67. Trockel MT, Menon NK, Rowe SG, Stewart MT, et al. Assessment of physician sleep and wellness, burnout, and clinically significant medical errors. JAMA Netw Open. 2020;3(12):e2028111.
68. Shanafelt TD, Boone SL, Dyrbye LN, et al. The medical marriage: a national survey of the spouses/partners of US physicians. Mayo Clin Proc. 2013;88(3):216–25. https://doi.org/10.1016/j.mayocp.2012.11.021.
69. Shanafelt TD, Hasan O, Hayes S, Sinsky CA, et al. Parental satisfaction of U.S. physicians: associated factors and comparison with the general U.S. working population. BMC Med Educ. 2016;16(1):228.
70. Gabbe SG, Melville J, Mandel L, and Walker E. Burnout in chairs of obstetrics and gynecology: Diagnosis, treatment, and prevention. American Journal of Obstetrics and Gynecology. 2002;186(4):601–12.
71. Golub JS, Johns MM 3rd, Weiss PS, Ramesh AK, Ossoff RH. Burnout in academic faculty of otolaryngology-head and neck surgery. Laryngoscope. 2008;118(11):1951–6. https://doi.org/10.1097/MLG.0b013e31818226e9. PMID: 18797419.
72. Johns MM, 3rd, and Ossoff RH. Burnout in academic chairs of otolaryngology: Head and neck surgery. Laryngoscope. 2005;115(11):2056–61.
73. Templeton K, Bernstein C, Sukhera J, Nora LM, et al. Gender-based differences in burnout: issues faced by women physicians. NAM Perspectives. Discussion Paper, National Academy of Medicine, Washington, DC, 2019.
74. Strous RD. Ethical considerations during times of conflict: challenges and pitfalls for the psychiatrist. Isr J Psychiatry Relat Sci. 2013;50(2):122–9.
75. Howe A, Smajdor A, Stocki A. Towards an understanding of resilience and its relevance to medical training. Med Educ. 2012;46(4):349–56.
76. Kemper KJ, Mo X, Khayat R. Are mindfulness and self-compassion associated with sleep and resilience in health professionals? J Altern Complement Med. 2015;21(8):496–503.
77. Balayssac D, Pereira B, Virot J, Collin A, et al. Burnout, associated comorbidities, and coping strategies in French community pharmacies–BOP study: a nationwide cross-sectional study. PLoS One. 2017;12(8):e0182956.

78. Sargent MC, Sotile W, Sotile MO, Rubash H, Barrack RL. Stress and coping among orthopaedic surgery residents and faculty. J Bone Joint Surg Am. 2004;86A(7):1579–86.
79. Shanafelt TD, Novotny P, Johnson ME, Zhao X, et al. The well-being and personal wellness promotion strategies of medical oncologists in the North Central Cancer Treatment Group. Oncology. 2005;68(1):23–32.
80. Dyrbye LN, Massie FS, Eacker A, et al. Relationship between burnout and professional conduct and attitudes among US medical students. JAMA. 2010;304(11):1173–80.
81. West CP, Shanafelt TD, Kolars JC. Quality of life, burnout, educational debt, and medical knowledge among internal medicine residents. JAMA. 2011;306(9):952–60.
82. Salzberg L. Physician well-being: improving office efficiency. FP Essent. 2018;471:16–9.
83. Pereira-Lima K, Gupta RR, Guille C, Sen S. Residency program factors associated with depressive symptoms in internal medicine interns: a prospective cohort study. Acad Med. 2019;94(6):869–75.

Part IV

Veteran and Military Families

Effects of Deployment on Military-Connected Children, Spouses, and Families

22

Kathrine S. Sullivan and Jessica Dodge

Introduction

While many aspects of military life can introduce stress into family systems, deployments are often described by military families as the most stressful [1]. Since the start of the Global War on Terror in 2001, over 2.7 million service members have experienced more than 3.3 million wartime deployments [2, 3]. The impact of deployment on service members has been extensively researched; these may include physical injuries, mental health symptomatology, substance use, and suicidality, problems which may be exacerbated by barriers to seeking treatment [4–7]. A smaller but growing body of evidence explores the impact that deployments have on the spouses, children, and families of service members [8–11]. As of 2017, 49.4% of service members are married and 39.5% have children [12]. Findings from empirical research with this population suggest that the majority of families weather the stressors of deployment successfully, but a subset of families may be struggling and at risk of adverse outcomes [13, 14].

Deployment is often described in the literature as a cyclical process rather than a discrete event, including 5 phases: (1) predeployment, (2) deployment, (3) sustainment, (4) redeployment, and (5) postdeployment or reintegration [15, 16]. A family's exposure to risk and access to protective factors are theorized to vary across this cycle. Though this perspective is often referenced when describing the impact of deployment on families, it is important to note that high operational tempo and other

K. S. Sullivan (✉)
Silver School of Social Work, New York University, New York, NY, USA
e-mail: kate.sullivan@nyu.edu

J. Dodge
Health Services Research and Development, Center for Clinical Management Research; Ann Arbor Veterans Affairs Hospital, Ann Arbor, MI, USA
e-mail: Jessica.Dodge@va.gov

C. H. Warner, C. A. Castro (eds.), *Veteran and Military Mental Health*,
https://doi.org/10.1007/978-3-031-18009-5_22

unique elements of recent conflicts have sped up and compounded this cycle. Among those who have deployed in service of the Global War on Terror, 43% did so multiple times [17]. Further, changes in technology have dramatically impacted how families experience the deployment cycle. More frequent communication between service members and their families during deployments may attenuate some of the stressors associated with separation but may also introduce new stressors as both service members and their families are more aware of the other's experiences [18, 19].

As the body of literature on this topic has grown significantly, an adequate treatment requires some specifications about scope. This chapter will describe the impact of deployment experiences on military-connected spouses, children, and families; this impact is considered distinct from the potential effects experienced during the reintegration period following deployment. While these are undoubtedly intertwined, deployment is time bound while reintegration is a subjective experience that can vary significantly in length depending on the adaptive capacities of the service member and their family [9]. Further, this chapter is written for civilian providers. While many military families receive health and mental health care from military providers, approximately 50% of military-connected families may receive some care from civilians [20, 21]. Services shift toward civilian providers particularly during deployments [22], and these providers may be less aware of the unique needs of this population. In order to explore the interrelated concepts discussed, a composite clinical case will be introduced below. Elements of this case will be presented throughout the chapter to amplify key points and illustrate the impact of treatment on outcomes described.

Vignette

The Fisher Family is a family of 5 (father-John (50), mother-Leslie (48), son-Byron (28), son-James (25), daughter-Jane (21)). They presented at a free family-based care clinic for service members/veterans and their families to process the loss of their eldest son, Byron (28), who died from an overdose of prescription medication. The 4 surviving members of the family came with the intention to process their grief together. The family participated in a 6-week resiliency-building family intervention that was designed as a preventative treatment for military families. While the primary reason for the visit was to process the loss of their son, unprocessed events and emotions that arose during John's military service emerged as treatment unfolded. The parents' goals for treatment were to gain coping skills to manage their recent loss. The children's goals were to develop communication skills to connect with each other and express how they were feeling.

Risk and Resilience Framework

The stress of deployment is not experienced in a vacuum but rather against a backdrop of other demands and in the context of the family's resources. This chapter employs a risk and resilience framework (see Fig. 22.1) to discuss the impact of

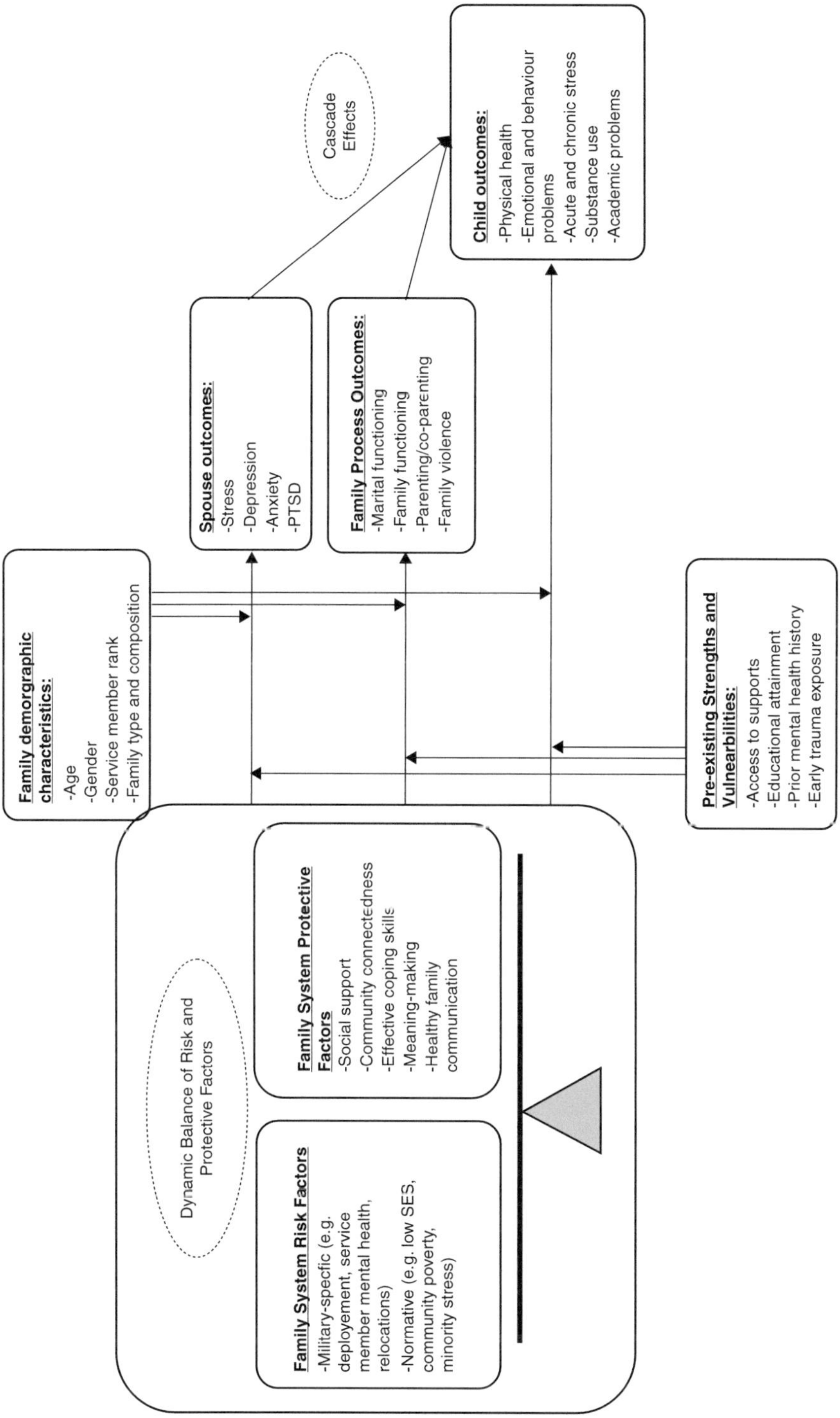

Fig. 22.1 Risk and resilience framework

deployment, in which resilience is defined as the dynamic balance between family-level risk and protective factors that determine whether a family is able to maintain or return to a previous level of functioning in the face of adversity [23–25].

Risk Factors

The deployment cycle is hypothesized to introduce risk, which may be exacerbated by a family's pre-existing vulnerabilities and counter-balanced by a family's internal and external resources. Risk factors may be military-specific or normative, referring to elements experienced by military and civilian families alike [26]. Beyond deployment, other relevant military-specific stressors could include the mental health of service members (discussed further below), experiences of relocation, un/underemployment of military spouses, and foreign postings [27–29]. Deployment itself can be experienced as an acute or a chronic stressor, represented as the number of prior deployments, cumulative days of deployment, or the percentage of a family's life that a service member has been deployed [9, 30–34]. Further, the timing of deployments in the family life cycle may compound risk. For example, deployments that coincide with a spouse's pregnancy can have negative outcomes that could influence the prenatal environment and have consequences for children in these families at birth [35]. Research has shown that deployment stressors are associated with elevated depression scores during pregnancy and in the post-partum period [36]. Normative stressors may include lower socioeconomic status [26, 37] and minority stress [38].

The case of the Fisher Family, they experienced both normative and military-specific risk factors that contributed to their clinical presentation. Their most pressing concern was the recent loss of their son, an experience which can impact military and civilian families alike. This normative stressor was experienced alongside several military-specific stressors. John served 20 years as a Marine and completed 4 combat deployments. During his combat tours, he witnessed the death of several close friends and took lives of the enemy. The family described how hard it was to live with John once he returned home. John's lack of communication, anger outbursts, and militant daily routines created conflict, but the family learned to cope through avoidance.

Protective Factors

Protective factors that counteract risk may be critical to understanding why many families successfully navigate the challenges that deployment presents [34, 39]. All military families possess a set of strengths that not all families in the general population possess. By definition these families have at least one employed parent with at least a high school education or equivalent, favorable pay and benefits, and access to high quality health and child care [40–42]. Beyond these factors, access to formal and informal sources of social support [30, 43–46], feeling connected to one's community [45, 47], effective coping mechanisms [48], the capacity to make meaning out of challenges [49, 50], and healthy family communication [33, 51] have all been shown to protect against adverse outcomes in this population.

In the example of the Fisher Family, Leslie and the children reported they coped well during John's deployments because they always lived close to family or had family visit regularly, which was an important source of social support. Further, there was a strong sense of love and commitment among the family that motivated each member to be open to different communication styles as well as to making collective meaning from their experiences. The family also had access to critical resources as a result of their military status. For example, John had a college degree that was paid for through his service, which contributed to the family's comfortable standard of living, and health insurance, which offered the possibility of seeking mental health services, though John was reluctant to pursue this option at the outset of family treatment.

Pre-existing Strengths and Vulnerabilities

A family's strengths and vulnerabilities that predate military service (e.g. educational attainment, pre-existing mental health problems, or prior traumatic experiences; [52]) may exacerbate or attenuate the relationship between this balance of risk and protective factors and the family's outcomes [26, 53, 54]. In some studies, for example, deployment experiences alone are not a significant predictor of adverse outcomes when considered alongside other stressors like parent mental health and community poverty [26].

The Fishers' extended family was a significant source of strength, which predated John's military service. Leslie reported that she never questioned whether their family would be there for her and the children during John's deployments, a sense of confidence that allowed her to access this critical source of social support during difficult times. Further, John shared that he had always experienced difficulty managing strong emotions, even during his childhood. Leslie observed that her husband's tendency toward isolation and occasional volatility was only exacerbated by combat exposure. She worried that he did not have the temperament to manage these experiences.

Outcomes Associated with Deployment

Experiences of deployment, considered in the context of the family's cumulative exposure to risk and protective factors, have been found to influence outcomes for military-connected spouses, children and families. The majority of these findings have suggested that deployment can have adverse consequences for a subset of military-connected family members. While there are potential stressors present at all stages of the deployment cycle, the most significant changes for spouses, children and families have been observed during deployment separations [33, 55].

Positive Outcomes

Though not regularly measured in quantitative studies, qualitative work suggests some positive outcomes from deployment. Adolescents in military families discuss opportunities for growth and development that arise particularly around the increased responsibilities they take on during the deployment of a parent [56]. Some military spouses express a sense of pride in the leadership role they play while their spouse is deployed [25]. Perhaps because they are physically distant from day-to-day stressors, recent findings suggest that service members have more positive views of their parenting and marital relationships during deployments [33]. Though these relationships have yet to be examined quantitatively, it is possible that positive outcomes associated with deployment are facilitated in families with greater access to resources.

Spouse Adverse Outcomes

The spouses of deploying or deployed service members may experience adverse outcomes across the deployment cycle. Rates of depression among some spouses appear to increase prior to deployment separations [57]. While service members are deployed, spouses may exhibit increased depression, anxiety, PTSD, or global distress [31, 33, 58]. Using health care records, an increased prevalence of diagnosed depression, anxiety disorders, sleep disorders, adjustment disorders and acute stress reactions were observed among spouses with a deployed service member [59]. Longitudinal explorations suggest that spouses' depression symptoms increase linearly during a deployment but level off and begin to return to pre-deployment levels as reunion with the deployed service member approaches [55].

A number of factors may impact these adverse outcomes. Perceived stress appears to be an important proximal factor, which may increase among spouses of deployed services members and is associated with increases in somatization and poorer physical and mental health [57, 60, 61]. Treatment seeking and stigma are also important considerations. Compared to spouses of non-deployed service members, experiencing a deployment is associated with increases in psychiatric service use and decreases in primary health care visits, implying less use of preventive care [22]. Despite this uptick in psychiatric care, several studies have identified low rates of treatment seeking compared to estimates of need in this population. In one sample, in which 79% of service members were deployed, only 41% of spouses screening positive for a mental health diagnosis actually sought specialty mental health treatment, citing logistical barriers like access to child care, difficulty getting an appointment, and concerns about stigma as barriers [58]. Spouses also report that concerns about harm that could come to their partner's career are a barrier to seeking treatment [57].

At the outset of treatment for the Fisher family, both John and Leslie presented with elevated symptoms of PTSD and depression. John wore sunglasses for the first two sessions to hide his grief. Leslie cried through most of the beginning sessions. John described feeling distant from his family and reported he did not know how to reconnect. John's isolation created significant stress for Leslie as she felt like the mediator between her husband and children, reporting that she never knew what was going to set John off. Leslie encouraged John to seek individual mental health treatment prior to pursuing family services. John complied and went to a nearby VA medical center but had such a bad experience getting an appointment that he vowed to never seek treatment again. John was easily upset when individual treatment was brought up in family sessions, but was compliant with family treatment because he did not want the tragic loss of his son to cause additional harm to his family.

Over the course of the family intervention, John was able to listen to his family's concern and was open to additional treatment at a local VA medical center. Additionally, the children expressed concern for their mother's overall mental health. Leslie regularly vocalized to her daughter how the disconnect between her children and husband made her sad. She cried frequently and expressed feelings of hopelessness about interactions with her husband on his bad days. Leslie was referred to an individual therapist through a veteran family support organization. Both John and Leslie were in individual treatment at their 10-month follow-up appointment and reported lower depression and post-traumatic stress symptoms.

Family Adverse Outcomes

Marital Functioning Conclusions about the impact of deployment on the health and stability of marital relationships has been mixed. In the context of the Global War on Terror, some findings suggest deployment does not impact relationship functioning [62], while other findings suggest the opposite [63]. In families with children, greater exposure to deployment has been associated with greater marital instability [2]. Longitudinal examination of these processes suggest that couples become less satisfied with their marriages across the deployment cycle, but more frequent communication during deployments may improve this trajectory [33]. Though younger couples may be at greater risk [64], overall there is little evidence that deployment exposure alone increases risk for divorce [65]. In contrast to these mixed results, findings are consistent regarding the adverse impact of PTSD symptoms, particularly in combat-exposed service members, on relationship functioning [62, 66].

Parenting There have also been mixed findings regarding the effect of deployment on parenting. With regard to the non-deployed parent, some research suggests deployment does not affect parental sensitivity [67], while others have found that parental responsiveness declines across the deployment cycle and continues to decline at reunion [55]. Satisfaction with the parenting relationship may also decline across the deployment cycle for non-deployed parents, while deployed parents report higher parenting satisfaction [33]. With regard to the deployed parent, disruption in primary caregiving relationships as a result of deployment separation may impact parenting, as children need consistent interaction in order to view caregivers as reliable sources of support and comfort [68]. Attachment may also be impacted by the physical and mental health of the deployed parent on their return [69].

Family Functioning Limited research on family functioning also suggests mixed effects. In longitudinal findings the deployment cycle has not been associated with significant changes in the family environment [33], but cumulative deployment exposure may adversely impact multiple elements of family functioning, including affective involvement, communication, and problem solving [2]. Another way to explore family-level impact is through examination of family violence outcomes associated with deployment. Each military branch operates a Family Advocacy Program (FAP) charged with preventing, investigating and addressing child maltreatment and intimate partner violence in military families [70]. Using FAP data, studies suggest increases in rates of maltreatment during periods of higher operational tempo [71–73] and spikes in maltreatment, and particularly neglect, during deployments [71, 74, 75]. Regarding intimate partner violence (IPV), some evidence points to a decrease in psychological and physical aggression across the deployment cycle [33], while other evidence has found a relationship between a history of deployment in the last year and an increased likelihood of spousal aggression [76]. This relationship may be accounted for by the consistently demonstrated link between PTSD symptoms and IPV perpetration [77].

At the outset of treatment, members of the Fisher family were isolated from one another. Communication between John and his children was stilted, and tension was high in early sessions. Though there was a history of violence in the family, there was no indication of current violence between John and Leslie or within the family as a whole. Through treatment, John learned and practiced active and reflective listening skills. John also shared some of the hardships he went through during his military service, which he had kept to himself in an effort to protect his family. The children were appreciative of this disclosure because they felt in the dark about what their father had been through. Additionally, through treatment, each member of the family was able to learn new emotion regulation skills. Through the awareness of how emotions can affect behavior, each member was able to practice different activities to help them calm down when they felt dysregulated.

Child Adverse Outcomes

Studies have taken a number of different methodological approaches to exploring mental, emotional, or behavioral health outcomes of military-connected youth and their relationship to deployment experiences, including school-based surveys that disaggregate outcomes for military and non-military-connected children [78–80], large-scale examination of pediatric health care records [32, 81], qualitative studies [82], as well as cross-sectional [30, 31, 83] and longitudinal survey research [33, 55]. One meta-analysis [8] and several reviews [9, 11, 38, 52, 84] suggest that parental deployment adversely impacts the adjustment and psychological well-being of children, though these associations may be small. Increases in mental health service utilization parallel increases in mental health concerns among military-connected youth [33]. In children ages 3–8 who experienced a parental deployment, mental and behavioral health visits increased by 11% overall, by 19% for behavioral disorders, and by 18% for stress disorders [81]; these increases were even greater for children whose parents were injured in combat [75]. Similar results were observed among military-connected youth ages 5–17, in which an excess of diagnoses including acute stress reaction/

adjustment, depression, and behavioral disorders were observed in children who experienced deployment. During parental deployment, increases in the use of prescription antidepressant and antianxiety medications have also been observed among military connected-youth [22]. While many factors may moderate these associations, findings consistently demonstrate that longer cumulative exposure to deployment and poor functioning of the at-home parent are associated with more negative mental health outcomes for youth [9, 32, 33, 78, 85].

Other critical outcomes for military-connected youth may also be impacted by deployment experiences. Physical health symptoms, including elevated heart rate and blood pressure, may increase during deployments [86]. Suicidality and substance use may also increase among adolescents both during and after deployments [33, 78, 87, 88]. Finally, modest negative relationships have been observed between deployment experiences and academic functioning [82, 83, 89, 90]. Deployment of a parent may also be associated with increases in other adverse experiences in school, including physical fighting, weapon-carrying and gang membership [91, 92].

Specific to the Fisher family, at the outset of treatment James would tear up when he talked about Byron and had taken time off work to grieve. Jane had a hard time putting into words how she felt, but was able to identify activities and people that offered her comfort. Both children described tension at home and difficulty communicating with their father. During treatment, both Jane and James were preparing to go back to school, which meant leaving the home. Soon after the death of her brother, Jane adopted an emotional support cat which she took with her when she left. In the wake of his brother's death, James began running on the beach with one of his friends. Running and talking with a close friend helped James feel more calm. Both decided they did not need any individual treatment at the end of family treatment. However, at 10-month follow-up, both wanted assistance in finding a full time therapist.

Interconnected Family Relationships and Developmental Cascades

While research often considers the discrete effects of deployment experiences on individuals or specific family relationships, theory suggests that these associations are not linear. Rather, family systems theory posits circular causality in which individual members of a family system and their relationships with one another have ongoing and reciprocal effects that reverberate through the system [93]. Developmental cascades capture the phenomenon of spreading effects across levels within a family system [94] and help to explain the "spillover" of stress associated with military family life between members of the system [95]. This concept has been observed in the critical role that at-home parents play in maintaining the wellbeing of military-connected youth across the deployment cycle. Increased anxiety, depression, perceived stress, and parenting stress in at-home parents consistently predicts increased adverse outcomes for children in military families [31, 83, 96, 97], suggesting that maintaining the health of at-home spouses may have a positive impact across military family systems.

While these effects are conceptualized as a family-level risk factor here, the impact of service member mental health parallels the cascade effects of spouse and family-level outcomes. Though an extensive review is beyond the scope of this chapter, a significant body of literature explores the impact of poor service member mental health, particularly PTSD, on parenting, intimate partner relationships, and individual child and spouse outcomes [33, 42, 66, 98]. Findings suggest adverse effects on parenting, marital or relationship functioning, family violence, and spouse psychological wellbeing, all of which likely have consequences for child outcomes [66, 98]. In particular, the numbing and avoidance symptoms of PTSD may be problematic for family functioning, as these symptoms may interrupt emotional expression that is critical to developing and maintaining close family relationships [66]. Spouses of combat veterans with PSTD may exhibit emotional distress in the form of stress, loneliness, somatic and psychiatric symptoms [99]. Similarly, children may exhibit increased fear, anxiety, behavior problems, and aggression, though findings among children are more mixed [99, 100]. Intimate relationships also appear to be adversely impacted by PTSD resulting in greater conflict and less intimacy [99]. Though studied less frequently, severity of depression symptoms among combat veterans may also be associated with increased family problems and intimate partner violence particularly during the reintegration period [100].

Demographic Moderators

A number of characteristics of military families may strengthen or attenuate the relationship between deployment experiences and adverse outcomes. For example, a meta-analysis of the relationship between deployment and adjustment among children concluded that the small association found was moderated by age. In this study, this relationship was detectable in early and middle childhood, but not in adolescence [8]. Other studies, however, have also found significant relationships between deployment experiences and adverse outcomes among older children and adolescents [30, 33]. Findings associated with child gender as a moderator are mixed. In one study, for example, girls exhibited increased externalizing behaviors during a parents' deployment compared to following their return, while boys exhibited the opposite pattern [31]. Other studies have suggested that boys may be more impacted during deployments [101]. Similarly the gender of the deployed parent may also be an important factor in understanding the strength and direction of the relationship between deployment and adverse outcomes, though evidence is similarly inconclusive [81, 102]. Service member rank may also moderate these relationships, although it is not clear whether these distinctions are related to the unique experiences of service members at different ranks or are ultimately a function of socioeconomic status which is closely tied to rank [37, 101]. Finally family type may also impact these relationships; dual military and single parent military families are rarely researched but their experiences during deployment may be significantly different [21].

Mechanisms

While the adverse impact of deployment on spouses, children and families has been relatively well documented, the mechanisms that underlie these associations are less well understood and may be of particular importance to clinical interventions.

Qualitative research with military spouses and children suggests a number of experiences associated with deployment may explain increases in adverse outcomes. For example, spouses reported increased stress associated with the challenges of single parenting as well fear and worry for the well-being of their loved one [103]. Further, increased demands on spouses' time during a deployment may prevent them from accessing protective factors, like exercise and social connections, that could counteract increased stress [104]. Qualitative work with military-connected adolescents also suggests that worry about their deployed parent, increases in responsibilities at home, and increased conflict or tension in family relationships may accompany parental deployment, which could explain adverse outcomes for some youth [46]. Further quantitative research is necessary in order to better understand these underlying mechanisms.

Interventions

Though an exhaustive treatment is outside the scope of the present chapter, there are several existing evidence-based interventions that address the unique needs of military families. Families OverComing Under Stress (FOCUS) is a preventative intervention that teaches resiliency skills surrounding the deployment cycle or transitions in military life [2, 105, 106]. After Deployment, Adaptive Parenting Tools (ADAPT) is an intervention designed for military parents with children ages 5–12 years old who have experienced a combat-related deployment [107]. Other programs include STRoNG Military Families [108, 109], HomeFrontStrong [110] and Strong Families Strong Forces [111], though these programs are only available in certain locations. Clinicians interested in referring to these programs or getting trained should visit program websites.

While the majority of programs focus on active duty families, some address the transition out of the service, including Sesame Street for Military Families: Transitions [112]. In addition, standard mental health treatments have also been evaluated in military populations, including behavioral couples therapy [113], or cognitive behavioral therapy for military children coping with deployments [114]. Further, several non-profits have started to provide free family-based services, including the Cohen Veterans Network [115]. See Table 22.1 for a list of free, national, in-person and remotely available resources for military families.

Treatment for the Fisher family included meeting with parents and children in separate sessions to build rapport and explore issues from different perspectives before bringing the whole family together. Once together, treatment was guided by the family's goals. Based on these goals, sessions focused on developing and practicing coping and communication skills. Coping skills included developing emotion regulation capacity and identifying activities that grounded each family member when feeling dysregulated. Communication skills included active listening, paraphrasing, and using I-statements to describe feelings.

Through this brief resiliency training, all members of the family were able to build on their greatest strength, love for and commitment to each other, as well as address areas of vulnerability, including communication and individual mental health. Brief preventative approaches to treatment can be particularly beneficial in military families because they can serve as an entry point into individual mental health care. Through this entry point, additional referrals to ongoing services were made.

Table 22.1 In-person and remotely available clinical resources for military families

In person military family resources	Remote military family resources
Give an Hour: A national network of mental health professionals who provide free mental health services for specific populations in need. Give an Hour has been serving military families since 2005 • www.givenanhour.org • Email: info@givenhour.org	**DoD family readiness council information page**: This page is a Facebook informational page where active duty families can learn about the Department of Defense Family Readiness Council, including getting a family needs assessment[a] www.facebook.com/DoDMFRC
The Fisher House Foundation: Builds comfort homes where military and veteran families can stay free of charge while a loved one is in the hospital. Homes are located at military and VA medical centers around the world • www.fisherhouse.org	**Operation We Are Here**: One-stop hub of resources for the military community and military supporters that offers a variety of resources for families • www.operationwearehere.com
Veterans Affairs Intimate Partner Violence (IPV) Assistance Program: This program is committed to helping Veterans and their partners who are impacted by IPV. Click on the link below to see what options are available in your location[b] • www.socialwork.va.gov/IPV/Index.asp	**Blue Star Families:** Bridges the gap between military family communities and the general public by providing free resources, services, and opportunities to more than 1.5 million military family members. Services are tailored more for active duty but they also offer support to veteran families as well • www.bluestarfam.org
Tragedy Assistance Program for Survivors (TAPS): Offers compassionate care to all those grieving the loss of a loved one who died while serving in our Armed Forces or as a result of his or her services[d] • National Military Survivor Helpline: 800-959-TAPS(8277) • www.taps.org	**National Military Family Association:** This association uses a grass roots approach to speak up on behalf of military families and empowers husbands, wives, and children of service members to understand and access their benefits[a] • www.militaryfamily.org
Cohen Veterans Network: Serves veterans and their families by providing high-quality, accessible, and integrated mental health care in person or through tele-health. Has clinics across the country[d] • www.cohenveteransnetwork.org	**Military OneSource**: Military OneSource (MOS) supplements existing family programs by providing a website and a worldwide, 24 h, seven-day-a-week information and referral telephone service to ALL active, Guard and Reserve Soldiers, deployed civilians and their families. Services are provided at no-cost • Call: 1-800-342-9647 • www.militaryonesource.mil

Families OverComing Under Stress (FOCUS): Provides resiliency training to military children and families who are active duty or in the reserve. It teaches practical skills to meet the challenges of deployment and reintegration, to communicate and solve problems effectively, and to successfully set goals together and create a shared family story[d] • www.focusproject.org	**Yellow Ribbon Reintegration Program**: Department of Defense-wide effort to promote the well-being of National Guard and Reserve members, their families and communities, by connecting them with resources throughout the deployment cycle. Through Yellow Ribbon events, Service members and loved ones connect with local resources before, during, and after deployments[c] • www.yellowribbon.mil
The Armed Services YMCA (ASYMCA): Has provided support services to military service members and their families for more than 140 years. It offers essential programs such as childcare, hospital assistance, spouse support services, food services, computer training classes, health and wellness services, and holiday meals, among many others[b] • www.asymca.org	**Penn State Clearing House**: Built for clinicians providing services to military families, the Clearinghouse Continuum of Evidence is an interactive, searchable database of evidence-based programs that address a wide variety of family and mental health issues, such as healthy parenting, financial literacy, nutrition and physical activity, stress, anxiety, and depression. • https://www.continuum.militaryfamilies.psu.edu/search
Family Readiness Systems: A network of agencies and services that promote the readiness and quality of life of all military families. Programs provide a range of services from financial management to child abuse prevention. Visit the website below for a list of contact points for all services[a, d] • https://www.militaryonesource.mil/family-relationships/family-life/keeping-your-family-strong/family-readiness-system	**Sesame Street for Military Families**: Sesame street has created several online programs for military families with young children covering a range of topics from leaving for or returning from a deployment to leaving the military altogether. Their website outlines the programs available by topic • www.sesamestreetformilitaryfamilies.org

[a] Services available for active duty only
[b] Veteran family focused
[c] National Guard and Reserve family focused
[d] Both in-person and remote or telehealth services available

Conclusions

Though limitations in current research exist, including a relative lack of longitudinal data and studies including multiple reporters from the same family, the existing literature suggests that the majority of military families are resilient, but that a significant subset is in need of additional supports from military and civilian communities alike. Families that have experienced longer or more deployments and families in which the at-home spouse has been adversely impacted may be at particularly elevated risk. Adverse impacts experienced at the individual level, by military-connected children or spouses, or at the family level have the potential to spread to other individuals or subsystems within a family. Thus, informed and timely prevention and intervention efforts to support the wellbeing of these individuals and families can have a compounding positive effect on military families as a whole. As a nation that benefits from their sacrifices, clinicians, researchers, and policy makers share a responsibility to respond effectively to the needs of military families experiencing deployment-related stressors.

Clinical Pearls

When working with military families, it is important to keep in mind several unique aspects of this population:

- A service member's military service may not be their main reason for seeking treatment. However, issues related to their service may still be present and important context for presenting problems.
- Military families may also seek treatment for reasons that are not specific to their family member's service. Military families experience many of the same stressors as the civilian population; the family should guide the focus of treatment.
- If a military-connected child is experiencing mental health issues, it may be important to assess the child's parents, considering the strong empirical relationship between parent and child mental health problems in this population.
- A complete biopsychosocial assessment that considers both normative and military specific risk and protective factors is critical when working with military spouses, children or families. As in work with civilian families, understanding the interplay between these factors will ultimately determine the focus of treatment.
- Military families have many strengths that can be leveraged to achieve positive treatment outcomes. These may include practiced resiliency through the experience of hardships and transitions during service, potentially stable income and housing, and free access to supports and services including health care and educational benefits (see Table 22.1).
- There is significant stigma and self-stigma around help seeking in the military culture, which extends to the spouses, children and families of service members. Civilian providers should be sensitive to the challenges stigma presents to seeking and following through with mental health services. During treatment, it may be necessary to reframe seeking mental health treatment as a strength in order to combat the effects of self-stigma.

References

1. Dimiceli EE, Steinhardt MA, Smith SE. Stressful experiences, coping strategies, and predictors of health-related outcomes among wives of deployed military servicemen. Armed Forces Soc. 2010;36(2):351–73. https://doi.org/10.1177/0095327X08324765.
2. Lester P, Aralis H, Sinclair M, Kiff C, et al. The impact of deployment on parental, family and child adjustment in military families. Child Psychiatry Hum Dev. 2016a;47(6):938–49. https://doi.org/10.1007/s10578-016-0624-9.
3. Tanielian T, Karney BR, Chandra A, Meadows SO, Team DLS. The deployment life study: methodological overview and baseline sample description. 2014. Available at https://www.rand.org/pubs/research_reports/RR209.html. Accessed January 10, 2020.
4. Hoge CW, Auchterlonie JL, Milliken CS. Mental health problems, use of mental health services, and attrition from military service after returning from deployment to Iraq or Afghanistan. JAMA. 2006;295(9):1023–32. https://doi.org/10.1001/jama.295.9.1023.
5. Hoge CW, Castro CA, Messer SC, McGurk D, et al. Combat duty in Iraq and Afghanistan, mental health problems, and barriers to care. N Engl J Med. 2004;351(1):13–22. https://doi.org/10.1056/NEJMoa040603.
6. Kim PY, Thomas JL, Wilk JE, Castro CA, Hoge CW. Stigma, barriers to care, and use of mental health services among Active Duty and National Guard soldiers after combat. Psychiatr Serv. 2010;61(6):582–8. https://doi.org/10.1176/ps.2010.61.6.582.
7. Milliken CS, Auchterlonie JL, Hoge CW. Longitudinal assessment of mental health problems among active and reserve component soldiers returning from the Iraq war. JAMA. 2007;298(18):2141. https://doi.org/10.1001/jama.298.18.2141.
8. Card NA, Bosch L, Casper DM, Wiggs CB, et al. A meta-analytic review of internalizing, externalizing, and academic adjustment among children of deployed military service members. J Fam Psychol. 2011;25(4):508–20. https://doi.org/10.1037/a0024395.
9. Creech SK, Hadley W, Borsari B. The impact of military deployment and reintegration on children and parenting: a systematic review. Prof Psychol Res Pract. 2014;45(6):452–64. https://doi.org/10.1037/a0035055.
10. de Burgh HT, White CJ, Fear NT, Iversen AC. The impact of deployment to Iraq or Afghanistan on partners and wives of military personnel. Int Rev Psychiatry. 2011;23(2):192–200. https://doi.org/10.3109/09540261.2011.560144.
11. White CJ, de Burgh HT, Fear NT, Iversen AC. The impact of deployment to Iraq or Afghanistan on military children: a review of the literature. Int Rev Psychiatry. 2011;23(2):210–7. https://doi.org/10.3109/09540261.2011.560143.
12. U.S. Department of Defense. 2017 demographics: profile of the military community. 2018. Available at http://download.militaryonesource.mil/12038/MOS/Reports/2017-demographics-report.pdf. Accessed January 10, 2020.
13. Cozza SJ, Lerner RM, Haskins R. Social policy report military and veteran families and children: policies and programs for health maintenance and positive development. Soc Policy Rep. 2014;28(3):3–17.
14. Park N. Military children and families: strengths and challenges during peace and war. Am Psychol. 2011;66(1):65–72. https://doi.org/10.1037/a0021249.
15. DeVoe ER, Ross A. The parenting cycle of deployment. Mil Med. 2012;177(2):184–90.
16. Pincus SL, House R, Christenson J, Adler LE. The emotional cycle of deployment: a military family perspective. US Army Med Dep J. 2001;4(4):9–18.
17. Institute of Medicine. Returning home from Iraq and Afghanistan: assessment of readjustment needs of veterans, service members, and their families. Washington: National Academies Press; 2013.
18. Paley B, Lester P, Mogil C. Family systems and ecological perspectives on the impact of deployment on military families. Clin Child Fam Psychol Rev. 2013;16(3):245–65. https://doi.org/10.1007/s10567-013-0138-y.
19. Wilson SR, Marini CM, Franks MM, Whiteman SF, et al. Communication and connection during deployment: a daily-diary study from the perspective of at-home partners. J Fam Psychol. 2018;32(1):42–8. https://doi.org/10.1037/fam0000333.

20. Huebner CR. Health and mental health needs of children in US military families. Pediatrics. 2019;143(1):e20183258. https://doi.org/10.1542/peds.2018-3258.
21. Lester P, Flake E. How wartime military service affects children and families. Futur Child. 2013;23(2):121–41. https://doi.org/10.1353/foc.2013.0015.
22. Larson MJ, Mohr BA, Adams RS, Ritter G, et al. Association of military deployment of a parent or spouse and changes in dependent use of health care services. Med Care. 2012;50(9):821–8. Retrieved from https://www.jstor.org/stable/41714565
23. Hawkins SA, Sulilvan K, Schuyler AC, Keeling M, et al. Thinking "big" about research on military families. Mil Behav Health. 2017;5(4):335–45. https://doi.org/10.1080/21635781.2017.1343696.
24. MacDermid Wadsworth SM. Family risk and resilience in the context of war and terrorism. J Marriage Fam. 2010;72(3):537–56. https://doi.org/10.1111/j.1741-3737.2010.00717.x.
25. Sullivan K. An application of family stress theory to clinical work with military families and other vulnerable populations. Clin Soc Work J. 2014;43(1):89–97. https://doi.org/10.1007/s10615-014-0500-7.
26. MacDermid Wadsworth SM, Cardin JF, Christ S, Willerton E, et al. Accumulation of risk and promotive factors among young children in US military families. Am J Community Psychol. 2016;57(1–2):190–202. https://doi.org/10.1002/ajcp.12025.
27. Blakely G, Hennessy C, Chung MC, Skirton H. A systematic review of the impact of foreign postings on accompanying spouses of military personnel. Nurs Health Sci. 2012;14:121–32. https://doi.org/10.1111/j.1442-2018.2011.00659.x.
28. Burrell LM, Adams GA, Durand DB, Castro CA. The impact of military lifestyle demands on well-being, army, and family outcomes. Armed Forces Soc. 2006;33(1):43–58. https://doi.org/10.1177/0002764206288804.
29. Harrell MC, Lim N, Castaneda LW, Golinelli D. Working around the military: challenges to military spouse employment and education. 2004. Available at https://www.rand.org/content/dam/rand/pubs/monographs/2004/RAND_MG196.pdf. Accessed January 10, 2020.
30. Chandra A, Lara-Cinisomo S, Jaycox LH, Tanielian T, et al. Children on the homefront: the experience of children from military families. Pediatrics. 2010a;125(1):16–25.
31. Lester P, Peterson K, Reeves J, Knauss L, et al. The long war and parental combat deployment: effects on military children and at-home spouses. J Am Acad Child Adolesc Psychiatry. 2010;49(4):310–20. https://doi.org/10.1016/j.jaac.2010.01.003.
32. Mansfield AJ, Kaufman JS, Engel CC, Gaynes BN. Deployment and mental health diagnoses among children of US army personnel. Arch Pediatr Adolesc Med. 2011;165(11):999–1005. https://doi.org/10.1001/archpediatrics.2011.123.
33. Meadows SO, Tanielian T, Karney B, Schell T, et al. The deployment life study: longitudinal analysis of military families across the deployment cycle. Rand Health Q. 2017;6(2):7. Available at http://www.ncbi.nlm.nih.gov/pubmed/28845345. Accessed January 9, 2021.
34. Sullivan K, Hawkins SA, Gilreath TD, Castro CA. Mental health outcomes associated with profiles of risk and resilience among military-connected youth. Fam Process. 2021;60(2):507–22.
35. Haas DM, Pazdernik LA. Partner deployment and stress in pregnant women. J Reprod Med. 2007;52(10):901–6.
36. Smith DC, Munroe ML, Foglia LM, Nielsen PE, et al. Effects of deployment on depression screening scores in pregnancy at an army military treatment facility. Obstet Gynecol. 2010;116(3):679–84. https://doi.org/10.1097/AOG.0b013e3181eb6c84.
37. Spera C. Spouses' ability to cope with deployment and adjust to Air Force family demands: identification of risk and protective factors. Armed Forces Soc. 2009;35(2):286–306. https://doi.org/10.1177/0095327X08316150.
38. Trautmann J, Alhusen J, Gross D. Impact of deployment on military families with young children: a systematic review. Nurs Outlook. 2015;63(6):656–79. https://doi.org/10.1016/j.outlook.2015.06.002.
39. Palmer C. A theory of risk and resilience factors in military families. Mil Psychol. 2008;20(3):205–17. https://doi.org/10.1080/08995600802118858.

40. Floyd L, Phillips DA. Child care and other support programs. Futur Child. 2013;23(2):79–97. https://doi.org/10.1353/foc.2013.0013.
41. Hosek J, MacDermid Wadsworth SM. Economic conditions of military families. Futur Child. 2013;23(2):41–59.
42. MacDermid Wadsworth SM, Bailey KM, Coppola EC. U.S. military children and the wartime deployments of family members. Child Dev Perspect. 2017;11(1):23–8. https://doi.org/10.1111/cdep.12210.
43. Bowen GL, Martin JA. The resiliency model of role performance for service members, veterans, and their families: a focus on social connections and individual assets. J Hum Behav Soc Environ. 2011;21(2):162–78. https://doi.org/10.1080/10911359.2011.546198.
44. Burrell LM, Durand DB, Fortado J. Military community integration and its effect on well-being and retention. Armed Forces Soc. 2003;30(1):7–24. https://doi.org/10.1177/0095327X0303000101.
45. Conforte AM, Bakalar JL, Shank LM, Quinlan J, et al. Assessing military community support: relations among perceived military community support, child psychosocial adjustment, and parent psychosocial adjustment. Mil Med. 2017;182(9):1871–8. https://doi.org/10.7205/MILMED-D-17-00016.
46. Huebner AJ, Mancini JA, Wade KE, McElhaney SJ, et al. Resilience and vulnerability: the deployment experiences of youth in military families. 2010. Available at https://www.researchgate.net/profile/Jay-Mancini/publication/228534218_Resilience_and_vulnerability_The_deployment_experiences_of_youth_in_military_families/links/0deec5280c42a36717000000/Resilience-and-vulnerability-The-deployment-experiences-of-youth-in-military-families.pdf. Accessed July 21, 2021.
47. Lucier-Greer M, O'Neal CW, Arnold AL, Mancini JA, Wickrama KKAS. Adolescent mental health and academic functioning: empirical support for contrasting models of risk and vulnerability. Mil Med. 2014;179(11):1279–87. https://doi.org/10.7205/MILMED-D-14-00090.
48. Weins TW, Boss P. Maintaining family resiliency before, during, and after military separation. In: Castro CA, Adler AB, Britt TW, editors. Military life: the psychology of serving in peace and combat, vol. 3. The military family. Westport: Praeger Security International; 2006. p. 13–38.
49. Everson RB, Darling CA, Herzog JR. Parenting stress among US Army spouses during combat-related deployments: the role of sense of coherence. Child Fam Soc Work. 2013;18(2):168–78. https://doi.org/10.1111/j.1365-2206.2011.00818.x.
50. Saltzman WR, Lester P, Beardslee WR, Layne CM, et al. Mechanisms of risk and resilience in military families: theoretical and empirical basis of a family-focused resilience enhancement program. Clin Child Fam Psychol Rev. 2011;14(3):213–30. https://doi.org/10.1007/s10567-011-0096-1.
51. McGuire A, Runge C, Cosgrove L, Bredhauer, et al. Timor-Leste family study: summary report. Brisbane: The University of Queensland Centre for Military and Veterans' Health; 2012.
52. Bello-Utu CF, DeSocio JE. Military deployment and reintegration: a systematic review of child coping. J Child Adolesc Psychiatr Nurs. 2015;28(1):23–34. https://doi.org/10.1111/jcap.12099.
53. Lavee Y, McCubbin HI, Patterson JM. The double ABCX model of family stress and adaptation: an empirical test by analysis of structural equations with latent variables. Sour J Marriage Family. 1985;47(4):811–25.
54. Lucier-Greer M, Arnold AL, Mancini JA, Ford JL, et al. Influences of cumulative risk and protective factors on the adjustment of adolescents in military families. Fam Relat. 2015;64(3):363–77. https://doi.org/10.1111/fare.12123.
55. Flittner O'Grady AE, Whiteman SD, Cardin JF, MacDermid Wadsworth SM. Changes in parenting and youth adjustment across the military deployment cycle. J Marriage Fam. 2018;80(2):569–81. https://doi.org/10.1111/jomf.12457.

56. Huebner AJ, Mancini JA, Wilcox RM, Grass SR, Grass GA. Parental deployment and youth in military families: exploring uncertainty and ambiguous loss. Fam Relat. 2007;56(2):112–22. https://doi.org/10.1111/j.1741-3729.2007.00445.x.
57. Warner CH, Appenzeller GN, Warner CM, Grieger T. Psychological effects of deployments on military families. Psychiatr Ann. 2009;39(2):56–63. https://doi.org/10.3928/00485713-20090201-11.
58. Eaton KM, Hoge CW, Messer SC, Whit AA, et al. Prevalence of mental health problems, treatment need, and barriers to care among primary care-seeking spouses of military service members involved in Iraq and Afghanistan deployments. Mil Med. 2008;173(11):1051–6. https://doi.org/10.7205/MILMED.173.11.1051.
59. Mansfield AJ, Kaufman JS, Marshall SW, Gaynes BN, et al. Deployment and the use of mental health services among U.S. Army wives. N Engl J Med. 2010;362(2):101–9. https://doi.org/10.1056/NEJMoa0900177.
60. Burton T, Farley D, Rhea A. Stress-induced somatization in spouses of deployed and non-deployed servicemen. J Am Acad Nurse Pract. 2009;21(6):332–9. https://doi.org/10.1111/j.1745-7599.2009.00411.x.
61. Padden DL, Connors RA, Agazio JG. Stress, coping, and well-being in military spouses during deployment separation. West J Nurs Res. 2011;33(2):247–67. https://doi.org/10.1177/0193945910371319.
62. Allen ES, Rhoades GK, Stanley SM, Markman HJ. Hitting home: relationships between recent deployment, posttraumatic stress symptoms, and marital functioning for Army couples. J Fam Psychol. 2010;24(3):280–8. https://doi.org/10.1037/a0019405.
63. McLeland KC, Sutton GW, Schumm WR. Marital satisfaction before and after deployments associated with the global war on terror. Psychol Rep. 2008;103(3):836–44. https://doi.org/10.2466/pr0.103.3.836-844.
64. Hogan PF, Furst Seifert R. Marriage and the military: evidence that those who serve marry earlier and divorce earlier. Armed Forces Soc. 2010;36(3):420–38. https://doi.org/10.1177/0095327X09351228.
65. Karney BR, Crown JS. Families under stress: An assessment of data, theory, and research on marriage and divorce in the military. 2007. Available at https://www.rand.org/content/dam/rand/pubs/monographs/2007/RAND_MG599.pdf. Accessed January 10, 2020.
66. Galovski T, Lyons JA. Psychological sequelae of combat violence: a review of the impact of PTSD on the veteran's family and possible interventions. Aggress Violent Behav. 2004;9(5):477–501. https://doi.org/10.1016/S1359-1789(03)00045-4.
67. Lester P, Liang L, Milburn N, Mogil C, et al. Evaluation of a family-centered preventive intervention for military families: parent and child longitudinal outcomes. J Am Acad Child Adolesc Psychiatry. 2016b;55(1):14–24.
68. Paris R, DeVoe ER, Ross AM, Acker ML. When a parent goes to war: effects of parental deployment on very young children and implications for intervention. Am J Orthopsychiatry. 2010;80(4):610–8. https://doi.org/10.1111/j.1939-0025.2010.01066.x.
69. Khaylis A, Polusny M, Erbes CR, Gewirtz A, Rath M. Posttraumatic stress, family adjustment, and treatment preferences among National Guard soldiers deployed to OEF/OIF. Mil Med. 2011;176(2):126–31.
70. Rentz ED, Martin SL, Gibbs DA, Clinton-Sherrod M, et al. Family violence in the military: a review of the literature. Trauma Violence Abuse. 2006;7(2):93–108. https://doi.org/10.1177/1524838005285916.
71. Gibbs DA, Martin SL, Kupper LL, Johnson RE. Child maltreatment in enlisted soldiers' families during combat-related deployments. JAMA. 2007;298(5):528–35. https://doi.org/10.1001/jama.298.5.528.
72. Martin SL, Gibbs DA, Johnson RE, Rentz ED, et al. Spouse abuse and child abuse by army soldiers. J Fam Violence. 2007;22(7):587–95. https://doi.org/10.1007/s10896-007-9110-2.
73. McCarroll JE, Fan Z, Newby JH, Ursano RJ. Trends in US army child maltreatment reports: 1990–2004. Child Abuse Rev. 2008;17(2):108–18. https://doi.org/10.1002/car.986.

74. Cozza SJ, Whaley GL, Fisher JE, Zhou J, et al. Deployment status and child neglect types in the U.S. army. Child Maltreat. 2018;23(1):25–33. https://doi.org/10.1177/1077559517717638.
75. Hisle-Gorman E, Harrington D, Nylund CM, Tercyak KP, et al. Impact of parents' wartime military deployment and injury on young children's safety and mental health. J Am Acad Child Adolesc Psychiatry. 2015;54(4):294–301. https://doi.org/10.1016/j.jaac.2014.12.017.
76. McCarroll JE, Ursano RJ, Liu X, Thayer LE, et al. Deployment and the probability of spousal aggression by U.S. army soldiers. Mil Med. 2010;175(5):352–6. https://doi.org/10.7205/MILMED-D-10-00048.
77. Marshall AD, Panuzio J, Taft CT. Intimate partner violence among military veterans and active duty servicemen. Clin Psychol Rev. 2005;25(7):862–76. https://doi.org/10.1016/J.CPR.2005.05.009.
78. Cederbaum JA, Gilreath TD, Benbenishty R, Astor RA, et al. Well-being and suicidal ideation of secondary school students from military families. J Adolesc Health. 2014;54(6):672–7. https://doi.org/10.1016/j.jadohealth.2013.09.006.
79. Gilreath TD, Wrabel SL, Sullivan K, Capp GP, et al. Suicidality among military-connected adolescents in California schools. Eur Child Adolesc Psychiatry. 2016;25(1):61–6. https://doi.org/10.1007/s00787-015-0696-2.
80. Sullivan K, Capp G, Gilreath TD, Benbenishty R, et al. Substance abuse and other adverse outcomes for military-connected youth in California: results from a large-scale normative population survey. JAMA Pediatr. 2015b;169(10):922–8. https://doi.org/10.1001/jamapediatrics.2015.1413.
81. Gorman GH, Eide M, Hisle-Gorman E. Wartime military deployment and increased pediatric mental and behavioral health complaints. Pediatrics. 2010;126(6):1058–66.
82. Mmari K, Roche KM, Sudhinaraset M, Blum R. When a parent goes off to war: exploring the issues faced by adolescents and their families. Youth Soc. 2009;40(4):455–75. https://doi.org/10.1177/0044118X08327873.
83. Flake EM, Davis BE, Johnson PL, Middleton LS. The psychosocial effects of deployment on military children. J Dev Behav Pediatr. 2009;30(4):271–8. https://doi.org/10.1097/DBP.0b013e3181aac6e4.
84. Hawkins SA, Schlomer GL, Bosch L, Casper DM, et al. A review of the impact of US military deployments during conflicts in Afghanistan and Iraq on children's functioning. Family Sci. 2012;3(2):99–108. https://doi.org/10.1080/19424620.2012.723017.
85. Mustillo S, MacDermid Wadsworth SM, Lester P. Parental deployment and well-being in children: results from a new study of military families. J Emot Behav Disord. 2016;24(2):82–91. https://doi.org/10.1177/1063426615598766.
86. Barnes VA, Davis H, Treiber FA. Perceived stress, heart rate, and blood pressure among adolescents with family members deployed in Operation Iraqi Freedom. Mil Med. 2007;172(1):40–3. https://doi.org/10.7205/MILMED.172.1.40.
87. Acion L, Ramirez MR, Jorge RE, Arndt S. Increased risk of alcohol and drug use among children from deployed military families. Addiction. 2013;108(8):1418–25. https://doi.org/10.1111/add.12161.
88. Reed SC, Bell JF, Edwards TC. Adolescent well-being in Washington state military families. Am J Public Health. 2011;101(9):1676–82. https://doi.org/10.2105/AJPH.2011.300165.
89. Chandra A, Martin LT, Hawkins SA, Richardson A. The impact of parental deployment on child social and emotional functioning: perspectives of school staff. J Adolesc Health. 2010b;46(3):218–23.
90. Engel RC, Gallagher LB, Lyle DS. Military deployments and children's academic achievement: evidence from Department of Defense Education Activity Schools. Econ Educ Rev. 2010;29(1):73–82. https://doi.org/10.1016/j.econedurev.2008.12.003.
91. Aranda MC, Middleton L, Flake E, Davis BE. Psychosocial screening in children with wartime-deployed parents. Mil Med. 2011;176(4):402–7.
92. Reed SC, Bell JF, Edwards TC. Weapon carrying, physical fighting and gang membership among youth in Washington State Military Families. Matern Child Health J. 2014;18(8):1863–72. https://doi.org/10.1007/s10995-014-1430-2.

93. Cox MJ, Paley B. Understanding families as systems. Curr Dir Psychol Sci. 2003;12(5):193–6. https://doi.org/10.1111/1467-8721.01259.
94. Masten AS, Cicchetti D. Developmental cascades. Dev Psychopathol. 2010;22(3):491–5. https://doi.org/10.1017/S0954579410000222.
95. Masten AS. Competence, risk, and resilience in military families: conceptual commentary. Clin Child Fam Psychol Rev. 2013;16(3):278–81. https://doi.org/10.1007/s10567-013-0150-2.
96. Allen ES, Rhoades GK, Stanley SM, Markman HJ. On the home front: stress for recently deployed Army couples. Fam Process. 2011;50(2):235–47. https://doi.org/10.1111/j.1545-5300.2011.01357.
97. Morris AS, Age TR. Adjustment among youth in military families: the protective roles of effortful control and maternal social support. J Appl Dev Psychol. 2009;30(6):695–707. https://doi.org/10.1016/j.appdev.2009.01.002.
98. Goff BSN, Crow JR, Reisbig AMJ, Hamilton S. The impact of individual trauma symptoms of deployed soldiers on relationship satisfaction. J Fam Psychol. 2007;21(3):344–53. https://doi.org/10.1037/0893-3200.21.3.344.
99. Dekel R, Monson CM. Military-related post-traumatic stress disorder and family relations: current knowledge and future directions. Aggress Violent Behav. 2010;15(4):303–9. https://doi.org/10.1016/j.avb.2010.03.001.
100. Sayers SL, Farrow VA, Ross J, Oslin DW. Family problems among recently returned military veterans. J Clin Psychiatry. 2009;10:e1–8.
101. Jensen PS, Martin D, Watanabe H. Children's response to parental separation during operation desert storm. J Am Acad Child Adolesc Psychiatry. 1996;35(4):433–41. https://doi.org/10.1097/00004583-199604000-00009.
102. Sullivan K, Benbenishty R, Astor RA, Cap G, et al. The impact of maternal and paternal deployment on depressive symptoms and well-being among military-connected youth. Mil Behav Health. 2015a;3(3):182–9. https://doi.org/10.1080/21635781.2015.1038402.
103. Runge CE, Waller M, MacKenzie A, McGuire ACL. Spouses of military members' experiences and insights: qualitative analysis of responses to an open-ended question in a survey of health and wellbeing. PLoS ONE. 2014;9(12):e114755. https://doi.org/10.1371/journal.pone.0114755.
104. Mailey EL, Mershon C, Joyce J, Irwin BC. "Everything else comes first": a mixed-methods analysis of barriers to health behaviors among military spouses. BMC Public Health. 2018;18(1):1013. https://doi.org/10.1186/s12889-018-5938-z.
105. Lester P, Mogil C, Saltzman W, Woodward K, et al. Families overcoming under stress: implementing family centered prevention for military families facing wartime deployments and combat operational stress. Mil Med. 2011;176(1):19–25. https://doi.org/10.7205/MILMED-D-10-00122.
106. Lester P, Saltzman WR, Woodward K, Glover D, et al. Evaluation of a family-centered prevention intervention for military children and families facing wartime deployments. Am J Public Health. 2012;102(S1):S48–54. https://doi.org/10.2105/AJPH.2010.300088.
107. Gewirtz AH, Pinna KLM, Hanson SK, Brockberg D. Promoting parenting to support reintegrating military families: after deployment, adaptive parenting tools. Psychol Serv. 2014;11(1):31–40. https://doi.org/10.1037/a0034134.
108. Rosenblum KL, Muzik M. STRoNG intervention for military families with young children. Psychiatr Serv. 2014;65(3):399. https://doi.org/10.1176/appi.ps.650302.
109. Rosenblum K, Muzik M, Waddell R, Thompson S, et al. Strong military families program: a multifamily group approach to strengthening family resilience. Zero Three. 2015;36(2):8–14.
110. Kees M, Nerenberg LS, Bachrach J, Sommer LA. Changing the personal narrative: a pilot study of a resiliency intervention for military spouses. Contemp Fam Ther. 2015;37(3):221–31. https://doi.org/10.1007/s10591-015-9336-8.
111. DeVoe ER, Ross AM, Paris R. Build it together and they will come: the case for community-based participatory research with military populations. Adv Soc Work. 2012;13(1):149–65.

112. Sherman MD, Monn A, Larsen JL, Gerwirtz A. Evaluation of a sesame street multimedia intervention for families transitioning out of the military. J Child Fam Stud. 2018;27:2533–40. https://doi.org/10.1007/s10826-018-1083-7.
113. Sayers SL. Family reintegration difficulties and couples therapy for military veterans and their spouses. Cogn Behav Pract. 2011;18(1):108–19. https://doi.org/10.1016/j.cbpra.2010.03.002.
114. Friedberg RD, Brelsford GM. Using cognitive behavioral interventions to help children cope with parental military deployments. J Contemp Psychother. 2011;41(4):229–36. https://doi.org/10.1007/s10879-011-9175-3.
115. Cohen Veterans Network Clinics. n.d.

Combat-Related Injuries and Bereavement: Effects on Military and Veteran Families and Suggested Interventions

23

Joscelyn E. Fisher, Rafael F. Zuleta, Kathryn R. Hefner, and Stephen J. Cozza

Introduction

Since 1973, after the end of the draft in the United States and the start of the all-volunteer military force, the number of military families, including dependent spouses and children has grown considerably. As of 2018, there were over 1.5 million dependent family members of active duty service members, and over 1 million dependent family members of Selected Reserve members [1]. Since the start of Operation Iraqi Freedom (OIF) and Operation Enduring Freedom (OEF), these families have continually faced difficult challenges associated with military life, including repeated combat deployments. Some of these families have also been affected by combat-related injuries, including *visible* (e.g., musculoskeletal injuries, amputations, burns) and *invisible* (e.g., posttraumatic stress disorder [PTSD], traumatic brain injury [TBI]) injuries, as well as bereavement. These profound stressors typically include short-term and long-term challenges that affect all members of the family and their relationships with each other.

This chapter provides information for U.S. physical and mental healthcare providers who treat military service members, veterans, and their families who are dealing with combat-related injuries or bereavement. Combat-related injuries have the capacity to undermine the health and well-being of all family members. In addition, combat deaths or other sudden deaths could result in prolonged grief in family members, as well as changes to family structure and relationships. These life-altering events often lead to transitions in lifestyle, moves from military installations, and disruptions in established support and services, including health care,

J. E. Fisher (✉) · R. F. Zuleta · K. R. Hefner · S. J. Cozza
Center for the Study of Traumatic Stress, Department of Psychiatry, Uniformed Services University of the Health Science, Henry M. Jackson Foundation for the Advancement of Military Medicine, Bethesda, MD, USA
e-mail: joscelyn.fisher.ctr@usuhs.edu; rafael.zuleta-miranda.ctr@usuhs.edu; khefner@emmes.com; stephen.cozza@usuhs.edu

C. H. Warner, C. A. Castro (eds.), *Veteran and Military Mental Health*,
https://doi.org/10.1007/978-3-031-18009-5_23

educational services, friendships, and a sense of community. It is important to be aware of the effects of visible and invisible injuries as well as bereavement on families in order to fully address the needs of patients. This chapter highlights how these events can affect the mental and physical well-being of patients and their families, and describes family-centered interventions that can assist families affected by military duty-related injury, illness, and death. *Resources* and *Actions to Take* are provided at the end of the chapter, in addition to several additional *Recommended Readings*.

Combat-Related Visible Injuries

Epidemiology

As of 2020, nearly 53,000 service members sustained non-fatal *visible* injuries in OEF, OIF, and Operation New Dawn (OND) [2]. Nearly 75% of all combat-related injuries from post-9/11 conflicts were attributed to explosive devices (e.g., improvised explosive devices, land mines) [3]. During 2001–2005, the most common combat-related injuries (54%) involved the extremities [4]. Injuries to the extremities required the longest average inpatient stay (nearly 11 days), were the most frequent cause of repeated hospitalizations, involved the greatest resource utilization during rehospitalization, and ultimately disabled 64% of those injured [5, 6]. Although considerable media attention was given to injuries resulting in amputations, they constituted a small portion of overall injuries (roughly 1,700 out of 52,000 wounded in action from 2002–2015) [7]. In addition to these *visible* injuries, service members and veterans may have experienced *invisible* injuries (described below), such as traumatic brain injury (TBI) and posttraumatic stress disorder (PTSD). The combination of both *visible* and *invisible* injuries can worsen functional outcomes [8, 9].

Injury Recovery Trajectory

Recovery from combat-related injuries has been conceptualized as involving an *injury recovery trajectory* that consists of four phases: acute care, medical stabilization, transition to outpatient care, and long-term rehabilitation and recovery [10]. During each phase, families face multiple emotional and logistical challenges (see Table 23.1). *Acute care* involves the immediate, often life-saving medical attention provided to the wounded service member in combat theater, as well as their transportation via the medical evacuation system. During *medical stabilization*, military spouses and children often relocate to military treatment facilities to be closer to their injured loved ones. However, not all family members may be able to move, so individual family members are sometimes geographically separated, disrupting

Table 23.1 Injury recovery trajectory

Phase	Explanation
1. Acute care	Initiated at the time of injury by military medics and includes care provided in combat hospitals
2. Medical stabilization	Incorporates definitive medical treatment in U.S. stateside military medical centers
3. Transition to outpatient care	Relocation of injured service members to treatment facilities closer to home, transition to different treatment teams, and possible medical discharge from military service
4. Long-term rehabilitation and recovery	Ongoing care of the service member/veteran in order to maximize treatment benefits and long-term functioning

Sources: Cozza [11], Cozza and Feerick [12], Cozza and Guimond [10], Holmes et al. [13]

daily routines and adding stress to the family system. *Transition to outpatient care* involves other challenges: finding new housing, working with new health care providers, enrolling children in new schools, and leaving military friends and communities behind. After the injured service member leaves the hospital, family members (both adults and children) may be required to take on new roles and responsibilities (e.g., new household tasks), which may be confusing, upsetting, or frustrating. *Rehabilitation and recovery* is usually the longest period in the injury recovery trajectory, during which the service member/veteran and their family learn to adapt to the injury and become accustomed to a new life. It may also involve ongoing caregiving provided by both adult and child family members.

Injury Communication

The confusion and distress that results from combat-related visible and invisible injuries can compromise communication between family members. *Injury communication* is a term used to describe the exchange and impact of information about the injury [10]. Effective injury communication requires that family members are able to discuss information about the injury, its consequences, and required treatments within the family (including using developmentally-appropriate language with younger children), as well as with those outside of the family (e.g., friends, community professionals, service providers). Principles of effective injury communication (Table 23.2) have been detailed in *Courage to Care—Courage to Talk* (see www.courage2talk.org, Center for the Study of Traumatic Stress), a public health campaign that focused on the importance of injury communication both within the family and between the family and healthcare providers.

As illustrated in the following vignette about SSGT Jones and his family, the *acute care* and *medical stabilization* phases of recovery are distressing and chaotic for families. Each creates challenges for cohesion and effective communication. (Note—All vignettes within this chapter are constructed from clinical experience, but do not represent actual people or families).

Table 23.2 Injury communication

What is meant by the term 'injury communication'?	Injury communication is an essential component of injured family care. In its broadest sense, 'injury communication' refers both to the exchange of information (provision and delivery of information related to the injury), and to the impact of information (the capacity of the family and family member to process information). Injury communication also refers to the impact on the family's behavior. Effective injury communication involves the timely, appropriate and accurate sharing of information from the moment of notification of injury throughout treatment
What is the goal of injury communication?	Its primary goal, to be achieved over time, is helping family members integrate the injury experience through a process of shared understanding. To this end, ongoing dialogue about the injury and its implications are extremely important
Why is injury communication important for clinical providers?	Injury communication is both a process and an opportunity for healthcare providers. In the process of communicating with families about combat injury, there are multiple opportunities to educate and help families understand the importance of connectedness and availability—both within the family and within one' community Understanding the impact of injury on children, especially from a developmental perspective enables providers to guide families on how best to communicate with children to sustain hope, connection to both parents, and continuity with family and community routines. Ultimately, effective injury communication helps injured families learn the skills of self-advocacy, leading to protection from isolation, a sense of connectedness, the capacity for appropriate and timely help-seeking, and family problem-solving. Providing quality communication and compassionate outreach that supports injury recovery, family function and health are important goals that healthcare providers can advance using the educational resources of the ***Courage to Care Courage to Talk*** campaign
What are the implications of effective injury communication for families and children of the injured service member?	Family members of the injured will need to effectively communicate with each other, as well as with numerous military and civilian healthcare and social support personnel including nurses, doctors of diverse specialties, social workers, psychologists, case managers, chaplains and support service staff. As participants in the communication process, the ***Courage to Care Courage to Talk*** campaign can provide families with tips on talking about war injury, talking with children, and talking with healthcare providers

Used with permission, Courage to Care—Courage to Talk, Center for the Study of Traumatic Stress

Vignette #1

SSGT Mark Jones is a 35-year-old Army noncommissioned officer who was injured by an IED while deployed to Iraq in 2004. His wife, Annette, and their three children, Stephanie (age 14), Sam (age 9), and Jackson (age 3), were living in Killeen, Texas near Fort Hood where Mark had been stationed before deployment. Annette was notified of the injury and made arrangements to fly to Landstuhl Regional Medical Center in Germany where Mark was medically evacuated. Annette left her children in the care of a neighbor until her 60-year-old mother could join the family from her home in Ohio. Mark was then transported to Walter Reed Army Medical Center in Washington, DC where he remained for 9 months while he underwent a series of surgeries (including bilateral lower extremity amputations) for multiple musculoskeletal injuries. Given her mother's own medical problems and need for treatment, Annette made the decision to relocate her two older children to live with her brother's family in rural Ohio, and to have Jackson join her at the Fisher House at Walter Reed, a hotel where family members often stay while visiting their hospitalized service members. Jackson accompanied his mother on visits to Mark in the hospital and was often perceived as a nuisance by nursing staff because of his "high energy" and disruptive behavior. When Annette was asked what she told her children about Mark's injury, she replied "I talked to Stephanie and Sam about his injuries. But I didn't know what to say to Jackson, since he is so young. I didn't think he would understand, so I just let him see for himself when he came to the hospital. He found out his Daddy lost his legs when he saw Mark in the bed."

Effect of Visible Injuries on Spouses and Children

The family's experience of a combat-related injury can be influenced by the type and severity of the injury, family composition, individual and family maturity, health or preexisting medical or psychological conditions, the ages of children, the course of medical treatment, and whether the injured regains satisfactory functioning [10, 13]. In addition, the effect of combat injury on the marital relationship can have far-reaching effects that reverberate throughout the family. For instance, disruption of the marital dyad, parenting, and parent-child relationships as a result of parental physical injury would likely affect child functioning [14–16]. Shared activities between a parent and child prior to the injury may no longer be possible, which can alter the way the parent connects with the child. It may be necessary for the injured parent to modify their previously-held vision of themselves as parents, as they acknowledge their bodily changes and loss of functioning [15]. In addition, the ability to co-parent effectively may be affected due to changes in parental responsibilities, disruption of household routines, strains in the marital relationship, and prolonged hospitalizations or rehabilitation [17, 18].

Few empirical studies have examined the burden of parental combat injury on military children. Hisle-Gorman et al. [19] described risks faced by young military children (3–8 years old) whose parents deployed and returned either uninjured or injured (both physically and psychologically) compared to children whose parents did not deploy. Children of deployed and uninjured parents were at elevated risk for child injuries, child maltreatment, and for increased mental health care visits compared to children whose parents did not deploy. Children with combat-injured parents were at even higher risk. A follow-up study [20] that included a broader age range of children also found that children of combat-injured parents had increased healthcare visits associated with maltreatment, child injuries, and mental disorders (including increased use of psychiatric medication), and decreased preventive care visits compared to children of non-deployed and deployed but uninjured parents. If the parent had PTSD, or comorbid PTSD and TBI, the impact on children's health was greater [20].

The following fictional vignette describing Mark, Annette, and their children highlights the challenges associated with *transition to outpatient care* and *long-term rehabilitation and recovery* (see Table 23.1). These challenges include discontinuity of healthcare, misuse of prescribed medication, and family conflict.

Vignette #2

Upon completion of medical treatment at Walter Reed and nearly 18 months after his injury, Mark was transferred to outpatient care at a VA Hospital in a rural area. Stephanie and Sam joined Mark, Annette, and Jackson there in a temporary three-bedroom apartment while the family looked for permanent housing that could accommodate Mark's physical needs. The family struggled with the transition in several ways. In contrast to appointments at Walter Reed, Mark now needed to be transported by Annette to appointments at the VA hospital which was 20 minutes from their apartment. Stephanie, who had become increasingly independent and thrived in school while living with her uncle, now had more babysitting responsibilities for her two younger siblings and caregiving responsibilities for her father. She had to manage these new responsibilities while attempting to make friends in a new high school. In contrast, Sam had struggled in school while living with his uncle due to the lack of the educational support services he had received from the Texas school district. Now that he was with the family, he also had become sullen and moody because his father was often sleeping and unable to engage him in the kinds of outdoor play that they had enjoyed prior to his injury. In fact, Mark's frequent sleeping generally affected his ability to parent effectively. One winter morning, Jackson was left under Mark's supervision while Annette was grocery shopping. Jackson left the apartment when Mark fell asleep after taking his prescribed pain medication. Child protective services was contacted when Jackson was found wandering unsupervised without a coat in the neighborhood.

Invisible Injuries

Invisible injuries, such as traumatic brain injury (TBI), post-traumatic stress disorder (PTSD), depression, and substance use disorders (SUDs), can be devastating in a different, but no less life-altering, manner compared to visible injuries. Invisible injuries can present unique challenges.

Traumatic Brain Injury

Epidemiology

According to the DoD, between 2000 and the first quarter of 2018, there were nearly 384,000 cases of traumatic brain injury (TBI), making it the "signature injury" of conflicts during this period [21–23]. Although large, this number may be an underestimate of the true total number of affected service members and veterans, as it can be difficult to identify and diagnose TBI, especially mild TBI [24].

Effect on Spouses and Children

TBI can affect the health, wellbeing, and functional capacity of the non-injured spouse, as roles and responsibilities that were previously conducted by their partner may have to be incorporated into the spouse's ongoing tasks [25]. Spouses of TBI patients are at higher risk for psychiatric disorders, such as depression and anxiety [25], and poor marital satisfaction resulting from TBI may also affect co-parenting [25].

These negative influences on the spouse's health and the couple's relationship can affect children [26]. Children may show increased externalizing behaviors, emotional issues, and post-traumatic symptoms following parental TBI [27]. Children report feelings of loss, isolation, and loneliness due to changes they perceive in their injured parent [28, 29]. A substantial number (42–79%) of children of TBI-affected service members/veterans experienced a decline in their overall health and behavior [30], particularly within the first 2 years following the TBI. Although 17–27% of children experienced declines in health and behavior that were associated with parental deployment, there were additional declines subsequent to the TBI [30]. The severity of the TBI and the amount of disruption to a family's organization are other factors that affect children [25, 26]. Furthermore, if an injured parent withdraws from other family members, demonstrates communication issues, exhibits low frustration levels, manages anger poorly, and presents difficulty regulating emotions and behaviors, these behaviors may distress and alienate a child who cannot comprehend what they are witnessing [31].

TBI can cause unique challenges for families compared to those caused by other physical and non-neurological impairments [26]. For instance, certain TBI symptoms, such as personality changes and unexpected emotional reactions, that can be particularly detrimental to interpersonal relationships [32]. TBI's effect on families may also be long-lasting (as described in Table 23.1), and it may not improve over time [25]. Those with poor financial and social support are at greater risk for these long-term effects, which is why facilitating access to practical resources (e.g., financial, housing, social, etc.) and professional services are essential for these families [25].

Posttraumatic Stress Disorder (PTSD) and Comorbidities

Epidemiology

PTSD symptoms and comorbidity with other disorders can affect how families function. The PTSD symptom clusters of re-experiencing, avoidance, negative cognitions and mood, and arousal each have negative effects on normative family processes that support resilience (see description below) [33]. Substance use disorders (SUDs) are highly comorbid with PTSD, as 46% of a national sample of US veterans who met lifetime criteria for PTSD also met lifetime criteria for an SUD [34], and 22% of Veterans treated for PTSD in the VA across the nation had a concurrent SUD diagnosis [35]. Similarly, depression is often comorbid with PTSD [36]. Although depression and SUDs have been shown to negatively affect marital and parent-child relationships [24, 37, 38], less is known about their specific effects in military families. In contrast, the effect of PTSD in military and veteran families has consistently been shown to be disruptive to family well-being.

Impact of PTSD on Spouses and Children

Spouses and partners of service members with PTSD report higher rates of distress, depression, and suicidal ideation, and poorer adjustment than spouses of service members without PTSD [39, 40]. In addition to affecting the psychological health of spouses, PTSD can negatively impact the relationship between the service member and spouse [41–46] by contributing to problems with intimacy, communication, intimate partner violence, reduced emotional and physical well-being, divorce, and relationship distress and marital satisfaction [43, 44, 47–50]. In particular, PTSD symptoms of avoidance, emotional numbing, and hyperarousal can negatively impact intimacy and are associated with relationship dissatisfaction, spousal abuse, and divorce [45, 51–54]. These effects on relationships appear to be specific to PTSD, rather than to trauma exposure, as divorce occurs at a higher rate in veterans suffering with PTSD compared to similarly trauma-exposed veterans without PTSD [48, 55].

PTSD can undermine parenting behaviors and parenting satisfaction [56–58]. Not only are parent-child relationships affected, but parental cooperation and coordination between parents can be negatively impacted. Given potential changes to previous ways of parenting, renegotiation of the co-parenting relationship may be required [47].

Children's emotional health can also be negatively affected by parental PTSD. General distress, depression, lower self-esteem, aggression, impaired social relationships, and school-related difficulties have been reported in children of service members with PTSD ([59]; reviewed in [57]). A child's reaction to a parent who has PTSD should be expected to vary by their age, maturity, temperament, and preexisting conditions. Children with preexisting medical, developmental, behavioral, or emotional conditions may experience greater distress or worsening of symptoms. Given the potential disruptions in lifestyle due to care for a parent with PTSD (e.g., geographical transitions, possible separations from established child care providers), children's healthcare may be neglected or inappropriately delayed. Parents and clinicians may need to use a lower threshold for referral to appropriate clinical resources for these more vulnerable children.

The following vignette of Lance Corporal Bradley and his family illustrates how military duty-related injuries and illnesses can affect the health and well-being of other family members (including children) across the injury recovery trajectory (see Table 23.1). Clinicians need to be attuned to evolving mental health needs in all family members.

Vignette #3

Lance Corporal Jim Bradley returned home to his wife, Mary, and their children, Mike (7) and Carrie (5) after a 6-month combat deployment. Many of his battle buddies were injured, and some didn't make it home. Images of his wounded and dismembered friends continue to pop into his mind at unpredictable moments, and, as a result, Jim is jumpy and irritable. In addition, he feels extremely guilty that he survived combat unscathed, while so many did not. Since returning home, he often wakes up multiple times per night from nightmares. One morning, Mike gleefully jumps on his father's bed wanting to "play," however, Jim is startled from his sleep and pushes Mike off the bed. Jim feels alienated from his family because they do not understand what is "wrong" with him. He sleeps in his office so Mary doesn't find out about his nightmares and he relies on alcohol to fall asleep. Jim begins drinking a six-pack every night, often takes a shot of vodka in the middle of the night to get back to sleep, and experiences anxiety in the morning when the alcohol has worn off. As a result, Jim craves alcohol during the day, and he starts sneaking sips of vodka from a flask. Mary notices the alcohol purchases on their credit card statements. She asks him to cut back on the alcohol and Jim gets angry. They begin arguing often and, during one physical altercation, Jim shoves Mary to the floor in front of the children. Several days later Mary is called by Carrie's kindergarten teacher who stated that Carrie had soiled herself in the classroom, asking "Have there been any new stresses in her life recently?" As a result, Mary demands that Jim seeks treatment or she will leave the house and take the children.

Combat-Related Bereavement

Epidemiology

During the ten years following September 11, 2001, 15,938 service members died while on active duty [60]. The causes of death varied, but most were sudden and violent, resulting from accidents, combat deaths, and suicide (34.0%, 31.5%, and 14.5%, respectively). Fifty-five percent of these deceased service members were married, and their surviving spouses ($n = 9{,}667$) were young at the time of bereavement (mean age = 32.8, SD = 9.3). Thirty-one percent of service members who died from 2001 to 2011 had children, totaling 12,641 bereaved children whose young age (mean age = 10.3 years, SD = 7.3) reflected the youth of their parents. In addition, children younger than 10 years old were 3.8 times more likely to experience a service member's death as a result of sudden and violent causes than children above the age of 10 [60].

Impact on Spouses and Children

The death of a service member often results in secondary losses for surviving family members, including changes in their way of life and their associated identities (e.g., military spouse, military child, military parent/sibling), loss of housing (e.g., needing to move from a military installation), and loss of connection to the military community [61]. For spouses and children, it can feel like an "involuntary discharge" when they relocate to the civilian world, leading to feelings of isolation, disconnectedness, loneliness, confusion, and disenfranchisement [60].

In addition to distress caused by these changes, family members bereaved by sudden and violent deaths (which are commonly the cause of military service members) are at higher risk for adverse psychological outcomes than those bereaved by other types of deaths [62]. Although intense acute grief is an expected response to bereavement, those who have been bereaved by sudden and violent deaths are at higher risk for a condition of persistent and impairing grief that can continue for years after the death [63]. This grief condition, referred to as Prolonged Grief Disorder in the DSM-5-TR [64] and previously variably referred to as *complicated grief*, *traumatic grief*, and *persistent complex bereavement disorder*, often co-occurs with depression and posttraumatic stress disorder, but is distinct from these conditions and responds to grief-specific treatments [65, 66].

Researchers at Uniformed Services University (USU), Center for the Study of Traumatic Stress (CSTS) conducted the National Military Family Bereavement Study (NMFBS; www.militarysurvivorstudy.org) to examine the impact of U.S. service member death on surviving family members. Fifteen percent of NMFBS participants endorsed grief symptoms consistent with prolonged grief disorder [11]. This proportion is similar to non-military family samples that were bereaved by sudden and violent deaths [62]. An analysis comparing healthcare data of military widows and a matched sample of non-bereaved military wives indicated two to fivefold increases in prevalence of depression, PTSD, and adjustment disorder, as well as increased healthcare utilization in widows in the 2 years after the death [67, 68]. A separate analysis of these data that examined physical health conditions indicated increases in prevalence of ill-defined conditions, in addition to mental health conditions in years 1 and 2 following bereavement. Health care utilization was highest for widows with comorbid ill-defined conditions and mental health conditions [69].

Information about bereaved military children is scarce. However, children are likely to be strongly affected by the deaths of loved ones, though they do not grieve in the same manner as adults. Instead of crying and displaying sad expressions that are typically shown by adults, a child's expression of grief may be unfocused and may include playing, talking, questioning, and observing, [70, 71]. In addition, many children may feel sad, cry, or become withdrawn, but others may express their emotions by regressing to earlier behaviors (e.g., bedwetting, temper tantrums, withdrawing), or displaying behavior problems [71]. Sometimes a loss may lead to anxiety, depression, and posttraumatic stress symptoms in children [72–74]. However, in a study of 360 parentally-bereaved children compared to 110 depressed children and 120 community controls, bereavement was associated with increased psychiatric symptoms in the first 2 years after death, but with fewer symptoms compared to children with clinical depression [75]. Some of these psychological symptoms may be related to changes in the child's care following the death of a parent due to the absence of the deceased parent and the grief of the surviving parent. A parent's mental health can affect the mental health of their children, as poorer adult outcomes are associated with poorer child outcomes [76], and higher family socioeconomic status and lower depressive symptoms of the surviving parent are associated with better child outcomes [75].

The following fictional vignette describing Shannon, a military widow, illustrates the challenges associated with military family bereavement and the need for clinicians to be attentive to family members who may require clinical intervention.

Vignette #4

Shannon was working at home in her office while her twin sons (age 2) were napping upstairs. She had been thinking about her recent text exchange with her husband, SGT Dave Williams, when the doorbell rang. She glanced out the window and noticed a government vehicle parked outside and two uniformed men standing by her door. Even before speaking with them, Shannon knew that Dave had been killed.

After the acute stress of speaking to the notification team and the chaplain, and then figuring out how to tell her young sons and family, Shannon was faced with numerous decisions that had to be made quickly during the next few days. Although she had help from the casualty assistance officer that was assigned to her, she needed to decide on details surrounding the dignified transfer of remains, the burial process, managing media requests, and obtain information about benefits and other financial, legal, and military paperwork. After several weeks, things settled down and the reality of life without Dave began to sink in. She decided that it might be easier to manage her twin sons if they were closer to her parents in rural Michigan. However, after the move, she missed the closeness she had had with other wives at Fort Drum, NY, where they had been stationed. She briefly dated a few men she had met at her new job, but after receiving cool responses from Dave's mother and sister about dating, she stopped. Shannon became increasingly isolated and her grief for Dave persisted. There were numerous times in which Shannon wasn't able to give full attention to either her children or her job. She started drinking alcohol more frequently at night once the children were in bed. Two years after Dave's death, Shannon continued to struggle with intense longing for Dave. She stopped reaching out to friends they had enjoyed as a couple, because it brought up too many painful memories.

Family-Centered Care in Families Facing Injury, Mental Disorders, and Death

Although combat-related visible and invisible injuries and bereavement are distinct experiences, each can powerfully impact military and veteran families by generating distress that can undermine parenting and other family processes. However, several theorists have detailed how family processes can be targeted to support resilience. For example, Family Resilience Theory [77] highlights the importance of shared beliefs, constructive communication, and healthy patterns of organization within families as being critical to overall family health in traumatic circumstances. Saltzman et al. [78] recommended targeting family resilience processes in traumatically-affected military families by encouraging understanding, support, and forgiveness among family members; improving communication and cohesion within the family; coordinating parental leadership; ensuring defined but adjustable roles and responsibilities; and developing shared goals and beliefs among adults and children. These family resilience processes can be differentially affected by certain symptoms or conditions. For instance, specific PTSD symptoms can negatively affect some of these processes rather than others. Table 23.3 summarizes these negative effects and highlights opportunities for intervention.

Table 23.3 Negative effects of PTSD symptom clusters on family resilience processes

	Re-experiencing	Avoidance	Negative cognitions and mood	Arousal
Emotional closeness	↓	↓	↓	↓
Communication		↓		↓
Safety and impulse control	↓		↓	↓
Family leadership		↓	↓	
Family hopefulness	↓		↓	
Supervision of children		↓		
Authoritative discipline of children		↓	↓	↓

Source: Adapted from Cozza [11]
Note: Down arrows indicate a negative effect of a PTSD symptom cluster on the indicated family resilience process
Reproduced with permission National Academies of Sciences, Engineering and Medicine [79]

Greater appreciation of these intrafamilial effects of PTSD and other combat-related stressors has fostered both theoretical and clinical appreciation of family-centered approaches to military and veteran families that have been affected [15, 80]. For instance, the National Academies of Sciences, Engineering, and Medicine published *Strengthening the Military Family Readiness System for a Changing American Society* [79], a report focused on the well-being of military families, including those affected by high-stress events, such as combat-related visible and invisible injuries and bereavement. One recommendation within that report was to increase access for military families to "effective, evidence-based and evidence-informed family strengthening programs, resources, and services" [79].

Several evidence-based family-centered strengthening programs have been developed for use in military communities. For example, Families OverComing Under Stress (FOCUS) [81] and After Deployment Adaptive Parenting Tools (ADAPT) [82] share common core components, including a strengths-based approach, and an emphasis on emotion regulation, communication, problem solving, and understanding and addressing children's developmental needs. In addition, ADAPT highlights several positive parenting practices, including parental limit setting and monitoring and involvement in school and other activities. Other programs, such as Strong Bonds [83] and Strength at Home [84] focus on strengthening couple functioning within families.

Additional family-centered interventions have been developed specifically for families affected by TBI or bereavement. Family Focused Therapy for TBI (FFT-TBI) [85] and Brain Injury Family Intervention (BIF) [86] share common intervention strategies, such as increasing knowledge about TBI, enhancing family communication, and improving problem solving, emotion regulation, and goal setting [85, 86]. The Family Bereavement Program (FBP) incorporates positive parenting strategies and individual and interpersonal strengthening activities to support family grief outcomes [87].

Although these family-centered strengthening programs differ in their emphases and details of their implementation, they share common goals centered on

Table 23.4 Family-strengthening goals to promote family resilience and well-being

1.	*Maintain a physically safe and structured environment*, protecting against interpersonal aggression among adults and children, and ensuring that children have adequate structure and support, have consistency in routines and rules, and are effectively monitored
2.	*Engage required resources*, accessing instrumental and social support within and outside the family to support adults and children, dyadic relationships and the family as a whole, and teaching family members how to effectively use their support opportunities (friends, extended family, teachers, coaches, faith-based communities, etc.)
3.	*Develop and share knowledge within and outside of the family*, building shared understanding about stressors, including service members' injury or illness, as well as modeling and teaching effective communication strategies among adults and children
4.	*Build a positive, emotionally safe, and warm family environment*, including effective stress reduction and emotional regulation strategies for parents to engage in and model for children, as well as engaging in activities that are calming and enjoyable for all
5.	*Master and model important interpersonal skills*, including individual and relational problem solving and conflict resolution and incorporating evidence-based strategies
6.	*Maintain a vision of hope and future optimism for the family*, engendering positive expectations among family members and creating a hope-filled family narrative
7.	*Utilize competent and authoritative parenting*, encouraging consequence-based strategies that promote mastery and minimizing harsh disciplinary practices
8.	*Incorporate trauma-informed approaches to care*, recognizing that families faced with stress and adversity are likely to be affected by trauma and loss experiences that uniquely impact adults and children within families, their relationships, and their development
9.	*Promote security among adults and children*, strengthening parent-child relationships that are known to contribute to individual and relational wellness for both adults and children, and focusing on effective conflict resolution between spouses or partners
10.	*Highlight the unique developmental needs of family members*, helping parents and other engaged adults in the family recognize and respond to their family members' needs effectively at each developmental stage

Sources: Compiled by the Committee on the Well-Being of Military Families. Source for Goal #5 is Dausch and Saliman [85], Gerwitz et al. [82]; source for Goal #6 is Saltzman et al. [78]
Reproduced with permission National Academies of Sciences, Engineering, and Medicine [79]

supporting family health and well-being, which were noted in a 2019 National Academies report (summarized in Table 23.4). Evidence-based approaches should serve as a foundation for clinical treatments offered to families affected by combat-related injury, illness, or bereavement. For example, in a family affected by PTSD, clinicians must ensure that adults and children understand the disorder and how it impacts behaviors and intrafamilial interactions (e.g., "It's not a good idea to jump on the bed and awaken Daddy because it frightens him."). As another example, clinicians can introduce problem-solving strategies, such as conflict resolution, within a family affected by TBI in order to minimize interpersonal arguments (e.g., "We know that talking about homework is stressful for Dad and Ebony, so let's wait until we are all calm to try to have that conversation."). Clinicians should also introduce skills for competent parenting (e.g., consequence-based discipline), ideas for activities that strengthen relationships (e.g., mutually enjoyable games or activities), and family hopefulness (e.g., "Although you miss your father, you are still a strong family that can manage.") into family-centered treatment strategies.

Conclusion

Because the health and well-being of each family member affects and is affected by the health and well-being of others in the family system, combat-related visible and invisible injuries and bereavement can each profoundly affect military and veteran families. As discussed in this chapter, combat-related injuries and combat-related bereavement are likely to affect family dynamics (e.g., roles and responsibilities, the functioning of the couple, parenting of children), social interactions with those outside the family, and logistical and practical concerns, such as residential moves and financial resources. It is vital that healthcare providers are aware of the challenges that these life-altering events can pose to family members of the identified service member or veteran patient. In addition, they must be familiar with the principles of family-centered care and the relevant and available interventions to treat their patients.

Additional Resources

- For resources related to injury communication visit *Courage to Talk*: https://www.courage2talk.org/
- *For Resources for Recovery* fact sheets for combat injured and ill families visit the Center for the Study of Traumatic Stress: https://www.cstsonline.org/fact-sheet-menu/fact-sheet-list
- For resources specific to bereaved military family see the *Stepping Forward in Grief* resource pagel: https://steppingforwardstudy.org/resources/
- For a comprehensive list of military family resources
  - The Rand Corporation's ***Additional Health-Related Resources for Service Members, Veterans, and Military Families***: https://www.rand.org/well-being/social-and-behavioral-policy/projects/veterans/resources.html
  - Military One Source: https://www.militaryonesource.mil/benefits-and-resources

Clinical Pearls

- Acknowledge that even though you are treating an individual patient, combat-related visible and invisible injuries are likely to affect all family members. Your patient's health and well-being are interconnected with the health and well-being of their family members.
- Ask your patients to describe their families: Who are their family members and how do patients relate to each of them?
- Document the entire family's military service histories, including combat-related injuries or traumatic losses.
- Expand your clinical focus to include the impact of visible and invisible injuries on functioning within interpersonal relationships (i.e., with adult and child family members), in addition to symptom resolution (i.e., reducing flashbacks or nightmares).

- Recognize that family relationships are dynamic and change over time. Sometimes they will improve, but they also may worsen. Do not assume that a marriage is "good" or "bad."
- Listen for indications that your patients' children or spouses are having difficulties and may need to be referred for interventions of their own.
- Become familiar with family processes (e.g., effective communication, problem solving, emotion regulation, goal setting) that support resilience, and encourage your patients and their families to incorporate such practices.
- Refer your patients and their families to family-centered interventions that are designed to encourage resilience processes and strengthen family well-being. These interventions will likely also support your patients' treatment progress.
- Screen bereaved patients for persistent and impairing grief symptoms (i.e., ongoing yearning or longing for the deceased) that indicates problems with grief adaptation and possibly the presence of prolonged grief disorder that requires evidence-based, grief-focused treatment.

Disclaimer The opinions and assertions expressed herein are those of the author(s) and do not reflect the official policy or position of the Uniformed Services University or the Department of Defense. The contents of this publication are the sole responsibility of the author(s) and do not necessarily reflect the views, opinions or policies of The Henry M. Jackson Foundation for the Advancement of Military Medicine, Inc. Mention of trade names, commercial products, or organizations does not imply endorsement by the U.S. Government.

References

1. Department of Defense. 2018 demographics: profile of the military community. 2018. Available at https://download.militaryonesource.mil/12038/MOS/Reports/2018-demographics-report.pdf. Accessed January 11, 2021.
2. Defense Casualty Analysis System. U.S. military casualties - OCO casualty summary by casualty type. 2020. Available at https://dcas-pki.dmdc.osd.mil/dcas/pages/report_sum_reason.xhtml. Accessed January 12, 2021.
3. Belmont PJ, Owens BD, Schoenfeld AJ. Musculoskeletal injuries in Iraq and Afghanistan: epidemiology and outcomes following a decade of war. J Am Acad Orthop Surg. 2016;24(6):341–8. https://doi.org/10.5435/JAAOS-D-15-00123.
4. Owens BD, Kragh JF, Wenke JC, Macaitis J, et al. Combat wounds in operation Iraqi freedom and operation enduring freedom. J Trauma Inj Infect Crit Care. 2008;64(2):295–9. https://doi.org/10.1097/TA.0b013e318163b875.
5. Masini BD, Owens BD, Jsu JR, Wenke JC. Rehospitalization after combat injury. J Trauma Inj Infect Crit Care. 2011;71(1):S98–S102. https://doi.org/10.1097/TA.0b013e3182218fbc.
6. Masini BD, Waterman SM, Wenke JC, Owens BD, et al. Resource utilization and disability outcome assessment of combat casualties from operation Iraqi freedom and operation enduring freedom. J Orthop Trauma. 2009;23(4):261–6. https://doi.org/10.1097/BOT.0b013e31819dfa04.
7. Fischer H. A guide to U.S. military casualty statistics: operation freedom's sentinel, operation inherent resolve, operation new dawn, operation Iraqi Freedom, and Operation Enduring Freedom. Congressional Research Service. 2015.
8. MacGregor A, Dougherty A, Galarneau M. Injury-specific correlates of combat-related traumatic brain injury in operation Iraqi freedom. J Head Trauma Rehabil. 2011;26(4):312–8. https://doi.org/10.1097/HTR.0b013e3181e94404.

9. MacGregor A, Tang J, Dougherty A, Galarneau M. Deployment-related injury and post-traumatic stress disorder in US military personnel. Injury. 2013;44(11):1458–64. https://doi.org/10.1016/j.injury.2012.10.009.
10. Cozza SJ, Guimond JM. Working with combat-injured families through the recovery trajectory. In: MacDermid Wadsworth S, Riggs D, editors. Risk and resilience in US military families. New York: Springer; 2011. p. 259–77.
11. Cozza SJ, Fisher JE, Mauro C, Zhou J, et al. Performance of DSM-5 persistent complex bereavement disorder criteria in a community sample of bereaved military family members. Am J Psychiatry. 2016;173(9):919–29. https://doi.org/10.1176/appi.ajp.2016.15111442.
12. Cozza SJ, Feerick MM. The impact of parental combat injury on young military children. In: Osofsky D, editor. Clinical work with traumatized young children. New York: The Guilford Press; 2011. p. 139–54.
13. Holmes AK, Rauch PK, Cozza SJ. When a parent is injured or killed in combat. Futur Child. 2013;23(2):143–62. https://doi.org/10.1353/foc.2013.0017.
14. Armistead L, Klein K, Forehand R. Parental physical illness and child functioning. Clin Psychol Rev. 1995;15(5):409–22. https://doi.org/10.1016/0272-7358(95)00023-I.
15. Cozza SJ, Holmes AK, Van Ost SL. Family-centered care for military and veteran families affected by combat injury. Clin Child Fam Psychol Rev. 2013;16(3):311–21. https://doi.org/10.1007/s10567-013-0141-3.
16. Gorman LA, Fitzgerald HE, Blow AJ. Parental combat injury and early child development: a conceptual model for differentiating effects of visible and invisible injuries. Psychiatry Q. 2010;81(1):1–21. https://doi.org/10.1007/s1126-009-9116-4.
17. Kelley SDM, Sikka A, Venkatesan S. A review of research on parental disability: Implications for research and counseling practice. Rehabil Couns Bull. 1997;41(2):105–21.
18. LeClere FB, Kowalewski BM. Disability in the family: the effects on children's well-being. J Marriage Fam. 1994;56(2):457–68. https://doi.org/10.2307/353112.
19. Hisle-Gorman E, Harrington D, Nylund CM, Tercyak KP, et al. Impact of parents' wartime military deployment and injury on young children's safety and mental health. J Am Acad Child Adolesc Psychiatry. 2015;54(4):294–301. https://doi.org/10.1016/j.jaac.2014.12.017.
20. Hisle-Gorman E, Susi A, Gorman GH. The impact of military parents' injuries on the health and well-being of their children. Health Aff. 2019;38(8):1358–65. https://doi.org/10.1377/hlthaff.2019.00276.
21. Defense and Veterans Brain Injury Center. Number of service members diagnosed with traumatic brain injury. 2018. Available at https://dvbic.dcoe.mil/dod-worldwide-numbers-tbi. Accessed on January 12, 2021.
22. DePalma RG, Hoffman SW. Combat blast related traumatic brain injury (TBI): decade of recognition; promise of progress. Behav Brain Res. 2018;340:102–5. https://doi.org/10.1016/j.bbr.2016.08.036.
23. Jackson GL, Hamilton NS, Tupler LA. Detecting traumatic brain injury among veterans of operations enduring and Iraqi freedom. N C Med J. 2008;69(1):43–7.
24. Tanielian T, Jaycox LH. Invisible wounds of war: psychological and cognitive injuries, their consequences, and services to assist recovery. Santa Monica, CA: RAND Corporation; 2008.
25. Verhaeghe S, Defloor T, Grypdonck M. Stress and coping among families of patients with traumatic brain injury: a review of the literature. J Clin Nurs. 2005;14(8):1004–12. https://doi.org/10.1111/j.1365-2702.2005.01126.x.
26. Urbach JR, Culbert JP. Head-injured parents and their children. Psychosomatics. 1991;32(1):24–33. https://doi.org/10.1016/S0033-3182(91)72108-7.
27. Pessar LF, Coad ML, Linn RT, Willer BS. The effects of parental traumatic brain injury on the behaviour of parents and children. Brain Inj. 1993;7(3):231–40. https://doi.org/10.3109/02699059309029675.
28. Butera-Prinzi F, Perlesz A. Through children's eyes: children's experience of living with a parent with an acquired brain injury. Brain Inj. 2004;18(1):83–101. https://doi.org/10.1080/0269905031000118500.

29. Charles N, Butera-Prinzi F, Perlesz A. Families living with acquired brain injury: a multiple family group experience. NeuroRehabilitation. 2007;22(1):61–76.
30. Brickell TA, French LM, Lippa SM, Lange RT. The impact of deployment and traumatic brain injury on the health and behavior of children of US military service members and veterans. Clin Child Psychol Psychiatry. 2018;23(3):425–41. https://doi.org/10.1177/1359104517740405.
31. Resnik LJ, Allen SM. Using international classification of functioning, disability and health to understand challenges in community reintegration of injured veterans. J Rehabil Res Dev. 2007;44(7):991–1006. https://doi.org/10.1682/jrrd.2007.05.0071.
32. Weinstein EA, Salazar AM, Jones FD. Behavioral consequences of traumatic brain injury. In: Jones FD, Sparacino LR, Wilcox VL, Rothberg JM, Stokes JW, editors. War psychiatry. Washington: TMM Publications; 1995. p. 319–51.
33. Cozza SJ. Family-focused intervention for PTSD: lessons from military families. In: Benedek DM, Wynn GH, editors. Complementary and alternative medicine for PTSD. Oxford: Oxford University Press; 2016. p. 179–202.
34. Pietrzak RH, Goldstein RB, Southwick SM, Grant BF. Prevalence and axis I comorbidity of full and partial posttraumatic stress disorder in the United States: results from wave 2 of the national epidemiologic survey on alcohol and related conditions. J Anxiety Disord. 2011;25(3):456–65. https://doi.org/10.1016/j.janxdis.2010.11.010.
35. Bowe A, Rosencheck R. PTSD and substance use disorder among veterans: characteristics, service utilization and pharmacotherapy. J Dual Diagn. 2015;11(1):22–32. https://doi.org/10.1080/15504263.2014.989653.
36. Rytwinski NK, Scur MD, Feeny NC, Youngstrom EA. The co-occurrence of major depressive disorder among individuals with posttraumatic stress disorders: a meta-analysis. J Trauma Stress. 2013;26(3):299–309. https://doi.org/10.1002/jts.21814.
37. Arria AM, Mericle AA, Meyers K, Winters KC. Parental substance use impairment, parenting and substance use disorder risk. J Subst Abus Treat. 2012;43(1):114–22. https://doi.org/10.1016/j.jsat.2011.10.001.
38. Whisman MA. Marital distress and DSM-IV psychiatric disorders in a population-based national survey. J Abnorm Psychol. 2007;116(3):638–43. https://doi.org/10.1037/0021-843X.116.3.638.
39. Calhoun PS, Beckham JC, Bosworth HB. Caregiver burden and psychological distress in partners of veterans with chronic posttraumatic stress disorder. J Trauma Stress. 2002;15(3):205–12. https://doi.org/10.1023/A:1015251210928.
40. Manguno-Mire G, Sautter F, Lyons J, Myers L, et al. Psychological distress and burden among female partners of combat veterans with PTSD. J Nerv Ment Dis. 2007;195(2):144–51. https://doi.org/10.1097/01.nmd.0000254755.53549.69.
41. Kessler RC. Posttraumatic stress disorder: the burden to the individual and to society. J Clin Psychiatry. 2000;61(suppl 5):4–12.
42. Klarić M, Fanciskovic T, Stevanovic A, Petrov B, et al. Marital quality and relationship satisfaction in war veterans and their wives in Bosnia and Herzegovina. Eur J Psychotraumatol. 2011;2(1):8077. https://doi.org/10.3402/ejpt.v2i0.8077.
43. Monson CM, Schnurr PP, Stevens SP, Guthrie KA. Cognitive-behavioral couple's treatment for posttraumatic stress disorder: initial findings. J Trauma Stress. 2004;17(4):341–4. https://doi.org/10.1023/B:JOTS.0000038483.69570.5b.
44. Renshaw KD, Rodrigues CS, Jones DH. Psychological symptoms and marital satisfaction in spouses of operation Iraqi freedom veterans: relationships with spouses' perceptions of veterans' experiences and symptoms. J Fam Psychol. 2008;22(3):586–94. https://doi.org/10.1037/0893-3200.22.3.586.
45. Riggs DS, Byrne CA, Weathers FW, Litz BT. The quality of the intimate relationships of male vietnam veterans: problems associated with posttraumatic stress disorder. J Trauma Stress. 1998;11(1):87–101. https://doi.org/10.1023/A:1024409200155.
46. Whisman MA, Sheldon CT, Goering P. Psychiatric disorders and dissatisfaction with social relationships: does type of relationship matter? J Abnorm Psychol. 2000;109(4):803–8. https://doi.org/10.1037//0021-843X.109.4.803.

47. Allen ES, Rhoades GK, Stanley SM, Markham HJ. Hitting home: relationships between recent deployment, posttraumatic stress symptoms, and marital functioning for Army couples. J Fam Psychol. 2010;24(3):280–8. https://doi.org/10.1037/a0019405.
48. Cook JM, Riggs DS, Thompson R, Coyne JC, Sheikh JI. Posttraumatic stress disorder and current relationship functioning among World War II ex-prisoners of war. J Fam Psychol. 2004;18(1):36–45. https://doi.org/10.1037/0893-3200.18.1.36.
49. Evans L, Cowlishaw S, Hopwood M. Family functioning predicts outcomes for veterans in treatment for chronic posttraumatic stress disorder. J Fam Psychol. 2009;23(4):531–9. https://doi.org/10.1037/a0015877.
50. Taft CT, Watkins LE, Stafford J, Street AE, Monson CM. Posttraumatic stress disorder and intimate relationship problems: a meta-analysis. J Consult Clin Psychol. 2011;79(1):22–33. https://doi.org/10.1037/a0022196.
51. Frederikson LG, Chamberlain K, Long N. Unacknowledged casualties of the Vietnam war: experiences of partners of New Zealand veterans. Qual Health Res. 1996;6(1):49–70. https://doi.org/10.1177/104973239600600104.
52. Lunney CA, Schnurr PP. Domains of quality of life and symptoms in male veterans treated for posttraumatic stress disorder. J Trauma Stress. 2007;20(6):955–64. https://doi.org/10.1002/jts.20269.
53. Monson CM, Taft CT, Fredman SJ. Military-related PTSD and intimate relationships: from description to theory-driven research and intervention development. Clin Psychol Rev. 2009;29(8):707–14. https://doi.org/10.1016/j.cpr.2009.09.002.
54. Solomon Z, Dekel R, Zerach G. The relationships between posttraumatic stress symptom clusters and marital intimacy among war veterans. J Fam Psychol. 2008;22(5):659–66. https://doi.org/10.1037/a0013596.
55. Jordan BK, Marmar CR, Fairbank JA, Schlenger WE, et al. Problems in families of male Vietnam veterans with posttraumatic stress disorder. J Consult Clin Psychol. 1992;60(6):916–26. https://doi.org/10.1037//0022-006x.60.6.916.
56. Berz JB, Taft CT, Watkins LE, Monson CM. Associations between PTSD symptoms and parenting satisfaction in a female veteran sample. J Psychol Trauma. 2008;7(1):37–45. https://doi.org/10.1080/19322880802125969.
57. Galovski T, Lyons JA. Psychological sequelae of combat violence: a review of the impact of PTSD on the veteran's family and possible interventions. Aggress Violent Behav. 2004;9(5):477–501. https://doi.org/10.1016/S1359-1789(03)00045-4.
58. Samper RE, Taft CT, King DW, King LA. Posttraumatic stress disorder symptoms and parenting satisfaction among a national sample of male Vietnam veterans. J Trauma Stress. 2004;17(4):311–5. https://doi.org/10.1023/B:JOTS.0000038479.30903.ed.
59. Rosenheck R, Nathan P. Secondary traumatization in children of Vietnam veterans. Hosp Community Psychiatry. 1985;36(5):538–9. https://doi.org/10.1176/ps.36.5.538.
60. Cozza SJ, Fisher JE, Zhou J, Harrington-LaMorie J, et al. Bereaved military dependent spouses and children: those left behind in a decade of war (2001-2011). Mil Med. 2017;182(3-4):1684–90. https://doi.org/10.7205/MILMED-D-16-00101.
61. Harrington-LaMorie J, Cohen J, Cozza SJ. Caring for bereaved military family members. In: Cozza SJ, Goldberg MN, Ursano RJ, editors. Care of military service members, veterans, and their families. Washington: American Psychiatric Publishing; 2014. p. 257–76.
62. Kristensen P, Weisæth L, Heir T. Bereavement and mental health after sudden and violent losses: a review. Psychiatry. 2012;75(1):76–97. https://doi.org/10.1521/psyc.2012.75.1.76.
63. Shear MK. Clinical practice: complicated grief. N Engl J Med. 2015;372(2):153–60. https://doi.org/10.1056/NEJMcp1315618.
64. American Psychiatric Association. (2022). Diagnostic and statistical manual of mental disorders (5th ed., text rev.). https://doi.org/10.1176/appi.books.9780890425787.
65. Middleton W, Raphael B, Burnett P, Martinek N. A longitudinal study comparing bereavement phenomena in recently bereaved spouses, adult children and parents. Aust N Z J Psychiatry. 1998;32(2):235–41. https://doi.org/10.3109/00048679809062734.

66. Prigerson HG, Horowitz MJ, Jacobs SC, Parkes CM, et al. Prolonged grief disorder: psychometric validation of criteria proposed for DSM-V and ICD-11. PLoS Med. 2009;6(8):e1000121. https://doi.org/10.1371/journal.pmed.1000121.
67. Cozza SJ, Harrington-LaMorie J, Fisher JE. U.S. Military Service deaths: bereavement in surviving families. In: Weiss EL, Castro CA, editors. American military life in the 21st century: social, cultural, and economic issues and trends. Santa Barbara: ABC-CLIO; 2019. p. 411–25.
68. Cozza SJ, Hefner KR, Fisher JE, Zhou J, et al. Mental health conditions in bereaved military service widows: a prospective, case-controlled, and longitudinal study. Depress Anxiety. 2019;37(1):45–53. https://doi.org/10.1002/da.22971.
69. Fisher JE, Krantz DS, Ogle CM, Zhou J, Zuleta RF, Strickman AK, Fullerton CS, Ursano RJ, Cozza SJ. Mental health, ill-defined conditions, and health care utilization following bereavement: a prospective case-control study. J Acad Consult Liaison Psychiatry. 2022;63(5):434–44. https://doi.org/10.1016/j.jaclp.2022.02.007. Epub 2022 Mar 5. PMID: 35257945.
70. Department of Defense. The impacts of deployment of deployed members of the Armed Forces on their dependent children. 2010. Available at https://download.militaryonesource.mil/12038/MOS/Reports/Report-to-Congress-on-Impact-of-Deployment-on-Military-Children.pdf. Accessed January 11, 2021.
71. McCown DE, Davis B. Patterns of grief in young children following the death of a sibling. Death Stud. 1995;19(1):41–53. https://doi.org/10.1080/07481189508252712.
72. Currier JM, Holland JM, Neimeyer RA. The effectiveness of bereavement interventions with children: a meta-analytic review of controlled outcome research. J Clin Child Adolesc Psychol. 2007;36(2):253–9. https://doi.org/10.1080/15374410701279669.
73. Finkelstein H. The long-term effects of early parent death: a review. J Clin Psychol. 1988;44(1):3–9. https://doi.org/10.1002/1097-4679(198801)44:1<3::AID-JCLP2270440102>3.0.CO;2-1.
74. Reinherz HZ, Giaconia RM, Hauf AM, Wasserman MS, Paradis AD. General and specific childhood risk factors for depression and drug disorders by early adulthood. J Am Acad Child Adolesc Psychiatry. 2000;39(2):223–31. https://doi.org/10.1097/00004583-200002000-00023.
75. Cerel J, Fristad MA, Verducci J, Weller RA, Weller EB. Childhood bereavement: Psychopathology in the 2 years postparental death. J Am Acad Child Adolesc Psychiatry. 2006;45(6):681–90. https://doi.org/10.1097/01.chi.0000215327.58799.05.
76. Saldinger A, Cain AC, Porterfield K, Lohnes K. Facilitating attachment between school-aged children and a dying parent. Death Stud. 2004;28(10):915–40. https://doi.org/10.1080/07481180490511993.
77. Walsh F. Strengthening family resilience. 2nd ed. New York: The Guilford Press; 2006.
78. Saltzman WR, Lester P, Beardslee WR, Laynce CM, et al. Mechanisms of risk and resilience in military families: theoretical and empirical basis of a family-focused resilience enhancement program. Clin Child Fam Psychol Rev. 2011;14(3):213–30. https://doi.org/10.1007/s10567-011-0096-1.
79. National Academies of Sciences, Engineering, and Medicine. High-stress events, family resilience processes, and military family well-being. In: Kizer KW, Le Menestrel S, editors. Strengthening the military family readiness system for a changing American society. Washington: National Academies Press; 2019. p. 203–32.
80. Wadsworth SM, Lester P, Marini C, Cozza SJ, et al. Approaching family-focused systems of care for military and veteran families. Mil Behav Health. 2013;1(1):31–40. https://doi.org/10.1080/21635781.2012.721062.
81. Lester P, Stein JA, Saltzman W, Woodward K, et al. Psychological health of military children: longitudinal evaluation of a family-centered prevention program to enhance family resilience. Mil Med. 2013;178(8):838–45. https://doi.org/10.7205/MILMED-D-12-00502.
82. Gerwitz AH, Pinna KL, Hanson SK, Brockberg D. Promoting parenting to support reintegrating military families: after deployment, adaptive parenting tools. Psychol Serv. 2014;11(1):31–40. https://doi.org/10.1037/a0034134.

83. Allen ES, Stanley SM, Rhoades GK, Markham HJ. PREP for strong bonds: a review of outcomes from a randomized clinical trial. Contemp Fam Ther. 2015;37(3):232–46. https://doi.org/10.1007/s.10591-014-9325-3.
84. Taft CT, Creech SK, Gallagher MW, MacDonald A, et al. Strength at home couples program to prevent military partner violence: a randomized controlled trial. J Consult Clin Psychol. 2016;84(11):935–45. https://doi.org/10.1037/ccp0000129.
85. Dausch BM, Saliman S. Use of family focused therapy in rehabilitation for veterans with traumatic brain injury. Rehabil Psychol. 2009;54(3):279–87. https://doi.org/10.1037/a0016809.
86. Kreutzer JS, Stejskal TM, Godwin EE, Powell VD, Arango-Lasprilla JC. A mixed methods evaluation of the brain injury family intervention. NeuroRehabilitation. 2010;27(1):19–29. https://doi.org/10.3233/NRE-2010-0578.
87. Sandler IN, Ayers TS, Wolchik SA, Tein JY, et al. The family bereavement program: efficacy evaluation of a theory-based prevention program for parentally bereaved children and adolescents. J Consult Clin Psychol. 2003;71(3):587–600. https://doi.org/10.1037/0022-006X.71.3.587.

Index

C. H. Warner, C. A. Castro (eds.), *Veteran and Military Mental Health*,
https://doi.org/10.1007/978-3-031-18009-5

D

N

O

MIX
Papier aus verantwortungsvollen Quellen
Paper from responsible sources
FSC® C105338

If you have any concerns about our products,
you can contact us on
ProductSafety@springernature.com

In case Publisher is established outside the EU,
the EU authorized representative is:
Springer Nature Customer Service Center GmbH
Europaplatz 3, 69115 Heidelberg, Germany

Printed by Libri Plureos GmbH
in Hamburg, Germany